An Occupational Therapist's
Guide to Home Modification Practice

An Occupational Therapist's
Guide to Home Modification Practice

Elizabeth Ainsworth, MOccThy, Grad Cert Health Sci
Queensland Department of Communities
Queensland, Australia

Desleigh de Jonge, MPhil (OccThy), Grad Cert Soc Sci
University of Queensland
Brisbane, Australia

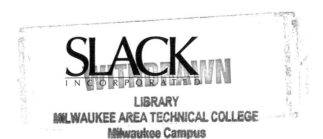

SLACK
INCORPORATED

ISBN: 978-1-55642-852-4

Photographs have been taken by Frank Brand.

The Instructor's Manual is also available from SLACK Incorporated. Don't miss this important companion to *An Occupational Therapist's Guide to Home Modification Practice*. To obtain the Instructor's Manual, please visit http://www.efacultylounge.com. In addition, be sure to check out Elizabeth Ainsworth's blog "Home Design for Living" at http://homedesignforliving.com.

Published by: SLACK Incorporated
                6900 Grove Road
                Thorofare, NJ 08086 USA
                Telephone: 856-848-1000
                Fax: 856-853-5991
                www.slackbooks.com

Contact SLACK Incorporated for more information about other books in this field or about the availability of our books from distributors outside the United States.

Library of Congress Cataloging-in-Publication Data

Ainsworth, Elizabeth,
  An occupational therapist's guide to home modification practice / Elizabeth Ainsworth, Desleigh de Jonge.
      p. ; cm.
  Includes bibliographical references and index.
  ISBN 978-1-55642-852-4 (alk. paper)
  1. Occupational therapy. 2. Home care services. 3. People with disabilities--Housing--Design and construction. I. de Jonge, Desleigh. II. Title.
  [DNLM: 1. Architectural Accessibility. 2. Disabled Persons--rehabilitation. 3. Environment Design. 4. Housing--standards. 5. Occupational Therapy. WA 795 A297o 2011]
  RM735.A635 2011
  615.8'515--dc22
                        2010020710

Printed in the United States of America

Last digit is print number: 10 9 8 7 6 5 4 3 2 1

DEDICATION

Dedicated to our families and friends, who have loved and supported us during this project, and to our clients, who provide inspiration and wisdom to expand our thinking and our practice and who challenge us to make a real difference in their lives.

CONTENTS

Section I: The Home, Community, and Societal Context of Home Modifications . . . 1

Section II: Delivery of Home Modification Services. 85

Section III: Home Modification Applications *287*

The Instructor's Manual is also available from SLACK Incorporated. Don't miss this important companion to *An Occupational Therapist's Guide to Home Modification Practice*. To obtain the Instructor's Manual, please visit **http://www.efacultylounge.com**. In addition, be sure to check out Elizabeth Ainsworth's blog "Home Design for Living" at **http://homedesignforliving.com**.

ACKNOWLEDGMENTS

We would like to thank John Bond and Brien Cummings at SLACK Incorporated for supporting and promoting our work.

We are also grateful for the generous support and assistance of the various knowledgeable authors and writers who contributed to the text.

Thanks are due to Karen Jacobs, Mary Ann Bruce, our colleagues at The University of Queensland, and the Queensland Department of Communities, who have provided encouragement and support to document this area of practice.

Additionally, we would like to thank Natalie MacDonald, former Director General, Queensland Department of Housing, for her support.

We would like to acknowledge members of the library staff of the Queensland Department of Public Works, who have worked tirelessly to provide us with information when compiling this publication: Wendy Wilkinson, Lizz Beven, Cecilie Williams, Mary Harlow, Therese Egan, Bob Lamb, Davydd McDonald, Robyne Sandison-Miller, Trudi Schuetz, Guy Vowles, Svea Sakellariou, Janelle Bartolo, Sannie Dragani, and Robyn Lather.

In assistance in the production of the text, we would like to thank David Hargreaves, Terry MacDermott, Carol Campbell, and Jenny Wilson, who have proofread the chapters; Frank Brand, Richard Kirk, Rod Hunter, and Paul Coonan for providing the photographs and drawings; and Professor Rob Imrie, Wally Dutcher, and Bill Krafft for supplying extra detail to enhance the chapters. We are also grateful to Ron and Beth Smith and Sally Ainsworth for participating in the photography sessions.

ABOUT THE AUTHORS

Elizabeth Ainsworth, MOccThy, Grad Cert Health Sci graduated in 1989 with a bachelor of occupational therapy (honors) degree and completed a master's in occupational therapy (contemporary clinical practice at the University of Queensland) and a graduate certificate in health science (occupational therapy at the University of Sydney) in 2000. She is the Principal Occupational Therapist in Housing and Homelessness Practice Improvement at the Queensland Department of Communities, leading a highly competent team of occupational therapists who specialize in working with older people and people with disabilities applying for or who live in social housing and who might experience barriers in the home environment. Elizabeth also provides home modification and universal design education and training in a private capacity to occupational therapy university undergraduate and postgraduate students and to occupational therapy clinicians working in a range of settings in the community. She is an active member of the Australian Network for Universal Housing Design (ANUHD) and the Australian Access Consultants Association (ACAA).

Desleigh de Jonge, MPhil (OccThy), Grad Cert Soc Sci graduated in 1978 with a bachelor of occupational therapy from the University of Queensland and completed a master's in philosophy from this university in 2001. She currently lectures in the School of Health and Rehabilitation Sciences at the University of Queensland and developed the curriculum on assistive technology and environmental design for the undergraduate, graduate entry, and postgraduate programs. Desleigh's national and international reputation in consumer-oriented analysis of assistive technologies, environmental design, and home modifications has earned her invitations to present at international conferences on assistive technology and home modification services and outcomes in the United States and Australia, and she has been published in national and international journals. Her teaching and research is focused on interventions and outcome measures that recognize consumer goals and priorities. She is a research associate of the Housing Policy Research Program at the University of Queensland's Social Research Centre and a member of the research team that recently completed an Australian Housing and Urban Research Institute (AHURI)-funded project on the role of home maintenance and modification services in achieving health, community care, and housing outcomes in later life. Desleigh is also a member of the Editorial Board for *Disability and Rehabilitation: Assistive Technology* and a member of the research review panel for the Home Modification Information Clearinghouse at the University of New South Wales.

Elizabeth and Desleigh have worked together during the past 11 years to provide training to occupational therapy students and practitioners. They have presented at national and international conferences on home modifications and universal design to a broad range of people from various backgrounds. This is the first book they have produced together.

Contributing Authors

Kathy Baigent, Dip OT, Dip Hlth Prom (Chapter 15)
Occupational Therapist, Housing and Homelessness
 Services
Queensland Department of Communities
Brisbane, Australia

Ruth Cordiner, DipCOT, Grad Cert OccThy (Chapters
 7, 15)
Occupational Therapist, Housing and Homelessness
 Services
Queensland Department of Communities
Brisbane, Australia

Shirley de Wit, BOccThy (Chapter 15)
Senior Occupational Therapist, Housing and
 Homelessness Services
Queensland Department of Communities
Brisbane, Australia

May Eade, BOccThy (Chapter 15)
Senior Occupational Therapist, Housing and
 Homelessness Services
Queensland Department of Communities
Brisbane, Australia

Andrew Jones, BA, MSW, GCE (Chapter 2)
Director, Australian Housing and Urban Research
 Institute (AHURI)
Queensland Research Centre
Research Program Director, Institute for Social
 Science Research
The University of Queensland
Brisbane St Lucia, Australia

Barbara Kornblau, JD, OT/L, FAOTA, ABDA, DAAPM,
 CDMS, CCM (Chapter 13)
Dean
School of Health Professions and Studie
University of Michigan—Flint
Flint, Michigan

Rhonda Phillips, BA, Grad Dip (Chapter 2)
Australian Housing and Urban Research Institute
 (AHURI)
Queensland Research Centre
Research Officer, Housing Policy Research Program
University of Queensland Social Research Centre
The University of Queensland
Brisbane, Australia

Jon Pynoos, MCP, PhD (Chapter 2)
UPS Foundation Professor, Gerontology, Policy and
 Planning
Co-Director, Fall Prevention Center of Excellence
Andrus Gerontology Center
University of Southern California
Los Angeles, California

Jon Sanford, M Arch, BS (Chapter 4)
Director, Center for Assistive Technology and
 Environmental Access
Co-Director, Rehabilitation Engineering Research
 Center on Workplace Accommodations
Research Architect, Rehabilitation Research and
 Development Center of Excellence
Associate Professor, College of Architecture
Atlanta VA Medical Center
Decatur, Georgia

Bronwyn Tanner, BOccThy, Grad Cert OccThy, Grad
 Cert Soc Planning, MPhil (Chapters 1, 5, 12)
Occupational Therapy Lecturer
James Cook University
Townsville, Queensland, Australia

The following is a list of general contributors to the book:

Carolyn Baum, PhD, OTR/L, FAOTA
Elias Michael Director, Occupational Therapy
Professor, Occupational Therapy and Neurology
Washington University School of Medicine
St. Louis, Missouri

Catherine Bridge, PhD
Associate Professor, Faculty of the Built Environment
University of New South Wales
New South Wales, Australia

Diane Bright, OTR MSc ID
Director
Alliance Therapy/Access Answers
Troy, Michigan

Paul Coonan, B Des St, B Arch
Assistant Director of Planning
Strategic Portfolio Management Communities
    Property Portfolio
Queensland Department of Communities
Queensland, Australia

Richard Duncan, BA, MRP
Executive Director
RL Mace Universal Design Institute
Chapel Hill, North Carolina.

Rod Hunter, F.Dip. Arch RMIT, Reg'd Architect
ACAA Accredited Access Consultant
Managing Director
Hunarch Consulting
Balwyn, Victoria, Australia

Richard Kirk, B Des St, B Arch
Director
Richard Kirk Architect
Brisbane, Queensland, Australia

Trish Lapsley, BOccThy
Private Practice Occupational Therapist
Brisbane, Queensland Australia

Mary Law, PhD, OT Reg (Ont.), FCAOT
Professor
School of Rehabilitation Science
Co-Founder
CanChild Center for Childhood Disability Research
McMaster University
Hamilton, Canada

Danise Levine, AIA
Assistant Director/Architect
IDEA Center
Buffalo, New York

Dory Sabata, OTD, OTR/L, SCEM
Clinical Assistant Professor
University of Kansas Medical Center
Department of Occupational Therapy Education
Kansas City, Kansas

Bevin Shard, Assoc Dip App Sc Building
Superintendent Representative
Department of Public Works
Brisbane, Queensland, Australia

Amelia Starr, B App Sc (OT)
Occupational Therapist and Access Consultant
NSW Government
AARC Australia
National Convenor, Australian Network for Universal
    Housing Design (ANUHD)
Strawberry Hills, New South Wales, Australia

Jonathan Ward, B Des St
Architectural Assistant
Richard Kirk Architect
Brisbane, Queensland, Australia

PREFACE

With the integration of people with disabilities into society, there has been increasing interest in modifying homes to enable them to live independently in the community. The aging population has also raised concerns about how well homes can support people's health and safety as they age. Occupational therapists require skills and knowledge to assess the modification needs of these consumers, including consideration of their current and future requirements and the nature and use of the home environment. Therapists also need to understand the technical aspects of the built environment, design approaches, and the application of a range of products and finishes to determine appropriate modification solutions.

In this book, we discuss the transactional approach to examining the person-occupation-environment interaction and provide therapists with a detailed understanding of the various dimensions of the home environment that impact on home modification decisions. We also examine the context of home modification services and the impact of various demographic, legislative, policy, and service delivery traditions on the development and delivery of home modification services. In particular, we review the current legislative environment and the funding schemes that facilitate service delivery. Additionally, we explore the roles and perspectives of each stakeholder in the home modification process, and we present a range of strategies to assist occupational therapists to achieve effective and positive service delivery outcomes. We examine, in detail, the home modification process, including a review of approaches to evaluating, measuring, and drawing the environment; identifying and evaluating interventions; applying design standards; and reporting and legal issues. To assist the reader in identifying bases for evidence-based practice and topics for future research and theory development, we provide an overview of the literature on evaluating home modification outcomes. The book concludes with a series of case studies that highlight the application of the home modification process in developing effective solutions for a range of consumer groups.

Our challenge has been to provide a textbook that not only presents the theory relating to the person-occupation-environment transaction, but also one that provides therapists with the information they need to examine and influence this transaction. This knowledge has been acquired through years of extensive clinical, educational, and research experience in home modification practice and in training undergraduate, graduate, and postgraduate occupational therapy students as well as novice and experienced practitioners. This book provides us with an opportunity to share our expertise and years of experience of working with older people and people with disabilities to identify their home modification requirements. In addition, our experience as supervising practitioners working in the field has enabled us to identify the essential learning needs of occupational therapists providing home modification services. To date, the small amount of the literature in this field has been based solely on expert opinion. This book emerges from a solid theoretical foundation to provide practical real-life applications and strategies. It also provides a framework for examining the efficacy of home modification practice, shaping future research using evidence in practice.

Home modification practice is of interest in many countries around the world today. This book capitalizes on this international interest by focusing on the theory, knowledge, and skills that cross borders. People who require modifications to their homes face similar issues across the world. Similarly, occupational therapists worldwide are concerned with optimizing occupational performance and ensuring that people can live safely, independently, and comfortably in their own homes. This book seeks to address these universal issues while acknowledging the legislative and funding contexts that shape service delivery in respective countries.

We have written this book to meet the needs of students and clinicians from a range of settings. It is often challenging for students when translating general theoretical principles, which are outlined in generic occupational therapy texts, into practice. Particularly difficult is balancing the many complexities when working in the home environment—how to work collaboratively with the consumer to develop a mutually acceptable outcome and how to balance the scientific, narrative, pragmatic, and ethical reasoning to develop an effective intervention. In this text, we discuss how to consider the personal, cultural, social, societal, temporal, and physical aspects of the home in decision making and provide students with a systematic process for identifying and evaluating home-based interventions. The practical application of theory, legislation, and standards is a strong focus of the information presented and will equip student occupational therapists to work with people with a broad range of disabilities and to implement an occupational therapy process in the home environment. It takes them systematically through the process in a detailed and practical way, which is often not provided in generic occupational therapy texts. This book also supports students on clinical placement and those new graduates who find themselves in practice with foundation knowledge and skills but who are keen to acquire a deeper understanding of how to deal with the complexities they face in various settings. Although students are provided with an overview of knowledge required for practice during university training, it is not until they are faced with real-world practice situations that they understand the importance of the information presented in class and are ready to integrate the detail that is provided in this text.

This text also provides practitioners with tools and resources for home modification practice. We have provided several comprehensive case studies to assist novice therapists to understand the range of issues they need to consider to conceptualize solutions. For experienced therapists, we have provided theory and practical detail that draws on research and international literature to affirm and refine their practice. The depth of this book also supports practicing therapists by providing a rich and detailed description of the issues they encounter in day-to-day practice. It draws on the expertise of clinicians with extensive experience in providing interventions in the home and reviews international legislative and service systems, research, and literature to support practice. The text also encourages experienced therapists to develop structures to systematically gather information on the outcomes of home modification practice in an effort to ensure good outcomes for clients, to refine occupational therapy intervention, and to build a body of evidence to support this field of practice.

This book provides a range of resources and tools, and it can be used as a teaching aid to support students, interns, and novice therapists or as a manual for more experienced home modification practitioners. The case studies also expose therapists to scenarios that they may not have encountered and broaden their knowledge base to inform future practice with a range of client groups. The book is unique in that it strongly focuses on the practical application of theory and research in day-to-day practice, working toward enabling people to stay in their homes and communities.

In identifying contributors for the book, one of our goals was to draw on the views of experts practicing in the field in order to bring a breadth of perspectives to the discussion about how to undertake home modification practice. Although occupational therapists might experience limitations in their home modification practice because of a lack of funding or the requirements of the service in which they work, we hope that the theory presented in this book will stimulate interesting and lively thinking and promote discussion about future research and practice in the field. An Instructor's Manual based on the content of this book has been developed for use by students and clinicians to enable them to further reflect on and learn from their practice.

Home modification practice is a dynamic and evolving area, and we see this book as a starting point for the future development of occupational therapy knowledge and skill. We welcome comments and contributions to further inform this area of practice.

Elizabeth Ainsworth, MOccThy, Grad Cert Health Sci
Desleigh de Jonge, MPhil (OccThy), Grad Cert Soc Sci

FOREWORD

This team of occupational therapists has compiled a book that is timely as occupational therapists seek to understand the issues of and acquire the skills necessary to address the issues of space and place in the lives of our clients. Stegner (1992) asked us to consider space as a container of experiences and reminds us that no space is a place until that which happens in it is remembered. Occupational therapists are the enablers that help clients maximize their experiences in their space: how to move in it, function in it, be safe in it, and, when there are problems, identify and remove barriers that compromise it. Hasselkus (2002) described our task—to come to understand the meaning of people's spaces and to fit our interventions into those meanings. She said that occupational therapy is what helps people achieve a life with meaning in their places as they strive for independence and participation. This book gives us the knowledge and tools to acquire the skills to help people preserve independence and meaning in their homes.

The book is extremely well conceptualized and well written. This writing team has taken the need to address these important issues to a new level. Their book provides information that creates a societal context for home modifications. They link home modifications to contemporary models of occupational performance and include the content that supports assessment, intervention, design standards, and legal considerations. In addition, there is a series of case studies, and they report the evidence that supports the effectiveness of home modification interventions.

The editors have extensive clinical experience in home modifications as well as providing training to undergraduate and postgraduate students and practicing clinicians on home modification practice. The Queensland State Government in Australia has a Department of Housing that serves people from various cultures and backgrounds. This department delivers integrated social housing to low-income households for the duration of their need, provides support for low- to moderate-income households in the private market, and helps build sustainable communities. During the past decade, this department has employed occupational therapists to provide housing needs assessments and home modifications to older people and people with a range of disabilities. The therapists have an important leadership role, influencing the values and practice of service delivery staff as they work with clients and providing advice on policy and procedure improvements to various service areas. Staff members have also contributed to developing strong partnerships with community agencies as part of their service delivery role. Many of the authors have contributed to and worked with the Department of Housing and thus bring their clinical experience and reasoning to their chapters.

This is a book that should be on the bookshelf in every clinic (after having been read by the clinicians) and should be a core text for students. It is an encyclopedia of housing issues and strategies. Occupational therapists' focus on housing is not restricted to aging but is central to the concept of participation for any person at any age who is limited by mobility, sensory, motor, cognitive, or psychological problems and needs the best environmental fit. The home is the place for roles and activities that define people's lives. Occupational therapists armed with knowledge and skills can make a difference in people's daily lives. I know this book can help us step up to leadership in this important area of practice—a practice that will meet society's as well as individuals' needs.

References

Hasselkus, B. R. (2002). *The meaning of everyday occupation.* Thorofare, NJ: SLACK Incorporated.
Stegner, W. (1992). The sense of place. In W. Stegner (Ed.), *Where the bluebird sings to the lemonade springs* (pp. 199-206). New York, NY: Random House.

Carolyn Baum, PhD, OTR/L, FAOTA
Elias Michael Director, Occupational Therapy
Professor, Occupational Therapy and Neurology
Washington University School of Medicine
St. Louis, MO

Section I
The Home, Community, and Societal Context of Home Modifications

This introductory section provides the underpinnings of home modification practice. It examines the importance of the home environment to the resident, the approaches to home modification service delivery, models of occupational therapy that guide practice, legislation impacting on the role of the occupational therapist, and the history and future of home modification services. This information provides the context for the rest of the book, which describes the practical delivery of occupational therapy services.

1

The Home Environment

Bronwyn Tanner, BOccThy, Grad Cert OccThy,
Grad Cert Soc Planning, MPhil

Occupational therapists play a key role in recommending home modifications in the home environment and yet, as a profession, we have given little consideration to this unique context. Drawing from the work of environmental psychology and gerontology, this chapter presents a framework for considering the experience of "home," describing the personal, temporal, social, cultural, societal, and physical dimensions created through person-environment transactions. The relationship between a person and his or her dwelling is unique and complex, and it is important that therapists understand and acknowledge the nature of this relationship if they are to successfully negotiate changes. In examining the experience of home for the individual, this chapter considers the implications that each dimension of home has for occupational therapists practicing within the field of home modifications.

CHAPTER OBJECTIVES

By the end of this chapter, the reader will be able to:
+ Describe the role of person-environment transactions in the creation of home as a place of action and meaning
+ Explain a framework that considers the various domains of the experience of home

+ Apply this framework when reflecting on his or her life experience and clinical practice
+ Interpret how the experience of home may impact on occupational therapy practice; in particular, on decisions made about changes to the home environment

INTRODUCTION

Anyone who has been traveling for some time and has been separated from those they love or has just had a hard day at the office knows the comforting thoughts of returning home. The use of the word *home* in our general vocabulary is so commonplace and unconscious that it almost defies definition because, in those four letters, so much meaning is contained. For decades, poets and songwriters have used the nostalgic and emotional response that this simple word evokes.

For many occupational therapists, their place of work and the focus of their intervention is their client's home environment. This is particularly true of therapists working in the field of home modifications; however, little information exists in our professional literature about this particular context and the impact our intervention has on the person's experience of home. In one sense, this is surprising considering the amount of time many clinicians spend in other people's homes. It is likely, however,

Ainsworth, E., & de Jonge, D.
An Occupational Therapists's Guide to Home Modification Practice (pp. 3-16)
© 2011 SLACK Incorporated

that this omission reflects the progression of our profession and its theoretical underpinnings—from a medical orientation focusing on the person, disease, and the effects of this on his or her function to a broader understanding that acknowledges the impact of context or environment on occupational performance. This increase in emphasis on context is evident when comparing the most recent American Occupational Therapy Association (AOTA) Practice Framework (2008) with the previous AOTA Uniform Terminology for Occupational Therapy (1994). The early document refers to contexts as being either temporal (chronological, development, life cycle, and disability status) or environmental (physical, social, and cultural). The more recent AOTA document contains a much richer and deeper understanding of the context and environment with cultural, personal, temporal, and virtual aspects being specific to the context and physical and social aspects being specific to the environment (AOTA, 2008). As this progression to a broader understanding of the impact of context on occupational performance has only significantly impacted practice within the past two decades, it is then perhaps not unusual that little information exists within our professional literature on the importance of the specific concept or context of home.

The concept of home has, however, been widely researched within other fields, and a proliferation of writing exists on this topic within the areas of sociology, anthropology, psychology, human geography, architecture, and philosophy. The concept of home and its meaning in theoretical, social, and cultural contexts has been the focus of several decades of research in the field of environmental psychology—and, more recently, gerontology—and this chapter aims to present a framework for understanding home based on this research.

DEFINING HOME

While there exists within the literature "pronounced conceptual and empirical diversity" about the "meaning of home" (Oswald & Wahl, 2005, p. 21), many researchers argue that "an emotional based relationship with the dwelling place is what defines the very nature and essence of home" (Moore, 2000, p. 210). In other words, when we talk about a house, we are speaking of a dwelling place, but when we talk of home, we are often speaking of a relationship between an "objective socio-physical setting" and a "subjective" individual (Oswald & Wahl, p. 22).

Within environmental psychology literature, much of the writing about the concept of home is based on the premise that people live in worlds of meaning. Throughout life, people interact with their social and physical environments and create "meaningful representations of the self within the environment" (Oswald & Wahl, 2005, p. 23). Depending on their individual needs, goals, histories, and experiences and their cultural or shared understanding, people attribute a variety of meanings to their environment and in doing so make sense of their life experiences (Rubinstein, 1989). The sense of home is essentially a relationship created between an individual and his or her environment in which the individual attaches psychological, social, and cultural significance to objects and spaces (Dovey, 1985; Hasselkus, 2002; Werner, Altman, & Oxley, 1985).

Home, then, is an experience created by a flowing together of people, spaces, and psychological processes out of which sense and meaning are created.

PERSON-ENVIRONMENT TRANSACTIONS: THE HEART OF HOME

When does a dwelling place become a home? For many people, it is when they "act on" the physical environment. They may personalize a space by putting up objects they value or creating new spaces, such as gardens. In acting on the environment, they establish a history of being "in place," and spaces take on a significance that they previously did not have for the individual. A relationship between a person and his or her dwelling place is created through the transactions that occur between the individual and the environment (Dovey, 1985). This idea of acting on and being acted upon is at the heart of a transactional approach to people and environments.

A transactional approach or framework interprets the interaction between a person and his or her environment or context as something that is dynamic and always changing. The person and context can only be understood when examined together as a unified system. Trying to gain knowledge or understanding about the person as separate from the context in which he or she lives and acts is seen as a meaningless exercise because the two elements (person and context) are interwoven and interdependent (Altman, Brown, Staples, & Werner, 1992). Within a transactional approach, the term *context* refers to much more than just the physical surroundings and encompasses personal, social, cultural, and political aspects.

To illustrate this, consider the case of an older, hospitalized woman who is being considered for discharge to her home following a stroke. In therapy, she is able to manage three to four steps easily with the assistance of one person. A predischarge visit to home reveals an entrance with two to three steps. As part of her discharge plan, education is provided to her husband as to how to provide assistance to her when using steps in the hospital. Based on her performance in the hospital, she is deemed to be safe to manage the steps at home and is discharged. When the community health team visits a few weeks after discharge, however, they find that she has not been able to leave the house as she is unable to use the two to three steps. Why is her performance at home different from what she was doing in the hospital? The change has not occurred in her physical abilities but in elements of the context. In the first place, the steps of her home have a higher rise than those in the hospital, creating a greater level of difficulty. This, however, was not the only reason. In the hospital, she was either assisted or supervised by a trained aide or therapist who provided her with encouragement and confidence when undertaking the task of climbing stairs. In her home context, her husband did not feel comfortable assisting her, partly because of a lack of experience but also because assisting his wife was not in line with his cultural expectations. Both husband and wife came from a cultural background where the wife was the one who gave assistance, and this had been her role up until her stroke. He therefore was neither comfortable nor willing to take on the role of her assistant, and she was unable to use the steps without his help. The approach taken in discharging this woman was to assume that the performance of the woman (managing two to three stairs) in the hospital would be the same in the home context. A transactional approach would not assume that a person's performance or behavior would be the same if the environment or context changed. A different context is highly likely to result in a different outcome as the nature of person-environment transactions is dynamic and interdependent.

In addition to seeing people and contexts as interrelated and interwoven, a key defining feature of a transactional perspective is the realization that person-environment transactions are both observable and unobservable. Transactions occur at the level of observable actions (activities, tasks, routines, rituals) and also through unobservable psychosocial processes by which people evaluate, interpret, and ascribe meaning to their experiences (Werner et al., 1985). An example of this is provided in a recent newspaper story (Dalton, 2008). An elderly woman was required to relocate from her home of many years to make way for a new freeway. The article related her distress in moving from the place where she had raised her children and lived happily with her husband until his death a few years previously. It ended happily with her relocation to another house within sight of her previous home. In the article, she related the story of her "duchesse," a large cedar dressing table in her bedroom. The duchesse was very precious to her, not just because her husband had built it but because it was a link to him after his death. She reported that, on his deathbed, her husband had told her that when she heard a noise coming from the duchesse, it would be him letting her know that he was there watching over her. She reported that following his death, on the nights when she heard a noise coming from the duchesse, she would converse with her husband. This woman had ascribed meaning to a simple timber storage cabinet well beyond its observed utilitarian use.

Recent writing in occupational therapy literature around the meaning of occupation illustrates a similar distinction between "doing" and "being" (Watson & Fourie, 2004, p. 20). Doing is the performance element of occupation—it is tangible and obvious. Being is the sense of personal existence, supported by beliefs and values. When one engages in an occupation—say, writing a chapter for a book on home modifications—the being part of the activity (the beliefs and values of the author) influences the doing (what is written), which in turn influences the being (ideas and thoughts are clarified and given structure and cohesion). As a result of this dynamic and evolving interaction between doing and being, the individual is engaged in "becoming" an author. Becoming, the third element of occupation, is the "lifelong journey of discovery and adaptation that is realized through doing and influenced by being" (Watson & Fourie, p. 20). It is important to realize that even the most mundane doing has elements of being. How we structure our daily routines, the way we make the bed and clean our teeth, and when we shower all have some connection to our sense of who we are; that is, the being side of occupation. Even small changes to these elements of "doing" can dramatically impact on "being." Pastalan and Barnes (1999) note that an older person's survival following relocation into a high-care residence is related to his or her success in setting up satisfactory routines (i.e., the doing of occupation). Failure to do this is a contributing factor in how long a person will live postrelocation (Pastalan & Barnes).

A transactional approach is at the heart of many of the occupational therapy frameworks that focus on occupational performance, such as the

Person-Environment-Occupational Model (Law, Cooper, Strong, & Stewart, 1996), the Ecological Model of Occupation (Dunn, Brown, & Youngstrom, 2003), the Person-Environment-Occupational Performance Model (Baum, Bass-Haugen, & Christiansen, 2005; Christiansen & Baum, 1997), and the Model of Human Occupation (Keilhofner, 2002). The most recent AOTA Practice Framework (2008) also acknowledges the dynamic nature of person-context interactions as well as the "subjective (emotional or psychological) and objective (physically observable) aspects of performance" (p. 628). However, in day-to-day practice, occupational therapists are often so focused on the observable, measurable aspects of people acting in their environments that they are at risk of giving little consideration to the unobservable meaning-making processes that occur within the home context.

Hasselkus (2002) highlights this point in her distinction between understanding "space" as a neutral, abstract entity and "place" as a structured world of meaning. She proposed that occupational therapists focus often on space—the functional ability of our clients to move through and manipulate space and their ability to perceive spatially and the general accessibility of the physical space—rather than place—the meaning that our clients give to that space (p. 27).

Within the context of home, a focus on the observable elements of person-environment transactions alone can impact significantly on the relationship that exists between a person and his or her home and can detract from the meaning of home to an individual (Hawkins & Stewart, 2002; Heywood, 2005; Tanner, Tilse, & de Jonge, 2008). It is therefore essential that occupational therapists working within the home environment, in particular those engaged in recommending alterations to that environment, have an understanding of the particular context that is home and the possible impact that they may have on this domain of significant personal meaning.

CONCEPTUAL MODEL OF HOME

In the literature, where the concept or meaning of home uses a transactional approach, researchers have frequently referred to the experience of home as occurring across three main domains (Hayward, 1975; Sixsmith, 1986; Smith, 1994). Sixsmith, for example, identified "three modes of experience—the personal home; the social home; and the physical home" with each home featuring "a unique and dynamic combination of person, social and physical

properties, and meanings" (p. 294). These experiences are also seen to occur "within a temporal matrix of past, present, and future" (Sixsmith, p. 295). In a recent review of the major approaches in environmental psychology and gerontology about the experience of home, Oswald and Wahl (2005) compiled a framework that also structured the meaning of home as occurring across the domains of the physical, social, and personal.

The AOTA Practice Framework (2008) defines contexts as "a variety of interrelated conditions within and surrounding the client that influence performance" and lists differing environments and contexts as physical, social, cultural, personal, temporal, and virtual (p. 642). These contexts relate to the three domains listed above in the following way. The physical domain of home relates directly to the physical context of the practice framework. The social domain of home relates to the social and cultural contexts. The personal domain of home encompasses the personal context as well as touching on temporal aspects.

Figure 1-1 is a diagrammatic representation of the conceptual model of home outlined in this chapter. It shows the three domains of experience (the physical, personal, and social) created out of the transaction occurring between the person and the environment, in a temporal context of past, present, and future. The following discussion will explore each of these domains and their relevance to occupational therapy practice, particularly in the area of home modifications.

THE PHYSICAL HOME

The physical home is concerned with the idea of real space—the raw material from which the dweller builds a home. This includes the design and layout of the dwelling and the space that exists between the physical structures, which is shaped by function, culture, and history (Sixsmith, 1986; Steward, 2000). The physical experience of home also encompasses issues of amenity, such as temperature regulation, air flow, and lighting (Despres, 1991).

As occupational therapists, we are perhaps most familiar with the physical elements of the home environment and, in particular, we are interested in the fit that occurs between the person and his or her abilities and the physical demand or press of the environment when an individual performs a task. This idea of person-environment fit is drawn from the work of M. Powell Lawton, an esteemed researcher and theorist in the area of aging and environment who is considered by many to be a key

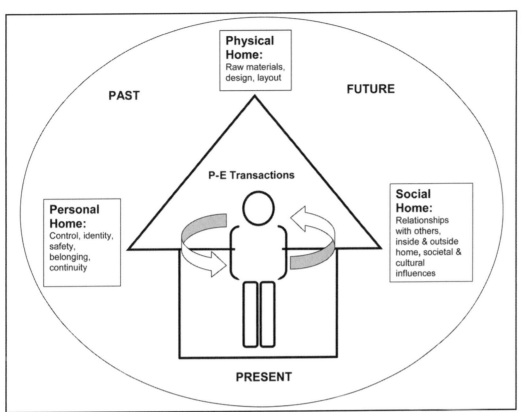

Figure 1-1. Conceptual model of home.

figure in the development of the home modifications field (Pynoos, Nishita, & Perelman, 2003). In attempting to address a neglect of the role of environment, particularly the physical environment, within the context of behavioral sciences generally and in gerontology specifically, Powell Lawton and Nahemow proposed an "Ecological Model of Environment and Ageing" in 1973 that was concerned with concepts of competence and environmental press (Powell Lawton, 1982).

Building on the earlier premise of Kurt Lewin, Powell Lawton and Nahemow's model proposed behavior as "the function of the competence of the individual and the environmental press of the situation" (Powell Lawton, 1982, p. 43) This behavior was "either...outwardly observable or an inner affective response" (Powell Lawton, p. 43). When a person was well adapted to his or her environment, he or she was considered to have achieved a state of balance between the press or demand of the external environment and his or her individual competency (Powell Lawton, p. 45; Figure 1-2).

One of the most common reasons for undertaking home modification is to reduce the demand of the physical environment, thus ensuring a better "fit" in which the person's abilities are well matched to what his or her environment requires. For example, removing a bathtub and installing a curbless shower recess reduces the demand or environmental press on an older person with limited range of movement and reduced muscle strength in the lower limbs. However, as indicated previously, it is important not to reduce the transaction between a person and his or her physical home environment to merely one of observable fit, as this relationship has been demonstrated to be far more subtle and complex.

There often exists between people and their physical home environments an innate understanding and awareness. Rubenstein (1989) found that older people "entexture" their physical environment to maximize their comfort by fine-tuning aspects of space, light, color, ambience, activity, and sound to suit the individual and his or her abilities (p. S51). Through the repeated routine use of a physical space, people develop an intimacy with the physical aspects of the home environment—a "physical insideness" (Dovey, 1985, p. 362). Often, this "profound sense of familiarity" is unconscious and only becomes apparent when threatened or destroyed (Dovey, p. 362).

The disruption of this "physical insideness" by changes to the physical structure and layout of a dwelling through home modifications can create distress for the individual even if physical amenity and accessibility is improved (Heywood, 2005; Tanner et al., 2008). The study by Tanner et al. told the story of

Figure 1-2. Press-competence model. (Copyright © 1973 by the American Psychological Association. Adapted with permission from Lawton, M. P. & Nahemow, L. [1973]. Ecology and the aging process. In C. Eisdorf, & M. P. Lawton [Eds.], *The Psychology of Adult Development and Aging* [pp. 619-674]. Washington, DC: American Psychological Association. No further reproduction or distribution is permitted without written permission from the American Psychology Association.)

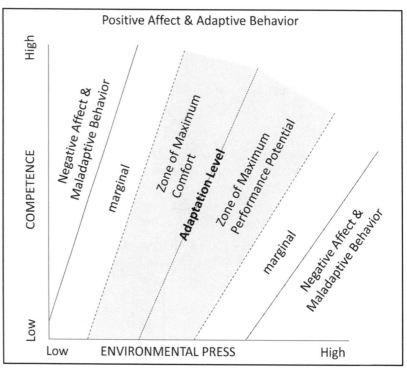

IMPLICATIONS FOR OCCUPATIONAL THERAPISTS

Olive, a widow who had lived in her home for 40 years. Olive had recently received a number of modifications to improve the overall accessibility of her home environment. The benefits of having an improved physical environment with less physical demand were tempered by her reaction to loss of familiar routines and habits. Because of the changes to the layout of her home to accommodate such improved access to the bathroom, toilet, laundry, and kitchen, Olive had to rearrange the way she did things on a daily basis. Simple routines and unconscious patterns of behavior were disrupted because of changes to room entrances and storage. She expressed a significant amount of distress about this and, in her own words, felt she had "lost her old home."

IMPLICATIONS FOR OCCUPATIONAL THERAPISTS

As indicated previously, the physical aspects of home are often the primary focus of the occupational therapist when considering how best to improve the fit between the individual and his or her home environment. The challenge for the therapist is to ensure that the physical aspects of the home environment are not considered separately from the individual and his or her goals and preferences. It is important that, when undertaking an assessment of the physical environment and identifying potential barriers or hazards to performance, the occupational therapist consider the innate understanding that exists between a person and his or her home. This includes gaining an understanding of the way the person has entextured or fine-tuned his or her home to suit individual needs and preferences. This will then enable a more comprehensive picture of the person-environment fit.

While a suitable physical environment has been identified by some researchers as an essential characteristic of a home (Smith, 1994), other studies have shown that the phenomenon of home is concerned minimally with physical structure and more with personal meanings (Hammer, 1999).

THE PERSONAL HOME

The concept of a personal home assumes that an emotionally based meaningful relationship exists between an individual and his or her dwelling place and that this experiential relationship is definitive in distinguishing a home from a house (Dovey, 1985; Moore, 2000). The personal home is a place of self-expression, identity, and personal control. It can be a central reference point in a person's life, encapsulating feelings of familiarity, security, and belonging (Despres, 1991; Dovey; Sixsmith, 1986). The personal home reflects the relationship, based on emotion and meaning, that develops between the person and his or her home environment.

Some common meanings of the personal home that have been identified in the literature and that will be explored include the following:

+ *Control*: Being at home means being in control and having mastery of the environment. This includes privacy, which is created by being able to control access to oneself (Despres, 1991; Smith, 1994);

+ *Safety and security*: Home is a haven and a place of regeneration, repose, and refreshment (Despres, 1991; Dovey, 1985; Sixsmith, 1986);

+ *Identity and expression of self*: Homes are personalized spaces, with many objects in the home being a reflection of an individual's identity (Despres, 1991; Dovey, 1985; Rubinstein, 1989; Sixsmith, 1986);

+ *Sense of belonging and continuity*: Home is where one has the experience of familiarity and is a symbol of continuity and connection between past, present, and future (Dovey, 1985; Mallett, 2004; Sixsmith & Sixsmith, 1991).

Control

The concepts of mastery and control are important when considering the relationship between the person and his or her home. Our homes are, perhaps, the only space in our lives in which we can expect to have control over what we do and whom we allow to enter. In this way, our homes are a personal territory; that is, places of privacy and security (Depres, 1991; Hayward, 1975; Tamm, 1999; Werner et al., 1985).

The perception of having control, particularly in the home environment, has been linked to higher levels of health and well-being and lower rates of hospitalization and mortality for older people (Schultz & Heckhausen, 1999). Control over access to one's home and one's person has been strongly linked to housing satisfaction among elderly residents (Kontos, 1998; Regnier, 2002).

For many older people and people with disabilities, relocation from home to residential care is often seen as a threat to the sense of self, independence, and control that having a home as a personal territory provides (Cooper & Hasselkus, 1992; Jones, de Jonge, & Phillips, 2008). Day (1985) has described home as "the last bulwark of independence" in older age (p. 53).

An outcome of home modifications is frequently the restoration of independence in the performance of personal and often intimate daily activities, such as showering and dressing. In increasing independence, privacy for the individual is also enhanced,

and the sense of home as a place of control is restored (Heywood, 2004a; Tanner et al., 2008). The impact of even small increases to privacy or control should not be underestimated. This was evident during a home assessment with Jill, a woman with cerebral palsy. Jill lived alone in her own unit but was assisted by visiting support workers in all activities of daily life. She used a motorized wheelchair for mobility and required assistance for all transfers in and out of her chair, showering, dressing, eating, and household tasks. As a result, Jill was always accompanied by a support worker for most of the activities normally undertaken with privacy. Of particular frustration to Jill was the supervision of showering, as this was an activity she enjoyed; however, because of safety concerns related to risk of inadvertently knocking the hot water tap with an uncontrolled movement, she always had someone present when showering. As a home modification, a temperature-regulating device to the hot water in the bathroom was installed. As a result of this modification, Jill could spend some time in the shower without the presence of a paid worker. Even though this modification did not alter Jill's functional performance in that she still needed assistance to wash, this small increase in privacy was extremely important to her in that it fostered a sense of home as a private space.

The issue of participation and control over the modification process is one that has been identified as a key area in the literature. A study into home adaptations in England and Wales found that wasteful adaptations, those resulting in poor outcomes because of a misdiagnosis of need, were "most often the result of limiting assessment to functional physical issues and leaving out psychological factors such as the need for dignity and sense of control. Wasteful adaptations were also typified by failure to heed the views of disabled people and families concerned" (Heywood, 2004a, p. 130).

The intrusion of outsiders, such as occupational therapists who recommend changes to the home environment, can alter the dynamic between the person and his or her home. This is particularly true where service delivery models are disempowering to the individual and so contribute to a loss of control (Heywood, 2004a). Studies into the role of professionals in home modifications show the importance of professional staff consulting, communicating, and listening to people with a disability when important decisions are being made about their housing (Heywood, 2004b, 2005; Nocon & Pleace, 1997; Pickering & Pain, 2003; Tanner et al., 2008). Ensuring that participants are actively engaged in the decision making around the intervention planned ensures the maintenance of perceived personal control and reinforces the meaning of home as a primary territory.

Safety and Security

The idea of home as a place of safety and security is linked with the issue of control. Home as a "haven," that is, a place for retreat, refreshment, and relaxation, is possible if one can control the intrusion of the public or "outside" and maintain a private or "inside" domain. In reality, dwelling places can, for many, fall short of the ideal of a place of safety or security. Children or adults in abusive relationships or older people in housing with physical features that they can no longer manage may not experience home as a haven or a place of safety.

The theme of home as a place of safety reinforces the importance of home modifications. People can often feel increasingly unsafe or threatened living in a home environment that provides physical barriers and challenges they can no longer manage. The purpose of modifying the home is often to improve the safety of the individual performing activities in his or her home environment by reducing the environmental demand. Home modifications both increase the actual safety of the person performing a specific task and the person's perceived sense of safety, security, and control. In reducing environmental press or demand, control of the environment is improved, and the experience of home as a place of security and safety is enhanced (Heywood, 2005; Tanner et al., 2008).

Identity and Self-Expression

Personalizing our dwelling places with objects that are individually significant is commonly how people express their identity in their home environments. In this way, home can be seen as an extension of self. There is a strong house-body metaphor as evidenced by the oft-reported feeling of personal violation when people are burglarized.

The value and meaning that people give to objects is unique and individual, and it is often difficult to understand the depth of feeling that people have for something you personally may not see as valuable. I recall one instance where, in following up on some home modifications that were completed, I spent a great deal of the time listening to and comforting the woman of the house. She was in tears over the carelessness of the tradesman who had damaged one of her garden gnomes. The amount of distress and grief that the loss of this ornament gave this woman was well beyond its monetary value (and my understanding!) but very real to her nonetheless.

In exploring the ways in which people attach meaning to their home environments, Rubenstein (1989) identified four aspects or stages in a continuum of relationship between people and objects or features of their physical environment.

The first stage of the continuum he called *accounting*, where one has an operating knowledge of objects or features that are at hand in the home (Rubenstein, 1989, p. S49). One is aware of the presence and location of various items such as cutlery, pencils, and gardening tools. Meaning is limited to basic utilitarian use or ownership. The second aspect is *personalization* in which environmental objects or features are endowed with meaning that is referent of events or aspects of one's life (Rubenstein, p. S49). Gifts that were given at Christmas or birthdays and objects bought on vacation are examples of this type of assigned meaning. There may not be an intense emotional involvement with the object, but there may be a story attached to them or they may give pleasure to the individual because of their associations.

The third stage Rubenstein (1989) called *extension*. In this process, the line between object and person becomes less distinct with a "more direct equation of the environmental feature with a part of self" (p. S49). Examples could be family photos, works of art, or other particularly precious objects, such as a wedding ring that means a great deal emotionally to the individual. As indicated previously, the value placed on the objects does not necessarily equate with monetary value. This was again brought home to me in the response of one client I visited who, when asked about what was most important or precious to her in her home, identified the tree in her front yard. The tree had been her first Christmas tree, in a pot on their dining room table when she, her husband, and young family first moved into their house more than 40 years ago. She very proudly proclaimed it was now a landmark in the district. The tree had become not only a referent of a life event (their first Christmas in their home) but also an extension of her self-identity, representing her life history in her home and community.

The fourth and final stage in Rubenstein's continuum is "embodiment" in which the "environmental feature becomes subjectively merged with the individual" (1989, p. S50). The environmental feature can also come to function as a prosthetic part of self. For me, this is illustrated in the story of an elderly lady I visited to assess her need for grab bars in her bathroom. She had lost her husband of many years about a year before my visit. When asked about her daily routine, she recounted her usual activities, which culminated with dinner in front of the TV in one of a pair of matching lounge chairs. The other chair had been her husband's, and prior to his death, they ritually had dinner every night in front of the TV watching the news and "chatting." After she told me this, she leaned over and whispered, "I still talk to him in his chair you know." For her, the chair represented or embodied the memory of a relationship that had lasted more than 50 years.

The endowment of symbolic meaning upon physical objects or features of the environment is an intensely personal and individual process. Home modifications, as changes to the physical environment, have the potential to inadvertently disrupt the symbolic environment of the home. Where home modifications are made without awareness and understanding of the significance of deeply embedded routines and rituals or the subjective meaning of various physical features in the home environment, they can equally undermine the sense of home and self-identity for an individual. Because the home environment is so closely linked to our idea of self and self-identity, suggestions of altering the physical appearance of the home in a way that is linked with disability or illness may be not be acceptable to the individual. Most occupational therapists who have recommended grab bars or assistive devices to clients can recall instances where recommendations were perceived negatively or rejected outright by the person because they projected an unwanted image of self or disrupted the aesthetic look of a bathroom (Hawkins & Stewart, 2002; Tamm, 1999; Tanner et al., 2008).

Sense of Belonging and Continuity

Because home is so closely tied to a sense of self and identity, it generates in many people a sense of belonging. "To be at home is to know where you are…to inhabit a secure center and to be orientated in space" (Dovey, 1985, p. 36). Associated with a sense of belonging is a sense of continuity, of connectedness with our past, present, and future in relationship to our home space (Dovey).

As well as assigning meaning to objects as representations of ourselves or our lives, we engage in personal rituals and routines that anchor us to dwelling places (Pastalan & Barnes, 1999, p. 82). As discussed previously with the story of Olive (Tanner et al., 2008), the performance of these daily tasks or rituals contributes to the creation of "insideness," a sense of familiarity and belonging that is "rooted in bodily routines" (Dovey, 1985, p. 38). Rowles (2000) uses the term *autobiographical insideness* to describe the relationship that develops over time

where a person becomes part of the place and the place becomes part of the person (p. 58S). This sense of the familiar becomes taken for granted. As a consequence, home becomes a place of relaxation because of the stability of routine behavior and experience (Dovey).

These daily routines and rituals, such as making the morning coffee, meals with family, sitting in a favorite chair to listen to favorite music, and hanging out the laundry, are usually highly individualized and provide us with comfort and a sense of control, belonging, and identity. They give us meaning in terms of who we are and what we do (Pastalan & Barnes, 1999). Rowles (2000) uses the term *choreography of being-in-place* to describe this complex arrangement of habitual actions, relationships, and environmental meanings (p. S59). When this daily choreography is disrupted through illness, accident, or loss of ability, the balance of a person's life is disturbed. Routines and rituals become disrupted, and there is the potential for a diminution of self and a loss of identity, self-esteem, and relationship to place and community (Pastalan & Barnes; Rowles).

The routines and rituals of daily life bring with them a temporal element that is an important consideration in understanding the meaning of home. Within a transactive perspective, home, as a physical, social, and personal experience, occurs within a temporal framework, reflecting the dynamic and changing nature of the meaning of "home" for individuals over time. Home is a place of the "lived experience" of time, which is often outside the here and now, or "clock" time (Zemke, 2004, p. 610). People's relationships to their homes have histories, futures, recurrences, and rhythms that affect their present experience and meaning (Dovey, 1985; Werner et al., 1985). The occupations occurring within the home have temporal aspects—"rhythm (patterns of tasks within the occupation), tempo (rate or speed of the process of occupation), synchronization (with other co-participants), duration, and sequence (ordering of task), which contribute to the patterns of daily occupations" (Zemke, p. 610).

As occupational therapists, we are often concerned with the minutia of activities of daily living in the here and now without truly understanding the depth of meaning that these life-centering activities give to the daily lives of the people with whom we work. Where home modifications are able to support the performance of daily rituals, they assist in sustaining a sense of place and a sense of self and identity.

For many older people who have lived in the same house for a number of years, homes become "storehouses of memories," providing a sense of identity

(Sixsmith & Sixsmith, 1991, p. 187). The significance of home can increase as people age because, due to reduced ability and energy, people spend increasingly more time at home (Haak, Ivanoff, Fange, Sixsmith, & Iwarsson, 2007; Sixsmith, 1986). Home becomes a way of "preserving independence and as a symbol of continuing individuality" (Sixsmith & Sixsmith, 1991, p. 189) with many older people preferring to remain at home as long as possible (Jones et al., 2008; Tanner et al., 2008).

Home modifications can play an important role in assisting the older person to age in place by reducing the demand of the environment. Heywood (2005) states that one of the key strengths of home modification is that it offers a way of maintaining a sense of "rootedness" or remaining in place (p. 545).

Though for older people the home of the past is important, for younger children with a disability, consideration of the continuity of home into the future is vital. Heywood (2004b) found that modifications carried out for children frequently lacked the vision of the child growing into the future. As a result, many modifications had become "completely unsuitable," particularly due to a lack of much needed space and provision for change (Heywood, p. 723). The needs of children to grow and develop "physically, intellectually, emotionally, and socially" (p. 722) must be incorporated into modification design to ensure a sense of home as a place of continuity and belonging.

Implications for Occupational Therapists

For many occupational therapists, the aspects of home as a place of deep personal meaning will align well with their individual orientation to home visiting and home modifications. This is because the professional frame of reference and associated model of practice from which an occupational therapist operates impacts directly on his or her understanding of the relationship of an individual to his or her environment and ultimately on his or her clinical reasoning and decision-making processes. Working from a client-centered approach automatically alerts the occupational therapist to the nuances of individual preferences and priorities and assists in keeping the individual in a position of control in his or her home environment supporting the unique relationship of the person to the home (Hawkins & Stewart, 2002).

Of primary importance is that occupational therapists respect clients' homes as personal territory—places of primary control, privacy, and security and arranged according to the personal preferences and personal meanings of the home dweller. All activities carried out in the home by occupational therapists should be participatory and collaborative, particularly any decision making about possible alterations or changes to the physical environment. The unique and personal value of objects within the home should be considered carefully.

In our busy, efficient schedules of home visiting, we can easily think only of clock time—the here and now—without consideration of the more subtle and temporal aspects contained within the home environment. Any assessment or intervention planned should be viewed not just in the present, but also within the context of past experiences and histories as well as future hopes and possibilities (Fisher, 1998). Changes to routines and rituals, each with their own unique temporal aspects, should be minimized and negotiated, with awareness of the importance of these activities in giving meaning to daily life.

Finally, it is important to remember that the relationship between a person and his or her dwelling place is unique and complex. Resistance to suggestions or recommendations by the occupational therapist may have its roots in aspects of the personal home that the individual may not be able to articulate. Embracing complexity for occupational therapists working in home modifications means looking beyond the home environment as merely a "conceptual space" that is geometric and objectively measured, in which people and things exist (Dovey, 1985, p. 35). Occupational therapists need to view home as a "lived space;" that is, a place that is dynamic and where the processes between the person and his or her environment occur "at the level of action and at the level of meaning" (Werner et al., 1985, p. 3).

THE SOCIAL HOME

The social home refers to the emotional environment created by relationships with others. In first consideration, the social home involves those relationships most significant to the individual such as a spouse or family who may often inhabit the same physical environment. The social home also extends further to those who may enter the home on occasion or are outside of the home space but still exert an influence, such as relatives, neighbors, friends, and community networks. The act of making a home is, however, in essence a cultural act. In establishing domestic arrangements, an individual is "expressing some of the most basic cultural notions about personhood and social life" (Rubenstein, 1989, p. S47). The social home therefore includes social influences, which are at some distance from the individual. These include cultural, political, and legal institutions, which influence the social experience of home through establishing norms, role expectations, shared cultural customs, and beliefs as well as behavioral standards, expectations, and opportunities (AOTA, 2008; Fisher, 1998).

With regard to the impact of modifications on the social home, studies have found that modifications can positively alter the relationships with others in the house by reducing the burden placed on caregivers who are often spouses or family members (Gitlin, Corcoran, Winter, Boyce, & Hauck, 2001; Heywood, 2004b; Lanspery & Hyde, 1997). An example of this is the caregiver who reported that she knew "what it was like to be in prison" prior to an access lift being installed in her house. Since the installation of the lift, she and her father (for whom she cares) have been "dirty stop outs…out nearly every day" with a greatly improved reported quality of life (Tanner et al., 2008, p. 205).

However, the converse can also be true. If the assessment of the client's home modification needs is done from a purely functionalist perspective, important aspects of the social home will be missed, and the client may resist recommendations that undermine his or her experience of the social home (Hawkins & Stewart, 2002). Heywood (2004b) reported examples of where the family structure had been weakened by a focus on the individual with a disability and not considering the family as a whole (p. 723).

As with the notion of autobiographical insideness, Rowles (2000) talks of social habituation that arises from daily common social interaction and the creation and maintenance within a neighborhood or community of social roles, with shared norms and implicit rules for behavior (p. 57S). For some, this experience of the social home can be the most important element in contributing to the essence of home for an individual.

An example of this is Betty, reported by Tanner and colleagues (2008). Betty was in her late 60s and lived in a larger, older house. She had great difficulty accessing her home environment, including the front steps and the bathroom. Minor modifications had been made; however, due to her functional limitations, she was unable to properly access the bath area and washed using a basin. When offered new accommodation that was fully accessible, within the same suburb, and less than a kilometer away from her current home, she chose to remain in an inconvenient and ill-suited physical dwelling.

The reason for this decision was to maintain her ongoing involvement with the local children who gathered in her front yard each morning to get on the school bus. As she said,

> By them (the children) being here the bus comes along up the road here, they walk across to catch it and I know they're safe.… It makes you feel you're doing something even though I'm not really doing anything…to most of the neighborhood children, I'm Nana. It doesn't matter whether they are related or not. I'm Nana. Even the 18- and 19-year-olds still refer to me as Nana. I've got a very large family! (Tanner et al., 2008, p. 203).

This valued social role and important social network would have been lost by the move, as the new accommodation was not on the school bus route (Tanner et al., 2008). This type of social relationship and connection with others is an integral part of the experience of home, particularly as one ages. Being able to contribute and do things for others has been found to be important in strengthening personal identity and a sense of being a valued part of society (Haak et al., 2007). An absence of relationships with others can result in loneliness and isolation for older people, and home can be experienced as "a prison" (Haak et al., p. 99). Thus, the location of the dwelling in terms of its ability to facilitate and sustain social networks and support valued social roles is an important aspect of the social home and should be considered in the assessment and recommendations of home modifications.

In considering changes to home layout and routines, societal norms for the home environment also need to be considered as these can have a significant impact on the level of acceptability of proposed changes. The social stigma associated with illness and disability can be a powerful deterrent to accepting the need for physical changes to the home that are symbolic of disability. For example, the installation of a ramp to the front entrance of a home may be rejected as it both stigmatizes the house as a "disabled" dwelling and is seen to reduce the economic value of the property. Additionally, it can also signal the vulnerability of the home dweller to potential home invasion.

Cultural norms about what is acceptable in the home can also impact the design of modifications, as many cultures have taboos and rituals regarding washing, food preparation, and social interaction. For example, in some communities, certain family members may be prohibited from interacting directly due to customary cultural laws. As family members can be residing in the same house, this can have significant implications for the design of home modifications around common use areas.

In most cultures, the cultural expectations about the use of home space can impact on the level of acceptance of suggested changes. Often, there is a division between private space (bedroom and bathrooms) and more public areas (lounge and dining rooms). Suggestions that breach this division may not be well received. For example, if following illness or trauma, a lounge room is more accessible than a bedroom and bathroom, the use of this more public space as a sleeping and bathing area may not be considered acceptable.

Implications for Occupational Therapists

The importance of the social home presents challenges to the assessment, decision making, and rationale for the delivery of home modification services. For the occupational therapist, assessment is often focused on the individual client and his or her level of function. As with the personal home, consideration of the social home requires the occupational therapist to think more broadly than traditional approaches. The social home demands a focus not just on the client and his or her immediate environment, but also on broader social networks, relationships, and roles both within the home and the wider community.

In assessing and designing for modification, the occupational therapy assessment must consider the needs and values of the caregiver or other family as well as those of the individual to ensure the best outcomes for home modification. Therapists may also be challenged by differing priorities of the individuals with whom they work as maintaining important social networks and roles within the wider community may be more important to the individual than comfort and accessibility in the physical environment. Understanding the cultural context of the individual is also an important factor that will impact on the design of modifications. Home modifications need to be viewed in the broader context of cultural and societal norms and customs as well as that of the individual's function.

Consideration of the social home will impact on the level of service delivery and the cost of modifications. Considering family and caregiver needs as well as those of the individual is likely to result in a more extensive modification with a higher cost. The importance placed on the valued social roles and social networks of an individual, particularly if living in an older dwelling, brings a complexity to discussions about economic viability of modifying the home. Heywood (2004b) states that "the complexity and range of human need is great and there

is a danger of underestimating it when considering the housing needs" of people with a disability (p. 724). Balancing the needs of the individual with the economic reality of service delivery will be a challenge; however, it is important, particularly for the occupational therapist, that the complexity of the social home is not underestimated as a powerful contributor to service quality and design.

CONCLUSION

In this chapter, we have explored, from a transactive perspective, a conceptual framework of home drawn from environmental psychology and gerontology literature. The aim of doing so was to provide a better understanding of the complex, dynamic, and unique relationship that is home and within which the process of home modification assessment and intervention takes place.

Home modifications have the potential to enhance the experience of home as a place of significant and unique personal and social meaning in a variety of ways. These include supporting the continuation of important personal rituals that link people to their home environment, providing a sense of place, self, and identity; enhancing control, safety, and security supporting home as a primary personal territory; and enhancing and fostering relationships and social networks by facilitating remaining at home. The potential also exists for home modifications to undermine the meaning and experience of home for an individual. This can occur if the physical aspects of accessibility and functionality are emphasized and the personal and social meanings of home held by the home dweller are neglected or disregarded and if models of service delivery are disempowering, contributing to a loss of control by individuals in decision making about their homes.

The challenge for the therapist is that much of the experience of home outlined in this chapter is not only unique and changing but also unobservable, un–self-conscious, and taken for granted until threatened. Just as a completed painting contains within it many layers of mostly hidden drawings and paint known only to the artist, so our homes, visible on one level as a physical structure, contain many hidden and unseen elements, known only to the home dweller.

In C. S. Lewis' classic tale *The Lion, the Witch, and the Wardrobe*, when Lucy enters the wardrobe, she finds an entire new world of Narnia awaiting her, a world that is both larger and more surprising than the banal world of an English house might lead one to expect (Lewis, 1991). Her brother Edmund, when entering the same wardrobe, merely finds a wardrobe. In a similar way, when we enter a person's home, we can be open to the wonder and complexity that is home and the world of meaning that exists for that individual, or we can limit our vision to ordinary expectations of visible, physical space. Having an understanding of the complex nature of person-environment relationships challenges the therapist to move beyond a simplistic, functionalist view of person-environment fit to one that embraces the complexity of what home means to an individual. Home modifications recommended by such a therapist have a much greater chance of benefiting individuals in their own unique world of meaning.

REFERENCES

Altman, I., Brown, B. B., Staples, B., & Werner, C. M. (1992). A transactional approach to close relationships: Courtship, weddings and place making. In W. B. Walsh, K. H. Craik, & R. H. Price (Eds.), *Person-environment psychology: Models and perspectives* (pp. 193-204). Hillsdale, NJ: Lawrence Erlbaum Associates.

American Occupational Therapy Association. (1994). Uniform terminology for occupational therapy--third edition. *American Journal of Occupational Therapy, 48*(11), 1047-1054.

American Occupational Therapy Association. (2008). Occupational therapy practice framework: Domain and process (2nd ed.). *American Journal of Occupational Therapy, 62*, 625-683.

Baum, C., Bass-Haugen, J., & Christiansen, C. H. (2005). Person-environment occupational performance: A model for planning interventions for individuals and organizations. In C. H. Christiansen and C. Baum (Eds.), *Occupational therapy: Performance, participation and well-being.* (pp. 242-266). Thorofare, NJ: SLACK Incorporated.

Christiansen, C. H., & Baum, C. (1997). Person-environment occupational performance: A conceptual model of practice. In C. H. Christiansen & C. Baum (Eds.), *Occupational therapy: Enabling function and well-being.* (2nd ed., pp. 46-71). Thorofare, NJ: SLACK Incorporated.

Cooper, B. A., & Hasselkus, B. (1992). Independent living and the physical environment. *Canadian Journal of Occupational Therapy, 59*(1), 6-15.

Dalton, T. (2008). House of memories. *Courier Mail*, January 12, 24-27.

Day, A. T. (1985). *We can manage: Expectations about care and varieties of family support among people 75 years and over.* Melbourne, Australia: Institute of Family Studies.

Despres, C. (1991). The meaning of home: Literature review and directions for future research and theoretical development. *Journal of Architectural and Planning Research, 8*(2), 96-115.

Dovey, K. (1985). Home and homelessness. In I. Altman & C. M. Werner (Eds.), *Home environments* (pp. 33-61). New York, NY: Plenum Press.

Dunn, W., Brown, C., & Youngstrom, M. J. (2003). Ecological model of occupation. In P. Kramer, J. Hinojosa, & C. B. Royeen (Eds.), *Perspectives in human occupation: Participation in life* (pp. 222-263). Baltimore, MD: Lippincott, Williams & Wilkins.

Fisher, A. G. (1998) Uniting practice and theory in an occupational framework. *American Journal of Occupational Therapy, 52*(7), 509-520.

Gitlin, L. N., Corcoran, M., Winter, L., Boyce, A., & Hauck, W. W. (2001). A randomized, controlled trial of a home environmental intervention: Effect on efficacy and upset in caregivers and on daily function of persons with dementia. *The Gerontologist, 41*(1), 4-14.

Haak, M., Ivanoff, S. D., Fange, A., Sixsmith, J., & Iwarsson, S. (2007). Home as the locus of origin for participation: Experiences among very old Swedish people. *Occupational Therapy Journal of Research: Occupation, Participation and Health, 27*(3), 95-103.

Hammer, R. (1999). The lived experience of being at home. *Journal of Gerontological Nursing, 25*(22), 10-19.

Hasselkus, B. R. (2002). *The meaning of everyday occupation.* Thorofare, NJ: SLACK Incorporated.

Hawkins, R., & Stewart, S. (2002). Changing rooms: The impact of adaptations on the meaning of home for a disabled person and the role of occupational therapists in the process. *British Journal of Occupational Therapy, 65*(2), 81-87.

Hayward, D. G. (1975). Home as an environmental and psychological concept. *Landscape, 20*, 2-9.

Heywood, F. (2004a). The health outcomes of housing adaptations. *Disability & Society, 19*(2), 129-143.

Heywood, F. (2004b). Understanding needs: A starting point for quality. *Housing Studies, 19*(5), 709-726.

Heywood, F. (2005). Adaptation: Altering the house to restore the home. *Housing Studies, 20*(4), 531-547.

Jones, A., de Jonge, D., & Phillips, R. (2008). *The role of home maintenance and modification services in achieving health, community care and housing outcomes in later life.* Melbourne, Australia: Australian Housing and Urban Research Institute.

Keilhofner, G. (2002). *A model of human occupation: Theory and application* (3rd ed.). Baltimore, MD: Lippincott, Williams & Wilkins.

Kontos, P. C. (1998). Resisting institutionalization: Constructing old age and negotiating home. *Journal of Aging Studies, 12*(2), 167-185.

Lanspery, S., & Hyde, J. (Eds.). (1997). *Staying put: Adapting the places instead of the people.* Amityville, NY: Baywood Publishing Company Inc.

Law, M., Cooper, B., Strong, S., & Stewart, D. (1996). The person-environment-occupation model: A transactive approach to occupational performance. *Canadian Journal of Occupational Therapy, 63*(1), 9-23.

Lewis, C. S. (1991). *The lion, the witch and the wardrobe.* London, England: HarperCollins.

Mallett, S. (2004). Understanding home: A critical review of the literature. *The Sociological Review*, 62-89.

Moore, J. (2000). Placing home in context. *Environmental Psychology, 20*, 207-217.

Nocon, A., & Pleace, N. (1997). Until disabled people get consulted: The role of occupational therapy in meeting housing needs. *British Journal of Occupational Therapy, 60*(3), 115-122.

Oswald, F., & Wahl, H. (2005). Dimensions of the meaning of home in later life. In G. D. Rowles & H. D. Chaudhury (Eds.), *Home and identity in late life: International perspective* (pp. 21-46). New York, NY: Springer Publishing Company Inc.

Pastalan, L. A., & Barnes, J. E. (1999). Personal rituals: Identity, attachment to place, and community solidarity. In B. Schwarz & R. Brent (Eds.), *Aging, autonomy and architecture: Advances in assisted living* (pp. 81-89). Baltimore, MD: The Johns Hopkins University Press.

Pickering, C., & Pain, H. (2003). Home adaptations: User perspectives on the role of professionals. *British Journal of Occupational Therapy, 66*(1), 2-8.

Powell Lawton, M. (1982). Competence, environmental press, and the adaptation of older people. In M. M. Powell Lawton, P. Windley, & T. Byerts (Eds.), *Aging and the environment* (Vol. 7, pp. 33-59). New York, NY: Springer Publishing Company.

Pynoos, J., Nishita, C., & Perelman, L. (2003). Advancements in the home modification field: A tribute to M. Powell Lawton. *Journal of Housing for the Elderly, 17*(1&2), 105-116.

Regnier, V. (2002). *Design for assisted living.* New York, NY: John Wiley & Sons, Inc.

Rowles, G. D. (2000). Habituation and being in place. *The Occupational Therapy Journal of Research, 20*(Suppl 2000), 52S-67S.

Rubinstein, R. L. (1989). The home environments of older people: A description of the psychosocial processes linking person to place. *Journal of Gerontology: Social Sciences, 44*(2), 545-553.

Schultz, R., & Heckhausen, J. (1999). Aging, culture and control: Setting a new research agenda. *The Journals of Gerontology, 54B*(3), 139-145.

Sixsmith, A. J., & Sixsmith, J. A. (1991). Transitions in home experience in later life. *Journal of Architectural and Planning Research, 8*(3), 181-191.

Sixsmith, J. A. (1986). The meaning of home: An exploratory study of environmental experience. *Journal of Environmental Psychology, 6,* 281-298.

Smith, S. G. (1994). The essential qualities of a home. *Journal of Environmental Psychology, 14,* 31-46.

Steward, B. (2000). Living space: The changing meaning of home. *British Journal of Occupational Therapy, 63*(3), 105-110.

Tamm, M. (1999). What does a home mean and when does it cease to be a home? Home as a setting for rehabilitation and care. *Disability and Rehabilitation, 21*(2), 49-55.

Tanner, B., Tilse, C., & de Jonge, D. (2008). Restoring and sustaining home: The impact of home modifications on the meaning of home for older people. *Journal of Housing for the Elderly, 22*(3), 195-215.

Watson, R., & Fourie, M. (2004). Occupation and occupational therapy. In R. Watson & L. Swartz (Eds.), *Transformation through occupation* (pp. 19-32). London, England: Whurr Publishers Ltd.

Werner, C. M., Altman, I., & Oxley, D. (1985). Temporal aspects of homes: A transactional perspective. In I. Altman & C. M. Werner (Eds.), *Home environments* (Vol. 8, pp. 1-32). New York, NY: Plenum Press.

Zemke, R. (2004). Time, space and the kaleidoscopes of occupation. *American Journal of Occupational Therapy, 58*(6), 608-620.

2

Approaches to Service Delivery

Desleigh de Jonge, MPhil (OccThy), Grad Cert Soc Sci;
Andrew Jones, BA, MSW, GCE; Rhonda Phillips, BA, Grad Dip;
and Jon Pynoos, MCP, PhD

Occupational therapists have long been interested in helping people to live well in their home environment but have not always had access to the funding, services, or resources to meet the home modification needs of their consumers. However, toward the end of the 20th century, a range of home modification services and resources were developed that enabled occupational therapists to access a selection of public and private services to address those needs. A number of factors have influenced the development and delivery of home modification services. This chapter aims to provide therapists with an understanding of those factors—the various demographic, legislative, policy, and service delivery traditions that have influenced, and will continue to influence, the development and delivery of home modification services—and the associated implications for occupational therapists and consumers of these services.

CHAPTER OBJECTIVES

By the end of this chapter, the reader will be able to:

+ Describe various demographic, legislative, policy, and service delivery traditions that have influenced the development and provision of home modification services

+ Describe the impact of health, community care, and housing service systems on the way home modification services are delivered and the associated implications for occupational therapists and consumers of home modification services

INTRODUCTION

As the demographics of societies change, governments and service providers seek to plan for and respond to the changing needs of the community. Advances in health care have resulted in increasing numbers of people surviving significant injuries and poor health conditions and living into old age. The soaring costs of health care and the aging population have impelled governments to establish strategic directions that allow older people and people with disabilities to continue to live in their own homes and communities. Policies such as de-institutionalization meant that people with disabilities were integrated back into the community in the latter part of the 20th century, and "aging-in-place" policies reflect a commitment to helping older people, as well as people with disabilities who are living longer, to remain in their communities. These recent demographic changes and policy developments have resulted in funding allocations across a

Ainsworth, E., & de Jonge, D.
An Occupational Therapists's Guide to Home Modification Practice (pp. 17-32)
© 2011 SLACK Incorporated

number of service systems—health, community care, and housing—to enable older people and people with disabilities to live safely and independently in the community. This funding also stimulated the development of a range of home modification services. These developments have had an effect on the workload of occupational therapists; whereas they have traditionally worked within the health system, they are now finding themselves increasingly in demand across a wide range of sectors.

Models of health have also had an influence on how health is conceived and funded and how services are delivered. Disability was viewed traditionally as an attribute of the person, which meant that health services were primarily focused on treating the person's disease or disorder. More recently, the social model of disability, which views disability as the inability of society to accommodate the diverse abilities in the community, has shifted the focus from addressing the limitations of the individual to addressing barriers in the environment. Furthermore, antidiscrimination and civil rights legislation, which acknowledges the rights of all people in the community, has led to the development of policies to ensure everyone has equitable access to community facilities and services. Consequently, revised building standards now ensure that people with disabilities can access public buildings. A growing interest in the design of residential buildings—to enable people to function well in their home environments across their lifespan—has also led to residential design standards and legislation being developed.

DEMOGRAPHICS

It is estimated that approximately 15.1% of Americans, which is 41.3 million people, have at least one type of disability, with more than half (22.7 million people) having two or more types of disability (Brault, 2008). Activity limitations are experienced by 15% of U.S. residents, or 37.7 million people, with 11.5 million people being unable to perform a major activity, 14.3 million being limited in the kind or amount of major activity they can perform, and 11.9 million being limited in activities other than their major activity (Kraus, Stoddard, & Gilmartin, 1996).

Internationally, there is an increasing number and proportion of older people, many of whom are aging with, or into, disability. The rise in the birth rate between 1946 and 1964 means that a large number of people are approaching retirement. This "wave" of baby boomers is expected to have an enduring

impact on societies for many decades to come—the result of a steady decline in fertility rates and increases in life expectancy (Freedman, 2007). In 1950, when baby boomers were first counted in the U.S. Census, people aged 65 and older made up just 8% of the population. In 2010, people aged 65 and older are projected to represent 13% of the total U.S. population; and, by 2030, this figure is expected to reach 19% (Vincent & Velkoff, 2010). Although the United States has a lower proportion of people older than 65 compared with many economically developed countries (National Institute on Aging, 2006), there are still enduring social and economic implications associated with this population trend. Figure 2-1 illustrates the impact of the Baby Boom Generation on the American population over time.

In the US, it has been reported that approximately 38% of older people in the community have some activity limitations resulting from chronic health conditions, with approximately 12% having limitations in a major activity (Kutty, 1999). Although activity limitations are not an inevitable consequence of aging and the prevalence of disability among older people has declined significantly in the latter part of the 20th century, older Americans have been found to have mobility impairments (33%), hearing impairments (33%), vision problems (20%), chronic disabilities (20%), and severe cognitive impairments (7% to 8%). Women, minorities, and people from lower socioeconomic groups are especially at risk (Freedman, Martin, & Schoeni, 2002). Figure 2-2 displays the growing rate of disability that occurs when people age.

The capacity of people to engage in daily activities and remain living in the community as they age or acquire a disability is also likely to be affected by the quality and nature of their living environment. Many people live in detached houses in the suburbs that are designed for young families with private transport. These dwellings have features that create hazards and barriers for occupants with disabilities or who are aging (Bridge, Parsons, Quine, & Kendig, 2002; Faulkner & Bennett, 2002). Housing is generally designed and constructed with little thought to the access, safety, independence, and location needs of the residents (Stone, 1998). Most housing in the United States (more than 90%) is inaccessible and unlikely to be replaced in the near future (Steinfeld, Levine, & Shea, 1998). Houses with stairs, narrow doorways and corridors, inaccessible toilets and bathrooms, and limited space "create" disability (Heywood, 2004; Oldman & Beresford, 2000) and can compromise the safety (Stone; Trickey, Maltais, Gosslein, & Robitaille, 1993), independence (Frain & Carr, 1996), and well-being (Heywood) of older residents

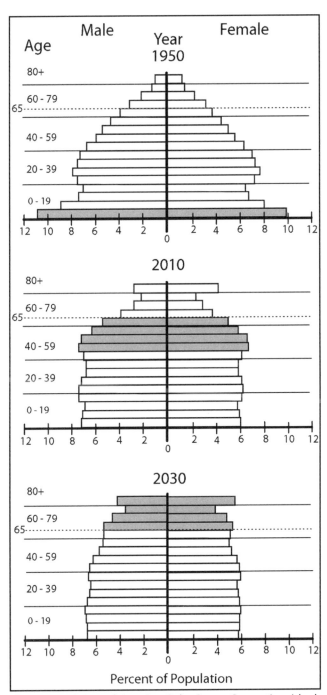

Figure 2-1. Aging of America; Baby Boom Generation (shaded). (Reprinted with permission from Bernard Steinman, MS, Research Assistant at the Fall Prevention Center of Excellence, Andrus Gerontology Center USC. Data Source: http://www.census.gov/prod/2010pubs/p25-1138.pdf.)

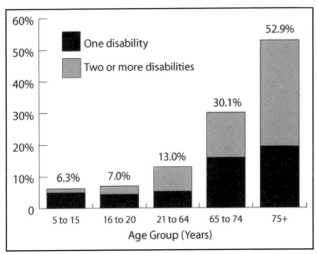

Figure 2-2. Disability and aging. (Reprinted with permission from Bernard Steinman, MS, Research Assistant at the Fall Prevention Center of Excellence, Andrus Gerontology Center USC. Data Source: http://www.census.gov/hhes/www/disability/GQdisability.pdf.)

that governments throughout the world are actively engaged in social and health reforms to ensure the ongoing health and well-being of older people and people with disabilities living in aging and unaccommodating homes in the community.

LEGISLATIVE AND POLICY DEVELOPMENTS AND DIRECTIONS

The emergence of the Civil Rights movement and antidiscrimination legislation in the 1960s and 1970s resulted in many governments committing to ensuring the acceptance and inclusion of people with disabilities in society. The subsequent development of accessibility standards for public buildings—for example, the Americans with Disabilities Act, 1990—then laid the foundation for recognizing the role of the built environment in affording people access to community facilities. In the residential sector, the movement toward de-institutionalization contributed to the emphasis on also creating housing environments that could accommodate people with disabilities as indicated in the United States by the Fair Housing Amendments Act, 1988. De-institutionalization shifted the focus from providing care in specialized settings to supporting people in their own communities. These policy initiatives have stimulated the development of other policies and services dedicated to building and modifying home environments to move people from congregate care to independent community living. In the United

and those with disabilities. These design features are costly to modify (Tabbarah, Silverstein, & Seeman, 2000) and can contribute to early institutionalization (Rojo-Perez, Fernandez-Mayoralas, Pozo-Rivera, & Rojo-Abuin, 2001). Because activity limitations are likely to increase as people age, it is not surprising

States, the 1999 Olmstead Decision requires that states provide services to older people and people with disabilities in the "most integrated setting appropriate," resulting in an increase in demand for community-based services and housing (Pynoos, Nishita, Cicero, & Caraviello, 2008, p. 85).

The concern around the world about the aging population and its impact on health and social services has resulted in a number of policy initiatives being proposed and implemented. In the United States, the role of housing in supporting older people in the community is gaining recognition from policymakers (Pynoos, Liebig, Alley, & Nishita, 2004). Older Americans are also beginning to exert political pressure through organizations such as the American Association of Retired Persons (AARP) and are increasingly recognized as having significant voting power (National Institute on Aging, 2006). These demographic, social, and policy changes have stimulated a rapid expansion in industries providing services for older people, including health care, aged care, financial services, and housing. These service industries have also become increasingly vocal, organized, and politically influential (Jones, de Jonge, & Phillips, 2008).

Although policy has concentrated on the residential environment, for the most part, the regulations have applied to multi-unit developments, omitting the vast array of single-family and smaller complexes where older people live. In several countries, however, there have been attempts to rectify this problem by concentrating on modifying existing units and building better housing in the first instance. Though home modification, as yet, does not have a high profile in policy development, it can make a general contribution to the implementation of aging policy and, more specifically, to health, community care, and housing policy for older people.

Home modifications can reduce the need for hospitalization of older people and the demand for expensive in-home and residential aged-care services (Mann, Ottenbacher, Fraas, Tomita, & Granger, 1999). Home modification can also play an important role in preventative health by reducing the incidence of accidents and falls among older people and reducing the mental and physical strain on caregivers (Heywood, 2005; Newman, 2003). Modifying the homes of older people can also reduce expenditure on social housing because it constitutes a less expensive form of housing assistance than direct social housing provision (Jones et al., 2008). Adaptations to the home can also help caregivers who form the backbone of personal care assistance for disabled people of all ages. There is even some preliminary evidence that home modifications, in conjunction with occupational and physical therapy, can reduce mortality (Gitlin, 2003).

In terms of promoting positive aging, home modification provides a means of facilitating healthy and independent living and allowing older people to continue to participate actively in home and community life. Appropriate housing is fundamental to an individual's well-being and social participation (Jones et al., 2008), and modifications can play an important role in enabling people to live independently and safely, to actively participate in household activities, and to maintain involvement with family and friends. When people choose to remain living in their own home for as long as possible, modifications, along with other community care services, can enable them to age in place. If people choose to relocate, they will have access to more suitable housing and locations, where the homes might be designed or adapted to better suit their requirements.

SERVICE DELIVERY SYSTEMS

Home modification services have often been described as a "complex patchwork" of services: various types of services have been developed and delivered though different service systems, each with their own particular goals, approaches, and interventions (Pynoos, 2001). This is largely because modification services have been developed and funded through a variety of programs and provided through an assortment of services with various aims. Occupational therapists generally work across different programs in an effort to stitch together a suitable modification solution for each client. It is often difficult, for both therapists and their clients, to comprehend the range of services available and what each can offer any given individual. Much of this complexity of home modification services is a result of being at the intersection of health, community care, and housing services and policies. Each of these has a different perspective on the goal of home modifications and tends to shape home modification practice through different policies and funding regimes. This is a challenge for occupational therapists; they have to operate effectively within and across programs to develop an approach to home modifications that transcends one particular program. In order to appreciate the impact of the service context on practice and to develop a holistic approach to home modification, each of these service environments needs to be examined.

THE HEALTH PERSPECTIVE

Home modifications and *home adaptations* are widely defined in health care contexts as "any permanent alteration to a building carried out with the intention of making [it] more suitable for a disabled person" (Heywood, 2004, p. 134). In this context, changes are made to the home environment "in order to accommodate a particular set of human abilities" (Bridge, 2005, p. 2). Like many interventions within health and rehabilitation settings, home modifications are viewed as a means of addressing or correcting problems specific to an individual (Wylde, 1998). Home modifications are provided as part of discharge planning following hospitalization (Auriemma, Faust, Sibrian, & Jimenez, 1999) or within a community health or health-funded in-home service.

Within a health context, home modifications are generally recommended by professionals to ensure that an individual with a particular impairment or health condition is safe and independent in his or her home (Auriemma et al., 1999) or to decrease the likelihood of admission to a hospital or care facility (Auriemma et al.; Gitlin, Miller, & Boyce, 1999). Health conditions, which are generally viewed as having a standard presentation and predictable pathology, are managed using practice guidelines or protocols of care. This can result in recommendations focusing on a specific health problem with less consideration being given to other difficulties, impairments, or aspirations the person might have (Tinker et al., 2004). The primary focus of interventions within the health context is often on remediation or correction of the health condition, with medications and interventions that remediate the condition taking precedence over other interventions. Home modifications, assistive devices, and an array of other interventions that promote the safety and independence of people with chronic conditions or long-term disabilities are frequently less of a priority within the health system. This factor is often reflected in the priority these services are given, along with the budget allocated for them.

Focus of the Health Perspective

Within a health perspective, the home environment is typically conceptualized as a discrete physical entity where modifications can be routinely recommended to accommodate specific functional impairments or health-related limitations. Frequently, an individual's functional ability is assessed in a clinical setting, and recommendations for modifications to the home environment can be made without undertaking an on-site visit (Pynoos, Tabbarah, Angelelli, & Demiere, 1998). When a home visit is undertaken, the focus is often on potential safety hazards or physical barriers to performing self-care activities. Consequently, the inside of the home, in particular the bathroom and bedroom, as well as an access point in and out of the home, receive most attention. Typically, modification recommendations in health-based services tend toward nonstructural changes, such as grab rails, shower seats, and other assistive devices (Pynoos et al.; Renforth, Yapa, & Forster, 2004). Structural changes, such as widening doorways, modifying bathrooms, and installing ramps, are less common because of the design and construction time involved, the financial cost, and the expertise and resources required in attaining these modifications (Auriemma et al., 1999; Pynoos et al.; Tabbarah et al., 2000). Moreover, because of regulatory and budget constraints, there is often little follow-up to ensure that modifications are working effectively—for example, there might be a problem with faulty equipment or poor installation, or the resident or caregiver might need training in how to use them.

With health-based services focused on ensuring that people with health conditions, injuries, or impairments are able to return home from the hospital and be safe and independent when performing self-care tasks in their home, practice and consumer outcomes are constrained in a number of ways. When function is defined in terms of impairments resulting from a specific injury or health condition, care protocols are developed for each of these. Consequently, the unique needs of the individual are often not well addressed. When people have similar injuries or conditions, the functional limitations—and the impact of these—can vary from one person to another. This generally necessitates a targeted assessment of each individual to assess his or her abilities and the performance of various activities. Furthermore, the particular priorities and preferences of individuals, their personal resources, and the strategies they use to address activity restrictions combine to influence the nature of difficulties identified and how these might be best addressed. With a focus on individual function, less attention is likely to fall on the environment—the challenges it presents when undertaking various activities or how it might be modified to promote further activity engagement. In addition, performance is generally evaluated in the hospital environment, which does not acknowledge the interaction between the individual, his or her activities, and the home environment. Consequently, the ability of a person to function on returning home can be either underestimated or overestimated because the familiarity of, or challenges within, the home environment have not been recognized.

Through policies and funding systems, health services can place constraints on occupational therapists and home modification outcomes for consumers. Therapists can be distracted from planning for an individual's capacity to operate effectively in the home and, instead, become preoccupied with maximizing function because of the status that these activities receive in the health system. The immediate focus on discharging the person from the hospital into a safe environment can mean that the long-term suitability of the home environment is not adequately addressed. Minimizing safety concerns and maximizing independence in self-care activities can often divert therapists' attention from determining the real extent of risk and maximizing engagement in meaningful occupations in the home. A focus on mobility and access into and within the home can result in inadequate attention being paid to access to the yard, neighborhood, and community. In addition, issues of personal concern, such as security, managing the ongoing maintenance of the home and garden (Jones et al., 2008), the social acceptability of the modifications, or the impact of the modifications on the meaning or value of the home (Heywood, 2004), tend not to be acknowledged or are undervalued.

Recent concerns about the prevalence of falls among older people living in the community and the resultant costs to the health system have directed attention to addressing hazards in the home environment. With approximately half of the falls occurring inside the home (Rogers, Rogers, Takeshima, & Mohammod, 2004), home modifications have been identified as one of a number of risk-management strategies to reduce the number of falls among the elderly (Gillespie, Gillespie, Cumming, Lamb, & Rower, 2001). A number of potential environmental hazards have been identified, including clutter, obstacles, loose rugs, lack of supports, and poor lighting (Clemson, Roland, & Cumming, 1997), and interventions are focused on removing these to promote safety. While falls risk and hazard identification have provided the foundation for many health-funded initiatives, there is little evidence to date that broadly targeted programs aimed at removing environmental hazards in the homes of older people in the community reduce the incidence of falls (Gillespie et al.). However, some success has been achieved with tailored programs targeted at the specific needs of people with increased falls risk, such as the frail elderly (Cumming et al., 1999) and those who have fallen previously (Close et al., 1999;

Nikolaus & Bach, 2003). This suggests that the individualized and holistic approach to environmental interventions favored by occupational therapists is likely to be more effective in reducing falls than those focused on hazard reduction alone. A meta-analysis of fall prevention interventions also indicates that multifactorial interventions that include medical risk assessment and management, physical activity, and home assessment and modification are likely to produce the largest reduction in falls among those at moderate to high risk (Rubenstein & Josephson, 2006). In this scenario, occupational therapists play a role as members of an interdisciplinary team. Regardless, as a profession, occupational therapists need to provide more evidence of the efficacy of their unique approach if their services expect to benefit from the funding being made available to reduce the incidence of falls among the elderly.

Traditionally, home modification services within health systems have largely focused on physical impairments. This has resulted in well-developed assessments, designs, resources, and services aimed at addressing physical impairments. Somewhat less attention has been given to addressing the sensory, cognitive, emotional, and social changes associated with aging. With the high prevalence of vision and hearing impairment among older people, there is a growing interest in making the home environment more manageable and safe for those with sensory impairments—for example, using modifications such as enlarged fittings, enhanced lighting, amplification devices, auditory signals, and contrasting colors (Auriemma et al., 1999). While it is important to address existing impairments through environmental interventions, further attention also needs to be directed to creating emotionally and socially supportive home environments that make it easier to carry out daily activities in the home. This would help to promote older people's self-confidence and self-esteem (Pynoos et al., 1998), and it would ensure that they maximize their engagement in daily activities, thus optimizing their general health and well-being. As a result of our less well-developed understanding of sensory, cognitive, emotional, and social issues in the home and associated environmental interventions, there are fewer assessments, designs, resources, and services dedicated to addressing these concerns within the health arena. Consequently, therapists can struggle to adequately address these needs with their clients, who, as a result, continue to struggle to manage in their home environment.

With the aging population and the rising incidence of dementia (Plassman et al., 2007), there is a growing interest in supporting older people with cognitive changes to remain living safely and independently in the community. The focus of health interventions is also to assist the caregivers, who are often responsible for supervising and assisting people in daily activities and managing those who are difficult or dangerous (Colombo, Vitali, Molla, Gioia, & Milani, 1998; Gitlin & Corcoran, 2000; Silverstein & Hyde, 1997). Home modifications might include nonstructural changes, such as reassigning rooms, installing fencing and gates, fitting safety locks on doors and cupboards, adding outlet covers and night lights, and improving lighting. A range of electronic devices have also been used, such as smoke detectors and movement monitoring and alarm systems (Silverstein, Hyde, & Ohta, 1993). Occasionally, structural changes such as an additional bathroom or bedroom are undertaken.

Use of Technologies

Increasingly, the potential of a range of new technologies is being recognized to help older people and people with disabilities to live safely in their homes and to assist in monitoring and managing people with complex health conditions in the community (Colombo et al., 1998). Generic technologies such as mobile phones, sensors, passive alarms, and remote video cameras are being used to enhance the safety and independence of older people (Tinker, 1999), and dedicated environmental controls, robotics, and communication and security technologies are being developed and integrated into the design of "smart homes" (Cowan & Turner-Smith, 1999; Tinker et al., 2004). These technologies have the potential to decrease adverse incidents in the home and to allow health conditions to be managed at home rather than in a health setting.

These technologies provide therapists with other tools to support people in their home environment, and the potential to save overall health care costs makes them attractive to those who fund services. However, these technologies can often be costly to purchase and support. Without a significant injection of funding into the already strained reserves of in-home services, they are likely to be overshadowed by low-tech options or remain a wonderful resource that is difficult to use. When budgets are allocated and prioritized, how will intangible and consumer-related benefits of environmental modifications hold up against the tangible financial benefits of in-home monitoring? These technologies also raise several ethical dilemmas (Tinker, 1999). Whose needs are being met through these technologies? What is their effectiveness in reducing the cost of health care delivery? What impact will they have on the concerns of well-meaning relatives who want assurance that their elderly relative is safe? What role will they play in enabling people to stay safely in their home environment? Homes are a place of privacy, and intrusive technologies could be resented by residents and impact negatively on the meaning of home (Heywood, 2004). Furthermore, there is the possibility that people would be at risk of increased isolation if they are managed and monitored remotely. On the positive side, new communication technologies could increase compliance with drug regimens and summon help quickly if a person has fallen. They can also put older people and people with disabilities in touch with people who otherwise may be unavailable to them and provide reassurance that problems will be relayed quickly to family members or service providers who can respond. Although there are many complexities to consider with the advent of these technologies, occupational therapists are well placed to implement them effectively and balance the other needs of the householder with the potential benefits of ongoing monitoring.

In summary, health care systems, policies, and programs are key contextual elements in developing and providing home modification services. Within this context, modifications largely have been associated with discharge planning following hospitalization, with care of people with disabilities or chronic health conditions in the home environment (including the older people with dementia and their caregivers), and with fall prevention. Though practices vary widely from one service to another, there are a number of prevailing characteristics of the health approach to home modifications. The primary focus is often on a particular health problem or condition, with home modification perceived as one of a suite of interventions designed to remediate the problem or address dysfunction. Key concerns center on safety and the capacity to independently perform self-care activities. Environmental interventions are generally minor, nonstructural modifications, and structural changes are used infrequently. With a focus on individual function, health-based services are less concerned with the long-term suitability of a residence; the social acceptability of modifications; and issues of identity, meaning, and lifestyle. While there is a growing appreciation of sensory, cognitive, emotional, and social issues and associated environmental interventions, assessments, designs, resources, and services aimed at addressing physical impairments are more highly developed. New technologies present increasing opportunities to assist, as well as manage and monitor, people in their homes; however, these need to be used judiciously to ensure they do not encroach on the rights and autonomy of the householder.

COMMUNITY CARE PERSPECTIVE

In recent decades, home modifications have emerged as one of a range of services provided by community care agencies. Others include home nursing, delivered meals, home help, transport, shopping assistance, allied health services, and respite care. Community care services are designed to directly assist older people and people with disabilities to remain living in their own homes and communities as well as support their families and caregivers in providing care (Steinfeld & Shea, 1993) and reduce admissions to residential care (Duncan, 1998; Stone, 1998). Modifications and associated services are seen as being essential in delaying reliance on personal assistance and avoiding an unwanted move (Gitlin et al., 1999). Within this service environment, home modifications have been defined as "adaptations to living environments intended to increase ease of use, safety, security and independence" (Pynoos et al., 1998, p. 3). While the main focus of health contexts is on home modifications to ensure safety and independence, the community care sector also provides maintenance and security services, acknowledging that older people and people with disabilities also need to maintain the dwelling and be safe and secure in their homes in addition to managing activities in and around the home. The way in which these services are delivered varies considerably from one location to another. However, modification assessments are generally undertaken by professionals working in either health or social services (Klein, Rosage, & Shaw, 1999) while maintenance and security assessments can be undertaken by a wide variety of individuals, including handymen, tradespeople, building contractors, social service organizations, and families themselves (Pynoos et al.). Although the modification work is primarily contracted out to builders and other tradespeople, some service providers employ their own trade staff. Some of these providers might be familiar with making modifications; however, many are untrained, thereby requiring specific instructions from the occupational therapist regarding what and where to install them.

A range of strategies are used in the community care context to enable people to remain living in their own homes; namely behavioral, nonstructural, and structural adaptations (Pynoos et al., 1998). Behavioral adjustments alter the way in which activities are carried out, while nonstructural adaptations involve reassigning spaces, installing grab bars, better lighting, or using special equipment or assistive devices. Structural changes involve installing ramps and step-less showers, widening doorways, and lowering countertops and cupboards (National Resource Center on Supportive Housing and Home Modification, n.d.; Pynoos et al.). Assistive devices are also used to address difficulties in performing many home-based activities. For example, in the United Kingdom, housing modifications or adaptations are classified as an assistive technology, defined as "any device or system that allows an individual to perform a task that they would otherwise be unable to do, or increases the ease and safety with which the task can be performed" (Cowan & Turner-Smith, 1999, p. 235). However, assistive devices are typically mobile and are not attached to the structure of the house (Pynoos et al.), whereas home modifications are generally permanent, secure, and fixed in place. Assistive devices are sometimes preferred by consumers and professionals, especially when they are uncertain about how to undertake structural changes (Pynoos et al.; Steinfeld et al., 1998), they are reluctant to commit to a permanent or costly modification (Pynoos & Nishita, 2003), or if they are renting and are uneasy about making changes to which a landlord might object or require them to remove if they leave.

Focus of Community Care Perspective

In community care, the focus shifts from the specific performance limitations of the person to an analysis of the fit between the person and his or her home environment. Lawton and Nahemow (1973) were the first to recognize the challenges or "press" provided by the environment and proposed that these were unique for each individual (see Figure 1-1 in Chapter 1). Practice models have subsequently developed over the past decade that have highlighted the limitations of focusing on either the person or his or her impairments or on the barriers in the environment, promoting the value of examining the interaction between the person and the environment (Rousseau, Potvin, Dutil, & Falta, 2001). The use of these models in the community sector also encouraged a shift from assessing narrowly defined self-care activities to examining an individual's capacity to manage in the home and the community (Peace & Holland, 2001). The focus is on establishing balance between environmental demands and individual competencies and adapting the home environment to match the capabilities of the person (Gosselin, Robitaille, Trickey, & Maltais, 1993; Rousseau, Potvin, Dutil, & Falta, 2002). In this approach, difficulties experienced by the person in the home are observed and analyzed, and identified environmental challenges are then addressed using environmental interventions tailored to meet the particular needs of the individual.

The role of the environment in supporting competence or creating incapacity is also reflected in the social model of disability, with its emphasis on the role of the environment in creating disability (World Health Organization [WHO], 2001). In the social model, disability is defined as "a dynamic interaction between health conditions and contextual factors" (WHO, p. 8). Problems in the home result from an inability of the home environment to accommodate the changing capacities of the person (Cowan & Turner-Smith, 1999; Tinker et al., 2004). Older people have been described as being "architecturally disabled" by inadequate design (Hanson, 2001), leading to an emphasis on reducing environmental barriers in the homes of older people and in residential design generally. However, the social model of disability does not restrict its view to purely physical aspects of the individual's immediate environment. It also acknowledges the "social and attitudinal aspects of the environment in which people live and conduct their lives" (WHO, p. 16). In addition, it recognizes the impact of society on an individual's capacity to engage in activities, describing the impact of formal and informal social structures, services, and overarching approaches or systems in the community on individuals (WHO).

Independence is a central concept in community care, both generally and with respect to home modification services (Clapham, 2005). It is commonly understood in this context to mean that the person is able to live at home rather than in residential care. Occupational therapists generally conceive independence to be the ability to perform a task without assistance; therefore, they seek to provide training or a device or to modify the environment in order to remove the person's reliance on others. However, for many people, independence holds a more nuanced association, including "being able to look after oneself," "not being indebted to anyone," and "the capacity for self-direction" (Clough, Leamy, Miller, & Bright, 2004, pp. 119-120). Independence reflects a "sense of being in control with respect to family, friends and formal care givers" (Heywood, Oldman, & Means, 2002, pp. 55-57). It is possible, then, that some people might consider their independence enhanced by the assistance of others, a home modification, or a move to residential care where they have ready access to caregiving, providing they retain control of when and how assistance is provided. In reality, this paradigm acknowledges the interdependence of people.

Place of Home Modification Services in Community Care

While home modification services have been established within community care systems in many countries, these services tend to be underdeveloped relative to other community care services as a result of limited funding and scarcity of trained providers (Pynoos et al., 1998). Because community care systems tend to prioritize those at risk of being institutionalized, services are prioritized and directed toward those defined by the service as having the least resources and the greatest level of need (Clapham, 2005). Consequently, health and safety concerns take precedence over independence and quality-of-life issues (Mann, Hurren, Tomita, Bengali, & Steinfeld, 1994), leaving home modification services fighting for resources in a system that provides so many essential and costly support services.

Although modifications are seen as part of the range of interventions with the potential to ensure safety and independence and assist people to remain in their homes and community, in reality it is less developed than the other services in the community care sector where providers are more familiar with the use of formal supports. The use of modifications is also hampered by a lack of understanding of the benefits of environmental interventions, restricted access to services and personnel with appropriate expertise, and the limited budgets available for such interventions. Balancing priorities and funding across maintenance, security, and modification services is also problematic when these services are competing for their share of inadequate budgets.

Coordinating the variety of services and service providers required for the successful implementation of modifications remains a prevailing issue in the provision of home modification services (Pynoos, 2004; Steinfeld et al., 1998). Modification services require health and social service providers to work with tradespeople, which can be complex given the differences in roles, knowledge, language, expertise, and expectations. Miscommunication and mistrust prevail if the various stakeholders are not afforded an opportunity to share knowledge and develop an understanding of each other's roles, language, expertise, and expectations. Community care services, which have invested in the development of trained home modification personnel, knowledge, and resources, are well placed to achieve good client outcomes. Services that require health and social service providers to contract out modifications to the private building sector are likely to experience difficulties in delivering quality services and outcomes. This is because of the difficulties in locating contractors with the necessary expertise, communicating requirements, and overseeing the work being undertaken.

In the community care sector, occupational therapists have access to a range of services and interventions to assist their clients to remain in their homes and communities. However, the ease with which these resources can be accessed depends largely on the structure of the funding and service system. The development of modification services over the past decade has resulted in a growing body of knowledge and an increasing number of designs and products being available. Recognition of the role of the environment in "disabling" people has resulted in the development of occupational therapy models and practice approaches that address the complexity of the interaction between the person, activities, and the environment. Occupational therapists are unique in their understanding of the activity engagement and the role of the environment and stand out among other health professionals in their capacity to provide home modification services. An understanding of environmental fit allows therapists to move from addressing problems to creating enabling homes and communities that recognize the uniqueness of each person and his or her environment. However, restricted funding and service policies often constrain practice in addressing essential issues and make it difficult for therapists to promote activity engagement within the home and community. For example, often the priority in hospital discharge is getting a person out as quickly as possible. As pointed out earlier, even though an occupational therapist assessment and home modification might be essential, these often do not occur, if at all, until the person is already back in his or her home, struggling with both his or her own limitations and that of the environment.

In summary, a key value underpinning community care and occupational therapy services is promoting independence. However, while these services define independence as enabling people to remain living in their own homes or reducing reliance on others for daily tasks, older people and people with disabilities generally think of it in terms of personal control. Recent developments in the community care sector have provided significant impetus for the development of home modification services. Although home modification services remain relatively underdeveloped when compared with other community care services, they have been established as being a legitimate part of the repertoire of community care services designed to enable people to remain living in the community. In community care, behavioral, nonstructural, and structural modifications are closely associated with maintenance and security services. Coordination difficulties persist in working across health, social, and construction sectors, and good intersectorial collaboration is likely to enhance the development of quality modification services. An understanding of the interaction between people and their living environment allows modification interventions to be tailored to the individual's unique individual circumstances and promote his or her active participation in the home and the community.

THE HOUSING PERSPECTIVE

Many people make changes to their home environments quite independent of health and community care systems. It is therefore useful to examine how people use generic services to make changes to their housing, commonly known as housing adjustments, to meet their changing needs and preferences. Throughout life, people encounter changes that necessitate them relocating or altering their existing housing—whether it is the composition of their family and household, their health and employment status, or their interests and lifestyle. People therefore access a range of housing services that thrive on assisting people to accommodate changes in their circumstances. Occupational therapists often need to work with these services or work with people who use these services to address their ongoing housing needs. In addition, therapists are increasingly recognizing a role for themselves within a diversity of housing services. Consequently, developing a broader view of housing adjustments can assist therapists in understanding home modifications as part of a continuum of housing issues and anticipating where occupational therapy can contribute to the delivery and further development of housing services.

From a housing perspective, people alter their housing or relocate when their existing home no longer meets their changed circumstances or lifestyle or reflects their tastes or projected image or identity. Though this view encompasses the notion of "accommodating a particular set of human abilities" (the health perspective; Bridge, 2005, p. 2) or "adapting living environments to increase ease of use, safety, security and independence" (the community care perspective; Pynoos et al., 1998, p. 3), it is more universal in scope in that it recognizes that people make many different types of changes to their housing throughout their lives. These changes are referred to in the housing literature as housing adjustments (Howe, 2003), housing careers (Kendig, 1984), or housing pathways (Clapham, 2005). Housing decisions made in response to a health condition or changing capacities are unlikely to be made in isolation and are likely to incorporate a range of goals.

Housing adjustments are described by Peace and Holland (2001) as the actual changes that individuals and households make to their housing in response to their particular needs, circumstances, and preferences at any point in time. Housing careers is a term that is used to describe the sequence of housing adjustments that an individual or household makes over a lifetime. It is recognized that there are widespread societal changes, including demographic changes and improvements in the standard of living, which are transforming established patterns of housing careers in many countries (Beer, Faulkner, & Gabriel, 2006). Housing pathways describe the "patterns of interaction…concerning house and home, over time and space" (Clapham, 2005, p. 27). The concept of housing careers primarily focuses on changes in the consumption of housing related to factors such as age, household structure, income and wealth, employment, and disability, while the notion of housing pathways places emphasis on the social meanings and relationships associated with housing (Jones et al., 2008). The pathways perspective views housing as being more than a set of physical characteristics—space, layout, condition, access, etc. It recognizes the meaning that a house might hold for the occupants, the patterns of interactions contained within it, and the lifestyle and identity the house affords its residents (Clapham).

In addition to providing shelter, a home has social, cultural, and personal dimensions that contribute to the meaning that dwelling holds for individuals (Fisher, 1998). Homes provide people with a safe place to engage in a range of roles and routines, express themselves through their possessions, and exercise autonomy and control over use of space and time (Peace & Holland, 2001). It is well recognized that housing contributes significantly to quality of life (Pynoos & Regnier, 1997). The significance of the home is even greater if people have lived there for many years (Pynoos & Regnier) or if they spend a considerable amount of time at home (Newman, 2003). For many people, it is both emotionally and financially the biggest single investment they make in their lives (Hanson, 2001). Hanson also found that the home is often the focus of "hopes, dreams, achievements and memories" (p. 37) and connects people into social networks with their neighbors, friends, and family. Increasingly, people are not just interested in finding a house. Many seek a community that offers them a distinctive mode of living or a particular lifestyle that enables them to express and define their identity (Clapham, 2005).

Focus of the Housing Perspective

The housing perspective provides a number of distinctive insights into housing decisions that have implications for development and delivery of home modification services. First, people use a broad range of strategies when addressing housing concerns. When making housing adjustments, some choose to move house in response to changes in their needs and preferences (Heywood et al., 2002; Stone, 1998), whereas others have a strong preference to continue to live in their current community (Peace & Holland, 2001). While home modification services are recognized as assisting people to adapt their homes to their changed circumstances (Tinker, 1999), there are some who are clearly better served by relocating to more suitable accommodation. It is important to recognize that housing adjustment, while common in the general community, is not widely supported in health and community care services except in determining when someone needs to move into supported accommodation. Many modification services tend to assume that people intend to or should remain in the current home and leave people to make decisions themselves about relocating and downsizing. Many people live in homes that constantly challenge their safety and independence and require a great deal of upkeep (Tinker). A home that was once a "castle" and a reflection of a person's identity and status in the community can become a "cage" or millstone, undermining identity and restricting freedom and lifestyle (Heywood et al.). Little support is offered to people with the often overwhelming and complex task of making a housing adjustment. While people who have made many moves during their lives are well placed to deal with the financial, legal, and real estate complexities they are likely to encounter, many are not sufficiently experienced or informed to successfully navigate these systems. Services with a housing perspective could provide an important way of enhancing the range of options available to people to make housing adjustments and "…enable people to take control of their pathway through the ability to make choices" (Clapham, 2005, p. 234). These services could also manage the complex systems involved in moving house for people with low income or limited skill or capacity.

Second, the housing perspective has also highlighted that people seek housing that reflects their identity and lifestyle aspirations. Very few people consider themselves to be "old" (Wylde, 1998), and even fewer regard themselves as "disabled" (Heywood et al., 2002; Wylde). Consequently, housing decisions are likely to be shaped by identity and lifestyle choice rather than perceptions of functional need. The health and community care approaches tend to favor professionally defined concepts of functional need, where services are provided to people; consequently, they are unlikely to acknowledge people's lifestyle and identity aspirations (Clapham, 2005). Concern has been raised about the negative impacts of home modifications on the meaning of home and the lack of attention to this dimension by home modification services (Messecar, Archbold, Stewart, & Kirschling, 2002). Adaptations to the home can have a negative impact on routines, self-image, connection with the home, and a sense of heritage (Heywood, 2005). Modifications can result in people being viewed as different and, of greater concern, can make them vulnerable to ridicule or violence (Fisher, 1998). For example, a person may be willing to put a grab bar in his or her own private bathroom adjoining the bedroom but not in another bathroom that might be used by guests, where it would bring attention to the disability and change the decor of their living space. This underscores the importance not only of choice but of identifying home modifications that are attractive and acceptable. When making changes in the home, it is therefore essential that all aspects of the home environment are considered, rather than focusing solely on the performance of specific self-care tasks (Heywood). Acceptance of interventions, such as assistive devices, has been shown repeatedly to be influenced by whether they support or undermine the older person's sense of personal identity (Harrison, 2004). Householders have been found to reject modification services if their perspectives and priorities differ from service providers (Gitlin, Luborsky, & Schemm, 1998) or if they anticipate that the changes will impact on their sense of independence and autonomy (Messecar et al.).

Third, when building or remodeling housing, there are opportunities to plan ahead to pay particular attention to areas such as entrances, pathways, lighting, kitchens, and bathrooms. This is an ideal time to bring together occupational therapists, remodelers, architects, and interior designers to work as a team to help people plan ahead in terms of thinking about aging in place and adding features that might help them stay in their homes. For example, when remodeling, a resident could install a zero-step entrance, a walk-in or roll-in shower instead of a conventional bath or shower/bath combination, and fit cabinets in the kitchen that are within easy reach or provide somewhere to sit down to prepare food. These types of features might be found in a universally designed house but can be incorporated into existing homes as well. In addition, rather than considering the dwelling's suitability solely for the resident, it should be seen as a place where others of varying abilities visit. This aspect incorporates the communal nature of housing and underlies the charter of the visitability movement, which has made inroads in both England and, to a lesser extent, the US.

In summary, from a housing perspective, people make adjustments to their housing throughout life in response to their changing circumstances. These adjustments can include making changes to the current dwelling or seeking alternative living environments. Increasingly, housing decisions are shaped by a quest for a particular lifestyle that allows people to express and define their identity. This perspective alerts occupational therapists to the need to consider people's housing concerns more broadly, to ensure that they are afforded adequate choice, and to ensure that they are provided with sufficient information and support that reflects their housing needs and preferences into the future. Furthermore, it reminds the profession to recognize people's aspirations and the personal nature of the home environment when undertaking modifications.

CONCLUSION

Recent demographic, legislative, policy, and service developments have resulted in a range of services being developed to promote people's safety, health, independence, and well-being in the home environment. Occupational therapists have an important contribution to make in enabling people to live well in the home and community and need to work effectively within and across health, community care, and housing systems to achieve good outcomes for their clients. Home modification services developed in the health care system are primarily concerned with ensuring safety and enabling independence through the use of minor or nonstructural modifications. Health-based services perceive the home as a physical entity that needs to be modified to accommodate functional deficits and, in so doing, therapists can overlook the long-term suitability of a residence, the social acceptability of modifications, and issues of identity, meaning, and lifestyle when designing interventions. Therapists working in this context need to be mindful of the personal, temporal, social, and cultural nature of the home environment when addressing physical aspects of the environment.

Within community care services, behavioral, nonstructural, and structural modifications are used in conjunction with a range of other services to support people to live safely and independently in the community. An understanding of the interaction between the person and his or her living environment allows modification interventions to be tailored to the individual's unique circumstances and promote his or her active participation in the home and the community. Therapists working in community care settings need to work across health, social, and construction sectors to develop good intersectorial collaboration and enhance the development of quality modification services.

Services developed within the housing sector acknowledge that people make adjustments to their housing throughout life in response to their changing circumstances. Within this sector, modifications are seen as part of a continuum of adjustments, which can also include seeking an alternative living environment that better suits the individual's identity and lifestyle aspirations. Within this perspective, occupational therapists are encouraged to consider people's broader housing concerns, to provide clients with sufficient information and support when making adjustments, and to help them think ahead in terms of the suitability of modifications to help them age in place.

Clients are likely to be seeking to maintain their safety, health, and well-being as well as their identity and lifestyle within the home and community, regardless of where they access home modification services. Therapists need to be aware of the context in which they work, the way this can shape their service delivery, and the importance of extending their service to acknowledge clients' broader needs or referring them to a service that is better suited to addressing their needs. Furthermore, professionals, such as occupational therapists and the organizations that represent them, have an important role to play in improving the policies that affect their practice and the lives of the clients they serve.

REFERENCES

Americans with Disabilities Act. (1990). ADA home page. Retrieved from http://www.usdoj.gov/crt/ada/adahom1.htm

Auriemma, D., Faust, S., Sibrian, K., & Jimenez, J. (1999). Home modifications for the elderly: implications for the occupational therapist. *Physical and Occupational Therapy in Geriatrics, 16*(2-4), 135-144.

Beer, A., Faulkner, D., & Gabriel, M. (2006). *21st century housing careers and Australia's housing future: Literature review.* Melbourne, Australia: Australian Housing and Urban Research Institute.

Brault, M. (2008). Disability status and the characteristics of people in group quarters: A brief analysis of disability prevalence among the civilian noninstitutionalized and total populations in the American Community Survey. Retrieved from http://www.census.gov/hhes/www/disability/GQdisability.pdf

Bridge, C. (2005). *Retrofitting, a response to lack of diversity: An analysis of community provider data.* Paper presented at National Housing Conference October 2005, Perth, Western Australia.

Bridge, C., Parsons, A., Quine, S., & Kendig, H. (2002). *Housing and care for older and younger adults with disabilities: Positioning paper.* Melbourne, Australia: Australian Housing and Urban Research Institute.

Clapham, D. (2005). *The meaning of housing.* Bristol, England: Policy Press.

Clemson, L., Roland, M., & Cumming, R. G. (1997). Types of hazards in the homes of elderly people. *Occupational Therapy Journal of Research, 17*(3), 200-213.

Close, J., Ellis, M., Hooper, R., Glucksman, E., Jackson, S., & Swift, C. (1999). Prevention of falls in the elderly trial (PROFET): a randomised controlled trial. *Lancet, 353*(9147), 93-97.

Clough, R., Leamy, M., Miller, V., & Bright, L. (2004). *Housing decisions in later life.* New York, NY: Palgrave Macmillan.

Colombo, M., Vitali, S., Molla, G., Gioia, P., & Milani, M. (1998). The home environment modification program in the care of demented elderly: Some examples. *Archives of Gerontology and Geriatrics, 27*(6), 83-90.

Cowan, D., & Turner-Smith, A. (1999). *The role of assistive technology in alternative models of care for older people.* London, England: The Royal Commission on Long Term Care.

Cumming, R. G., Thomas, M., Szonyi, G., Salkeld, G., O' Neill, E., & Westbury, C. (1999). Home visits by an occupational therapist for assessment and modification of environmental hazards: a randomized trial of falls prevention. *Journal of American Geriatric Society, 47*(12), 1397-1402.

Duncan, R. (1998). Blueprint for action: The National Home Modifications Action Coalition. *Technology and Disability, 8*(1-2), 85-89.

Faulkner, D., & Bennett, K. (2002). *Linkages among housing assistance, residential (Re), location and the use of community health and social care by old-old adults: Shelter and non-shelter implications for housing policy development.* Melbourne, Australia: Australian Housing and Urban Research Institute.

Fisher, A. G. (1998). Uniting practice and theory in an occupational framework. *American Journal of Occupational Therapy, 52*(7), 509-520.

Frain, J. P., & Carr, P. H. (1996). Is the typical modern house designed for future adaptation for disabled older people? *Age and Ageing, 25*(5), 398.

Freedman, V. A. (2007). Demographic reflections on the aging baby boom and its implications for health care (commentary). In K. Warner Schaie & P. Uhlenberg (Eds.), *Social structures: Demographic changes and the well-being of older persons* (pp. 80-90). New York, NY: Springer Publishing Company.

Freedman, V. A., Martin, L. G., & Schoeni, R. F. (2002). Recent trends in disability and functioning among older adults in the United States: A systematic review. *Journal of the American Medical Association, 288*(24), 3137-3146.

Gillespie, L. D., Gillespie, W. J., Cumming, R. G., Lamb, S. H., & Rower, B. H. (2001). *Interventions for preventing falls in the elderly.* Oxford, England: The Cochrane Library.

Gitlin, L. N. (2003). Next steps in home modifications and assistive technology research. In N. Charness & K. W. Schaie (Eds.), *Impact of technology on successful aging* (pp. 188-202). New York, NY: Springer.

Gitlin, L. N., & Corcoran, M. (2000). Making home safer: Environmental adaptations for people with dementia. *Alzheimer Care Quarterly, 1*(1), 50-58.

Gitlin, L. N., Luborsky, M. R., & Schemm, R. L. (1998). Emerging concerns of older stroke patients about assistive devices. *The Gerontologist, 38*(2), 169-180.

Gitlin, L. N., Miller, K. S., & Boyce, A. (1999). Bathroom modifications for frail elderly renters: outcomes of a community-based program. *Technology and Disability, 10*(3), 141-149.

Gosselin, C., Robitaille, Y., Trickey, F., & Maltais, D. (1993). Factors predicting the implementation of home modifications among elderly people with loss of independence. *Physical and Occupational Therapy in Geriatrics, 12*(1), 15-27.

Hanson, J. (2001). From "special needs" to "lifestyle choices": Articulating the demand for "third age" housing. In S. Peace & C. Holland (Eds.), *Inclusive housing in an ageing society* (pp. 29-54). Bristol, England: Policy Press.

Harrison, M. (2004). Defining housing quality and environment: Disability, standards and social factors. *Housing Studies, 19*(5), 691-708.

Heywood, F. (2004). The health outcomes of housing adaptations. *Disability and Society, 19*(2), 129-143.

Heywood, F. (2005). Adaptation: Altering the house to restore the home. *Housing Studies, 20*(4), 531-547.

Heywood, F., Oldman, C., & Means, R. (2002). *Housing and home in later life.* Buckingham, England: Open University Press.

Howe, A. (2003). *Housing an older Australia: More of the same or something different? Keynote address.* Melbourne, Australia: Australian Housing and Urban Research Institute. Retrieved from http://ahuri.ddsn.net/downloads/2003_Events/HFAA/Anna_Howe_keynote.pdf

Jones, A., de Jonge, D., & Phillips, R. (2008). *The impact of home maintenance and modification services on health, community care and housing outcomes in later life: Positioning paper.* Melbourne, Australia: Australian Housing and Urban Research Institute.

Kendig, H. (1984). Housing careers, life cycle and residential mobility: Implications for the housing market. *Urban Studies, 21*(3), 271-283.

Klein, S. I., Rosage, L., & Shaw, G. (1999). The role of occupational therapists in home modification programs at an area agency on aging. *Physical and Occupational Therapy in Geriatrics, 16*(3-4), 19-37.

Kraus, L., Stoddard, S., & Gilmartin, D. (1996). *Chartbook on disability in the United States, 1996. An InfoUse Report.* Washington, DC: US National Institute on Disability and Rehabilitation Research.

Kutty, N. K. (1999). Demand for home modifications: A household production function approach. *Applied Economics, 31*(10), 1273-1281.

Lawton, M. P., & Nahemow, L. (1973). Ecology and the aging process. In C. Eisdorfer & M. P. Lawton (Eds.), *Psychology of adult development and aging* (pp. 619-674). Washington, DC: American Psychological Association.

Mann, W. C., Hurren, D., Tomita, M., Bengali, M., & Steinfeld, E. (1994). Environmental problems in homes of elders with disabilities. *The Occupational Therapy Journal of Research, 14*(3), 191–211.

Mann, W. C., Ottenbacher, K. J., Fraas, L., Tomita, M., & Granger, C. V. (1999). Effectiveness of assistive technology and environmental interventions in maintaining and reducing home care costs for the frail elderly: A randomized control trial. *Archives of Family Medicine, 8,* 210-217.

Messecar, D. C., Archbold, P. G., Stewart, B. J., & Kirschling, J. (2002). Home environmental modification strategies used by caregivers of elders. *Research in Nursing and Health, 25,* 357-370.

National Institute on Aging. (2006). *Dramatic changes in U.S. aging highlighted in new census, NIH report: Impact of baby boomers anticipated.* Retrieved from http://www.nia.nih.gov/NewsAndEvents/PressReleases/PR2006030965PlusReport.htm

National Resource Center on Supportive Housing and Home Modification. (n.d.). Home modification. Retrieved from http://www.homemods.org/pages/various/homemods.htm

Newman, S. (2003). The living conditions of elderly Americans. *The Gerontologist, 43*(1), 99-109.

Nikolaus, T., & Bach, M. (2003). Preventing falls in community-dwelling frail older people using a home intervention team. *Journal of the American Geriatric Society, 51,* 300-305.

Oldman, C., & Beresford, B. (2000). Home sick home: Using housing experiences of disabled children to suggest a new theoretical framework. *Housing Studies, 15*(3), 429-442.

Peace, S. M., & Holland, C. (2001). *Inclusive housing in an ageing society: Innovative approaches.* Bristol, England: Policy Press.

Plassman, B. L., Langa, K. M., Fisher, G. G., Heeringa, S. G., Weir, D. R., Ofstedal, M. B., et al. (2007). Prevalence of dementia in the United States: The aging, demographics, and memory study. *Neuroepidemiology, 29,* 125-132.

Pynoos, J. (2001). *Meeting the needs of older people to age in place: Findings and recommendations for action.* San Diego, CA: The National Resource Center for Supportive Housing and Home Modification.

Pynoos, J. (2004). On the forefront of the ever-changing field of home modification. *Rehabilitation Management, 17*(3), 34, 35, 50.

Pynoos, J., Liebig, P., Alley, D., & Nishita, C. M. (2004). Homes of choice: Towards more effective linkages between housing and services. *Journal of Housing for the Elderly, 18*(3-4), 5-39.

Pynoos, J., & Nishita, C. M. (2003). The cost and financing of home modifications in the United States. *Journal of Disability Policy Studies, 14*(2), 68-73.

Pynoos, J., Nishita, C. M., Cicero, C., & Caraviello, R. (2008). Aging in place, housing and the law. *The Elder Law Journal, 16*(1), 77-105.

Pynoos, J., & Regnier, V. (1997). Design directives in home adaptation. In S. Lanspery & J. Hyde (Eds.), *Staying put: Adapting the places instead of the people* (pp. 41-54). Amityville, NY: Baywood.

Pynoos, J., Tabbarah, M., Angelelli, J., & Demiere, M. (1998). Improving the delivery of home modifications. *Technology and Disability, 8,* 3-14.

Renforth, P., Yapa, R. S., & Forster, D. P. (2004). Occupational therapy predischarge home visits: A study from a community hospital. *British Journal of Occupational Therapy, 67*(11), 488-494.

Rogers, M. E., Rogers, N. L., Takeshima, N., & Mohammod, M. I. (2004). Reducing the risk for falls in the homes of older adults. *Journal of Housing for the Elderly, 18*(2), 29-39.

Rojo-Perez, F., Fernandez-Mayoralas, G., Pozo-Rivera, F. E., & Rojo-Abuin, J. M. (2001). Ageing in place: Predictors of the residential satisfaction of the elderly. *Social Indicators Research, 54*(2), 173-208.

Rousseau, J., Potvin, L., Dutil, E., & Falta, P. (2001). A critical review of assessment tools related to home adaptation issues. *Occupational Therapy in Health Care, 14*(3-4), 93-104.

Rousseau, J., Potvin, L., Dutil, E., & Falta, P. (2002). Model of competence: A conceptual framework for understanding the person-environment interaction for persons with motor disabilities. *Occupational Therapy in Health Care, 16*(1), 15-36.

Rubenstein, L. Z., & Josephson, K. R. (2006). Falls and their prevention in elderly people: What does the evidence show? *Medical Clinics of North America, 90*(5), 807-824.

Silverstein, N. M., & Hyde, J. (1997). The importance of a consumer perspective in home adaptation of Alzheimer's households. In S. Lanspery & J. Hyde (Eds.), *Staying put: Adapting places instead of people* (pp. 91-111). Amityville, NY: Baywood.

Silverstein, N. M., Hyde, J., & Ohta, R. (1993). Home adaptation for Alzheimer's households: Factors related to implementation and outcomes of recommendations. *Technology and Disability, 2*(4), 58-68.

Steinfeld, E., Levine, D., & Shea, S. (1998). Home modifications and the fair housing law. *Technology and Disability, 8*, 15-35.

Steinfeld, E., & Shea, S. (1993). Enabling home environments: Identifying barriers to independence. *Technology and Disability, 2*(4), 69-79.

Stone, J. H. (1998). Housing for older persons: An international overview. *Technology and Disability, 8*(1-2), 91-97.

Tabbarah, M., Silverstein, M., & Seeman, T. (2000). A health and demographic profile of non-institutionalized older Americans residing in environments with home modifications. *Journal of Aging and Health, 12*(2), 204-228.

Tinker, A. (1999). *Ageing in place: What can we learn from each other?* The Sixth F. Oswald Barnett Oration, September 9, 1999, Melbourne, Australia.

Tinker, A., McCreadie, C., Stuchbury, R., et al. (2004). *Introducing assistive technology into the existing homes of older people: Feasibility, acceptability, costs and outcomes.* London, UK: Institute of Gerontology.

Trickey, F., Maltais, D., Gosslein, C., & Robitaille, Y. (1993). Adapting older persons' homes to promote independence. *Physical and Occupational Therapy in Geriatrics, 12*(1), 1-14.

U.S. Department of Housing and Urban Development. (2007). FHEO Programs. Retrieved from http://www.hud.gov/offices/fheo/progdesc/title8.cfm

Vincent, G. K., & Velkoff, V. A. (2010). The next four decades-The older population in the United States: 2010 to 2050. Retrieved from http://www.census.gov/prod/2010pubs/p25-1138.pdf

World Health Organization (2001). *International classification of function, disability and health.* Geneva, Switzerland: Author.

Wylde, M. A. (1998). Consumer knowledge of home modifications. *Technology and Disability, 8*(1-2), 51-68.

Models of Occupational Therapy

Desleigh de Jonge, MPhil (OccThy), Grad Cert Soc Sci

Models provide a framework for thinking and clinical decision making. They also provide a framework for defining our scope of concern and role, identifying and understanding issues or problems, determining appropriate evaluation and intervention strategies, and evaluating outcomes. A number of models have been developed over the years that assist occupational therapists in understanding the difficulties individuals have with performance and the factors that impact on it. Each model conceptualizes performance, the environment, and the interaction between them in different ways, all of which have an impact on how occupational therapists engage with issues and implement occupational and environmental interventions. This chapter reviews three key models used by occupational therapists when undertaking home modifications and examines how each shapes home modification practice and outcomes. In particular, the chapter describes the rehabilitation model, the occupational performance model, and ecological models and examines how each contributes to our understanding of how people engage in meaningful occupations in the home and community. Also examined is the evolution of occupational therapy practice models and their relevance and integrity in light of recent politico-sociocultural trends, such as the shift to a social model of disability and the development of consumer-driven services.

Chapter Objectives

By the end of this chapter, the reader will be able to:

+ Describe how models have shaped occupational therapy practice in the area of home modifications

+ Describe how the rehabilitation model, occupational performance model, and two ecological models (namely, the person-environment-occupation model and the person-environment-occupational-performance model), structure practice

+ Identify the strengths and limitations of each of these models with respect to home modification practice

Introduction

As a profession, occupational therapy continues to evolve in response to scientific advancements, as well as philosophical shifts in society and within particular service contexts. Changes in the scope and focus of the profession are clearly evident in the successive models developed to guide and describe occupational therapy practice. Models reflect our thinking and shape our practice (Reed & Sanderson, 1999) and can be described as being conceptual or procedural in nature. Conceptual models are

Ainsworth, E., & de Jonge, D.
An Occupational Therapists's Guide to Home Modification Practice (pp. 33-48)
© 2011 SLACK Incorporated

usually presented in a graphic form, overviewing concepts and describing the relationships between the identified elements. In contrast, procedural models specify a procedure for attending to issues and elements. To illustrate the function of each of these models, imagine you were to plan a trip using a map. A map is like a conceptual model, outlining the boundaries of the geographical area to be explored, various places of interest, their spatial relationships, and their means of connection. Because many of us travel with a finite amount of time and financial resources in mind, we also need to develop a travel schedule (procedural model) so that we can visit all of the important landmarks and plan a methodical and efficient route of travel. Although you might be able to undertake your trip using only one of these approaches, your understanding of the destination and relevant resources is enhanced by using both a map and a schedule.

The same is true when using models in practice. Therapists need both conceptual and procedural models to practice effectively. However, some models are predominantly conceptual, requiring therapists to develop their own plan of action. This is true for many occupational therapy models. Other models are largely procedural, requiring therapists to rely on their own understandings of the elements of concern and interrelationships. Many frames of reference, practice, and service models provide this structure. Effective practice relies on therapists having an understanding of all of the elements of concern and their interactions as well as a plan of operation. However, it is also essential that the procedural model reflects the focus and goals of the conceptual model. There is little point in having a map of the whole of Europe if you confine your trip to Italy. It would also be difficult to convince people you have seen Europe if you have traveled only from Rome to Florence, and it would be challenging to navigate between and within small villages if your map only has the major highways marked. Without an appropriate map, your travel experience would not reflect your intentions, nor would it live up to your expectations. Equally, therapists need to ensure that their actions echo their stated focus and goals. This requires that they have sufficient understanding of the issues they are dealing with (conceptual model) and that these are reflected in an appropriate plan of action (procedural model).

Therapists tend to use different models—either implicitly or explicitly—depending on their primary area of practice, where and when they were trained, and the models they relate to personally. Additionally, service environments and reimbursement schedules, which also have an impact on the focus and scope of practice, can influence therapists' choices of model or shape the way they are operationalized. As a consequence, therapists often choose models that fit well with the service context, or they focus on aspects of the model that fit well with the service or reimbursement requirements.

Many therapists are not aware of the models or other influences shaping their practice. These therapists generally operate intuitively on internalized understandings (Reed, 1998) or use well-practiced and routine approaches to address issues. As a result, they select and use assessment tools and interventions without necessarily being aware of the beliefs and attitudes directing these decisions. Whether or not they are conscious of the models directing their actions, therapists hold their own views of people and a particular understanding of the cause and impact of impairment or disability. These views delineate the therapists' scope of concern, determine the nature of services they offer, and dictate how they work with consumers, define and evaluate needs, and focus their interventions. Without a clearly identified model to define the scope of practice and provide a systematic approach, practice is reliant on personal experience and trial and error (Krefting, 1985). Practice is then "hit or miss" and is dependent on therapists sharing practice wisdom or building appropriate experience.

Therapists who are conscious of their practice framework can explain their unique contribution to the team, describing their expertise or justifying their approach. When they find themselves in conflict with consumers or other service providers, who might have different understandings or expectations, they can understand the situation and are able to explore the other person's perspective, articulate their own, and identify common goals. Therapists who acknowledge or reflect on their model of practice remain alert to the scope of concern of the profession and select assessment and intervention approaches that address these concerns. With a clear and well-articulated model of practice, therapists are able to prioritize clients' specific needs over service imperatives and processes. These therapists are also able to recognize and respond to conceptual developments and new knowledge in an area of practice. There is harmony between what they say they do and what they actually do because their procedures are well aligned with their conceptual model.

It is therefore important that therapists are aware of the concepts shaping their practices and driving their decision making. In an effort to illustrate the impact of models on the nature of services provided and the outcomes achieved, each model will be examined in turn using one case study. The way in which each model shapes service delivery and determines outcomes will be described and analyzed with particular reference to their capacity to respond to consumer concerns and to deal with important aspects of the home environment.

Mrs. Hume is an 82-year-old woman who lives on her own in a four-bedroom detached house in an older inner-city suburb. She has lived in this neighborhood for 60 years, having raised her family in the two-story house her husband built soon after they were married. When her husband died 5 years ago, her widowed 80-year-old sister moved in. Mrs. Hume has three children—a daughter who lives 10 miles away in the same city, a son who lives in a nearby city, and another son who has moved interstate. She has rheumatoid arthritis and has been admitted to the hospital following a recent flare-up of her condition. Medication has been re-evaluated, and her condition has settled. She has been referred to occupational therapy to assist in her return home.

Before reading any further, take a few moments to reflect on this case and, as her occupational therapist, write down what you would offer Mrs. Hume.

+ What would be your main focus?
+ How would you determine need?
+ How would you address needs?
+ How would you work with Mrs. Hume?
+ How do you view the home environment?
+ What outcomes are you expecting from your interventions?

The way therapists regard Mrs. Hume, relate to her and her home environment, and define and address her needs reveals much about the model of practice from which they work. As you read through this chapter, you may recognize aspects of models evident in your approach with Mrs. Hume. Through the discussion of each of these models, you should come to appreciate the impact of your current conceptualizations on the nature of the services you provide, the procedures you use, and the subsequent outcomes you could achieve for Mrs. Hume. In addition, you will be able to reflect on contemporary views of disability, the environment, and client-centered practice, and how well these understandings are reflected in your current practice.

THE REHABILITATION MODEL

Occupational therapy, originally embedded in a humanistic tradition (Schwartz, 2003), has been strongly influenced by the medical science and biomedical models of practice. Following World War II and the emergence of rehabilitation medicine, occupational therapy joined other allied health professionals in providing medical care to returning soldiers. By the 1970s, with the proliferation of scientific knowledge and expansion of the health care industry, and as a result of the Rehabilitation Act of 1954, occupational therapy was well established in rehabilitation services (Schwartz).

The rehabilitation model is founded on extensive knowledge of the structure and function of the human body and the impact of injury and disease. This has had an enduring influence on the way people with disabilities are viewed and their needs defined within rehabilitation services. Within this model, people are regarded as human organisms consisting of a series of complex systems, with the underlying structures and functions that are common to all humans. Traditionally, medical specialists and rehabilitation professionals have defined their scope of concern or responsibilities in terms of a particular body system; for example, cardiologists are responsible for matters concerning the circulatory system and neurologists focus on the neural system. Similarly, allied health professionals have tended to define their roles in terms of functional systems: physiotherapists are primarily concerned with neuromuscular function, psychologists with mental function, and speech pathologists with voice and speech function (Seidel, 1998). The initial focus of rehabilitation was to restore an individual's function when his or her capacity had been altered or limited by a physical or mental impairment that could not be remediated by surgery or medical intervention (Seidel). However, this model has continued to evolve in response to social changes, such as deinstitutionalization and the Independent Living Movement (Schwartz, 2003), resulting in a shift to promoting independence. Consequently, occupational therapists have focused on restoring the individual's ability to function independently in daily activities.

Within this model, impairment is defined as the "loss or abnormality of psychological, physiological or anatomical structure or function" (World Health Organization [WHO], 1980, p. 47), and disability is viewed as a restriction or lack of ability to perform an activity in a manner or within the range considered "normal" (Seidel, 1998). Assessment is therefore focused on identifying specific symptoms and signs of abnormality and quantifying the person's functional capacities in various areas, such as neuromuscular, mental, or cardiovascular, as well as independence in daily activities. The rehabilitation model requires the combined and coordinated use of medical, social, educational, and vocational measures to train or retrain an individual to the highest possible levels of function (WHO). Interventions involve retraining and the use of remedial activities to restore function, compensatory techniques to support the completion of tasks and activities, as well as assistive devices and environmental adaptations to accommodate lost function.

In a rehabilitation model, the degree to which maximum function and independence can be achieved is believed to be dependent on the individual's level of motivation. The therapist is perceived to be an expert who brings specialist knowledge about the physiology and pathology of impairment to the process and educates the individual about appropriate remediation and adaptive strategies (Dewsbury, Clarke, Randall, Rouncefield, & Sommerville, 2004). Therapists advise clients on how to regain lost function and recommend suitable compensatory techniques, assistive devices, or environmental adaptations to promote independence. Typically, assistive devices are recommended more frequently than environmental adaptations because these interventions are both less costly and less complex to implement (Auriemma, Faust, Sibrian, & Jimenez, 1999; Pynoos, Tabbarah, Angelelli, & Demiere, 1998; Tabbarah, Silverstein, & Seeman, 2000). Within this model, the environment is seen as a static physical entity that can be modified to accommodate an individual's identified functional impairment. The focus is largely on aspects of the environment that create barriers to independence in specific self-care activities, such as mobility, bathing, and toileting. The outcomes generally sought by therapists and services using a rehabilitation approach are for the person to regain maximum function and independence. Consequently, outcome measures focus on evaluating the person's degree of independence and functions believed to underpin independence. Because independence is defined as being able to complete tasks without assistance (Tamaru, McColl, & Yamasaki, 2007), many outcome measures seek to determine the extent to which individuals can complete tasks on their own.

Addressing Home Modification Needs Using a Rehabilitation Framework

In light of the previous description of the rehabilitation model, how would a therapist using this model address Mrs. Hume's home modification needs? The following questions will be used to guide this analysis:

+ What would be the therapist's primary focus?

+ How would a therapist using this model define Mrs. Hume's needs?

+ What evaluation processes would Mrs. Hume experience?

+ What interventions or services would be available to Mrs. Hume?

+ How would the therapist work with Mrs. Hume?

+ How would the environment be addressed in this model?

+ What outcomes would Mrs. Hume expect to achieve?

The extensive scientific and medical knowledge underlying the rehabilitation model would ensure that Mrs. Hume receives the very best medical care. This means that her condition would be actively managed by health professionals and that she could expect reduced inflammation, pain, and long-term damage to her joints. She would be under the care of a rheumatologist for the management of her condition and would be referred to other specialists as required. She is likely to be receiving the service of a physiotherapist to maximize her range of movement and muscle strength, and she is likely to be referred to an occupational therapist to maximize her function and independence in activities associated with daily living. She may also be referred to a hand therapist—or possibly a physiotherapist or occupational therapist—for splints to protect her joints. Within the rehabilitation model, Mrs. Hume would be identified primarily in terms of her health condition and would be provided services in line with protocols for that condition. Evaluation would commonly focus on defining her level of function, including measures of range of movement, grip strength, and independence. Mrs. Hume is also likely to receive ongoing evaluations of her physical and functional capacity as successive health professionals establish a baseline and periodically re-evaluate her condition to note improvements in her response to medications and remedial exercise and activities.

The goal of interventions would be to achieve maximum function, and Mrs. Hume is likely to be given exercises, taught compensatory joint protection strategies, and provided with splints and assistive devices to allow her to complete the activities of daily living considered "normal" for adults her age—for example, all adults are expected to be independent in toileting. Assistive devices, such as reachers and tap turners, would commonly be recommended based on her diagnosis of rheumatoid arthritis (Mann & Lane, 1995) or in response to particular activity difficulties. Specific barriers to completing self-care activities in the home—for example, low toilet and standard tap and door fittings—would result in recommended environmental modifications, such as grab rails or lever taps. The therapist might or might not make a home visit, largely because potential environmental barriers could be determined from Mrs. Hume's known impairments, from identified functional capacities and performance difficulties in daily activities, and through discussion with Mrs. Hume about features in the home. Mrs. Hume would receive advice from the therapist about appropriate remedial strategies and suitable assistive devices and modifications. Lack of compliance with recommended interventions would be attributed to Mrs. Hume's lack of motivation or understanding of her condition and the purpose of the interventions. The therapist would then seek to educate Mrs. Hume about her condition and the benefits of adhering to recommendations. It is anticipated that the recommended interventions would allow Mrs. Hume to function independently in self-care activities. Follow-up evaluations might be undertaken to confirm that she is completing tasks independently. Current independence measures actually would show a drop in Mrs. Hume's independence score if additional support strategies were introduced to activities.

Implications of Using the Rehabilitation Model for Home Modifications

The extensive knowledge of body structures and functions that underlies the rehabilitation model allows therapists using this model to reduce the amount of residual impairment resulting from an injury or health condition and promote high levels of function and independence. Having grown out of a medical model, the rehabilitation model uses a "medical" or individual model of disability, which sees disablement as a personal problem resulting from disease, trauma, or other health condition and requiring care and individual treatment by medical professionals (WHO, 2001). Consequently, much of the evaluation process is focused on determining the degree of impairment or deficits the person has. Measures of function either rely on personal interpretations of normal function or refer to data that detail the maximum or average for any given age group. However, little is known about the strength or range of movement requirements for everyday tasks (Badley, 1995; Law & Baum, 2005), and assessment results might over- or underestimate the specific requirements of particular tasks for any given

individual in his or her environment (Dunn, 2005). A deeper understanding of the specific difficulties someone experiences in daily activities would ensure that interventions are more appropriately tailored to the individual.

There are often a number of people involved in providing care and addressing specific deficits, all of which can leave the affected person feeling overwhelmed, fragmented, and disempowered. A focus on presenting physical problems can also mean that social and emotional needs are not acknowledged well within this model (Seidel, 1998). Evaluation and treatment protocols tend to focus on specific functions and do not allow the therapist to develop an understanding of the real person—their concerns and priorities. Rehabilitation goals of maximizing function and independence often take precedence over the client's unique concerns and goals. Whereas therapists are concerned with ensuring that people can function without help, clients might be more worried about having control over their daily activities and making lifestyle decisions (Clough, Leamy, Miller, & Bright, 2004; Heywood, Oldman, & Means, 2002). Consequently, devices or modifications recommended by a rehabilitation therapist to promote independence in the shower, for example, might not be acceptable because the client might be more interested in conserving time and energy to engage in his or her chosen activities rather than being exhausted by routine self-care tasks. When clients do not embrace the interventions on offer, it is often perceived that they lack motivation or understanding. However, because goals and interventions are largely determined by the professional with specific reference to their client's performance deficits (Law, 1998), they might not be well suited to the client's requirements, preferences, or lifestyle.

It is often difficult for clients to shape and direct intervention in the rehabilitation model because therapists are usually the ones who have extensive knowledge of the injury or health condition, its pathology, and how it can be remediated. In addition, clients usually have little knowledge of the interventions available and are reliant on the expertise of the therapist for recommendations. Although it would be useful to use this opportunity to educate the client about alternative options and their relative benefits, the focus instead is on increasing compliance (Law, 1998), assuming that once the person understands why the intervention is considered necessary he or she will automatically accept it.

In the rehabilitation model, restoration of function is usually the primary focus of treatment, with remediation strategies, such as assistive devices and environmental modifications, receiving less attention. In the hierarchy of rehabilitation interventions, these strategies are frequently seen as part of discharge planning, and there is insufficient time to effectively plan and implement the intervention before the person is discharged. With interventions focused primarily on a client's specific performance difficulties, little attention is given to how the environment can support and promote further engagement in activities. The restricted view of the environment as a physical entity means that its personal, cultural, and social aspects are often overlooked. Consequently, interventions might not be tailored as well as they could be to the home environment and could create challenges for the client and others instead.

The outcomes of rehabilitation are generally defined and evaluated by service providers (Law, 1998) and are traditionally focused on achieving a specific performance standard or complete independence. It is difficult to measure the success of modification outcomes, especially in terms of independence achieved, using the standardized tests currently in use because many measures of independence assign a penalty for using any assistance, including a device. For example, when using the Functional Independence Measure (FIM; Uniform Data System for Medical Rehabilitation, 1997), people can only achieve the highest score of 7 if they do not use a device or have any assistance to complete the task (Cook & Hussey, 2002). In addition, rehabilitation outcome measures do not recognize the impact of the impairment on the person's daily life. Consequently, the FIM does not assess the value of activities for the individual or the quality or acceptability of performance.

OCCUPATIONAL PERFORMANCE MODELS

In an effort to differentiate itself from other health care professions and to articulate its unique scope of concern, occupational therapy developed its own models and frameworks for practice. These models aimed to unify the profession that had been fractured by an explosion of new knowledge about the internal workings of the body and psyche and increasingly specialized practice structured around medical conditions. An overemphasis on techniques and the use of modalities prompted the profession to re-examine its direction and to reconnect with its original philosophy, beliefs, and focus on occupation (Schwartz, 2003). *Occupational performance*, a term first coined in the American Occupational Therapy Association's

(AOTA) grant report in 1973, became the unique and central concern of the profession because it focused on individuals' abilities to accomplish tasks related to their roles and developmental stage (AOTA, 1973; Reed, 2005). The Occupational Performance Model (OPM) was one of the earliest models to evolve from this shift in direction. It grew out of a series of AOTA task forces and committees in the 1970s and the writings of leaders in the profession about that time, such as Llorens, Mosey, and Reilly (Kielhofner, 2004; Llorens, 1989; Pedretti, 1996). Although originally described as a frame of reference for practice and educational design (AOTA, 1973, 1974), the OPM detailed the profession's domains of concern, focus, and areas of expertise and has had a substantial and enduring influence on practice, especially in physical rehabilitation (Turpin, in press).

The OPM recognizes humans as active beings who are able to influence their physical and mental health and their physical and social environment through participation in purposeful activity or occupation (Pedretti, 1996). It is concerned with developing, restoring, and maintaining an individual's ability to perform everyday activities, tasks, and roles, in a satisfying manner, appropriate to the person's developmental stage, culture, and environment (AOTA, 1973, 1974; Mosey, 1981; Pedretti). Occupational performance is dependent on intact neurophysiological development and integrated functioning of the performance components including sensorimotor, cognitive/cognitive integration, and psychosocial/psychological subsystems. Failure or disruption in performance areas—activities related to daily living (ADLs) and work/productive activities or play/leisure—are believed to result from deficits in task learning experience, performance components, and/or an unsupportive life space or context. Figure 3-1 displays a graphical representation of the OPM as presented by Pedretti.

In the OPM, assessment focuses on examining performance in ADLs, work/productive activities, and play/leisure, traditionally expressed in terms of level of engagement and independence. Capacity in performance components is also assessed because these are presumed to support occupational performance. Therapists generally access biomedical, psychiatric, or developmental models to understand and address specific performance component difficulties. The aim of intervention is to achieve a balance and optimum occupational performance with a focus on resuming previous occupational roles or to assume new and satisfying roles with a particular focus on achieving independence in performance areas. To this end, a continuum of interventions is used, including adjunctive methods, enabling

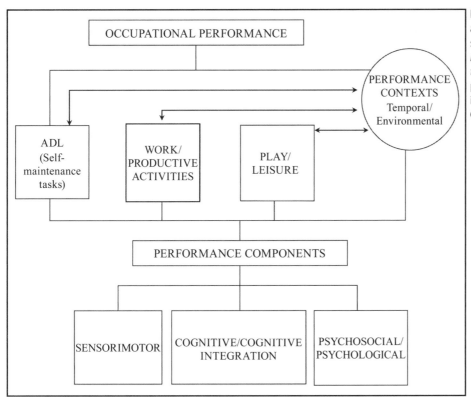

activities, purposeful activity, and occupational performance and roles.

Adjunctive methods include exercise, positioning, sensory stimulation, splints, and selected physical agent modalities, while enabling activities include simulated activities, such as stacking cones and practice boards as well as assistive devices. These methods primarily focus on assessing and remediating performance components but with the ultimate goal of facilitating and preparing for occupational performance. Assistive devices, such as wheelchairs, and environmental control systems are used to accommodate performance deficits and enable independence in daily activities. Purposeful activities—activities that are relevant and meaningful to the client—allow the therapist to assess and remediate deficits in performance areas and prepare the client for the final stage of the treatment continuum—resuming occupational roles in his or her real environment. Although remediating performance components is a central concern in developing interventions, treatment stages overlap and occur simultaneously rather than in a strictly progressive fashion.

Therapists use their expert knowledge of performance components to remediate or compensate for performance "defects" and facilitate occupational performance. To ensure that treatment remains focused on the client's occupational performance context, the therapist consults with the client to determine his or her valued roles and preferred activities. The context is acknowledged as important to successful occupational performance; however, the temporal context is primarily related to "the individual's age, developmental stage or phase of maturation, and stage in important life processes, such as parenting, education, or career" and disability status—for example, acute, chronic, terminal, improving, or declining (Pedretti, 1996, p. 5). Three environmental contexts are identified: physical, social, and cultural.

> The physical environment includes homes, buildings, outdoors, furniture, tools, and other objects. The social environment includes significant others and social groups. The cultural environment includes customs, beliefs, standards of behavior, political factors, and opportunities for education, employment, and economic support (Pedretti, 1996, p. 5).

The outcomes sought by therapists in this model would include optimum functioning in performance components because these are believed to provide the foundation for performance in ADLs and work and play/leisure activities. Other appropriate outcomes would be independence in these activities and the resumption or acquisition of developmentally appropriate roles.

Addressing Home Modification Needs Using an OPM Framework

The focus of the therapist working with Mrs. Hume in an OPM framework would be primarily on restoring and maintaining her ability to perform daily activities and roles. The therapist would assess how her condition impacted on her specific performance components, such as her sensorimotor performance, and identify activities and roles she was unable to undertake satisfactorily, with a particular interest in establishing her level of independence in daily activities. Primarily, the therapist would be concerned with assessing performance components as well as evaluation of everyday activities that allow Mrs. Hume to look after herself and manage in the home environment (Hittle, Pedretti, & Kasch, 1996). An evaluation of Mrs. Hume's joints and skin quality, range of movement, strength, hand function, sensation, and endurance would be completed using observation and formal testing procedures (Hittle et al.). The therapist would assess her performance in a number of discrete tasks, such as self-care, home management, work activities, and exercise behaviors, through interview and observation. The attention given to work or leisure, education, and social activities would vary depending on reimbursement schedules and the priorities of the service organization and the consumer. A home evaluation would be undertaken with the purpose of assisting the client in "making modifications to simplify work, save energy and protect joints from undue stress" (Hittle et al., p. 647).

Drawing on his or her knowledge of biomechanics and rehabilitation, the therapist would optimize Mrs. Hume's function by:

+ Remediating lost range of movement and muscle strength through the use of adjunctive methods such as exercise and selected physical agent modalities

+ Maintaining her abilities through the use of splints, enabling activities such as tabletop tasks and purposeful activity such as ADLs and household activities

+ Compensating for lost function using joint protection and energy conservation techniques and assistive devices, such as built-up and extended handles, reachers, book stands, bowl holders, special clothing, raised toilet seats, grab rails, and modifying fixtures and fittings in the environment (Hittle et al., 1996)

The therapist would develop goals and tailor interventions in light of Mrs. Hume's unique situation and interests, focusing attention on activities of most concern to Mrs. Hume and relevant to her life stage and living situation. The home environment would be reviewed in terms of its ability to support occupational performance. Aspects of the physical environment, such as features of the building, furniture, fixtures, and fittings that can no longer be managed, would be identified and removed, replaced, or modified. Consideration would also be given to other people in the environment and to how roles may need to be reassigned or modified to assist Mrs. Hume in daily activities. Family members and caregivers would be educated about Mrs. Hume's condition so that they can support her by undertaking more difficult activities. Cultural aspects of the home and community, such as customs and behavior standards, would be acknowledged when evaluating activities and roles and recommending changes.

At the completion of the treatment process, it would also be anticipated that Mrs. Hume's motor performance would have improved and that she could complete activities independently. These improvements would then result in her resuming valued roles and being generally satisfied. Injury, decreased occupational performance, or further deformity or disability would be considered unfavorable, or unintended, outcomes.

Implications of Using the OPM Model for Home Modifications

The occupational performance model offers occupational therapists a vehicle for defining their unique scope of practice. Much of the knowledge about body structures and functions gained by the profession during its alignment with the rehabilitation model provided the foundation for understanding and addressing function and skill development as it impacts on occupational performance. This focus on occupational performance allows therapists to consider sensorimotor, cognitive/cognitive integration, and psychosocial/psychological performance in the context of the person's everyday activities, tasks, and roles and in relation to his or her developmental stage, culture, and environment. However, its emphasis on remediating performance components as a means of improving occupational performance reflects an individual model of disability. Similar to the rehabilitation model, this model sees disability as primarily resulting from specific incapacities of the individual. Although the environment is seen as the context of occupational performance and a mechanism for supporting atypical performance, it is not clearly identified as contributing to disability.

Traditionally, the OPM has been operationalized using a bottom-up approach where evaluation and intervention focus on deficits in performance components that are presumed to be the foundation for successful occupational performance. This often results in therapists focusing their energies on remediating performance components without due consideration of the demands of various activities and the environment (Holm, Rogers, & Stone, 1998). However, improvements in generic abilities might not always generalize to daily activities, and not all tasks require optimum function (Holm et al.; Weinstock-Zlotnick & Hinjosa, 2004). Furthermore, many performance deficits cannot be fully remediated, especially for people with chronic health conditions or permanent disabilities (Holm et al.). Consequently, some clients are discharged from therapy with residual occupational performance difficulties that require further adjustment and accommodation. Managed care, time-limited hospitalizations, and defined reimbursement schedules have also resulted in therapists having reduced contact with clients and less opportunity to remediate performance components (Baum & Law, 1997). This requires that greater consideration be given to enabling the client to undertake everyday activities before performance components have been fully remediated.

An alternative, top-down approach has been proposed as a means of addressing some of these concerns. A top-down approach redirects the therapist's attention to first identifying valued occupations and then determining the performance deficits contributing to performance difficulties (Baum & Law, 1997). Once the capacities impacting directly on occupational performance have been identified, a more focused evaluation of performance components is undertaken (Holm et al., 1998). When evaluations and interventions are structured around clients' valued activities and roles, there is greater potential for them to be actively involved in the process and for their priorities to be addressed. Clients are still reliant on the therapist's expertise to advise on appropriate adjunctive and enabling activities and assistive devices, but the client's unique occupational performance needs are prioritized in the process.

At times, therapists experience difficulty attending to or prioritizing occupational performance issues because these issues may be perceived as being outside the scope of the service or not recognized within reimbursement schedules. In these situations, it is important that therapists remain mindful of the clients' priorities and target evaluation and interventions to address these, even if performance in valued activities is not being addressed directly. For example, if a therapist is primarily responsible for making splints for Mrs. Hume, it is very important that these splints are constructed with her primary occupational performance and roles in mind. It is also crucial that therapists see themselves as part of a continuum of care and refer clients to therapists in other services who have the focus and resources to address the client's specific occupational performance concerns. When occupational performance is addressed in a holistic way, all of the factors impacting on performance can be identified and the full range of suitable interventions determined. Even if the therapist is not in a position to provide the solutions, the client can be empowered to investigate assistance from elsewhere or purchase preferred solutions themselves. If therapists are addressing only a defined part of occupational therapy's scope of concern, they need to ensure that clients understand what it is they can and cannot attend to. This is particularly important when consumer priorities are in conflict with the service focus. In such cases, clients should be redirected to services that are better aligned to their specific needs. It is also important that therapists work within the service to advocate for policy and service delivery changes that better reflect clients' occupational performance needs.

Like other early models of occupational performance, the OPM does not reflect a well-developed understanding of the environment (Rogers & Holm, 2009). In the OPM, the environment has been conceptualized as the context or backdrop to occupational performance and in the graphic sits external to, but in interaction with, performance areas. While this model urges therapists to consider clients' life stages and disability status as well as the physical, social, and cultural environment when assessing performance components and developing interventions, the role of the environment in creating or increasing disability is not recognized. Furthermore, the dynamic nature of the environment and its interaction with the person and his or her occupations are concepts that are also not understood. Consequently, this model does not use the environment effectively as an intervention for addressing occupational performance issues.

The outcomes measured in the OPM place emphasis on measuring improvements in motor performance and independence. These professional assessments do not necessarily acknowledge the importance of various activities to clients or their satisfaction with their performance of various valued activities. The specific difficulties or improvements experienced by clients in everyday activities are also not registered on standardized ADL assessments, especially on measures of independence that penalize the use of assistive devices. The effectiveness of specific interventions in addressing occupational performance concerns in the home and their impact on the home environment are also overlooked because the need to assess the efficacy of interventions once they are in place is not prioritized in this model.

ECOLOGICAL MODELS

A number of ecological models have been developed in recent years in recognition of the importance of the role of the environment to occupational performance. The Ecology of Human Performance (EHP; Dunn, Brown, & McGuigan, 1994), the Person-Environment-Occupation-Performance (PEOP; Christiansen & Baum, 1997), and the Person-Environment-Occupation (PEO; Law et al., 1996) models consider occupational performance to be the primary interest of occupational therapists and recognize the dynamic and reciprocal interaction between the person, occupation, and the environment. All three models are founded on the notion of "goodness of fit," where occupational performance is optimized by a match between the person's skills and abilities and the occupational and environmental affordances and demands. The models also reflect the values of the disability movement, where the environment is viewed as an agent in creating disability and value (Brown, 2009).

While these models have a number of elements in common, there are also some distinct differences (Baum, Bass-Haugen, & Christiansen, 2005). These differences largely lie in the components, definitions, and structure of the models (Brown, 2009). The EHP and PEO models are largely conceptual and serve as a means of integrating information and understanding how things work as a whole. They require therapists to draw on other theories and frameworks to understand specific factors contributing to occupational performance issues and then guide the selection of assessment and interventions (Brown, 2009). The PEOP model integrates a range of existing theories from occupational science, neuroscience, environmental science, and other biological and social sciences to provide a more detailed description of aspects of the person and his or her occupation and environment that contribute to occupational performance and participation. It also details a process for addressing concerns (Baum et al.), which makes it easier for therapists to use. A graphical representation of the PEOP is provided in Figure 3-2.

The ecological models build on the traditional occupational therapy concepts of people as unique, occupational beings and also incorporate theories of environment-behavior to provide a richer description of the environment and its relationship with people and their occupations. In particular, the PEO and PEOP models highlight the dynamic nature of occupational performance and the transactional relationship between the person, his or her occupation, and the environment (Baum & Christiansen, 2005; Stewart et al., 2003). These elements are considered to interact reciprocally and continuously across space and time to constrain or facilitate occupational performance (Figure 3-3; Baum et al., 2005; Law et al., 1996).

The focus of these models is on optimizing occupational performance and participation by enhancing the congruence between the person, his or her occupation and roles, and the environment. Both models incorporate a top-down approach, where the person is considered within the context of his or her goals, roles, and occupations (Baum & Christiansen, 2005). Need is defined in terms of the person's specific concerns, with particular attention paid to identifying the nature and extent of occupational performance issues. Therapists use both objective and subjective methods to evaluate performance, participation, and the person-environment-occupation fit and to understand the value and acceptability of the performance to the person (Law et al., 1996).

These models recognize the uniqueness of each person and situation and use a client-centered approach to examine occupational performance strengths and weaknesses focusing on aspects of the person, occupation, and environment that could enhance performance. Each person is viewed holistically and is acknowledged as bringing unique personal attributes, capacities, and life experiences to the collaboration. Each model encourages therapists to use a broad range of intervention strategies aimed at making changes in the person, occupation, and the environment; however, it is recognized that changes in any one of these areas will have an impact on the others.

Drawing on theories of the environment from several disciplines, these models describe the environment as having cultural, socioeconomic, institutional or societal, physical (natural and built environment), and social elements, which, in dynamic interaction with the person and their occupations, can enhance or diminish occupational performance. Each model considers these environmental domains from a person, household, neighborhood, and community perspective (Law et al., 1996),

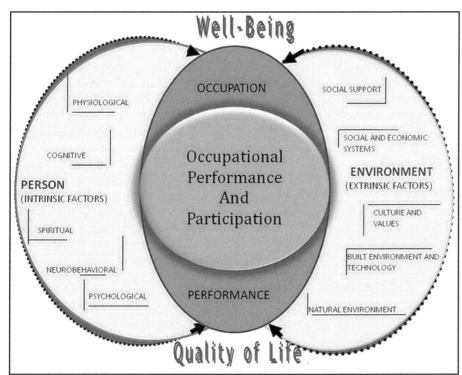

Figure 3-2. The Person-Environment-Occupation-Performance Model. (Reprinted with permission from Baum, C. M., & Christiansen, C. H. (2005). The person-environment-occupation-performance model: An occupation-based framework for practice. In C. H. Christiansen, C. M. Baum, & J. Bass-Haugen (Eds.), *Occupational therapy: Performance, participation and well-being* (3rd ed., pp. 243-266). Thorofare, NJ: SLACK Incorporated.)

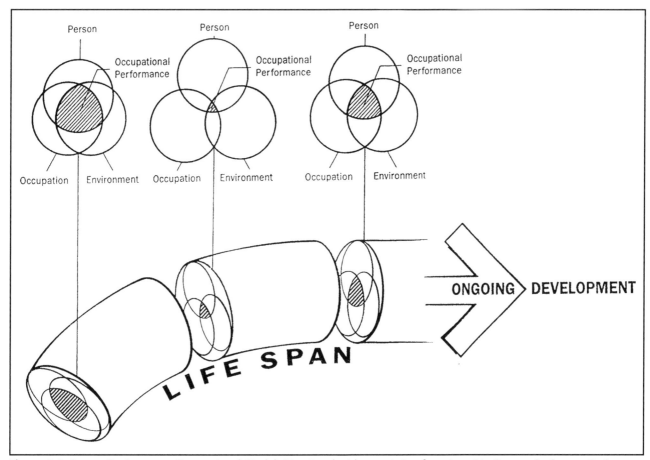

Figure 3-3. Person-Environment-Occupational Model. (Reprinted with permission from Law, M., Cooper, B., Strong, S., Stewart, D., Rigby, P., & Letts. L. (1996). The person-environment-occupation model: A transactive approach to occupational performance. *Canadian Journal of Occupational Therapy, 63,* 9-23.)

with the PEOP model demonstrating its application in dealing with individuals, organizations, and population- or community-based issues. The expected outcome of these models is that the person is well-supported to engage in everyday life and can undertake the roles, responsibilities, and interests that meet his or her intrinsic needs for self-maintenance, expression, and fulfillment.

Addressing Home Modification Needs Using an Ecological Framework

In using an ecological model, in the case of Mrs. Hume, the therapist first recognizes the uniqueness of her experience of her condition and how this, in combination with her occupations and roles and the environments in which she lives, works, and recreates, impacts on her occupational performance. Mrs. Hume's occupational performance is likely to vary throughout the day, from one day to another, and into the future, depending on her capacities, the demands of her roles and occupations, and how the context constrains or enables performance. The therapist will seek to optimize Mrs. Hume's occupational performance by enhancing the congruence between her, her occupations and roles, and the relevant environments. Using a top-down approach and discussion, the therapist will identify the nature and extent of occupational performance concerns in collaboration with Mrs. Hume. He or she will obtain an occupational history and profile and observe and analyze performance using standardized performance and occupational and environmental assessment tools. The therapist will identify Mrs. Hume's occupational performance goals and, together with her, will evaluate the quality of her performance to determine its acceptability and to ensure valued occupations are prioritized.

These models recognize Mrs. Hume's life experience, values, interests, personal attributes, and strengths and build on existing strategies and supports to develop interventions. The therapist will explore a range of alternative interventions with Mrs. Hume, including skill development, alternative ways of undertaking tasks, and changes to the environment. Consultation with Mrs. Hume follows with a view to extending her involvement in occupations and roles and increasing her participation, where appropriate, in activities in the home and community. The therapist will work closely with Mrs. Hume to explore and evaluate various options to ensure that they fit with her requirements,

preferences, personal style, and the way tasks are undertaken. In addition, the therapist will discuss the intervention options with Mrs. Hume to ensure that they will work within the cultural, socioeconomic, institutional, physical, and social aspects of her home environment and community. Therapists using these models are aware that any change to the person, occupation, or environment is likely to impact . Hence, care is taken to examine these possibilities prior to recommending them and then to monitor unexpected outcomes following implementation. The occupational performance outcomes sought by Mrs. Hume form the foundation for evaluation, using tools that assess her satisfaction with her current performance as well as more objective measures of performance quality. In addition, measures of Mrs. Hume's participation in the household, neighborhood, and wider community would also be used. The therapist might encourage Mrs. Hume to write to her local council requesting improved accessibility to, and additional seating in, the shopping mall. Alternatively, the therapist might make representation to management of the local mall or local business community to advocate for better access or additional seating for older people and people with disabilities. The therapist might also join community or industry groups to advocate for more appropriate housing and better access to community facilities and services for older people and people with disabilities.

Implications of Using an Ecological Model for Home Modifications

Ecological models acknowledge the complexity and variability of occupational performance and the dynamic transaction between the person, occupation, and environment. This closely reflects the reality of practice and enables therapists to analyze and explain occupational performance in terms of the "fit," rather than attributing problems to the individual. These models also recognize the uniqueness of each person, the way tasks are performed, and the personal nature of the home environment, allowing therapists to understand and tailor interventions to specific situations. Each model shifts the therapist's focus from evaluating the detail of each of the elements to trying to understand the whole transaction. The elements in the models are also conceptualized and described broadly so that they can be adapted and expanded to fit various situations and practice settings.

Both the PEO and PEOP models allow therapists to recognize each person as holding a variety of roles simultaneously and shift the focus from improving the performance of specific activities to enabling people to engage in a broad range of valued occupations. Using a holistic view of the person also allows the therapist to acknowledge the experience and knowledge that each person brings to the collaboration. The models encourage therapists to gain a deeper understanding of clients' perceptions of issues and performance and to work with their clients to identify priorities, as well as existing strengths and supports, that can be used to promote occupational performance.

An understanding of the inevitable variability of performance ensures that therapists develop solutions that are flexible enough to support performance across the day, the week, and into the future. By providing a range of alternative intervention options aimed at improving the person's capacity and skill to find another way to perform the activity or modifying the environment, the therapist provides choices and assists clients to build a repertoire of useful strategies to use in different situations. These models also require therapists to look beyond just the home environment and to ensure that performance is supported in all the environments in which the person operates. It also enables the therapist to work with clients to deal with the complexity of the home environment and to determine how interventions might impact on the cultural, socioeconomic, institutional, physical, and social aspects of the home environment and the community. With an understanding of the complexity of the home environment and the uniqueness of each person, therapists appreciate the need for follow-up to ensure that the interventions have no unexpected outcomes. The perceptions of the person are central to evaluating the success of the intervention, which ensures that the solution is not only evaluated in terms of effectiveness but also in terms of how well the solution reflects the goals and wishes of the client and fits the unique person-environment-occupation transaction. Finally, these models encourage therapists and the profession to look beyond the individual household and situation to examine how services, systems, and policies can be mobilized to further promote occupational engagement and performance, encouraging therapists to become involved in communities and systems to ensure all members of the community can fully participate in society (Brown, 2009).

CONCLUSION

Therapists use models, either implicitly or explicitly, to define their scope of concern and role, identify and understand issues or problems, determine appropriate evaluation and intervention strategies, and evaluate outcomes. Conceptual models overview concepts and describe the relationships between the identified elements, and procedural models specify a procedure for attending to issues and elements. Therapists need both conceptual and procedural models to operate effectively because practice requires therapists to have an understanding of all of the elements of concern and their interactions as well as a plan of action. However, therapists need to be aware of the models they draw on in practice and ensure that their actions echo their stated focus and goals. Each model presented in this chapter conceptualizes the person, occupational performance, environment, and interaction between these in different ways, all of which have an impact on how occupational therapists engage with issues and implement environmental interventions.

The rehabilitation model provides therapists with knowledge of body structures and functions and allows them to reduce the amount of residual impairment resulting from an injury or health condition and to promote function and independence. However, without a deeper understanding of the particular difficulties an individual is experiencing in daily activities, interventions are not tailored to the specific needs of the individual and may result in changes that are ineffective or unacceptable in the home environment.

In shifting the focus of therapy to occupational performance, the OPM provides occupational therapists with a unique role and allows them to consider the impact of impairments on everyday life. A bottom-up approach, however, can cause therapists to be overly preoccupied with remediating performance components, leaving less time to address occupational performance concerns in the natural environment. Furthermore, although this model acknowledges the environment as the context of performance, it does not recognize its role in furthering or preventing disability.

The ecological models, with their understanding of the dynamic transaction between the person, occupation, and environment, provide an excellent framework for addressing the complexities that individuals encounter when undertaking everyday activities in the home and community.

In acknowledging the uniqueness of each person and his or her occupational roles and environment, these models allow therapists to collaborate with clients to tailor interventions to their specific needs. Recognition of the environment as a means of limiting and creating occupational performance opportunities also enables therapists to actively use the environment to promote participation within the home and community. Ecological models also encourage therapists to move beyond working with individuals to becoming agents of change within the community, thus ensuring equitable participation for all.

REFERENCES

American Occupational Therapy Association. (1973). *Project to delineate the roles and functions of occupational therapy personnel.* Rockville, MD: Author.

American Occupational Therapy Association. (1974). *A curriculum guide for occupational therapy educators.* Rockville, MD: Author.

Auriemma, D., Faust, S., Sibrian, K., & Jimenez, J. (1999). Home modifications for the elderly: Implications for the occupational therapist. *Physical and Occupational Therapy in Geriatrics, 16*(2-4), 135-144.

Badley, E. M. (1995). The genesis of handicap: Definition, models of disablement and the role of external factors. *Disability and Rehabilitation, 17,* 53-62.

Baum, C. M., Bass-Haugen, J., & Christiansen, C. H. (2005). Person-environment-occupational performance: A model for planning interventions for individuals and organizations. In C. H. Christiansen, C. M. Baum, & J. Bass-Haugen (Eds.), *Occupational therapy: Performance, participation and well-being* (3rd ed.) (pp. 373-392). Thorofare, NJ: SLACK Incorporated.

Baum, C. M., & Christiansen, C. H. (2005). Person-environment-occupational performance: An occupation-based framework for practice. In C. H. Christiansen, C. M. Baum, & J. Bass-Haugen (Eds.), *Occupational therapy: Performance, participation and well-being* (3rd ed., pp. 243-266). Thorofare, NJ: SLACK Incorporated.

Baum, C. M., & Law, M. (1997). Occupational therapy practice: Focusing on occupational performance. *American Journal of Occupational Therapy, 15*(4), 277-288.

Brown, C. E. (2009). Ecological models in occupational therapy. In E. B. Crepeau, E. S. Cohn, & B. A. Boyt Schell (Eds.), *Willard and Spackman's occupational therapy* (11th ed., pp. 435-445). Philadelphia, PA: Wolters Kluwer Lippincott Williams & Wilkins.

Christiansen, C. H., & Baum, C. M. (1997). Person-environment occupational performance: A conceptual model for practice. In C. H. Christiansen & C. M. Baum (Eds.), *Occupational therapy: Enabling function and well-being* (2nd ed., pp. 46-71). Thorofare, NJ: SLACK Incorporated.

Clough, R., Leamy, M., Miller, V., & Bright, L. (2004). *Housing decisions in later life.* New York, NY: Palgrave Macmillan.

Cook, A., & Hussey, S. (2002). *Assistive technologies: Principles and practice* (2nd ed.). St. Louis, MO: Mosby.

Dewsbury, G., Clarke, K., Randall, D., Rouncefield, M., & Sommerville, I. (2004). The anti-social model of disability. *Disability and Society, 19*(2), 145-158.

Dunn, W. (2005). Measurement issues and practices. In M. Law, C. Baum, & W. Dunn (Eds.), *Measuring occupational performance: Supporting best practice in occupational therapy* (pp. 21-32). Thorofare, NJ: SLACK Incorporated.

Dunn, W., Brown, C., & McGuigan, A. (1994). The ecology of human performance: A framework for considering the impact of context. *American Journal of Occupational Therapy, 48,* 595-607.

Heywood, F., Oldman, C., & Means, R. (2002). *Housing and home in later life.* Buckingham, UK: Open University Press.

Hittle, J. M., Pedretti, L. W., & Kasch, M. C. (1996). Rheumatoid arthritis. In L. W. Pedretti (Ed.), *Occupational therapy: Practice skills for physical dysfunction* (pp. 639-660). St. Louis, MO: Mosby.

Holm, M. B., Rogers, J. C., & Stone, R. G. (1998). Treatment of performance contexts. In M. E. Neistadt & E. Crepeau (Eds.), *Willard and Spackman's occupational therapy* (9th ed.) (pp. 471-520). Philadelphia, PA: Lippincott-Raven Publications.

Kielhofner, G. (2004). The development of occupational therapy knowledge. In G. Kielhofner (Ed.), *Conceptual foundations of occupational therapy* (3rd ed., pp. 27-63). Philadelphia, PA: F. A. Davis.

Krefting, L. H. (1985). The use of conceptual models in clinical practice. *Canadian Journal of Occupational Therapy, 52*(4), 173-178.

Law, M. (1998). *Client-centered occupational therapy.* Thorofare, NJ: SLACK Incorporated.

Law, M., & Baum, C. M. (2005). Measurement in occupational therapy. In M. Law, C. Baum, & W. Dunn (Eds.), *Measuring occupational performance: Supporting best practice in occupational therapy* (pp. 3-20). Thorofare, NJ: SLACK Incorporated.

Law, M., Cooper, B., Strong, S., Stewart, D., Rigby, P., & Letts. L. (1996). The person-environment-occupation model: A transactive approach to occupational performance. *Canadian Journal of Occupational Therapy, 63,* 9-23.

Llorens, L. A. (1989). Health care system models and occupational therapy. *Occupational Therapy in Health Care, 5*(4), 25-37.

Mann, W. C., & Lane, J. P. (1995). *Assistive technology for persons with disabilities* (2nd ed.). Bethesda, MD: American Occupational Therapy Association.

Mosey, A. C. (1981). *Occupational therapy: Configuration of a profession.* New York, NY: Raven Press.

Pedretti, L. W. (1996). Occupational performance: A model for practice in physical dysfunction. In L. W. Pedretti (Ed.), *Occupational therapy: Practice skills for physical dysfunction* (pp. 3-12). St. Louis, MO: Mosby.

Pynoos, J., Tabbarah, M., Angelelli, J., & Demiere, M. (1998). Improving the delivery of home modifications. *Technology and Disability, 8,* 3-14.

Reed, K. (1998). Theory and frame of reference. In M. E. Neistadt & E. B. Crepeau (Eds.), *Willard and Spackman's occupational therapy* (9th ed., pp. 521-524). New York, NY: Lippincott-Raven.

Reed, K. (2005). An annotated history of the concepts used in occupational therapy. In C. H. Christiansen, C. M. Baum, & J. Bass-Haugen (Eds.), *Occupational therapy: Performance, participation, and well-being* (3rd ed., pp. 567-626). Thorofare, NJ: SLACK Incorporated.

Reed, K., & Sanderson, S. N. (1999). *Concepts of occupational therapy.* Philadelphia, PA: Lippincott, Williams & Wilkins.

Rogers, J. C., & Holm, M. (2009). The occupational therapy process. In E. B. Crepeau, E. S. Cohn, & B. A. Boyt Schell (Eds.), *Willard and Spackman's occupational therapy* (11th ed., pp. 478-518). Philadelphia, PA: Wolters Kluwer Lippincott Williams & Wilkins.

Schwartz, C. B. (2003). The history of occupational therapy. In E. B. Crepeau, E. S. Cohn, & B. A. Boyt Schell (Eds.), *Willard and Spackman's occupational therapy* (10th ed., pp. 5-14). Philadelphia, PA: Lippincott Williams & Wilkins.

Seidel, A. C. (1998). Theories derived from rehabilitation perspectives. In M. E. Neistadt & E. B. Crepeau (Eds.), *Willard and Spackman's occupational therapy* (9th ed., pp. 536-542). New York, NY: Lippincott-Raven.

Stewart, D., Lette, L., Law, L., Acheson Cooper, B., Strong, S., & Rigby, P. J. (2003). The person-environment-occupation model. In E. B. Crepeau, E. S. Cohn, & B. A. Boyt Schell (Eds.), *Willard and Spackman's occupational therapy* (10th ed., pp. 227-234). Philadelphia, PA: Lippincott, Williams & Wilkins.

Tabbarah, M., Silverstein, M., & Seeman, T. (2000). A health and demographic profile of non-institutionalized older Americans residing in environments with home modifications. *Journal of Aging and Health, 12*(2), 204-228.

Tamaru, A., McColl, M. A., & Yamasaki, S. (2007). Understanding "independence": Perspectives of occupational therapists. *Disability and Rehabilitation, 29*(13), 1021-1033.

Turpin, M. (in press). Occupational performance and adaptation models. In M. Turpin & M. Iwama (Eds.), *Using occupational therapy models in practice: A fieldguide*. Oxford, UK: Elsevier.

Uniform Data System for Medical Rehabilitation. (1997). *Functional independence measure* (Version 5.1). Buffalo, NY: Buffalo General Hospital, State University of New York.

Weinstock-Zlotnick, G., & Hinjosa, J. (2004). Bottom-up or top-down evaluation: Is one better than the other? *American Journal of Occupational Therapy, 58*(5), 594-599.

World Health Organization. (1980). *The international classification of impairments, disabilities and handicaps* (ICIDH). Geneva, Switzerland: Author.

World Health Organization. (2001). *International classification of function, disability and health*. Geneva, Switzerland: Author.

Legislation, Regulations, Codes, and Standards Influencing Home Modification Practice

4

Elizabeth Ainsworth, MOccThy, Grad Cert Health Sci;
Desleigh de Jonge, MPhil (OccThy), Grad Cert Soc Sci;
and Jon Sanford, M Arch, BS

This chapter provides an overview of the international legislative framework relevant to promoting the rights of people with a disability through access to the built environment. Human rights and disability discrimination legislation has shaped community values, design and building practice, and service delivery to ensure that people with disabilities are afforded equitable access within the community. In particular, the building regulations, codes, and standards that incorporate access and mobility requirements have sought to address discrimination that might occur because of barriers in public facilities and spaces. Although these regulations have focused primarily on public facilities, they are not without impact on housing. Legislation relating to the design of accessible housing is emerging. With an enhanced understanding of the relevance and application of client rights and building legislation, occupational therapists will be better equipped to promote the inclusion of people with disabilities into everyday life and to empower them to claim their rightful place in society.

CHAPTER OBJECTIVES

By the end of this chapter, the reader will be able to:

+ Describe the development of international human rights and the implications for people with disabilities

+ Discuss disability discrimination and building legislation and their impact on the design of public and private built environments

+ Understand the relevance and application of rights-based legislation and building legislation to the design and modification of the home environment

+ Understand the application of the complaints and remedial processes that are used in relation to rights-based legislation and building legislation

INTERNATIONAL LEGISLATIVE FRAMEWORK

Integrating people with disabilities into the community and enabling them to live in homes they can call their own requires an understanding of the international rights-based legislation that has evolved over time. While people with disabilities were once seen as being dependent on welfare, social assistance, or charity, they are now regarded primarily as citizens with equal rights and obligations. The following discussion briefly describes recent changes

Ainsworth, E., & de Jonge, D.
An Occupational Therapists's Guide to Home Modification Practice (pp. 49-66)
© 2011 SLACK Incorporated

in the definition and models of disability, how these have influenced the development of legislation, and service delivery to people with disabilities.

Definition of Disability

The definition of disability has changed significantly in recent decades. Prior to the end of the 20th century, disability was defined using a medical model that attributed disability to health conditions. Disability was seen as a problem within the person, a result of an individual's physical or mental limitations. A traditional definition of disability, widely promulgated by the World Health Organization (WHO), described disability as "any restriction or inability resulting from a disturbance or loss of bodily or mental function associated with disease, disorder, injury, or trauma, or other health-related state" (WHO, 1980, p. 143).

In the last decade of the 20th century, a number of new models of disability began to emerge based on Nagi's work (1965, 1976) that defined disability as the outcome of an interaction between impairment and environmental factors (Institute of Medicine [IOM], 1991, 1997; National Center for Medical Rehabilitation Research, 1993). Though social models of disability differed slightly on the relationship among medical conditions, impairments, functional limitations, and the effects of the interaction of the person with the environment, they generally agreed that disability was a function of the interaction of the person with the environment (Brandt & Pope, 1997). Social models of disability continued to develop and evolve as people with disabilities, their advocates, and organizations supporting them sought to use these to stimulate change in society (Office of the United Nations High Commissioner for Human Rights, 2006; Swain, 2004).

As a result, WHO (2001) has adopted a social definition of disability. The new *International Classification of Functioning Disability and Health* (ICF) not only defines disability as the interaction of body function and structure with contextual (that is, environmental and personal) factors but has extended it to include the activity and participation outcomes that result from this interaction. The environment is viewed as either a barrier or facilitator to activities and participation in social roles (WHO). Simply put, for an individual with an impairment (e.g., cannot ambulate), the typical home environment (e.g., stairs) can pose barriers to everyday activity (for example, getting in and out of the house) and participation in social roles (e.g., neighbor interaction), whereas home modifications (e.g., ramp) can facilitate those outcomes.

Importance of Social Models of Disability

Social models of disability have encouraged a shift in focus, from flaws or deficits in the individual—as described in the medical model or individual model of disability—to activity restrictions or barriers created by a society that excludes people from participating in everyday life in the community (Harrison & Davis, 2001; Oliver, 1990, 1996). These models describe disability as a complex phenomenon created, in part, by features of the physical, economic, and political environment and not simply a manifestation of a person's impairment (Australian Institute of Health and Welfare, 2003; Dickson, 2007; Harrison & Davis; Samaha, 2007). The environment is seen to facilitate participation that enables the fulfillment of roles appropriate to age, gender, and social and cultural identity. Alternatively, it can contribute to isolation, limiting achievement of daily activities and restricting participation in social, cultural, and community activities (WHO, 2001).

The social models of disability provide frameworks for the formulation of appropriate recommendations to create reasonable and necessary environments that provide appropriate access for people with a disability (Kornblau, Shamberg, & Kein, 2000). It challenges occupational therapists to reconsider their individualistic and medical approaches to occupational performance problems and encourages them to identify and eliminate social and environmental barriers to performance and participation (Whalley Hammell, 2001).

Though social models of disability have facilitated a shift from focusing on individual deficits to examining disabling environments and practices, they are under increasing scrutiny. Like the medical model and other theorizations of disability, these models by no means provide a comprehensive description of the experience of disability and are reductionist in nature (Imrie, 1996). In particular, social models have a tendency to ignore how impairment, in and of itself, has the potential to debilitate—regardless of the environmental and social conditions (Imrie & Hall, 2001a; Shakespeare & Watson, 2001).

Although it is undeniable that environments and social practices can alienate and disable people, addressing these issues alone might not eliminate the difficulties people with impairments experience (Shakespeare & Watson, 2001). Further, environmental design and social manipulations cannot always prevent the personal experience of physical and intellectual restrictions (Imrie & Hall, 2001a). It is therefore important to take appropriate action to address impairment in conjunction with removing environmental barriers and disabling practices (Shakespeare & Watson). Whatever model of disability is used, it is critical that all of the dimensions of the person's experiences are considered, including those of a physical, psychological, cultural, social, and political nature, rather than simplifying disability and operating within a medical or social model (Shakespeare & Erickson, 2000).

DISABILITY LEGISLATION

The social models of disability, with their recognition of the environment's influence on the experience of disability, have led to worldwide legislation aimed at protecting the rights of people with disabilities. The creation of a variety of international declarations and national legislative acts protects the human rights and civil rights of people with disabilities throughout the world (Hurst, 2004).

Human Rights Protections

Human rights are those rights that are inherent in an individual's humanity. They sit above human-made laws and exist whether there are national laws to uphold them or not (Hurst, 2004). The universal establishment of human rights is regarded as the single most important political development influencing social change.

The rights of people with disabilities have been the subject of much attention in the United Nations (UN; Office of the United Nations High Commissioner for Human Rights, 2006). Through the creation of various declarations, rules, and conventions, people with disabilities are now recognized as legitimate citizens in society. The first indicators of international concern regarding the rights of people with disabilities were described in the *UN Declaration on the Rights of Mentally Retarded Persons* (1971) and in the *UN Declaration on the Rights of Disabled Persons* (1975). Although these declarations did not detail the monitoring mechanisms or the reporting obligations of the international community, they served as the framework for human rights protections for people with disabilities worldwide. As a result, they are regarded as the most important milestones in the development of equal rights for people with disabilities (Imrie & Hall, 2001a).

The 1975 *UN Declaration on the Rights of Disabled Persons* clearly called for national and international action to protect the rights of individuals with disabilities. It specifically stated that

Disabled persons have the right to live with their families or with their foster parents and to participate in social, creative or recreation activities. No disabled person shall be subjected, as far as his or her residence is concerned, to differential treatment other than that required by his or her condition or by the improvement which he or she may derive there from. If the stay of a disabled person in a specialized establishment is indispensable, the environment and living conditions therein shall be as close as possible to those of the normal life of a person of his or her age (UN, 1975).

In the following decades, the UN, through various activities, continued to promote human rights for people with disabilities. The UN General Assembly proclaimed 1981 the International Year of the Disabled. In 1982, the General Assembly adopted the World Program of Action Concerning Disabled Persons, which established a world strategy to promote equality and full participation by people with disabilities in social life and development. In 1983, the UN declared the ensuing 10 years to be the UN Decade of Disabled Persons (1983-1992).

Because of the experience gained during the Decade of Disabled Persons, the UN adopted a resolution entitled *Standard Rules on the Equalization of Opportunities for People With Disabilities* in 1993. The purpose of the resolution was to ensure that people with disabilities could exercise the same rights and have the same obligations as others (Degener & Quinn, 2000; Mooney Cotter, 2007). It established broad principles to guide nation states in developing domestic antidiscrimination and equal opportunities legislation (Imrie & Hall, 2001a).

While the *Standard Rules on the Equalization of Opportunities for People With Disabilities* are considered to be the key moral imperative for change on a worldwide basis (Degener & Quinn, 2000), they were, nonetheless, nonbinding. As a result, disability rights activists and scholars have pressed for the adoption of a new worldwide convention on the elimination of discrimination against people with disabilities (Degener & Quinn). In response, the UN Convention on the Rights of Persons with Disabilities and its Optional Protocol were adopted on December 13, 2006, at the UN headquarters in New York and were opened for signature and ratification on March 30, 2007. The convention is considered the first comprehensive human rights treaty of the 21st century (UN, 2008).

The convention marks a "paradigm shift" in attitudes and approaches to people with disabilities—moving them from being viewed as "objects" of charity requiring medical treatment and social protection to "subjects" with rights, who are capable of claiming those rights (UN, 2008). Further, the convention emphasizes that people with disabilities can make decisions about their lives based on their free and informed consent as well as being full and active members of society (UN). Unlike the *Declaration on the Rights of Mentally Retarded Persons* (1971) and the *Declaration on the Rights of Disabled Persons* (1975), the convention boldly sets out a plan of action for countries to enact laws and take other measures to improve disability rights and to eliminate legislation, customs, and practices that discriminate against people with disabilities.

The UN declarations have also highlighted the rights of people with disabilities to have access to the physical environment. The move to incorporate accessibility requirements into the various declarations, rules, and conventions is considered one mechanism by which people's citizenship can become a tangible outcome. The most recent UN Convention on the Rights of People with Disabilities (2008) details specific requirements with respect to accessibility to the built environment. However, it does not describe what accessibility should look like or how it should be created, leaving it up to the various nations that sign and ratify the convention to detail specifications and develop mechanisms for implementation and monitoring compliance. As a result, there continues to be a great deal of political diversity and complexity in providing appropriate access, conditioned by country-specific social, institutional, and political attitudes and values (Imrie & Hall, 2001a). Some countries have legislation in place to ensure there is appropriate access to public buildings; however, the convention does not stipulate how nations should meet their responsibilities in terms of access to adequate housing. Further work is needed at an international level to ensure that well-designed housing is available for people with disabilities (Imrie & Hall, 2001b). Nations might use a range of strategies, including the following:

+ Building publicly funded housing and accommodation programs

+ Ensuring building regulation and certification through national, state, or local government programs

+ Enforcing antidiscrimination laws

+ Introducing industry incentives

+ Providing education and awareness training (Ozdowski, 2005)

Disability Discrimination Legislation and Civil Rights

Though changes to the built environment go some way to providing people with disabilities access to facilities and services in the community, they cannot fully eradicate misconceptions and disablist attitudes in society. Such values and structures are better influenced through the pursuit of civil rights for people (Imrie, 1996). One of the basic human rights is freedom from discrimination, and antidiscrimination legislation ensures that this right, through civil rights laws—or others, such as social welfare laws, constitutional laws, or criminal laws—can be enforced (Hurst, 2004).

Historically, people with disabilities have been excluded from, or marginalized in, the community through discrimination. Disability discrimination means treating a person with a disability less favorably, for a reason related to that person's disability, without justification (Hendricks, 1995; Williams & Levy, 2006). To ameliorate disability discrimination, many countries have enacted legislation to mandate that people with disabilities be afforded the right to fully participate in all aspects of society. Although many countries have some form of disability discrimination legislation, the enforcement method, strength, and effectiveness of this legislation varies considerably (Gleeson, 2001). In an analysis of international disability discrimination legislation, Degener and Quinn (2000) identified that the scope of the terminology and definitions differs substantially between countries. They identified that some of the most comprehensive disability discrimination laws exist in Australia, Canada, Hong Kong, the Philippines, the United Kingdom, and the United States. Their analysis included employment, provision of goods and services, and transport. Additional areas specified included housing (Canada and Australia), education (United States and Australia), land possession (Australia), access to premises (Canada, United Kingdom, and Australia), and telecommunications (United States and Australia).

The strength of disability rights legislation can be attributed to different forces in different countries. In the United States, the empowerment and influence of disability advocacy groups, such as Vietnam veterans returning from war championing the need for change (Barnes, Mercer, & Shakespeare, 1999), was instrumental in moving welfare reform toward civil rights law (Degener & Quinn, 2000; Waddington & Diller, 2007). In the United Kingdom, civil rights laws focused less on individual rights and more on the achievement of social-policy gains (Gleeson, 2001). Because there is no written constitution in

Britain, the rights-based advocacy model, Gleeson points out, has not been adopted. Whereas the widespread politicization of people with disabilities and an advocacy group approach has been used successfully in the United States to bring about legislative change, other countries, such as the United Kingdom where various disability groups have not been as unified and effective in influencing change (Imrie, 1996), have relied on charities to drive the process (Gleeson). In contrast, Australia and New Zealand have secured improved civil rights and social structural change, largely through initiatives in state-government policy regimes (Gleeson).

The United States was one of the first countries to adopt antidiscrimination legislation and civil rights laws, starting with scattered equality provisions in various laws (Degener & Quinn, 2000). Legislation within the United States began with general civil rights legislation in 1964. This seminal piece of legislation did not specifically target people with disabilities, but instead served as the basis for a series of disability-specific laws that covered both U.S. federal government and the country as a whole (Fletcher, 2004; Peterson, 1998). The push for civil rights legislation in the U.S. continued with the development of more comprehensive laws, such as the Americans with Disabilities Act (ADA) in the 1990s. Table 4-1 outlines the history of the development of U.S. legislation, regulations, and standards.

The ADA (1990) represents not only the centerpiece of U.S. civil rights legislation related to people with disabilities, it is also a landmark piece of legislation throughout the world. The intent of this legislation is to ensure that people with a disability equal opportunity, full participation, independent living, and economic self-sufficiency, and it is considerably more extensive in its coverage than other U.S. legislation (Department of Employment, Education, Training, and Youth Affairs, 1997). Not only does it give people with disabilities the same protection as other groups, it also seeks to integrate people with disabilities into the social mainstream and to break down barriers created by prejudice (Waddington & Diller, 2007). The ADA requires planners to consider access as being more than a technical or design issue and to understand its role in social injustice (Imrie, 1996). As rights-based legislation, it has heightened society's awareness of the built environment and the part it has played, and continues to play, in isolating and alienating people with disabilities (Imrie). Further, it has increased the visibility of people with disabilities in society; it has provided them with legal and often moral means of influence; and it has transformed some aspects of service provision for people with disabilities (Imrie & Hall, 2001a).

TRANSLATING LEGISLATION INTO REGULATIONS

In the United States, when Congress passes a piece of legislation, it becomes a law. Laws dictating social policy alone, such as the ADA (1990), are generally insufficient to achieve accessibility. Consequently, building laws and state legislation that allow states to enforce building codes (including accessibility provisions) have also been promulgated to protect the rights of individuals with disabilities. There are also design guidelines to assist developers to fulfill the requirements of these laws. These guidelines then serve as the basis for nominating the standards that detail the technical information. Figure 4-1 illustrates the relationship between laws, guidelines, and standards.

The ADA is a comprehensive but complex law and is considered to have a "patchwork quilt" of regulations associated with it (Ostroff, 2001). For example, the Architectural Barriers Act (ABA) of 1968 was initially developed to ensure access to facilities designed, built, altered, or leased with federal funds. This law was one of the first efforts to ensure access to the built environment; although, unlike the ADA, it did not have its basis in equal rights.

Under the ABA and ADA, the Access Board develops and maintains accessibility guidelines. These guidelines specify minimum or baseline design criteria for regulations and standards to fulfill the requirements of these laws, but they are not enforceable unless a recognized agency adopts them as regulations. Prior to 2004, the ADA and ABA had separate guidelines. For example, the *Minimum Guidelines and Requirements for Accessible Design* (MGRAD; Architectural and Transportation Barriers Compliance Board, 1981) was first issued in 1982 as the accessibility guidelines for the ABA. Similarly, the *Americans with Disabilities Act Accessibility Guidelines* (ADAAG, 1991) was developed by the Access Board to support civil rights legislation (ADA) by addressing accessibility to all public facilities, regardless of whether they receive federal funding (Nishita, Liebig, Pynoos, Perelman, & Spegal, 2007). These were periodically revised and, in 2004, were combined to form a uniform set of guidelines— the *ADA-ABA Accessibility Guidelines*—to cover both acts and to be more compatible with the American National Standards Institute (ANSI) A117.1 (2003), the model accessibility code that is referenced in most U.S. building codes. By 2009, all federal agencies, with the exception of the Department of Housing and Urban Development, had adopted the ADA-ABA Accessibility Guidelines as mandatory to

Table 4-1. Developments in United States Legislation, Standards, and Design Documentation

LEGISLATION	*STANDARDS AND DESIGN DOCUMENTATION*
1964—Civil Rights Act **1966**—30 states pass the accessibility legislation to use A117.1 **1968**—NCABRH report—Design for All Americans—establishes groundwork for future accessibility legislation **1968**—Architectural Barriers Act (ABA) (Public Law 90-480)—those buildings and facilities designed, constructed, altered, or leased with federal funds required to be fully accessible	**1961**—ANSI A117.1 Making Buildings Accessible For and Usable by the Physically Handicapped (American National Standards Institute)—voluntary access standards unless adopted by state or local governments **1965**—Formation of the National Commission on Architectural Barriers to Rehabilitation of the Handicapped (NCABRH)
1973—49 states pass accessibility legislation to use ANSI A117.1 **1973**—Rehabilitation Act **1978**—Rehabilitation Act amended—authorizes the Access Board to establish minimum accessibility guidelines under the ABA and to ensure compliance with requirements.	**1973**—Access Board created under Section 504 of the Rehabilitation Act 1973
1988—Fair Housing Amendments Act—expands the coverage of the Civil Rights Act **1968** to cover families with children and people with disabilities; access required for multifamily dwellings consisting of four or more units both public and private	**1980**—ANSI A117.1 revision **1982**—*Minimum Guidelines and Requirements for Accessible Design* (MGRAD)—Architectural and Transportation Barriers Compliance Board issues minimum guidelines under the ABA that form the basis for enforceable standards **1984**—Uniform Federal Accessibility Standards (UFAS)—Four federal agencies jointly adopt standards to enforce the ABA, based on MGRAD and cover newly constructed or renovated buildings built with federal funding, including public housing **1986**—ANSI A117.1 revision
1990—Americans with Disabilities Act (Public Law 101-336)—extends civil rights protection to people with disabilities; prohibits discrimination in the full and equal enjoyment of goods, services, facilities, privileges, advantages, or accommodations of any place of public accommodation (Title III) and state or local government (Title II). New building construction and alterations to be accessible—publicly and privately funded. Access requirements applicable to common areas; multiunit accommodation.	**1991**—*Americans With Disabilities Act Accessibility Guidelines* (ADAAG)—covers access in new construction and alterations to places of public accommodation and commercial facilities covered by the ADA; also applicable to state and local government facilities. Guideline serves as the baseline of standards used to enforce the ADA; the Access Board issued supplements to ADAAG covering state and local government facilities (1998), children's environments (1998), play areas (2000), and recreation facilities (2002). **1991**—*Fair Housing Accessibility Guidelines* (FHAG) (Housing and Urban Development)—guides design requirements for multifamily housing. **1992**—CABO/ANSI A117.1 revision **1998**—CABO/ANSI A117.1 revision **2003**—ICC/ANSI A117.1 revision **2004**—*Americans With Disability Act and Architectural Barriers Act Accessibility Guidelines* (ADA/ABA Guidelines)—the Access Board jointly updates its guidelines under the ADA and ABA to make them more consistent. Enforcing agencies under the ADA and ABA adopt new standards based on these updated guidelines.

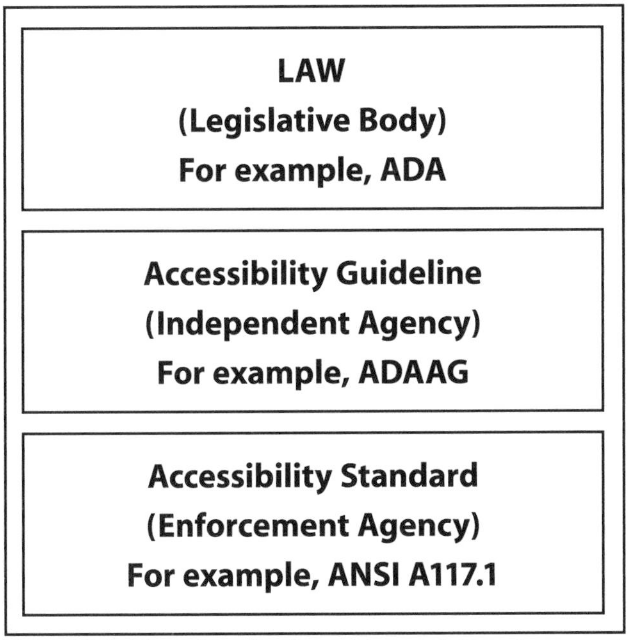

Figure 4-1. Hierarchy of enforceable regulations to support legislation.

ensure building accessibility in the public and private sectors.

Guidelines developed to reinforce the ADA and ABA serve as a baseline for the development of standards. Standards provide the technical information required to make spaces or elements accessible. This includes detailing specifications, such as dimensions, materials, and slope or gradient requirements (Bowen, 2009). In 1984, the Uniform Federal Accessibility Standards (UFAS, 1988) was developed to enforce the ABA and Section 504 of the Rehabilitation Act (1973) for buildings constructed with federal funding, including public housing. UFAS was the result of combining accessibility standards developed by four separate federal agencies to comply with the Architectural and Transportation Barriers Compliance Board's MGRAD (1981). Similarly, in 1994, the ADA standards were developed by the Department of Justice to enforce the ADA legislation and to ensure equal access in and out of commercial buildings and places of accommodation. The ADA standards have their basis in the ADAAG developed by the Access Board.

Recently, the Access Board has combined both the ADA and ABA Guidelines into one unified set of guidelines (ADA-ABA Guidelines, 2004). By 2009, some of the federal agencies vested with enforcing the ABA adopted the new ADA-ABA guidelines. However, by 2009, neither enforcing authority for the ADA had adopted the new version of the ADAAG as *ADA Accessibility Standards*. As a result, the new guidelines are not mandatory unless adopted by

these authorities. Because federal laws (ADA) and regulations take precedence over state and local laws and regulations, state/local laws/regulations have to meet the minimum requirements of the federal laws, although they can specify higher standards (Rogerson, 2005).

There is a complex array of legislation covering various building types in the United States. For example, building works addressed by various pieces of legislation include the following:

+ Construction or alteration of state and local government and commercial facilities (ADA)

+ Access to buildings constructed, leased, or funded by the federal government (ABA)

+ Access to public spaces in multifamily housing (ADA)

+ Construction or renovation of public housing (Rehab Act)

+ Construction or modifications to federally funded, designed, leased, or altered accommodation (ADA)

+ Construction and modifications to multifamily housing through specific housing legislation (Fair Housing Amendments Act, FHAA)

Each of these laws has associated guidelines and standards that address design requirements of the specific facilities covered by the legislation (Table 4-2).

IMPLEMENTING AND MONITORING ACCESS REQUIREMENTS

There are various mechanisms for implementing and monitoring compliance with legislation and building regulations. As discussed in the previous section, the design of guidelines and standards is fundamental to ensuring building and facilities allow equitable access. These standards and guidelines assist designers, developers, and builders in the design and building of accessible facilities. Building on the requirement of Section 504 of the 1973 Rehabilitation Act, the ADA requires that government entities receiving federal funds ensure access to all new facilities and develop plans to correct deficiencies in existing facilities. To promote accessibility, there is training in ADA requirements, design guidelines and standards, and technical assistance via toll-free hotlines and publications (Ostroff, 2001). To check compliance, builders can undertake activities, including engaging experts to review plans, changing contract documents with design and

Table 4-2. Types of Facilities Addressed by Various Laws, Guidelines, and Standards

LAW	GUIDELINES	STANDARD	TYPE OF FACILITIES
ADA (civil law)	1991—ADAAG 2004—ADA-ABA Guidelines	1992,1998, 2003—ANSI A117.1	Construction or alteration of facilities in both public (state and local government facilities) and private (places of public accommodation and commercial facilities) sectors, including places of public accommodation and commercial, state, and local government buildings and public spaces within multifamily housing
ABA (building law)	1981—MGRAD	1988—UFAS	All buildings constructed by or on behalf of the US leased by the federal government or financed by federal dollars
504 Rehab Act (civil law)		UFAS	New construction or renovation to a building using assistance from the federal government, including public housing
Fair Housing Act 1968 (building law)	1991—Fair Housing Accessibility Guidelines (FHAG)	ANSI A117.1	Sale, rental, and financing of private and public housing as well as the physical design of multifamily housing—four units or more or as few as two attached units that are not owner-occupied
Fair Housing Amendments Act 1988 (building law)	1991—Fair Housing Accessibility Guidelines (FHAG)	ANSI A117.1	Residential structures of four or more units. Newly constructed multifamily dwelling units
Visitability (selected states)			Private single-family residences (NEW)

construction firms to ensure proper responsibility, and completing construction site inspections and post-construction inspections.

In most countries, the two main ways authorities can monitor compliance are through preconstruction approval and a postconstruction complaints-based process. Preconstruction approval requires that plans are submitted to an authority for endorsement (the issuance of a building permit that allows construction to take place) before building can commence (Richard Duncan, personal communication, July 23, 2009). This ensures that the design complies with local or state building codes (not necessarily civil rights laws) prior to construction. A postconstruction complaints-based process, which generally follows compliance with the provisions of the civil rights laws and their guidelines, allows complaints about a facility's inaccessibility to be filed with a suitable authority once the problems have been identified. Enforcing disability discrimination law is often the task of public administrative agencies and the courts (Degener & Quinn, 2000), though complaints and lawsuits can be brought by private individuals, groups, and other private entities.

Some countries, such as Australia, have a national building code that requires all new public facilities and major renovations to comply with referenced access standards. This code mandates that plans be endorsed as complying with accessibility requirements prior to construction. Such a process ensures that all public buildings meet essential accessibility requirements and that the design and building industry is clear about their responsibility to provide accessibility. This requirement also reduces the likelihood of a postconstruction complaint relating to discrimination; however, it does not preclude it. The disability discrimination legislation is used to deal with postconstruction-based complaints.

Disability discrimination legislation takes precedence over building codes and regulations and provides broader mandates for inclusion than building codes and standards; lawsuits involving accessibility issues are usually based on human or civil rights legislation (Ringaert, 2003). A building might be built according to a building code and/or standard, but if it excludes a targeted user or protected class of people, certain entities could sue because human or civil rights legislation would indicate that a person could not be discriminated against in the built environment on the basis of that person having a disability (Ringaert).

In the United States, there are no preconstruction approval processes for ADA compliance; rather, the ADA is enforced after construction when a complaint is filed. Individuals who believe they have been discriminated against may file a complaint with the relevant federal agency or federal court (Disability Rights Education and Defense Fund, 2008). Enforcement agencies encourage informal mediation and voluntary compliance (Disability Rights Education and Defense Fund). Yee and Golden (2007) describe enforcement of the law as playing a large role in the ADA's success in raising public awareness of the rights of people with disabilities. The Disability Rights Section of the Civil Rights Division of the U.S. Department of Justice is given the lead federal role in enforcing the legislation; and they investigate complaints lodged by the public, undertake periodic compliance reviews, and bring civil enforcement action (Mooney Cotter, 2007; Yee & Golden). However, the Department of Justice is authorized to bring a lawsuit where there is a pattern or practice of discrimination in violation of the legislation (Mooney Cotter). In enacting the ADA, Congress encouraged the use of alternative means of dispute resolution, including mediation, to resolve disputes. The ADA mediation program was established in 1994. If mediation is unsuccessful, the various parties can pursue all legal remedies provided under the legislation, including private lawsuits (Mooney Cotter).

Under the provisions of the ADA, existing structures that have been built prior to the ADA's enactment also need to have accessibility improvements when possible. In the United States, barriers have to be removed only when it is readily achievable or structurally practicable. Readily achievable means that the changes are easily accomplished and can be carried out with little difficulty or expense. Examples include the simple ramping of a few steps or the installation of grab bars where only routine reinforcement of the wall is required. In determining whether an action to make a public accommodation accessible would be readily achievable, the overall size and cost of the proposed changes to the development are considered. Full compliance is considered structurally impracticable only in those circumstances where the incorporation of accessibility features.

In the United Kingdom, the Disability Discrimination Act (DDA) of 1995 (Equality and Human Rights Commission, 1995) is a civil law that gives an individual the right to take action against an organization if the person with a disability feels that he or she has been discriminated against on the basis

of disability. Unlike other countries, the DDA gives only general guidance as to what might be required to fully meet the requirements of the act and has no specific compliance document. As a result, it also allows the requirements of the DDA to alter in line with changes in national best practice guidelines with regard to disability.

In the United Kingdom, the Commission for Equality and Human Rights has a role to eliminate discrimination against people with disabilities and to promote equality of opportunity (Sawyer & Bright, 2007). It advises the government on the working of disability legislation, sponsors test cases with a view to establishing case law, and writes codes of practice relating to the legislation (Sawyer & Bright). The Commission for Equality and Human Rights sponsors an independent conciliation service to enable disputes to be settled without the need for recourse in courts (Sawyer & Bright). To assist potential claimants to decide whether to bring a claim, there is a question-and-reply procedure that sets out a framework to raise questions and obtain information from service providers (Williams, 2005). In England and Wales, people can bring civil proceedings to a county court. They can seek an application from a county court and have up to 6 months from the time they have been discriminated against in which to submit their claim. If the claim is small (less than £5000), proceedings take place without a solicitor, and a fee is payable. In Scotland, there are three types of court action, depending on the amount to be claimed. There are various guidelines relating to the fees payable, the process to be used, and whether it is appropriate to use a lawyer.

The DDA in the United Kingdom is considered by some to be more progressive in some areas than the ADA; it has introduced a wide range of regulations to ensure accessibility and that reasonable adjustments are made (Imrie & Hall, 2001b). New design and planning benchmarks are emerging (Gooding, 1996; Imrie & Hall). Access auditing of public premises has also increased over time, and businesses are questioning the implications of the DDA for their service (Gooding; Imrie & Hall).

In Australia, access to the built environment is monitored through the DDA (1992) through a postconstruction complaints-based process. The DDA requires that action plans be developed by the operators or owners of the public premises and lodged with the Human Rights and Equal Opportunities Commission to ensure that complaints are not submitted postconstruction. The Australian DDA recognizes that equitable access for people with disabilities could cause unjustifiable hardship for the owner or operator of the premises. The DDA does not require that access be provided in the built environment if it would impose unjustifiable hardship on the person who would have to provide the equitable access. The Federal Court or Federal Magistrates Service determines what constitutes unjustifiable hardship. Issues considered in the claims of unjustifiable hardship can include cost to the proprietor; technical limits; topographical restrictions; the positive and negative effect on other people; safety, design, and construction issues; and the benefit for people with disabilities.

The Canadian Charter of Rights and Freedoms with the federal and provincial human rights legislation is a different approach to the complaints-based human rights approach followed in Australia and the United States (Department of Employment, Education, Training, and Youth Affairs, 1997). The Canadian Human Rights Act (1985) emphasizes the need to accommodate people with disabilities unless doing so causes undue hardship (Mallory Hill & Everton, 2001). Case law has shown that upholding this accommodation is a right and not a privilege (Mallory Hill & Everton). Undue hardship is measured against health, safety, and cost (Mallory Hill & Everton). The Canadian Human Rights Commission is responsible for human rights issues and their application at the federal level. Separate provincial and territorial human rights commissions are responsible for enacting the provisions of the Human Rights Code within each province and municipality (Mallory Hill & Everton).

Private Housing Legislation

Similar legislative and regulatory mechanisms exist in the residential sector, although there are few accessibility regulations that cover residential facilities and even fewer that comprehensively regulate the design and modification of private housing specifically for people who are older or who have disabilities (Hyde, Talbert, & Grayson, 1997). Nonetheless, there is a growing movement in some countries to extend accessibility regulations to private housing. A number of countries have adopted disability discrimination legislation, which has proven useful in situations where complaints have been made by people with disabilities who have not been able to access the common areas of multifamily complexes. Countries such as Canada, which has specifically omitted residential design and construction from national legislation, have left residential accessibility up to local jurisdictions (Clarke Scott, Nowlan, & Gutman, 2001; Mallory Hill & Everton, 2001; Rogerson, 2005). The United States is one of the few countries in the world with civil rights legislation that covers private (multifamily) housing (Starr, 2005). Further, the ABA and the Rehabilitation Act (1973) require a small percentage (5%) of housing constructed with public funds to have accessible dwelling units, and these are generally made available only to people who are eligible for publicly funded housing (Maisel, Smith, & Steinfeld, 2008).

Specifically, in the United States, the Fair Housing Act (FHA), originally passed as Title VIII of the Civil Rights Act of 1964, prohibits discrimination in the sale, rental, and financing of private and public housing as well as the physical design of newly constructed multifamily housing based on race, color, religion, gender, or national origin (FHA, 1968). Title VIII was amended in 1988 by the Fair Housing Amendments Act (FHAA), which expanded the coverage of the act to prohibit discrimination based on disability or family status. The FHAA significantly expanded the scope of the original legislation and strengthened its enforcement mechanisms to cover public and private multifamily housing (accommodation with more than four units; FHAA, 1988). Consequently, under this legislation, property owners are required to allow a tenant with a disability to undertake modifications within certain guidelines to accommodate his or her individual need (Newman & Mezrich, 1997). However, tenants would be required to pay for the alterations, comply with the building codes, and, if requested, return the property to its original condition when they leave (Lawlor & Thomas, 2008).

To reinforce the FHAA (1998), the U.S. Department of Housing and Urban Development (HUD) released technical requirements for multifamily housing in 1991. The FHAG are designed to help builders comply with accessibility requirements as required by the government (International Code Council, 2007). It refers regularly to ANSI A117.1 (2003) and guides developments that may or may not have elevators.

The FHAG cover newly constructed multifamily homes constructed by builders, private property owners, and publicly assisted landlords (Imrie, 2006). Exempt properties include newly constructed townhouses or less than four housing unit complexes and properties constructed in locations with unusual terrain or other site characteristics that limit accessibility (Mooney Cotter, 2007; Newman & Mezrich, 1997; Nishita et al., 2007).

Builders constructing four or more owner-occupied dwelling units in buildings with one elevator or more have to make all units accessible or have to ensure accessibility to ground-floor units only if there is no elevator (Imrie, 2006; Newman & Mezrich, 1997). Accessible design required in newly constructed housing (rather than in existing housing) includes accessible common-use areas—for example, via at least one accessible entrance; doors that are wide enough for wheelchairs to pass through; and kitchens and bathrooms that allow a person using a wheelchair to maneuver. It also includes other adaptable features within the housing—for example, an accessible route to and through the dwelling, light switches, thermostats, and other controls in accessible locations, and reinforcement in bathroom walls for future installation of grab rails (U.S. Department of Justice, 2005). The owner of newly constructed buildings must be an active participant in making the building accessible and usable by people with disabilities compared with the more passive role played by owners of existing properties (Newman & Mezrich).

Under the FHAG, access to public spaces in multifamily housing—for example, exterior spaces, elevators, corridors, and interior common spaces—is mandated by the technical requirements for public spaces in the ADA/ABA Guidelines. If a facility does not comply with these requirements, residents with disabilities can request reasonable modifications to common interior or exterior areas at the property owner's expense (Newman & Mezrich, 1997).

One goal of the FHAA (1988) is to facilitate home modifications in rental housing (Steinfeld, Levine, & Shea, 1998) by providing people with disabilities the right to reasonable accommodation. This means that a landlord cannot prevent a tenant from adding home modifications to a housing unit to increase its accessibility (National Association of Home Builders [NAHB] Research Center, 2007), though these changes must be negotiated. There is a requirement that tenants pay for these modifications themselves and that they use a licensed contractor to complete the work. At the end of their tenancy, they must return the area to its original condition, again at the cost of the tenant who installed the original modifications (NAHB Research Center; Steinfeld et al.). However, there might be modifications made to the interior of the home that do not have to be removed if they do not affect the next tenant's use of the apartment (Steinfeld et al.). The section of the bill that deals with retrofitting existing multiunit dwellings calls for "reasonable accommodation" for people with disabilities, but it is vague on the responsibility of the owner to pay for changes even in the common areas (Pynoos & Nishita, 2006, p. 284).

As previously indicated, federal U.S. law requires access for people with mobility and other impairments to all new multifamily residences and to a small percentage of single family homes constructed with public funds (Maisel et al., 2008). Consequently, current housing policy in the United States does not address the vast majority of single-family homes (as well as duplexes, townhomes, and triplexes) in which most people live (Maisel et al.). As a result,

"visitability" legislation has been developed and implemented in the United States over the past two decades, most of it occurring at state and local levels (Spegal & Liebig, 2003). The visitability movement seeks to increase the supply of housing that people with disabilities can visit or live in for a short term. Design features include the incorporation of a zero-step entrance, wide doorways, and at least a bathroom on the main floor of the home (Maisel et al.).

Visitability programs have also begun to spread throughout the United States, using mandates, incentives, and voluntary-based codes to encourage visitable design to be adopted in new housing. To date, visitability legislation has been created in at least 27 U.S. cities (Maisel et al., 2008). There is little known about the outcomes of these programs because of the following:

+ Not all locations use the term *visitability* in their enactments

+ There is no pattern of organizations accountable for the oversight of the ordinances

+ Agencies responsible for the implementation of the approach are not specified

+ There is no one method of keeping track of how many homes have been built (Spegal & Liebig, 2003)

The extent to which visitability is adopted depends on local municipalities "buying" into the idea and ensuring it is included in local ordinances or building codes. Much of the approach is being adopted unevenly, depending on the political stance of the various states. Visitability is continuing to face opposition because of concerns about cost and consumer perception (Kochera, 2002).

Because of the fragmented adoption of visitability on the state and local level, the visitability movement has inspired the creation of the Inclusive Home Design Act that was first introduced into the U.S. Congress as a bill in 2003, reintroduced in 2005, and then again in 2007 (now known as HR 4202) (Maisel et al., 2008). Although Congress has not yet passed the bill, it has the potential to ensure that single-family homes receiving assistance from the federal government incorporate visitable features (Maisel et al.).

The U.S. Supreme Court Olmstead decision (1999) has also affected accessible housing because it requires states to administer services, programs, and activities for people with disabilities in "integrated" settings (Maisel et al., 2008). The decision has led to more homes being made accessible, with some states using funding from federal grant programs for home modifications for people moving from institutions into the community (Maisel et al.).

IMPLEMENTING AND MONITORING ACCESS REQUIREMENTS

The FHAA (1988) established administrative enforcement mechanisms to enable the HUD attorneys to bring actions before administrative law judges on behalf of people experiencing housing discrimination. HUD has an Office of Program Compliance and a Disability Rights Office of Fair Housing and Equal Opportunity. Complaints filed with HUD are investigated by the Office of Fair Housing and Equal Opportunity (FHEO; Mooney Cotter, 2007). The Department of Justice can take over the role of the department in seeking resolution on behalf of aggrieved people if it proceeds as a civil action (Mooney Cotter).

Similar to disputes in the public sector, disability discrimination legislation also takes precedence over building codes and regulations in residential settings (Ringaert, 2003). Consequently, a building constructed according to a building code and/or standard may still result in a complaint or lawsuit if a person is discriminated against in the built environment based on that person having a disability (Ringaert).

EVALUATION OF CURRENT LEGISLATION AND STANDARDS

The rights-based approach to access policy used in the United States has also been identified as having limitations (Gooding, 1994; Higgins, 1992; Imrie, 1996; Young, 1990). First, this type of approach reinforces the individual conceptualization of disability, emphasizing the problem as belonging to the individual rather than a problem being the norms embedded in society (Higgins; Imrie). Second, it presumes that the current situation that works for the majority is the ideal, and therefore it should be available and acceptable to all (Higgins; Imrie). Third, it is underpinned by a form of legal individualism that ignores or denies the structural inequalities that perpetuate discrimination against people's disabilities (Imrie). The onus remains with the "victim" to establish harm has been done in each situation (Imrie; Young). Rights legislation also attempts to provide equal protection to distinctly unequal groups and does not recognize the potential value of positive discrimination in addressing structural disadvantages (Gooding; Imrie). While legislation can contain overt discrimination, it cannot eradicate it fully (Doyle, 1995; Imrie & Hall, 2001a). Consequently,

the political and economic power of people with disabilities needs to be restored to enable them to influence government and corporate attitudes and practice (Imrie & Hall, 2001b).

There is a great deal of diversity and complexity in the way discrimination and civil rights legislation and building legislation regulations, codes, and standards have been developed, operationalized, and monitored across the world. Consequently, international legislative frameworks have also had varying meaningful impacts on design practice and people with disabilities. For example, the civil status of people with disabilities is markedly different between the United States and the United Kingdom. Despite this difference, there continues to be a struggle for this group in both countries to gain strong and binding antidiscrimination legislation that influences service delivery and the design of the built environment (Imrie, 1996). Access issues in the United States are regarded as matters of social justice, a problem relating to a person's civil liberties (Imrie). In the United Kingdom, the government sees access as a technical or compensatory matter that can be dealt with through redistributive measures (Imrie), and U.K. developers have noted that people with disabilities have limited financial impact on their services and are reticent to build in features that meet their needs (Harrison & Davis, 2001).

Almost all of the countries and territories have not yet made the access requirements of people with disabilities and elderly people an integral part of development plans relating to different features of the built environment (UN, 1995). There are separate approaches to formulating access legislation distinct from existing relevant laws, by-laws, codes, rules, and regulations in countries and territories such as China, the Islamic Republic of Iran, Hong Kong, Japan, the Republic of Korea, and Vietnam (UN). In contrast, Australia, Malaysia, and Singapore adopted an integrated approach in formulating their respective access legislation by incorporating access standards for people with disabilities into relevant existing building regulations (UN).

Another issue is that various pieces of legislation do not address the issues of creating livable and usable living spaces (Imrie & Hall, 2001b). There is evidence of failure to incorporate access considerations in urban and rural development projects and a focus on access to buildings rather than the overall development (Imrie, 2006). While access legislation of Malaysia and Singapore applies to all types of buildings, including domestic buildings, legal instruments of other countries and territories apply to public buildings only (UN, 1995).

The use and enforcement of access law worldwide is inconsistent and uneven within and between regulatory authorities (Centre for Housing Research, 2007; Mazumdar & Geis, 2001; Newman & Mezrich, 1997; Switzer, 2001). There is a perception that there have been inadequate staffing and budgetary resources at various government levels to implement and enforce the legislation (Hinton, 2003; Mazumdar & Geis). Further, there is evidence that there is a high level of ignorance about how and when to use the regulations, particularly among those people who are in roles of enforcement (Barnes, 2007; Centre for Housing Research; Steinfeld et al., 1998). For example, confusion exists in relation to how building regulations interface with disability discrimination legislation, resulting in design responses that are often limited or confused (Imrie & Hall, 2001a). Builders and owners are required to have an understanding of how their buildings meet the broad civil rights requirements of the law and, yet, many have never studied law or civil rights interpretations (Salmen, 2001). There is a view that even when owners understand the law, they might not understand their responsibilities (Steinfeld et al.).

Ambiguities, exemptions, and get-out clauses characterize access statutes, thus diminishing their coverage and effectiveness (Barnes, 2007; Imrie & Hall, 2001a; Milner & Madigan, 2001; Newman & Mezrich, 1997). For example, the ADA has get-out clauses such as "undue hardship," "readily achievable," and "unreasonable financial costs," which can be used to justify not making built environments accessible (Imrie, 1996). This and other legislation have stipulations on reasonable provision of access for people with disabilities that are vague and open to interpretation—that is, there appears to be multiple interpretations of the word *reasonable*, which is used frequently in legislation in this area (Imrie & Hall).

The complaint process relies on people with disabilities contacting the relevant authorities. However, they often do not understand the intent and application of the legislation, regulations, and standards and experience a great deal of difficulty in navigating the complaints system. The complaints process can often be protracted and poorly articulated or promoted. At times, people with disabilities do not have the emotional energy to cope with the process and can fear negative or inadequate responses to their requests, making them feel even more disempowered (Frank, 2005; Newman & Mezrich, 1997). Further, some legal systems, such as those in the United States, are adversarial in nature, influencing people's perceptions of or reactions to the complaint process (Mazumdar & Geis, 2001).

Finally, agencies and groups participating in formulating access legislation has varied greatly between countries (Nielsen & Ambrose, 1998; UN, 1995). Consequently, legislation has tended to form without a comprehensive understanding of the needs of all disabled people (Milner & Madigan, 2001; UN). There is an emphasis on adults in wheelchairs and a focus on the medical conception of disability that is abstract and generalized (Imrie & Hall, 2001a). There is also a generalization of access requirements across groups of people (Imrie & Hall). Building regulations also fail to take account of the diverse and changing needs of people with disabilities (Imrie & Hall). Attitudes toward people with disabilities are still being framed by the concept of the "undeserving poor," or buildings are being designed to provide minimum standards of access (Imrie, 2003). Architects have been described as making accessibility a legal rather than a moral imperative (Mazumdar & Geis, 2001). Consequently, attitudinal and architectural barriers continue to exist that limit the participation of people with disabilities in society (Switzer, 2001).

Private Homes

To support disability rights, civil rights legislation has included provisions for the removal of physical barriers to activity and participation as well as the designation of authorities to enforce those accessibility requirements. As pointed out at the beginning of this chapter, the jurisdiction for these regulations is primarily public facilities. There are few regulations that cover residential facilities and even fewer that comprehensively regulate the design and modification of private housing, specifically for people who are older or who have disabilities (Hyde et al., 1997). Nonetheless, there is a growing movement in some countries to extend accessibility regulations to private housing. In some countries, in the absence of specific legislation, the design guidelines and standards produced for public buildings are often used as a guide when modifying private homes. As explained in the chapter on design standards (Chapter 12), this can be problematic if designers, builders, and occupational therapists are not familiar with the limitations associated with the use of these standards. This can include, for example, the potential mismatch between the functional ability of the person and the responsiveness of the accessible design (Sanford & Megrew, 1999).

Worldwide, approaches to ensuring housing accessibility are continuing to develop. For example, in Europe, housing accessibility has been secured by three main strategies:

1. Mainstreaming, whereby all new dwellings must meet accessibility standards (for example, Denmark, Sweden, Norway, the Netherlands)

2. Exclusive legislation, which is applied to only certain categories of users such as wheelchair users (for example, United Kingdom, Austria, Germany, Portugal, Luxembourg)

3. A progressive approach in which increasing degrees of accessibility and adaptability are stipulated for different building types and users (for example, Italy; Nielsen & Ambrose, 1998)

Although many countries have adopted various requirements for new housing, such as the United States, these requirements are typically intended for new multifamily housing (Kochera, 2002). Countries with multifamily accessibility policies include Italy, the Netherlands, France, Spain, Greece, and Sweden (Kochera). The United Kingdom is an exception to this because the design requirements have been extended to single-family homes (Kochera). This includes providing basic visitability features in all newly constructed residential homes built on or after October 25, 1999, such as single-family homes, regardless of the needs of the occupants (Kochera). While it is easy to provide incentives and regulations for new stock, most older people and people with long-term disabilities live in established housing and cannot readily afford to purchase new dwellings. Following are examples of countries that have building regulations requiring accessibility in private homes (Imrie, 2006):

+ Norway: Building regulations require an accessible entry and external approach to the common entrance of a building that has more than four dwellings; toilets in all new dwellings regardless of whether they are single-family homes or multiunit developments.

+ Sweden: Building regulations state that there must be wheelchair access to all units in a residential building of three stories or more, including an accessible path of travel from the pavement to the building entrance, accessible thresholds, and the provision of a lift (there is no requirement for this in single-family homes).

+ Denmark: Building regulations stipulate that single-family homes that are self-built have to be constructed to minimum levels of accessibility including having a no-step entrance.

+ Australia, Willoughby Council, New South Wales: New developments with more than nine dwellings to incorporate adaptable housing design (AS4299); this is similar for multiunit developments for Waverley and Ryde Councils in New South Wales.

+ Japan: All new housing, both public and private, to be built to universal design standards.

The U.S. approach to accessible housing is poor and underdeveloped. No single U.S. law or program regulates comprehensively for the design and adaptation of housing specifically for people who are older or who have disabilities, although a patchwork of federal programs and mechanisms support the implementation of home modifications (Hyde et al., 1997; Milner & Madigan, 2001). Regulations and design standards typically focus on the needs of wheelchair users with little consideration for the diverse needs of the population of people with disabilities. Little research exists on the changes in wheelchair size and shape and the impact of the introduction of new technology to improve the mobility of the equipment and comfort of the user, let alone the needs of the broader population of people with disabilities whose access needs might differ significantly from the wheelchair user. Inevitably, future adaptations to homes designed specifically for wheelchair users are necessary to ensure better accessibility within the home and to cater to the needs of a broader range of people with disabilities (Imrie, 2006).

A progressive approach, with use of increasing degrees of accessible and adaptable design for different building types and people with disabilities, can ensure housing accessibility. For example, Italy has various laws and ministerial decrees, rather than a building code or building regulations. It stipulates three levels of accessibility: accessible (access to a building, including common areas, through the entry and use spaces within the building safely and independently); visitable (access to the principle spaces within buildings and to where there is at least one accessible toilet); and adaptable design (modification to the built environment at little cost; Christophersen, 2001; D'Innocenzo & Morini, 2001). This progressive approach has developed from the movement to integrate people with disabilities into the community. Details and technical prescriptions have been added gradually to existing regulations over the years, resulting in professionals needing to keep in mind the design requirements of people with disabilities while developing solutions (D'Innocenzo & Morini). Initially, public buildings were introduced to access regulations; now, that has been extended to include public residential buildings and neighborhoods (D'Innocenzo & Morini). Different design approaches for different building types were selected based on the needs and priorities of the neighborhood. People's varying differences have been driving a "policy of differences" for design practice rather than designing to suit "the average man" (D'Innocenzo & Morini, p. 15.20). Though there are gaps in the practice of this progressive design approach in Italy, a strong societal belief that every person has the right to access his or her own house and external built environments has emerged (D'Innocenzo & Morini).

Regulations, incentives, and information have been the three mechanisms used to promote adaptable housing for people of all ages and abilities in Europe (Nielsen & Ambrose, 1998). However, statutes in relation to providing accessible housing vary in form and content and are stronger in social-housing schemes or where the government has significant influence over the construction process (Imrie, 2006). The legal basis for ensuring access to housing is generally ineffectual, with limited means of enforcement (Imrie). Consequently, some view nonlegislative means as the fastest way to improve building practice (Nielsen & Ambrose). There is a perception that regulations increase cost, stifle design creativity and innovation, and decrease responsiveness to the market (Imrie). However, although there is a clear demand for accessible housing, there has been a poor market response. Some believe nonlegislative approaches, such as voluntary guidelines, branding of universal designs, and information campaigns, to be the least successful strategies for encouraging the development of more accessible housing in communities (Centre for Housing Research, 2007). The countries that have been most successful in producing a market response, such as the United States, Japan, and Norway, have systematically combined regulatory, incentive, and collaborative capacity building strategies (Centre for Housing Research). Countries where populations have been growing older faster have had regulations for new housing in place for a considerable length of time (Centre for Housing Research).

IMPLICATIONS FOR OCCUPATIONAL THERAPISTS

Occupational therapy services will continue to be in demand to provide home modification advice as people with disabilities struggle with environments that require design improvements. Therapists understand that people with disabilities constitute a diverse population that does not suit a "one-size-fits-all" design approach. They have an awareness of the limitations of the access standards that are used as the basis for public building and private home design and have an important role in informing builders and developers about the individual design needs of clients.

An understanding of human rights and building legislation will equip therapists with knowledge and information that can be shared with people with disabilities who might need to negotiate with builders and government authorities about inappropriate design solutions in the public and private sectors. Therapists can encourage and empower people with disabilities to advocate for their own needs and provide their perspective on improvements needed during design and planning processes. Occupational therapists are also well suited to influencing the values and perspectives of builders and advocating for better-designed environments within the community by educating builders and designers about the diverse needs of people with disabilities, discussing the implications of designs, and challenging builders and designers to build more universally. Therapists are also well placed to contribute to the evaluation of the effectiveness of various built environments and the impact of the environment on occupational performance, health, safety, independence, quality of life, and home and community participation outcomes. They also hold a professional responsibility to monitor and respond to proposed legislative changes and to support calls for improvements to legislation, guidelines, and standards.

CONCLUSION

This chapter has provided an overview of the international legislative framework relevant to promoting the rights of people with a disability through access to the built environment. There has been information given on the social models of disability, their advantages, and their limitations for people with disabilities.

This chapter has described how human rights and disability discrimination legislation has attempted to shape community values, design and building practice, and service delivery to ensure people with disabilities are afforded equitable access within the community. Information has been provided on the ADA as a landmark piece of legislation in the civil rights struggle for people with disabilities in the United States. In some countries, such as the United Kingdom, building regulations and standards that incorporate access and mobility requirements have sought to address discrimination that might occur from barriers in public facilities and spaces. Very few countries have required their legislation to include mandatory accessible design of private homes.

This chapter has highlighted that the emergence of home environments that do not further disable people is far from being realized. While disability discrimination, civil rights, and building legislation in various countries have influenced the design of public buildings, they have not made private accessible housing available to everyone requiring it, nor have they eliminated attitudinal barriers (Switzer, 2001). Current legislation around the world is not likely to make a dramatic change to the housing circumstances of people with a disability. Rather, significant action is required to transform attitudes and value systems toward people with disabilities to positively influence housing quality and design (Imrie, 2006). Occupational therapists are well qualified and experienced to make a valuable contribution to transforming these attitudes and values. They can influence the values and perspective of builders as they work in collaboration to design a more comprehensive use of dwelling spaces by people with diverse needs. As well, they have a valuable role to advocate for people with disabilities and to empower them to influence design and construction practice in the community.

REFERENCES

American National Standards Institute. (2003). *ICC/ANSI A117.1-2003: Accessible and Usable Buildings and Facilities*. New York, NY: Author.

Americans With Disabilities Act. (1990). ADA Home Page. Retrieved from http://www.usdoj.gov/crt/ada/adahom1.htm

Americans With Disabilities Act Accessibility Guidelines. (1991). ADA accessibility guidelines for buildings and facilities (ADAAG). Retrieved from http://www.access-board.gov/adaag/html/adaag.htm

Americans with Disabilities Act and Architectural Barriers Act Accessibility Guidelines. (2004). ADA and ABA accessibility guidelines for buildings and facilities. Retrieved from http://www.access-board.gov/ada-aba/final.cfm

Architectural Barriers Act. (1968). The Architectural Barriers Act (ABA) of 1968. Retrieved from http://www.access-board.gov/about/laws/aba.htm

Architectural and Transportation Barriers Compliance Board. (1981). Minimum guidelines and requirements for accessible design. *Federal Register, 46*(11), 4270-4304.

Australia Disability Discrimination Act. (1992). Disability Discrimination Act 1992. Retrieved from http://www.dredf.org/international/Ausdda.html

Australian Institute of Health and Welfare. (2003). *Disability: The use of aids and the role of the environment*. Canberra, Australia: Author.

Barnes, C. (2007). Education, citizenship and social justice. Retrieved from http://esj.sagepub.com/cgi/reprint/2/3/203

Barnes, C., Mercer, G., & Shakespeare, T. (1999). *Exploring disability: A sociological introduction*. Cambridge, UK: Polity Press.

Bowen, I. (2009). Access basics: The laws, the regulations, the standards (and where they come from): The Americans With Disabilities Act and Section 504. Retrieved from http://ada-one.com/pdf/AccessBasics.pdf

Brandt, E., & Pope, A. M. (Eds.). (1997). *Enabling America: Assessing the role of rehabilitation science and engineering*. Washington, DC: National Academy Press.

Canadian Human Rights Act. (1985). Canadian Human Rights Act (R.S., 1985, c. H-6). Retrieved from http://laws.justice.gc.ca/en/h-6/index.html

Centre for Housing Research. (2007). *Housing and disability: Future proofing New Zealand's housing stock for an inclusive society*. Prepared by CRESA/Public Policy & Research/Auckland Disability Resource Centre for Centre for Housing Research, Aotearoa, New Zealand, and the Office of Disability Issues.

Christophersen, J. (2001). Accessible housing in five European countries: Standards and built results. In W. F. E. Preiser & E. Ostroff (Eds.), *Universal design handbook* (pp. 13.1-13.14). New York, NY: McGraw Hill.

Civil Rights Act. (1964). Teaching with documents: The Civil Rights Act of 1964 and the Equal Employment Opportunity Commission. Retrieved from http://www.archives.gov/education/lessons/civil-rights-act

Clarke Scott, M. A., Nowlan, S., & Gutman, G. (2001). Progressive housing design and home technologies in Canada. In W. F. E. Preiser & E. Ostroff (Eds.), *Universal design handbook* (pp. 36.1-36.15). New York, NY: McGraw Hill.

Degener, T., & Quinn, G. (2000). A survey of international, comparative and regional disability law reform. Retrieved from http://www.dredf.org/international/degener_quinn.html

Department of Employment, Education, Training, and Youth Affairs. (1997). *Comparison of international provisions on disability discrimination in education*. Canberra, Australia: Author.

Department of Housing and Urban Development. (1991). Fair housing accessibility guidelines. *Federal Register, 56*(44), 9472-9515.

Dickson, E. (2007). *Equality of opportunity for all? An assessment of the effectiveness of the Anti-Discrimination Act 1991 (Queensland) as a tool for the delivery of equality of opportunity in education for people with impairments*. Unpublished thesis. T. C. Beirne School of Law, University of Queensland.

D'Innocenzo, A., & Morini, A. (2001). Accessible design in Italy. In W. F. E. Preiser & E. Ostroff (Eds.), *Universal design handbook* (pp. 15.1-15.23). New York, NY: McGraw Hill.

Disability Rights Education & Defense Fund. (2008). A comparison of ADA, IDEA, and Section 504. Retrieved from http://www.dredf.org/advocacy/comparison.html

Doyle, B. (1995). *Disability, discrimination and equal opportunities: A comparative study of the employment rights of disabled persons*. London, UK: Mansell.

Equality and Human Rights Commission. (1995). *The law about disability discrimination*. Retrieved from http://www.equalityhumanrights.com/your-rights/disability/the-law-about-disability-discrimination

Fair Housing Act. (1968). United Stated Department of Justice Civil Rigths Division: Fair Housing Act. Retrieved from http://www.usdoj.gov/crt/housing/title8.php

Fair Housing Amendments Act. (1988). FHEO programs. Retrieved from http://www.hud.gov/offices/fheo/progdesc/title8.cfm

Fletcher, V. (2004). American access. *Green Places*, February, 24-25.

Frank, J. J. (2005). Barriers to the accommodation request process of the Americans with Disabilities Act. *Journal of Rehabilitation, 71*(2), 28-39.

Gleeson, B. (2001). Disability and the open city. *Urban Studies, 38*(2), 251-265.

Gooding, C. (1994). *Disabling laws, enabling acts*. London, UK: Pluto Press.

Gooding, C. (1996). *Blackstone's guide to the Disability Discrimination Act 1995*. London, UK: Blackstone Press.

Harrison, M., & Davis, C. (2001). *Housing, social policy and difference: Disability, ethnicity, gender and housing*. Bristol, UK: The Policy Press.

Hendricks, A. (1995). The significance of equality and non-discrimination for the protection of the rights and dignity of disabled persons. In T. Degener & Y. Koster-Dreese (Eds.), *Human rights and disabled persons: Essays and relevant human rights instruments* (pp. 40-62). Leiden, the Netherlands: Martinus Nijhoff Publishers.

Higgins, P. C. (1992). *Making disability: Exploring the social transformation of human variation*. Springfield, IL: Thomas.

Hinton, C. A. (2003). The perceptions of people with disabilities as to the effectiveness of the Americans With Disabilities Act. *Journal of Disability Policy Studies, 13*(4), 210-220.

Hurst, R. (2004). Legislation and human rights. In J. Swain, S. French, C. Barnes, & C. Thomas (Eds.), *Disabling barriers—Enabling environments* (pp. 297-230). London, UK: Sage Publications.

Hyde, J., Talbert, R., & Grayson, P. J. (1997). Fostering adaptive housing: An overview of funding sources, laws and policies. In S. Lanspery & J. Hyde (Eds.), *Staying put: Adapting the places instead of the people* (pp. 223-236). Amityville, NY: Baywood Publishing Company Inc.

Imrie, R. (1996). *Disability and the city: International perspectives*. New York, NY: St. Martin's Press.

Imrie, R. (2003). Architects' conceptions of the human body. *Environment and Planning D: Society and Space, 21*, 47-65.

Imrie, R. (2006). *Accessible housing: Quality, disability and design*. London, UK: Routledge Taylor and Francis Group.

Imrie, R., & Hall, P. (2001a). An exploration of disability and the development process. *Urban Studies, 38*(2), 333-350.

Imrie, R., & Hall, P. (2001b). *Inclusive design: Designing and developing accessible environments*. London, UK: Spon Press.

Institute of Medicine. (1991). *Disability in America: A national agenda for prevention* (A. M. Pope & A. R. Tarlov Eds.). Washington, DC: National Academy Press.

Institute of Medicine. (1997). *Enabling America: Assessing the role of rehabilitation science and engineering* (E. N. Brandt & A. M. Pope Eds.). Washington, DC: National Academy Press.

International Code Council. (2007). *Improving the accessibility of buildings for people with disabilities*. Retrieved from http://www.iccsafe.org/safety/Pages/accessibility-1.aspx

Kochera, A. (2002). *Accessibility and visitability features in single family homes: A review of state and local activity*. Retrieved from http://assets.aarp.org/rgcenter/il/2002_03_homes.pdf

Kornblau, B., Shamberg, S., & Kein, R. (2000). Occupational therapy and the Americans With Disabilities Act (ADA). *American Journal of Occupational Therapy, 54*(6), 622-625.

Lawlor, D., & Thomas, M. (2008). *Residential design for ageing in place*. Hoboken, NJ: John Wiley.

Maisel, J. R., Smith, E., & Steinfeld, E. (2008). *Increasing home access: Designing for visitability*. Retrieved from http://assets.aarp.org/rgcenter/il/2008_14_access.pdf.

Mallory Hill, S., & Everton, B. (2001). Accessibility standards and universal design developments in Canada. In W. F. E. Preiser & E. Ostroff (Eds.), *Universal design handbook* (pp. 16.1-16.17). New York, NY: McGraw Hill.

Mazumdar, S., & Geis, G. (2001). Interpreting accessibility standards: Experiences in the US courts. In W. F. E. Preiser & E. Ostroff (Eds.), *Universal design handbook* (pp. 12.1-12.8). New York, NY: McGraw Hill.

Milner, J., & Madigan, R. (2001). The politics of accessible housing in the UK. In S. M. Peace & C. Holland (Eds.), *Inclusive housing in an ageing society: Innovative approaches* (pp. 77-100). Bristol, UK: The Policy Press.

Mooney Cotter, A. (2007). *This ability*. Hampshire, UK: Ashgate Publishing Ltd.

Nagi, S. Z. (1965). Some conceptual issues in disability and rehabilitation. In M. B. Sussman (Ed.), *Sociology and rehabilitation* (pp. 100-113). Washington, DC: American Sociological Association.

Nagi, S. Z. (1976). An epidemiology of disability among adults in the United States. *Milbank Memorial Fund Quarterly, 54*, 439-468.

National Association of Home Builders Research Center. (2007). *Safety first: A technical approach to home modifications: Rebuilding together training workshop student guide*. Upper Marlboro, MD: Author.

National Center for Medical Rehabilitation Research. (1993). *Research plan for the National Center for Medical Rehabilitation Research*. Washington, DC: National Institutes of Health.

National Commission on Architectural Barriers to Rehabilitation of the Handicapped. (1967). *Design for all Americans: A report of the National Commission on Architectural Barriers to Rehabilitation of the Handicapped*. Retrieved from http://www.eric.ed.gov/ERICWebPortal/search/detailmini.jsp?_nfpb=true&_&ERICExtSearch_SearchValue_0=ED026786&ERICExtSearch_SearchType_0=no&accno=ED026786

Newman, S. J., & Mezrich, M. N. (1997). Implications of the 1988 Fair Housing Act for the Frail Elderly. In S. Lanspery & J. Hyde (Eds.), *Staying put: Adapting the places instead of the people* (pp. 237-252). Amityville, NY: Baywood Publishing Company, Inc.

Nielsen, C. W., & Ambrose, I. (1998). *Lifetime adaptable housing in Europe*. Retrieved from https://iospress.metapress.com/content/clcxwwxappgwdhpg/resource-secured/?target=fulltext.pdf

Nishita, C. M., Liebig, P. S., Pynoos, J., Perelman, L., & Spegal, K. (2007). Promoting basic accessibility in the home: Analyzing patterns in the diffusion of visitability legislation. *Journal of Disability Policy Studies, 18*(1), 2-13.

Office of the United Nations High Commissioner for Human Rights. (2006). *Standard rules on the equalization of opportunities for persons with disabilities*. Retrieved from http://www2.ohchr.org/english/law/opportunities.htm

Oliver, M. (1990). *The individual and social models of disability*. Paper presented at Joint Workshop of the Living Options Group and the Research Unit of the Royal College of Physicians. Retrieved from http://www.leeds.ac.uk/disability-studies/archiveuk/Oliver/in%20soc%20dis.pdf

Oliver, M. (1996). *Understanding disability, from theory to practice*. London: Macmillan.

Ostroff, E. (2001). Universal design practice in the United States. In W. F. E. Preiser & E. Ostroff (Eds.), *Universal design handbook* (pp. 12.1-12.8). New York, NY: McGraw Hill.

Ozdowski, S. (2005). *Submission to the VBC/ABCB consultation on accessible housing*. Retrieved from http://www.humanrights.gov.au/disability_rights/accommodation/housesub.htm

Peterson, W. (1998). Public policy affecting universal design. *Assistive Technology, 10*, 13-20.

Pynoos, J., & Nishita, C. M. (2006). Home modifications. In R. Schulz, L. S. Noelker, K. Rockwood, & R. Sprott (Eds.), *The encyclopedia of aging* (4th ed., pp. 528-530). New York, NY: Springer.

Rehabilitation Act. (1973). The Rehabilitation Act Amendments of 1973, as amended. Retrieved from http://www.access-board.gov/enforcement/Rehab-Act-text/intro.htm

Ringaert, L. (2003). Universal design of the built environment to enable occupational performance. In L. Letts, P. Rigby, & D. Stewart (Eds.), *Using environments to enable occupational performance* (pp. 97-116). Thorofare, NJ: SLACK Incorporated.

Rogerson, F. (2005). *A review of the effectiveness of Part M of the building regulations*. Dublin, Ireland: National Disability Authority.

Salmen, J. P. S. (2001). US accessibility codes and standards: Challenges for universal design. In W. F. E. Preiser & E. Ostroff (Eds.), *Universal design handbook* (pp. 12.1-12.8). New York, NY: McGraw Hill.

Samaha, A. D. (2007). *What good is the social model of disability?* Retrieved from http://lawreview.uchicago.edu/issues/archive/v74/74_4/Samaha.pdf

Sanford, J. A., & Megrew, M. B. (1999). Using environmental simulation to measure accessibility for older people. In E. Steinfeld & S. Danford (Eds.), *Measuring enabling environments* (pp. 183-206). New York, NY: Plenum Press.

Sawyer, A., & Bright, K. (2007). *Access manual: Auditing and managing inclusive built environments*. London, UK: Blackwell Publishing Ltd.

Shakespeare, T., & Erickson, M. (2000). Different strokes: Beyond biological determinism and social constructionism. In H. Rose & S. Rose (Eds.), *Alas poor Darwin* (pp. 229-247). New York, NY: Harmony Books.

Shakespeare, T., & Watson, N. (2001). The social model of disability: An outdated ideology? In S. N. Barnartt & B. M. Altman (Eds.), *Research in social science and disability, Vol. 2. Exploring theories and expanding methodologies* (pp. 9-21). New York, NY: Elsevier Science Ltd.

Spegal, K., & Liebig, P. (2003). *Visitability: Trends, approaches and outcomes*. Los Angeles, CA; University of Southern California: The National Resource Centre on Supportive Housing and Home Modification.

Starr, A. (2005). *Churchill fellowship report*. Canberra, Australia: The Winston Churchill Memorial Trust of Australia.

Steinfeld, E., Levine, D. R., & Shea, S. M. (1998). Home modifications and the fair housing law. *Technology and Disability, 8,* 15-35.

Supreme Court of the United States. (1999). OLMSTEAD V.L.C. (98-536) 527 US 581. Washington, DC: Author.

Swain, J. (2004). International perspectives on disability. In J. Swain, S. French, C. Barnes, & C. Thomas (Eds.), *Disabling barriers—Enabling environments* (pp. 54-60). London, UK: Sage Publications.

Switzer, J. V. (2001). The Americans With Disabilities Act: Ten years later. *Policy Studies Journal, 29*(4), 629-632.

Uniform Federal Accessibility Standards. (1988). *Uniform federal accessibility standards* (UFAS). Retrieved from http://www.access-board.gov/ufas/ufas-html/ufas.htm

United Kingdom Disability Discrimination Act. (1995). *Disability Discrimination Act 1995*. Retrieved from http://www.opsi.gov.uk/acts/acts1995/1995050.htm

United Nations. (1971). *Declaration on the rights of mentally retarded persons*. Retrieved from http://www2.ohchr.org/english/law/res2856.htm

United Nations. (1975). *United Nations declaration on the rights of disabled persons*. Retrieved from http://www2.ohchr.org/english/law/res3447.htm

United Nations. (1993). *The standard rules on the equalization of opportunities for persons with disabilities*. Retrieved from http://www.un.org/esa/socdev/enable/dissre00.htm

United Nations. (1995). *The promotion of non-handicapping environments for disabled and elderly persons in the Asia and Pacific Region—Chapter 1*. Retrieved from http://www.unescap.org/esid/psis/disability/decade/publications/z15008cs/z1500802.htm

United Nations. (2008). *Convention on the rights of persons with disabilities*. Retrieved from http://www.un.org/disabilities/default.asp?navid=12&pid=150

United States Access Board. (1984). *Uniform Federal Accessibility Standards*. Retrieved from http://www.access-board.gov/ufas/ufas-html/ufas.htm

United States Department of Justice. (2005). *A guide to disability rights laws*. Retrieved from http://www.ada.gov/cguide.htm

United States Supreme Court. (1999). OLMSTEAD V. L. C. (98-536) 527 U.S. 581 (1999) 138 F.3d 893.

Waddington, L., & Diller, M. (2007). *Tensions and coherence in disability policy: The uneasy relationship between social welfare and civil rights models of disability in American, European and International employment law*. Retrieved from http://www.dredf.org/international/waddington.html

Whalley Hammell, K. (2001). Changing institutional environments to enable occupation among people with severe physical impairments. In L. Letts, P. Rigby, & D. Stewart (Eds.), *Using environments to enable occupational performance* (pp. 35-54). Thorofare, NJ: SLACK Incorporated.

Williams, P. J. G. (2005). The Disability Discrimination Act 2005. *Access by Design. Centre for Accessible Environments, 103,* 6-7.

Williams, P. J. G., & Levy, D. (2006). New DDA duties of property owners and managers. *Access by Design. Centre for Accessible Environments, 106,* 6-9.

World Health Organization. (1980). *The international classification of impairments, disabilities and handicaps (ICIDH)*. Geneva, Switzerland: Author.

World Health Organization. (2001). *The international classification of function, disability and health: ICF*. Geneva, Switzerland: Author.

Yee, S., & Golden, M. (2007). *Achieving accessibility: How the Americans with Disabilities Act is changing the face and mind of a nation*. Retrieved from http://www.dredf.org/international/paper_y-g.html

Young, I. M. (1990). *Justice and the politics of difference*. Princeton, NJ: Princeton University Press.

History and Future of Home Modification Services

Bronwyn Tanner, BOccThy, Grad Cert OccThy, Grad Cert Soc Planning, MPhil

The development of home modification (HM) as a strategy to respond to the needs of people with a disability and an aging population is linked to trends in both the population and demographics of the developed world and changes in social, political, and legislative outlooks. This chapter will review the way in which HM services have been established internationally and will investigate issues facing HM service delivery in past, current, and future contexts. Essential to effective service delivery is an understanding of the roles, perspectives, and responsibilities of key stakeholders in the HM process. To be an effective part of the HM service delivery process, the occupational therapist requires an understanding of the various perspectives of each stakeholder. This chapter will explore the role and perspectives of each stakeholder, as well as provide a range of strategies to assist the occupational therapist to achieve effective and positive service delivery outcomes.

CHAPTER OBJECTIVES

By the end of this chapter, the reader will be able to:

+ Identify factors influencing the development of HM services
+ Discuss HM policy and service systems currently operating internationally
+ Describe and contrast roles and perspectives of key stakeholders in HM service delivery and implications for effective and efficient service provision
+ Outline strategies for occupational therapists working within a HM service when working with other key stakeholders
+ Identify possible future directions in HM services and strategies for the occupational therapist to assist in effective and efficient service development and provision

INTRODUCTION

The growth of HM service delivery in recent times is a reflection of the changes in thinking about the role of the environment in health and function. The International Year of the Disabled Person in 1981 and the United Nations Decade of Disabled Persons (1983–1992) heralded a period of social and political activity worldwide that resulted in a paradigm shift in how functioning (and disability) was understood. By 2002, the World Health Organization (WHO) had issued a new *International Classification of Functioning, Disability, and Health*, which no longer emphasized the medical model of disability but instead acknowledged the impact of contextual factors on individual function. The impact of the social construction model of disability has resulted

Ainsworth, E., & de Jonge, D.
An Occupational Therapists's Guide to Home Modification Practice (pp. 67-84)
© 2011 SLACK Incorporated

in changes to legislation, policy, and service delivery for people with a disability, with many services focused on supporting equitable, independent, and community-based lifestyles (Bricknell, 2003; Steinfeld & Danford, 1999; WHO, 2001; Zola, 1997).

In the past two decades, after the changes in disability-related legislation and the flow on to policy and service provision, aged care policy in many developed countries has increasingly focused on assisting older people who have care needs to remain living in community settings. The growing importance of home to the health, well-being, and independence of older people has also been recognized with the term *aging-in-place*, which is frequently used within policy contexts. This term is most commonly used to describe the process of being supported in order to remain at home as individual abilities decline. Community care and aging-in-place have become cornerstones of policy and practice in many Western countries dealing with an increasingly aging population, with a range of programs and strategies being implemented to promote safety, independence, health, and well-being at home (Faulkner & Bennett, 2002).

The paradigm shift toward the social model of disability has strongly influenced the move toward community-based care for both people with a disability and older people. The Independent Living Movement, which gained momentum in the United Kingdom and the United States in the late 1970s to early 1980s, led to changes in legislation and policy to enable people with a disability to have some choice about living in the community rather than in residential care (Hurstfield, Parashar, & Schofield, 2007). A number of other factors have also contributed to this shift to community- and home-based care for people with a disability and older people, including the increasing concern and recognition that existing policy frameworks in aged care have been insufficient to respond to the increasing growth of the older population into the future (Gray, 2001). As well, there is a recognition of the cost-effectiveness of policies that assist older people and people with a disability to remain in their communities rather than to reside in more specialized institutionalized environments (Andrews, 2002; Heumann & Boldy, 1993; Hurstfield et al.). There has also been an increasing understanding and recognition of the diversity of the older population and recognition of the rights of older people, the majority of whom prefer to remain in a familiar home and community (Faulkner & Bennett, 2002). Finally, there is the recognition of the need for changes in attitudes, policies, and practices so that the economic and social contributions of people with a disability and older people are supported and that "people everywhere are able to

age with security and dignity and continue to participate in their societies as citizens with full rights" (Australian Institute of Health & Welfare, 2003, p. 275; Faulkner & Bennett; Hurstfield et al.).

HOME MODIFICATION SERVICE DEVELOPMENT

Existing Housing and Need for Modifications

Despite the well-established preference of most older people to age at home and the acknowledgment of the role of the environment as a major factor in enabling or disabling the achievement of both daily activities and community participation, it is only recently that there has been a shift in focus from purpose-built housing and institutional settings for older people and people with a disability to existing housing and community environments (Lanspery, Callahan, Miller, & Hyde, 1997; Pynoos, Cohen, Davis, & Bernhardt, 1987).

Evaluations of community care programs have highlighted that housing, more often than economic circumstances, influenced the capacities of older people or people with a disability to live in the community (Kendig & Gardner, 1997). Studies have also shown that the trend in community care policy to promote independent living and individual choice is dependent on a good supply of suitable housing (L. Watson, 1997).

As the population ages, modifying current housing stock to meet the needs of older people to age in place will be increasingly important; however, historically, HM is given little acknowledgement as a means of facilitating aging-in-place or supporting community living for people with a disability within a strategic policy context. While there is increasing realization of the importance of housing design in supporting older people or people with a disability, strategic direction in many countries tends to emphasize the need for new housing to meet the need of this population (Andrews, 2002; Smith, Rayer, & Smith, 2008). Initiatives that address improvements in the design of newly built housing to accommodate the needs of people as they age or people with a disability are vitally important to address the lack of accessible and adaptable housing in the community. Unfortunately, the importance of modification of existing housing as a way of meeting the needs of older people and people with a disability has been overlooked or omitted from many strategic policy and planning initiatives. This omission emphasizes the lack of recognition that HM receives at a strategic policy level. In part, the problem lies with the fact that HM lies in "no mans' land" in between housing policy, which focuses on the building of "bricks and mortar," and health services and community care, which emphasize personal care (Jones, de Jonge, & Phillips, 2008; Pynoos, Liebig, Overton, & Calvert, 1997).

As noted in Chapter 2, housing stock worldwide has not been designed or constructed to accommodate the needs of older people or people with a disability in terms of accessibility, safety, independence, and location (Stone, 1998). For example, in the United States, one study estimated that more than 90% of the 100 million housing units are not accessible, nor are they likely to be replaced in the near future (Nishita, Liebig, Pynoos, Perelman, & Spegal, 2007; Steinfeld, Levine, & Shea, 1998), and the proportion of housing stock being built with stairs increased 182% between 1970 and 1993 in the United States (Wylde, 1998). The reliance on new building development to meet the needs of older people or people with a disability is tenuous considering it is widely acknowledged that "development, design and building processes are inattentive to the needs of disabled people" (Imrie & Hall, 2001, p. 3). Of the more than 60 countries that have accessibility legislation worldwide, very few of these consider accessibility to new private residences as part of the legislative framework. Even in countries where the concept of "visitability" (basic accessibility features in newly constructed residential homes) is legislated, provisions have been "beset by problems of vagueness and ambiguity and rarely used to their full potential" (Imrie, 2006, p. 15), and it is acknowledged that there is a "long way to go in increasing the number of homes that are accessible and supportive" (Nishita et al., p. 13). Given this situation, there is a clear role for modification of existing housing as a strategy to support community living for older people and people with a disability. However, in many developed countries, HM services, while on the increase, continue to lack appropriate recognition at a legislative and policy level (Jones et al., 2008).

Legislative Support for Home Modification Service Development

The establishment, design, and delivery of a HM service varies between countries and, like accessibility in the built environment, is influenced by the type, nature, and direction of legislation and policy in existence in a particular country. Legislation and flow on policy directly affect the way HM services are resourced, including the amount of funding available, eligibility criteria, and the type and level of modification that is provided (Jones et al., 2008).

In many non-Western or developing countries, there are minimal legislative and policy frameworks in place and minimal welfare support for people with a disability. This lack of legislative support results in few resources or infrastructure to support modification of home environments for older people or people with a disability (Imrie, 2006).

Though many developed countries have legislation and policy in place that supports full participation and equity for people with disabilities and aging-in-place for older people, the outworking of these principles is complex, and there is often no overarching framework that legislates the provision of HM services. In countries such as the United States, New Zealand, and Australia, disability issues are considered within a human rights legislative framework rather than a rehabilitative or health framework as in Sweden.

Sweden provides a clear example of how legislative and policy frameworks support consistent and comprehensive HM service development. Sweden's legislation in relation to older people and people with a disability establishes a framework for the development of services including HM services (Lilja, Mansson, Jahlenius, & Sacco-Peterson, 2003). By law, local authorities are obliged to provide grants for housing modification services to anyone who has a disability irrespective of financial or housing situation (Petersson, Lilja, Hammel, & Kottorp, 2008). Policy arising from the legislation ensures that people with a disability do not bear the cost of reducing environmental barriers to their activities of daily living. As a result, all costs of modifications are covered, based on the person's self-assessment, an occupational therapist's assessment, technical advice, and alignment with legal guidelines. Under this legislative framework, HMs are considered essential elements of health care, and consistent provision of HMs is supported through policy and practice frameworks (Lilja et al.).

As outlined in Chapter 4, human rights legislation, such as the Americans with Disability Act (ADA; U.S. Department of Justice, 2010) and the Fair Housing Amendments Act (FHAA—housing specific amendments to the Civil Rights Act of 1968; U.S. Department of Housing and Urban Development [HUD], 2007; U.S. Department of Justice, 2009), enshrines the right of people with a disability to equitable and nondiscriminatory access to housing and housing services. However, supporting a person with care needs to live in the community very often requires a diverse array of services including home help, home maintenance, personal care and assistance, assistive technology, and HMs. Many of these services vie for the same funding, and HM service does not receive distinctive treatment (Lilja et al., 2003; Pynoos, Nishita, & Perelman, 2003). In many countries such as the United States, the United Kingdom, and Australia, there is a historic fragmentation of housing, health, and community care in policy areas, with the result that there is a lack of coordinated policy development and consequent service provision to support community-based living (Faulkner & Bennett, 2002; L. Watson, 1997). This lack of specific acknowledgement of HM services within policy and the associated poor integration of related areas at a policy level significantly affect the development and funding of HM services, with public funding for HM services being limited. In the United States and Australia, HM service delivery has been frequently described as being less than ideal, with lack of sufficient funding, poor coordination of services, and lack of geographic coverage of services cited as some of the main barriers to effective service delivery (Duncan, 1998a; Jones et al., 2008; Pynoos, 2001; Pynoos, Tabbarah, Angelli, & Demiere, 1998; Smith et al., 2008; Tabbarah, Silverstein, & Seeman, 2000; Trickey, Maltais, Gosselin, & Robitaille, 1993).

Funding and Home Modification Services

As indicated previously, funding arrangements for HM services are directly linked to provisions within the legislation of a particular country. Both Sweden and the United Kingdom have legislation that ensures a specific allocation of funds for HM services. Within the United Kingdom, the Mandatory Disabled Facilities Grant requires local authorities to fund a range of modifications to the homes of eligible people with a disability. However, even within countries that legislate for funding of HMs, problems exist. Within the United Kingdom, the Mandatory Disabled Facilities Grant is criticized as being poorly publicized, and the grant is distributed in a reactive rather than proactive way, resulting in poor uptake (Awang, 2002). Unlike Sweden, where funds are available irrespective of individual financial circumstance, in the United Kingdom, funding is limited to people on pensions and with low incomes, and there are differing levels of service across different geographical areas. In both the United Kingdom and Sweden, concerns exist as to the impact of an aging population on the viability of the current schemes with an increasing gap existing between need and available resources. Sweden is considering requiring financial contributions from the individual user to address this gap (Lilja et al., 2003).

Within counties such as the United States and Australia, where there is no legislative mandate for funding HM services, the cost of modification is often borne by the individual. For example, in the United States, the FHAA of 1998 requires that landlords allow for modification to properties where needed by the renter (U.S. Department of HUD, 2007). It does not, however, make provision for funding (Steinfeld et al., 1998). Consequently, many people pay for modifications out of their own pockets, often taking out loans, because the cost can be significant (Duncan, 1998b). A similar situation exists in Australia where there is no overarching policy framework for HM services and uneven levels of HM service provision across the country (Jones et al., 2008).

In both the United States and Australia, funding is available for HMs; however, it is generally considered to be difficult to access and insufficient to meet existing needs (Smith et al., 2008). Both countries have described the organization and provision of HM services as a "complex patchwork of programs" (Jones et al., 2008; Pynoos et al., 2003). Programs are often funded from a variety of diverse sources (federal, state, local, and community), resulting in fragmentation, inflexibility, and administrative burden, and there is an absence of integrated information systems about HM services (Jones et al.; Smith et al.).

In the United States, several federal departments have programs that provide funding for HM through both loans and grants, including the Department of HUD, the Department of Energy, the Administration on Aging, the Social Security Administration, and the Department of Veterans Affairs (Duncan, 1998b; Smith et al., 2008). Other sources exist at state and community levels in both public and private sectors; however, typically, people pay out of their own pockets for modifications because HMs are a low priority in many of the funded programs (Duncan; Pynoos et al., 1998).

In both the United States and Australia, even federally funded programs differ from state to state with regard to requirements and resources available, and funding is often in a block grant with a range of other essential services related to community care vying for priority (Duncan, 1998b; Jones et al., 2008). In many countries, such as Australia, the United Kingdom, and the United States, there has been a call to reconsider the current approach to the organization and provision of HM services. There is a clearly identified need to establish clear policy goals and benchmarks for service delivery to address the great disparity that exists in levels of service provision within various countries (Duncan; Jones et al.; Pynoos et al., 2003).

Future Policy Direction

The comparison between a country such as Sweden that has an apparently cohesive and well-established system of HM service delivery and that of the United States or Australia where HM services are "patchwork" highlights the importance of a strongly articulated policy framework regarding the development of provision of HM services. In both the United States and Australia, the need for clearly identified national goals and objectives regarding the development and provision of HM services has been acknowledged and strongly advocated (Duncan, 1998a; Jones et al., 2008; Pynoos, 1993; Pynoos et al., 1998).

Because HM services exist at the junction of housing, health, and community care policy, their existence, purpose, and benefits are poorly articulated and recognized (Jones et al., 2008; Pynoos et al., 1998). Better and stronger connections are therefore needed between HM service as a strategy in each of the policy areas of housing, health, and aging, and better integration between these areas needs to occur (Faulkner & Bennett, 2002; Jones et al.; Pynoos et al.). Jones et al. propose that a national program be established with "a set of objectives concerning housing, health and community-care outcomes, linked to a national strategy for older people and whole-of-government aging policy" (p. 136). They also propose a lead agency across federal and state levels of government, coordinating a range of services delivered at a regional or local level, with "national benchmarks for levels of provision of services, terms of eligibility and user charges and development of professional and technical expertise" (Jones et al., p. 137). It is argued that restructuring HM services in this way would establish HM services as a recognized and effective strategy within a broader comprehensive and effective approach to the provision of accessible and appropriate housing for older people and people with a disability.

HOME MODIFICATION SERVICE DESIGN AND DELIVERY

Defining Home Modification Services

It is useful at this point to examine what can broadly be considered to be part of a HM service and how the differing policy areas can affect service design. In many countries, HM services can consist of two main types of service: HMs and home repairs.

HMs include structural modifications (changes to the structure of the home, such as widening doorways and remodeling bathrooms) and nonstructural modifications (the installation or alteration of fittings and fixtures, such as grab rails and ramps; Jones et al., 2008). Home repairs involve mending damaged elements of the home, such as steps and roofs, and maintenance work, such as lawn mowing and installation or replacement of smoke alarms. In addition, a HM service can be a direct service that will carry out the necessary work or an indirect service that offers information and advice, referral, project management, and funding (Jones et al.).

As described in Chapter 2, where the HM service is situated in terms of the health, community care, and housing policy domains will influence the type and orientation of the service provided (Jones et al., 2008). A HM service that is primarily associated with the health domain will often have an emphasis toward addressing a specific health problem, particularly if related to discharge from a hospital or health facility. The most common modifications for this type of service will be nonstructural, such as the installation of grab rails or prescription of assistive devices that address a particular functional concern related to the health condition of the person. Less emphasis will be put on broader issues of access outside of the home, the general repair and maintenance of the home, and community access (Jones et al.).

For a HM service located in the community care policy domain, the emphasis will be on enabling a person to remain in his or her home environment for as long as possible. In this way, there is likely to be an emphasis on home repair and maintenance as well as modification to delay either the need for personal assistance or a move to residential care (Jones et al., 2008). Generally, this type of HM service has a broader view of the person and his or her home than a health-based service. Interventions, modifications, or repairs aim at improving the "fit" between the person's competencies and the overall demand of home and community. The expansion of community care programs has provided momentum for HM service development in recent years, and it is within this context that many HM services are based (Jones et al.).

A less common arrangement is a HM service located within the housing policy context. In this situation, rather than viewing HMs as relating specifically to a health issue or supporting an individual to remain at home, the HM service is viewed from the broader perspective of housing choice (Jones et al., 2008). Often, HMs for health or support reasons occur in situations of urgency; for example, to enable a person to return home from the hospital or to delay admission to care. HM services operating within a housing perspective are more focused on lifestyle choice and adjustment to changes in circumstances and preferences (Jones et al.). In this way, HMs can be viewed as a way of enhancing "the range of options available to people in later life to create housing and living arrangement that meet their needs and reflect their identity and lifestyles" (Jones et al., p. 14).

Jones et al. (2008) consider a number of advantages for future HM service development in viewing HMs within a housing policy perspective. This broader perspective allows for a more universal approach to HM service design and delivery, encompassing not only the health, safety, and independence aspects of the health and community care approaches, but also preventative and proactive responses to lifestyle issues associated with aging (Jones et al., p. 137). Acknowledging HM services within a housing policy framework also links HM services to the wider issues of accessible design of new dwellings and to the professional and technical expertise of the housing and building industries.

Barriers to Effective Home Modification Service Delivery

Though on the increase, the actual prevalence of HM is low, and there exists a significant unmet need. Out of all households with at least one member with a physical activity limitation in the United States, only about 38% had HMs present (Nishita et al., 2007). In Australia, existing data suggest that approximately 16% of people 65 years and older have a HM, with the incidence higher in privately owned dwellings than in rental dwellings (Bricknell, 2003).

It has been identified that the process of HM service delivery can be troublesome and time consuming and can result in ineffective and poor outcomes (Heywood, 2004a; Pynoos, Sanford, & Rosenfelt, 2002; Tanner, Tilse, & de Jonge, 2008). While a lack of an overarching specific policy framework, fragmented systems of funding and service delivery, and a general lack of funding to meet existing need have been identified as major barriers to effective development of HM services in countries such as the United States and Australia, several other associated difficulties also affect service delivery.

Across many countries, a lack of information about both the existence and benefits of HM services is identified as a major barrier to effective service delivery (Jones et al., 2008; Pynoos et al., 1998; Tanner et al., 2008). While a lack of profile of HM services is related to the low priority they

have in many bulk funding programs, in countries with mandatory grants for HMs such as the United Kingdom, there is still often a lack of information available to potential users of this service. Agencies with HM grant money do not receive funding for publicity and generally fail to promote availability, particularly if there is a high demand for services (Awang, 2002). Awang found that for the U.K. population of older people included in their study who had received HMs, "half the participants entered the system purely by chance and none of the participants had been aware that adaptation services and grant assistances existed" (p. 6).

Compounding this is the lack of awareness and knowledge of the advantages of HMs by consumers, support services, and industry providers. Home care agencies are generally thought to underuse HMs to resolve unsafe situations in a person's home, often because of the unknown cost and lack of knowledge about possible solutions and the process of getting the work done (Pynoos et al., 1998; Smith et al., 2008). The health system and associated services tend to prioritize medical equipment and personal care services over modifications to the home environment. A lack of knowledge on the part of potential service users as well as health and building professionals about the benefits of HMs has been cited as a key issue to overcome in improving both the uptake and quality of HMs (Steinfeld et al., 1998). Education programs that are directed at a range of stakeholders have been strongly recommended as a way of overcoming the lack of awareness and knowledge. Education and advocacy are required for potential service users as well as policymakers, funding bodies, and health and building professionals (Duncan, 1998a; Jones et al., 2008).

Another significant barrier to the effective delivery of HM services is the lack of available professionals with expertise in the area of HM. This includes occupational therapists and building professionals. Occupational therapists are increasingly being recognized as playing an important role in HM service process and delivery, particularly in the areas of assessment, follow-up, and evaluation of completed work (Pynoos et al., 2002, 2003). The role of the occupational therapist has been promoted as one of understanding and meeting consumers' goals so that the individual is enabled, enhanced, and empowered to make choices, solve problems, and maintain control (Pickering & Pain, 2003; Pynoos et al., 2003). However, chronic shortages of occupational therapists in many countries have resulted in significant waiting times for HM assessment (Jones et al., 2008). Difficulty in locating skilled building professionals who have an understanding and knowledge of HM is also a key barrier to the successful delivery of a HM service (Jones et al.). Delays in getting work started and completed have been noted in a number of studies as well as issues regarding poor follow-up and evaluation of completed work (Nocon & Pleace, 1997; Stark, 2004; Tanner et al., 2008).

As indicated previously, HM services lie at the intersection of health, community care, and housing sectors. This affects not just policy but also the range of individuals (stakeholders) who are involved in the delivery of this complex, multifield service. A HM service brings together a wide range of people holding differing priorities, professional orientations, and knowledge. A poor understanding of and poor communication between the various stakeholders in the service delivery process have the potential to create a great number of barriers to effective service delivery. A good understanding of how services and the individuals involved operate will help to improve existing service delivery and assist in the design of new programs (Pynoos, 1993). Understanding the perspectives of each of the key stakeholders and how they may affect other members of the service delivery team is essential to effective HM service delivery and outcomes.

KEY PEOPLE IN HOME MODIFICATION SERVICE DELIVERY

Though there is some diversity in the policy and procedures that impact on the organization and operation of programs within and between countries, commonly, HM programs use a combination of employed staff (such as a program coordinator and employed tradesmen/handymen to carry out minor work) and subcontractors who are usually licensed professionals (including occupational therapists) operating under contract (Pynoos et al., 1997). While the role, level, and nature of involvement of each of these key players will differ between services, there is a general consistency in the type of people (stakeholders) who are usually involved in the delivery of a HM service (Pynoos et al., 2002).

Working with other professions is commonplace for many occupational therapists; however, most therapists work within multidisciplinary teams, usually made up of others who are also involved in the health sector. HM programs tend to differ from more traditional health care or social service programs primarily in the types of people involved in service delivery and in the types of skills needed to carry out the service. HM programs straddle both health care and housing sectors and require skilled professionals from both areas.

Because of the cross-sector nature of HM service delivery, problems can arise at various stages in the process, and a lack of understanding of the role and contribution of various stakeholders involved can contribute to a less-than-effective outcome (Heywood, 2004a). By examining the role and contribution of each stakeholder in the delivery of a HM service, some strategies can be identified that will facilitate effective service delivery and outcomes.

The key people involved in the delivery of HMs commonly include the following:

+ The person (home dweller) and his or her significant others (this can be family, friends, or caregivers)
+ The referring agency
+ The organization managing and/or providing funding for the service
+ Construction and building professionals
+ Design professionals
+ The health professional, most often an occupational therapist

How effective a service is depends on the dynamic interplay between stakeholders in key areas of the values, knowledge, and perspectives that they bring to the process, the culture that each profession or organization operates within, and the balance of power and control related to decision making.

The Home Dweller or Householder

Understanding the perspective of the home dweller is fundamental to the successful outcome of HM service delivery. As discussed in Chapter 1, the service delivery will occur in this person's home environment—a context full of personal meaning and significance. This context is both an area of primary control for the home dweller and a reflection or even an extension of his or her self-identity (Dovey, 1985; Despres, 1991; Sixsmith, 1986).

As people, we make sense of our physical world by giving meaning and order to our surroundings, and this creates a sense of "insideness" with particular contexts, especially places of significant meaning, such as a home (Dovey, 1985; Rowles, 2000). The priorities of the home dweller therefore may not be the same as those of other stakeholders who lack this sense of insideness, and HMs can be rejected by home dwellers if the proposed change is incongruent with their self-image or their idea of home. An example of this is where parents of a child with a disability may decline modifications that they feel makes their home less home-like and more institutional (Hawkins & Stewart, 2002).

Consideration of the perspectives and values of significant others (e.g., family members) in the design and delivery of HM services is also important, particularly where others' use of space will be affected (Heywood, 2004a). This can be problematic (e.g., in an intergenerational family) where use of equipment such as an over-toilet frame can impede toilet training of a young child, or when the significant other's needs for space are not considered.

Implications for Service Delivery

Inclusion of the home dweller and significant others in decision making about changes to the physical environment is of paramount importance. The issue of participation and control over the modification process is one that has been identified as a key area in the literature (Heywood, 2004a, 2005; Nocon & Pleace, 1997; Pickering & Pain, 2003; Tanner et al., 2008). Poor outcomes in HM services have been identified as being related to poor understanding of the individual's need and limiting assessment to a functional understanding of the person without consideration of issues of control, participation, or the needs of significant others (Heywood).

A small qualitative study showed that levels of participation in decision making around HM impacted on levels of client satisfaction and also on client behavior (Tanner et al., 2008). While small and nongeneralizable, this study also showed that where people did not feel involved in the decision making around modifications to their home, they altered the recommendations with the contractor without consulting the occupational therapist or service provider. It is therefore essential that those involved in the HM process understand the importance of home as a place of privacy, identity, and primary control. Treating someone else's home as a workplace and not involving him or her in the process from the beginning will most likely result in an unsatisfactory outcome (Heywood, 2004a; Nocon & Pleace, 1997; Tamm, 1999).

Strategies for the Occupational Therapist

Occupational therapists entering a person's home need to be conscious of the assumptions that they bring with them with regard to their role, particularly in the area of decision making in a person's home. Client-centered philosophy encourages occupational therapists to think of their relationship to the individual with whom they are working as a partnership where individuals have opportunities to define and prioritize their own areas of need and have a role in jointly planning for intervention. This approach assists in keeping the individual in a position of control in his or her home environment, supporting the unique relationship of the person to his or her home (Hawkins & Stewart, 2002).

It is essential that the occupational therapist be committed to a participatory decision-making process. The occupational therapist needs to ensure that the home dweller is actively engaged in the decision making around the intervention planned. Communication needs to be clear and choices around options provided (Heywood, 2004a). This approach will help reinforce the meaning of home as a primary territory with a perceived degree of personal control (Smith, 1994; Tanner et al., 2008).

If the person is accustomed to a passive role with health or other professionals, the home dweller may not feel confident to voice his or her opinion or to take an active role in decision making. The occupational therapist needs to be sensitive to this dynamic and support the person to give his or her views and opinions not only in their own interactions but in interactions between the person and other stakeholders, such as building and design professionals. Because the occupational therapist is the person who gathers assessment information about the individual, he or she is often in a good position to argue the case for an individual to a funding body or organization and may be well placed to negotiate better outcomes for an individual.

Heywood (2004a) states that the foundation of quality outcomes in HM is a full understanding of the needs of the home dweller. This understanding must extend beyond a functional perspective of need to one that includes the need to restore or maintain the individual's dignity and to recognize his or her values and those of significant others (Heywood, 2004a, 2004b).

The literature has identified that often there is a difference in values between the home dweller and the professionals, such as occupational therapists entering the home environment (Heywood, 2004a; Nocon & Pleace, 1997). Often, older people do not perceive environmental barriers as hazards to the same extent as a visiting therapist (Pynoos et al., 2002). Negotiation between what is important to the home dweller and what the therapist perceives as needing to be addressed requires sensitivity, and the resultant outcome may be affected by a number of issues.

Concern over the cost of modifications and the energy required to carry out or organize the work have been identified as barriers that prevent some home dwellers from carrying out HMs (Steinfeld & Shea, 1993). Others may reject suggestions on the basis that they imply a degree of disability or frailty that they do not accept. The image of disability made evident by modifications such as ramps, grab rails, and stair lifts may not be tolerable to the person, and it may require time and ongoing discussion for suggested changes to be accepted (Heywood, 2004b; Wylde, 1998).

The occupational therapist working within the home environment also needs to display a high level of cultural competence and sensitivity. A therapist who is culturally competent will be aware of, have knowledge of, and be sensitive to the cultural background of the individual and cultural issues that may impact on the values and practices of the individual and influence his or her decision-making processes regarding any proposed intervention (Fitzgerald, Mullavey-O'Brien, & Clemson, 1997; R. M. Watson, 2006).

The Referring Agency

It has been recognized in a number of studies that access to information about HM services is generally poor (Awang, 2002; Tanner et al., 2008; Wylde, 1998). In some instances, a lack of information and publicity has been used to prevent an over demand for HM services (Awang). Referrals to HM programs frequently come from other agencies and workers in the area who may have more knowledge of what is available than the individual. Referring agencies can be a source of valuable information about the person and his or her history, family, and current level of function.

The referring agency may or may not have accurate information about what the HM service delivery can and will supply and eligibility for the service. An outcome of misinformation can be the raising of expectations that may not be able to be met. It is therefore important that referring services or agencies have accurate and updated information about the HM program.

Implications for Other Stakeholders

Promotion of the HM service to referring agencies is essential in ensuring that unmet need is addressed and appropriate referrals are made. Referral agencies need to have up-to-date information about services offered, funding available, and eligibility criteria. It has been identified that enhancing communication and knowledge and improving interagency referral systems are the most effective strategies in improving the coordination of services for the individual (Jones et al., 2008; Pynoos, 1993).

Strategies for the Occupational Therapist

As indicated previously, referring agencies may be a good source of initial information about the referred individual. Communication with the relevant person within the referring agency prior to a home visit may be a useful strategy for the occupational therapist to gain valuable background information. This initial contact also provides a good opportunity to clarify what expectations both the individual and the referring body have of the HM service and to clarify what the HM service is able to offer. It may also be appropriate to organize a joint home visit with the referring agency, particularly if they are frequent visitors or well known to the individual concerned.

Keeping the referring agency informed throughout the HM process is important in maintaining good networks and communication. This can be done by forwarding written reports for their information as well as providing less formal feedback regarding the proposed intervention and timeframes.

Requesting feedback from agencies that frequently refer to the HM service is also valuable in evaluating the effectiveness of HM service delivery, including the input of the occupational therapist.

The Administrating/Funding Organization

The administrating organization may often be a local or state organization that administers state or federal funds. Many not-for-profit service organizations administer a range of community-based services, of which home repair and modifications may only be one of many services they coordinate. As indicated previously, funding for HM may be administered through a block grant, with many other services vying for the same bucket of funds, so the way an organization prioritizes funding and decision making around services can impact significantly on the type of HM service that is offered.

Many organizations that administer HM services are by nature bureaucracies; that is, organizations based on rationalism, hierarchy, and impersonal rules. The characteristics of bureaucratic organizations include the enforcement of rule-bound procedures, the focus on written rather than verbal discourse, and the use of experts with specialized and technical languages of discourse (Dovey, 1985). Bureaucracies tend to have a "centralised order imposed across diverse particular cases according to typical situations," and this "typical situation" approach to meeting individual need has been the experience of people within HM service delivery, sometimes with negative outcomes (Crozier, 1964, cited in Dovey, p. 56; Heywood, 2004b; Tanner et al., 2008). As well as being limited in their response to individual need, the bureaucratic organization model is, nonparticipatory by nature, with little scope for service users or recipients to shape or determine service delivery (Awang, 2002).

The majority of service organizations have policies and practices regarding eligibility criteria, which also define the population they are able to serve and the limit of their service. For example, an organization may decide to use allocated funds for minor modifications only and in this way provide service to a larger number of people than if they did major, more costly modifications. This, however, will place limits on the amount and type of modification that can be recommended. Difficulty also arises where home repairs are required in addition or prior to modifications being carried out. Such work may not be seen as part of the organization's service criteria and therefore may limit the access that some people have to the service.

Implications for Other Stakeholders

For the home dweller or householder, dealing with a bureaucratic organization can be overwhelming, often due to complexity of forms, people, and processes that need to be negotiated to get an outcome (Awang, 2002). The typical situation approach of bureaucracies also means that, in the application of rules and regulations, the individual becomes invisible and may not be granted power to influence outcomes. There is an inherent tension between the bureaucratic organization delivering the HM service and the home dweller or service recipient around the issues of power and control. Culturally, a bureaucracy is service oriented and inflexible, with little scope to allow the users or recipients of the service control or power in decision making (Awang). These negative experiences of organizational service delivery can undermine the experience of home for the person and be profoundly disempowering for the individual, resulting in negative health effects (Dovey, 1985; Heywood, 2004b).

Strategies for the Occupational Therapist

The role of the occupational therapist within HM service delivery has been promoted as one of understanding and meeting the individual's goals so that the individual is enabled, enhanced, and empowered to make choices, solve problems, and maintain control (Pickering & Pain, 2003; Pynoos et al., 2003). It is therefore crucial that the occupational therapist endeavors to keep the individual in the center of the assessment and decision-making process within the organizational framework.

It is important that the organization's restrictions and limitations do not in turn compromise the assessment process for the occupational therapist (Heywood, 2004b). The occupational therapy assessment should reflect as much as possible a full understanding of the needs of the home dweller rather than being restricted to what the organization will or won't fund or what organizational processes typically promote. Because of their focus on the individual, therapists are well placed to speak up for the individual and promote a full understanding of his or her needs within the organizational framework. If necessary, the occupational therapist should push the boundaries of bureaucratic administration if it is important to address the needs of the individual. It is also important that the home dweller is fully aware of the options that are available to him or her and is informed of ways his or her needs can be met through other systems or services.

The occupational therapist can also contribute to change where there is a need for a broadening of policy, systems, and structures. Putting concerns in memos, gathering data and statistics about unmet need, and gathering support from others to lobby for change are all ways that may be effective in bringing about improved service delivery.

Design and Construction Professionals

HM services usually involve two main types of professions—the occupational therapist who focuses on the fit between the person and his or her dwelling and the design and building professional who are involved in the design and completion of modification work (Jones et al., 2008). Invariably, the HM process requires the expertise of the construction industry no matter what the extent of modification. The services of a design professional are usually only required in the case of major modifications where changes proposed will alter the design and layout of the home.

Each profession has an embedded culture, which includes the norms, values, beliefs, traditional knowledge, skills, and core practices that guide and shape professional behavior and identity (R. M. Watson, 2006). It is into this culture that new professionals are socialized through education, training, and work experiences. Understanding the cultural orientation of a profession is important in understanding how professional reasoning and decision making occurs.

The building profession has a culture that is strongly embedded in a regulatory environment. It is an industry that is prescribed, regulated, and inspected and rightly so, given the issues of safety that are involved. This perspective is extremely valuable to the HM interaction because the building professional is able to advise what is possible and not possible, in accordance with various codes and regulations within a home environment. The downside of this, however, is that standard responses to an individual's needs can become entrenched and documents such as public access standards can be given a higher priority than is practicable or advisable in a unique and dynamic individual situation (Pynoos et al., 2002).

Accessibility codes are typically designed to determine minimal legal guidelines for public access and have a stereotypical view of the end user, for example, a user of a wheelchair. They have very little to do with the needs, aspirations, desires, and uniqueness of a particular individual and do not cater to the many variations of individual function of people who have a disability (Danford & Steinfeld, 1999; Imrie & Hall, 2001). For example, current public access standards in many countries are not based on research for older people, and assuming that designing for wheelchair use will be suitable or appropriate for the older person with a range of mobility needs is an untested hypothesis that has not been evidenced in research. In fact, research in the United States has shown that some modifications to the existing accessible standards "may promote more disability among older adults than it ameliorates" (Pynoos et al., 2002, p. 16; Sanford & Megrew, 1995).

Architectural or technical aspects are emphasized by building professionals with the home dwelling considered as a "piece of hardware" and the personal and social aspects of home disregarded (Imrie, 2006, p. 14). In this way, technical knowledge dominates the construction professional's decision making and actions. Many building professionals have time and money constraints and can be financially vulnerable particularly if they are subcontractors. Tradition also plays a strong role in the builder's work, with many being resistant to changing the way they do their work (Burns, 2004).

Current literature suggests that the construction industry in many countries does not respond well to the needs of people with a disability and that formal education of building professionals on the needs of people with a disability is "more or less non-existent" (Imrie & Hall, 2001, p. 6; Burns, 2004; Imrie, 2006). Imrie and Hall assert that "inattentiveness to and exclusion of the needs of (people with a disability) are evident at all stages of the design and development of the built environment" (p. 6). The house building industry has been characterized by a lack of innovation and a "poorly developed sense of customer focus when compared to other service sectors" (Burns, p. 768). This lack of interest or willingness to be innovative has resulted in a standardization of house design where "certain household types and certain bodies are targeted" (Burns, p. 769). The drive for standardization has been linked to the rise of large-scale corporate property development

in which standardized fittings and fixtures are commonplace and the construction "revolves around industry standards, which are inattentive to bodily diversity or differences" (Imrie & Hall, p. 9). Older people and people with a disability often have requirements that are not met by standard housing designs and thus provide builders with challenges to their traditional designs and techniques (Burns).

Within the professional culture of the design professions, such as architecture or interior design, designing for the needs of people with a disability has not been a significant feature of design theory or a major part of the design and development process (Goldsmith, 1997; Imrie & Hall, 2001). The focus of the design process tends to be aesthetics and technical cleverness more than the user or functionality of the building (Goldsmith) with "the concern of the decorative and the ornamental" remaining a "powerful part of the design professions" (Imrie & Hall, p. 12). Where the needs of people with a disability have been incorporated into a project, "there is the tendency to reduce disability to a singular form of mobility impairment, that of the wheelchair user" (Imrie & Hall, p. 10).

Within the architectural profession, there have been and continue to be challenges to the dominant design culture. Imrie and Hall (2001) use the terms *social architecture* or *social design* to describe a trend that proposed to "recognise the multiplicity of needs of building users" and the need to accommodate them in building projects (p. 12). This movement has sought to recenter the design process on the user of the building and to incorporate a broader and more holistic understanding of the needs of users of the buildings. The core values of social design align with environmental and social justice and human rights; however, Imrie and Hall report that the movement has had little impact on the thinking of the design professions in relation to people with a disability.

Inclusive design and universal design are similarly social movements that have, in recent times, gained prominence in both the United Kingdom and the United States. Inclusive design, like the social design movement, is concerned with the "sustainability, flexibility and adaptability" of buildings to accommodate the diversity of building users, placing the user of the building in the center of the design process (Milner & Madigan, 2004, p. 734). Universal design is concerned with making products and environments as usable as possible to the broadest range of users. Applied to housing, universal design far exceeds the minimum specification of access standards, seeking to create homes that are "useable by and marketable to people of all ages and abilities" (Mace, 1998, p. 22). This type of design process is in contrast to the compensatory approach in which elements of accessibility are added on to previously inaccessible or standard designs (Imrie & Hall, 2001).

Implications for Other Stakeholders

Building and design professionals are essential to the HM process, and the technical knowledge they bring, when combined with professional knowledge of the occupational therapist and the lived experience of the client, can and should result in good outcomes. Where the technical knowledge of the design and construction professional dominates without consideration of the unique person-environment dynamic at play, the outcomes can be less than satisfactory (Pynoos et al., 2002; Tanner et al., 2008). It is therefore important that the technical knowledge of the design and construction professionals is used in a way that ensures that the outcome is compliant with relevant building codes and regulations but is also focused on individual need.

A resistance to innovation and change on the part of the construction professional can cause problems within the HM process. Remembering a strong tie to tradition, the phrase "it's not possible" may really mean "that's not the way it is usually done." Similarly, the idea of a collaborative partnership between the client, the therapist, and the builder may be an unfamiliar concept to the construction professional who is more familiar with an authoritative hierarchical work culture.

Strategies for the Occupational Therapist

Though professional orientation and culture differs between stakeholders within the HM service delivery, they are complementary, and consideration of each stakeholder's perspective is important in establishing good communication, understanding, and effective outcomes.

Clear and ongoing communication is the best strategy to facilitate a good working arrangement. It is helpful for the therapist to have a basic understanding of building terminology to be able to understand to some extent the construction issues involved with the modification process. Asking questions and getting clarification is important. Often, therapists need to work through alternative solutions on site with the building professional so that they can fully understand the regulatory requirements and engage in problem-solving to explore how performance requirements might be met differently. Therapists also need to communicate their recommendations clearly both when speaking and writing. Because visual communication dominates the construction industry, clear, unambiguous drawings should accompany any HM recommendations.

The therapist also has a responsibility to ensure that the individual and his or her needs remain the focus of the work carried out. Professional tradespeople and builders can have significant influence over the individual home dweller due to their technical knowledge base, and it is important that the building process with its regulatory culture does not subvert the home dweller's needs. Most occupational therapists operate from a client-centered perspective, meaning that they perceive their role to be one of collaboration with the person in receipt of their services, with their intervention designed to meet goals stated by the individual. The therapist needs to ensure that the individual, as the expert of his or her life, is recognized and that his or her thoughts, ideas, and wishes are not overwhelmed by the technical discourse of the building and design professional.

While there is excellent scope for collaboration, differences in professional culture can also lead to situations of conflict, and good conflict resolution skills are an important part of the occupational therapist's repertoire. Assertive communication that provides, in plain language, the professional reasoning that informs the opinions and decisions regarding occupational therapist recommendations is essential to ensure good understanding and communication. Often, conflict can arise over differing views regarding areas of responsibility within the HM process. Detailed practice policy and procedures that outline the HM process are useful tools in clarifying areas of responsibility for different stakeholders. The occupational therapist can play a valuable role in the development of good practice and procedural documents within a HM service.

Consulting Occupational Therapist

As students and new graduates, we undergo a professional enculturation, which orients us to the particular nuances and culture of our chosen field. Culture is not a static experience, however, and the culture of a profession is dynamic and changing (R. M. Watson, 2006). The culture of the profession enables us to engage in the joint production of meaning within our professional community (R. M. Watson). It provides us with both self-understanding and shapes our professional identity through shared beliefs and values (R. M. Watson).

Central to the occupational therapy profession is the belief in the power of occupation as a purposeful and meaningful activity to the person who engages in it (American Occupational Therapy Association [AOTA], 2008). At the heart of this engagement is the relationship between the therapist and the client.

While the importance of the client/therapist relationship has been recognized since the earliest days of occupational therapy, there has been a gradual change in more recent times from a culture of the professional as expert to one of client centeredness where the client is seen as a partner with the therapist (Duggan, 2005).

Within the HM area, occupational therapists are interested in the enhancement of the occupational performance of the individual, and they accomplish this by improving the fit between that individual, his or her occupation, and his or her home environment through making physical changes to that environment. The values and beliefs that therapists bring with them regarding the client/therapist relationship will affect the provision of HM service in all aspects from assessment to evaluation. When entering each person's home, therapists need to be conscious of the assumptions that they bring with them with regard to their role, particularly in the area of decision making regarding changes to that person's home. The occupational therapist needs to be particularly aware of the impact of organizational culture on their service delivery. An authoritarian, bureaucratic organization (such as a hospital or government department) may impact on the values and beliefs that therapists bring to the HM interaction. Is the home dweller seen as an active participant or a passive receiver? Where does the power lie in the decision-making process—with the expert professional or with the home dweller who is an expert in his or her own life?

Client-centered philosophy encourages occupational therapists to think of their relationship with the individual as a partnership where individuals have opportunities to define and prioritize their own areas of need and have a role in jointly planning for intervention. This approach assists in keeping the individual in a position of control in his or her home environment, supporting the unique relationship of the person to his or her home (Hawkins & Stewart, 2002).

Occupational therapists are increasingly being recognized as playing an important role in HM service process and delivery, particularly in the areas of assessment, follow-up, and evaluation of completed work (Pynoos et al., 2002, 2003). Occupational therapists come to the role of assessment and intervention with a theoretical background that guides decision making. The profession's models of practice also guide therapists by providing a basis for understanding the dynamic interaction between people, their occupations, and their environments.

As well as their theoretical knowledge, occupational therapists use assessments, measurements, knowledge of functional anatomy, anthropometrics, and understanding of disease processes as tools to gather data about the situation. However, the use of professional reasoning is essential to a good outcome. Occupational therapists engaging in professional reasoning use their knowledge of the functional impacts of health conditions (scientific reasoning), the understanding of the client's life story and their perspectives as experts in their own life (narrative reasoning), and considerations of the practical limitations and ethical considerations of the situation (pragmatic and ethical reasoning) to determine the best outcome for a client (Boyt Schell, 2003). Working with clients and their goals and desires, therapists are able to construct a view of the future using their theoretical knowledge, technical knowledge, and interactive professional reasoning processes.

Implications for Other Stakeholders

As indicated previously, the occupational therapist's role in the HM process is to ensure that a full understanding of the needs of each home dweller is gathered and that this understanding drives the decision making and intervention planning.

Of primary importance is the therapist's relationship with the home dweller as a partner in the intervention process. The therapist therefore needs to be supportive of the individual, ensuring that his or her views and opinions are heard. A limitation to this may be the amount of time the therapist is able to allocate to ongoing involvement in the HM process. As a contracted professional, occupational therapists may only be involved in the assessment and planning stages of the process with limited time provided to engage with the individual home dweller.

Though there are significant differences between the professional cultures of occupational therapists and construction and design professions, there is great scope for complementary and harmonious interaction. The key is effective and ongoing communication between all stakeholders that ensures that each person's knowledge and expertise is used throughout the HM process.

FUTURE CHALLENGES FOR HOME MODIFICATION SERVICE DELIVERY
Strategic Policy Direction

Awareness of the benefits of HMs has been increasing; however, there are still significant challenges to the viability and usefulness of HM service delivery. Emphasis at a legislative and strategic policy level is on implementing change in new construction as seen by the increase in visibility legislation, particularly across the United States, including legislation such as the proposed Inclusive Home Design Act (Smith et al., 2008). While this move toward inclusive design is gaining momentum at an international level, significant issues still face those living in existing inaccessible and unsafe housing.

At a strategic policy level, there is a need for greater recognition of the importance of HM to community living for people with a disability and for our increasingly aging population. In many countries, HM services are intrinsically linked to health and community care policy areas. For example, a recent report from the Office for Disability Issues in the United Kingdom (Heywood & Turner, 2007) highlighted four main ways in which the provision of housing modifications and equipment produces savings to health and social care budgets. These were savings in the cost of residential care through enabling people to remain in their homes and reducing the cost and need for in-home care services; savings through the prevention of accidents with associated high costs of hospital and residential care admissions; savings through prevention of waste brought about because of underfunding of modification services, which resulted in delays in implementation and provision of inadequate or ineffectual solutions; and finally savings through achieving better outcomes for the same expenditure by improving the quality of life of recipients and caregivers and family members (Heywood & Turner). Though the report found evidence of the preventive and therapeutic role of HMs, it also highlighted the ongoing issue of underfunding for HMs and increasingly restrictive eligibility criteria related to this, reducing the availability of HMs to many people who would benefit (Heywood & Turner).

As indicated previously, Jones et al. (2008) consider that there is a strong case for reconsidering the current approach to the organization of HM services and suggest that the future of HM service delivery may lie in the recognition that HM services are a major contributor to the housing policy area, rather than being seen primarily under the banner of health and community care policy areas. Aligning HM services with strategic housing policy links the HM service to the areas of accessible and inclusive housing and national strategies for housing, while still maintaining links to the health and community sectors (Jones et al.). In this way, strategic policy direction that provides a coordinated, funded service delivery response across public and private housing and also links housing into health and aged care services may be more achievable.

Service Design and Delivery Direction

At a service level in the United States and Australia, many of the issues facing HM service delivery today were being raised more than a decade ago. First, while there is an increase in the organizations and programs funded to provide HM services, there is a lack of a systematic approach to the organization of such services, with limited policy development, few benchmarks for service delivery, and great disparities in the level of service provision (Jones et al., 2008; Pynoos et al., 1998). Resourcing is considered to be insufficient to meet demand, and lack of funding results in delays in work being carried out (Jones et al.; Pynoos et al.). Services and service recipients are often overwhelmed by the cumulative impact of numerous building, health, disability, and legal requirements (Awang, 2002; Jones et al.), which are in themselves barriers to accessing and delivering an effective HM service.

While levels of expertise have developed over the past decade, there are still shortages in skilled professionals from both the health and construction sectors that contribute to delays in service provision. A lack of awareness about the advantages of HM continues to exist both within the community and service sectors, resulting in unreliable referral processes (Jones et al., 2008; Pynoos et al., 1998).

Though many issues exist, research has shown overwhelmingly that HM services are well-received, and positive outcomes such as improved independence, heightened confidence and well-being, greater security, prevention of accidents, and improved quality of life are generally reported (Heywood & Turner, 2007; Jones et al., 2008; Petersson et al., 2008). There is, however, a clear need for the development of a research evidence base to underpin HM services development and delivery, particularly in the areas of the need and demand for HM services; the outcome and cost-effectiveness of HM as an intervention; and the identification of particular factors that impact on service provision and outcomes, including the supply of expert professionals (Heywood & Turner; Jones et al.).

Implications for the Occupational Therapist

Involvement with HM services delivery presents new challenges to occupational therapists both in the knowledge base they need to acquire and in the professional sectors with whom they collaborate. Effective HM service delivery relies on ensuring that the individual and his or her unique and particular needs remain central to the assessment and decision-making process, and the occupational therapist has a key role in ensuring that this occurs.

While the focus of occupational therapy has traditionally been on the individual receiving his or her service, therapists are increasingly being challenged to step outside of their conventional clinical roles and become involved in HM service delivery as agents of change. First and foremost, occupational therapists are well placed to observe the effect of policy and procedural issues on individual service delivery. Poor communication and information about HM service delivery and complex application procedures and forms are key barriers to effective HM service delivery against which therapists can advocate for change. Establishing and undertaking formal evaluation processes, seeking and recording individual client feedback, and providing reports of concerns to the relevant people within organizational structures are all strategies that can be undertaken by individual therapists.

A lack of awareness of the benefits of HMs is another identified barrier that occupational therapists can assist in addressing. Therapists can play a key role in the education of both community and service sectors regarding the benefits of HM through both formal presentations about the HM service to consumer and referral agencies and through informal professional networking.

Building an evidence base for intervention in this area is also an important role for the profession. Quality research into the outcomes of HMs from the perspective of the home dweller and evaluating the effectiveness of HM service delivery are areas that occupational therapists are well equipped to address. Engaging in formal evaluation of environmental interventions can yield important data that can be formulated into reports, publications, or professional presentations. Linking with agencies or institutions that may be interested in undertaking formal research, such as universities, is also advantageous for therapists in terms of professional development as well as building a much needed evidence base for practice.

CONCLUSION

This chapter has provided an overview of the development of HM services and has also identified barriers to effective service delivery. A key element of effective HM service delivery is the interaction and collaboration between key stakeholders in the HM process. While collaborating with others to achieve a positive outcome for an individual is usual

practice for occupational therapists, the HM area can provide a new challenge. Unlike more traditional areas of occupational therapist practice, HM programs straddle both health care and housing sectors and require skilled professionals from both areas. Having insight into the perspectives of all stakeholders involved in the HM process and understanding how these may impact on occupational therapy service delivery is essential for ensuring good outcomes for the home dweller. Occupational therapists need to be aware of the direction of future trends in HM policy, service design, and delivery so that they can be involved in shaping and directing future outcomes. Building a strong evidence base for effective HM intervention is an important area for occupational therapy involvement.

REFERENCES

American Occupational Therapy Association. (2008). Occupational therapy practice framework: Domain and process (2nd ed.). *American Journal of Occupational Therapy, 62*, 625-683.

Andrews, K. (2002). *National strategy for an ageing Australia: An older Australia, challenges and opportunities for all.* Canberra, Australia: Department of Health and Ageing, Commonwealth Government of Australia.

Australian Institute of Health and Welfare. (2003). *Australia's welfare 2003.* Canberra, Australia: Author.

Awang, D. (2002). Older people and participation within disabled facilities grant processes. *British Journal of Occupational Therapy, 65*(6), 261-268.

Boyt Schell, B. A. (2003). Clinical reasoning: The basis of practice. In E. B. Crepeau, E. S. Cohn, & B. A. B. Schell (Eds.), *Willard & Spackman's occupational therapy* (10th ed., pp. 131-139). Sydney, Australia: Lippincott, Williams & Wilkins.

Bricknell, S. (2003). *Disability: The use of aids and the role of the environment.* Canberra, Australia: Australian Institute of Health and Welfare.

Burns, N. (2004). Negotiating difference: Disabled people's experiences of house builders. *Housing Studies, 19*(5), 765-780.

Danford, G. S., & Steinfeld, E. (1999). Measuring the influences of physical environments on the behaviours of people with impairments. In E. Steinfeld & G. S. Danford (Eds.), *Enabling environments: Measuring the impact of environment on disability and rehabilitation* (pp. 111-137). New York, NY: Plenum Publishers.

Despres, C. (1991). The meaning of home: Literature review and directions for future research and theoretical development. *Journal of Architectural and Planning Research, 8*(2), 96-115.

Dovey, K. (1985). Home and homelessness. In I. Altman & C. M. Werner (Eds.), *Home environments* (Vol. 8, pp. 33-61). New York, NY: Plenum Press.

Duggan, R. (2005). Reflection as a means to foster client-centred practice. *Canadian Journal of Occupational Therapy, 72*(2), 103-112.

Duncan, R. (1998a). Blueprint for action: The national home modifications action coalition. *Technology and Disability, 8*, 85-89.

Duncan, R. (1998b). Funding, financing and other resources for home modifications. *Technology and Disability, 8*, 37-50.

Faulkner, D., & Bennett, K. (2002). *Linkages among housing assistance, residential (re)location and the use of community health and social care by old-old adults: Shelter and non-shelter implications for housing policy development.* Sydney, Australia: Australian Housing and Urban Research Institute.

Fitzgerald, M. H., Mullavey-O'Brien, C., & Clemson, L. (1997). Cultural issues from practice. *Australian Occupational Therapy Journal, 44,* 1-21.

Goldsmith, S. (1997) *Designing for the disabled: The new paradigm.* London, UK: Architectural Press.

Gray, L. (2001). *Two year review of aged care reforms.* Canberra, Australia: Department of Health and Aged Care, Commonwealth Government of Australia.

Hawkins, R., & Stewart, S. (2002). Changing rooms: The impact of adaptations on the meaning of home for a disabled person and the role of occupational therapists in the process. *British Journal of Occupational Therapy, 65*(2), 81-87.

Heumann, L. F., & Boldy, D. P. (Eds.). (1993). *Aging in place with dignity: International solutions relating to the low income and frail elderly.* Westport, CT: Praeger Publishers.

Heywood, F. (2004a). Understanding needs: A starting point for quality. *Housing Studies, 19*(5), 709-726.

Heywood, F. (2004b). The health outcomes of housing adaptations. *Disability & Society, 19*(2), 129-143.

Heywood, F. (2005). Adaptation: Altering the house to restore the home. *Housing Studies, 20*(4), 531-547.

Heywood, F., & Turner, L. (2007). *Better outcomes, lower costs: Implications for health and social care budgets of investment in housing adaptations, improvements and equipment: a review of the evidence.* Norwich, UK: Office of Disability Issues, Department for Work and Pensions.

Hurstfield, J., Parashar, U., & Schofield, K. (2007). *The costs and benefits of independent living.* Norwich, UK: Office of Disability Issues, Department for Work and Pensions.

Imrie, R. (2006). *Accessible housing: Quality, disability and design.* London, UK: Routledge.

Imrie, R., & Hall P. (2001). *Inclusive design: Designing and developing accessible environments.* London, UK: Spon Press.

Jones, A., de Jonge, D., & Phillips, R. (2008). *The role of home maintenance and modification services in achieving health, community care and housing outcomes in later life.* Queensland, Australia: Australian Housing and Urban Research Institute.

Kendig, H., & Gardner, I. L. (1997). Unravelling housing policy for older people. In A. Borowski, S. Encel, & E. Ozanne (Eds.), *Ageing and social policy in Australia* (pp. 175-191). Melbourne, Australia: Cambridge University Press.

Lanspery, S., Callahan, J. J. J., Miller, J. R., & Hyde, J. (1997). Introduction: Staying put. In S. Lanspery & J. Hyde (Eds.), *Staying put: Adapting the places instead of the people* (pp. 1-22). Amityville, NY: Baywood Publishing Company, Inc.

Lilja, M., Mansson, I., Jahlenius, L., & Sacco-Peterson, M. (2003). Disability policy in Sweden: Policies concerning assistive technology and home modification services. *Journal of Disability Policy Studies, 14*(3), 130-135.

Mace, R. L. (1998). Universal design in housing. *Assistive Technology, 10,* 21-28.

Milner, J., & Madigan, R. (2004). Regulation and innovation: Rethinking "inclusive" housing design. *Housing Studies, 19*(5), 727-744.

Nishita, C. M., Liebig, P. S., Pynoos, J., Perelman, L., & Spegal, K. (2007). Promoting basic accessibility in the home: Analysing patterns in the diffusion of visibility legislation. *Journal of Disability Policy Studies, 18*(1), 2-13.

Nocon, A., & Pleace, N. (1997). Until disabled people get consulted: The role of occupational therapy in meeting housing needs. *British Journal of Occupational Therapy, 60*(3), 115-122.

Petersson, I., Lilja, M., Hammel, J., & Kottorp, A. (2008). Impact of home modification services on ability in everyday life for people aging with disabilities. *Journal of Rehabilitative Medicine, 40,* 253-260.

Pickering, C., & Pain, H. (2003). Home adaptations: User perspectives on the role of professionals. *British Journal of Occupational Therapy, 66*(1), 2-8.

Pynoos, J. (1993). Toward a national policy on home modifications. *Technology and Disability, 2,* 1-8.

Pynoos, J. (2001). *Meeting the needs of older persons to age in place: Findings and recommendations for action.* Los Angeles, CA: The National Resource Center for Supportive Housing and Home Modification, Andrus Gerontology Center, University of Southern California.

Pynoos, J., Cohen, E., Davis, L., & Bernhardt, S. (1987). Home modifications: Improvements that extend independence. In V. Regnier & J. Pynoos (Eds.), *Housing the aged: Design directives and policy considerations* (pp. 277-303). New York, NY: Elsevier.

Pynoos, J., Liebig, P., Overton, J., & Calvert, E. (1997). The delivery of home modification and repair services. In S. Lanspery & J. Hyde (Eds.), *Staying put: Adapting the places instead of the people* (pp. 171-191). Amityville, NY: Baywood Publishing Company, Inc.

Pynoos, J., Nishita, C., & Perelman, L. (2003). Advancements in the home modification field: A tribute to M. Powell Lawton. *Journal of Housing for the Elderly, 17*(1&2), 105-116.

Pynoos, J., Sanford, J. A., & Rosenfelt, T. (2002). A team approach to home modifications. *OT Practice, 8,* 15-19.

Pynoos, J., Tabbarah, M., Angelli, J., & Demiere, M. (1998). Improving the delivery of home modifications. *Technology and Disability, 8,* 3-14.

Rowles, G. D. (2000). Habituation and being in place. *The Occupational Therapy Journal of Research, 20*(Suppl. 2000), 52S-67S.

Sanford, J. A., & Megrew, M. B. (1995). An evaluation of grab bars to meet the needs of elderly people. *Assistive Technology, 7*(1), 36-47.

Sixsmith, J. (1986). The meaning of home: An exploratory study of environmental experience. *Journal of Environmental Psychology, 6,* 281-298.

Smith, S. G. (1994). The essential qualities of a home. *Journal of Environmental Psychology, 14,* 31-46.

Smith, S. K., Rayer, S., & Smith, E. A. (2008). Aging and disability: Implications for the housing industry and housing policy in the United States. *Journal of the American Planning Association, 74*(3), 289-306.

Stark, S. (2004). Removing environmental barriers in the homes of older adults with disabilities improves occupational performance. *The Occupational Therapy Journal of Research: Occupational, Participation and Health, 24*(1), 32-39.

Steinfeld, E., & Danford, G. S. (1999). Theory as a basis for research on enabling environments. In E. Steinfeld & G. S. Danford (Eds.), *Enabling environments: Measuring the impact of environment on disability and rehabilitation* (pp. 11-33). New York, NY: Kluwer Academic/Plenum Publishers.

Steinfeld, E., Levine, D., & Shea, S. (1998). Home modifications and the fair housing law. *Technology and Disability, 8,* 15-35.

Steinfeld, E., & Shea, S. (1993). Enabling home environments: Identifying barriers to independence. *Technology and Disability, 2*(4), 69-79.

Stone, J. H. (1998). Housing for older persons: An international overview. *Technology and Disability, 8*(1-2), 91-97.

Tabbarah, M., Silverstein, M., & Seeman, T. (2000). A health and demographic profile of non-institutionalised older Americans residing in environments with home modifications. *Journal of Aging and Health, 12*(2), 204-228.

Tamm, M. (1999). What does a home mean and when does it cease to be a home? Home as a setting for rehabilitation and care. *Disability and Rehabilitation, 21*(2), 49-55.

Tanner, B., Tilse, C., & de Jonge, D. (2008). Restoring and sustaining home: The impact of home modifications on the meaning of home for older people. *Journal of Housing for the Elderly, 22*(3), 195-215.

Trickey, F., Maltais, M. A., Gosselin, C., & Robitaille, Y. (1993). Adapting older persons' homes to promote independence. *Physical and Occupational Therapy in Geriatrics, 12*(1), 1-14.

U.S. Department of Housing and Urban Development. (2007). *FHEO programs*. Retrieved from http://www.hud.gov/offices/fheo/progdesc/title8.cfm

U.S. Department of Justice. (2009). *Fair Housing Act*. Retrieved from http://www.justice.gov/crt/housing/title8.php

U.S. Department of Justice. (2010). *ADA home page*. Retrieved from http://www.ada.gov

Watson, L. (1997). High hopes: Making housing and community care work. Joseph Rowntree Foundation. Retrieved from http://www.jrf.org.uk

Watson, R. M. (2006). Being before doing: The cultural identity (essence) of occupational therapy. *Australian Occupational Therapy Journal, 53*, 151-158.

World Health Organization (2001). ICIDH-2: *International classification of functioning and disability*. Geneva: Author.

Wylde, M. A. (1998). Consumer knowledge of home modifications. *Technology and Disability, 8*, 51-68.

Zola, I. K. (1997). Living at home: The convergence of aging and disability. In S. Lanspery & J. Hyde (Eds.), *Staying put: Adapting the place instead of the people* (pp. 25-40). Amityville, NY: Baywood Publishing Company Inc.

Section II
Delivery of Home Modification Services

This second section focuses on the home modification process, including evaluating client need, measuring the person and the environment, and documenting this information for stakeholders involved in the process. There is information about identifying suitable interventions, the influence of design approaches and standards on practice, and sourcing and evaluating products and designs. This section also challenges occupational therapists to consider ethical and legal issues that might arise in home modification practice. Also provided is detail on the importance of evaluating client and service outcomes. This information will inform the development of occupational therapists' knowledge, skills, and abilities in using modified home environments to enable occupational performance and facilitate roles and participation in the home and community.

The Home Modification Process

Elizabeth Ainsworth, MOccThy, Grad Cert Health Sci
and Desleigh de Jonge, MPhil (OccThy), Grad Cert Soc Sci

This chapter describes the home modification process as undertaken by occupational therapists. Overall, the process involves screening and prioritizing referrals, evaluating occupational performance in the home environment, planning and negotiating interventions, and monitoring and evaluating outcomes. More specifically, occupational therapists arrange appointments, visit clients, listen to clients' stories of their experiences in the home, gather information, evaluate occupational performance, research interventions, negotiate and recommend intervention options, seek technical advice, and evaluate the effectiveness of the interventions in relation to client outcomes. At each stage of the process, occupational therapists adopt a dynamic occupation-based and client-centered approach, which is influenced by specific models of practice and guided by professional reasoning. Such practice ensures that the health and level of participation of each client is maintained or enhanced through engagement in occupation or valued daily activities.

CHAPTER OBJECTIVES

By the end of this chapter, the reader will be able to:

+ Describe the process occupational therapists use when undertaking a home modification

+ Explain the contribution of the occupational therapist, the client, and other stakeholders to the home modification process

INTRODUCTION

The home environment provides the context for many roles and activities and is an important setting for occupational therapists to examine when seeking to promote a person's occupational performance (Stark, 2003). With careful planning, people can remain in their own homes and continue to participate in community life (Law & Baum, 2005). Occupational therapists work with older people and people with disabilities to promote their engagement in life activities in the home and community. In this work, therapists develop an understanding of the interaction between the following:

+ The clients' physical, cognitive, neurobehavioral, and psychological capacities

+ Their physical, social, cultural, personal, and temporal contexts

+ The activities, tasks, and roles that clients identify as important (American Occupational Therapy Association [AOTA], 2008; Law & Baum, 2005)

Occupational therapists take a specific approach to home modification practice that is guided by a range of models of practice, the client-centered and

Ainsworth, E., & de Jonge, D.
An Occupational Therapists's Guide to Home Modification Practice (pp. 87-112)
© 2011 SLACK Incorporated

collaborative approach, and by professional reasoning. Of significance to the occupational therapy process is the importance that clients assign to their homes and the value associated with completing the home modification assessment in this environment.

Recently, ecological or transactional models in occupational therapy have recognized the dynamic relationship between the person, environment, and occupations and regard occupational performance (the ability of a person to carry out activities of daily life) as a result of the transaction between the client, the activity, and the environment or context (Brown, 2009). The focus of home modifications intervention, using these models, is to optimize occupational performance. Occupational therapists establish a picture of the person's occupational performance by gathering information about his or her occupational history, patterns of living, interests, values, needs, and priorities to develop an occupational profile (AOTA, 2008). Then, by observing how the client performs activities relevant to desired occupations, the therapist evaluates occupational performance, taking note of the effectiveness of performance and performance patterns (AOTA). The various ecological transactional models that guide this process provide the theoretical basis, or underlying concepts, that guide evaluation and the selection of environmental interventions for use to optimize occupational performance (Stark, 2003).

Occupational therapists use a client-centered and collaborative approach to ensure that they develop a deep appreciation of the client's experience and how each is managing the occupations of everyday life in the home and community. A client-centered and collaborative approach allows therapists to work in partnership with clients throughout all stages of the home modification process, including evaluation, planning, and negotiating interventions, and monitoring and measuring the outcomes (Law, Baptiste, & Mills, 1995). It honors the contributions of both the client and the occupational therapist (AOTA, 2008; Law, 1998). Clients bring their stories to the process, identifying and sharing their concerns and priorities, while therapists contribute their knowledge of occupational performance and the person-environment-occupation transaction (AOTA; Law, 1998).

Professional reasoning skills are used by therapists as they listen to clients and observe them interacting with their environment to plan, direct, perform, and reflect on the care of clients (Boyt Schell & Schell, 2008). A framework of scientific, narrative, pragmatic, and ethical reasoning is used during the home modification process to frame issues and guide problem solving and decision making.

This framework also guides therapists in selecting and negotiating interventions in collaboration with the client (Boyt Schell, 2003; Crabtree, 1998).

Throughout the home modification process, therapists remain mindful that the home is a private living space and that clients attach meaning to the home, the spaces, and the objects within it (Gitlin, in press). Interventions can have a significant impact on the home environment, which can influence clients' acceptance and adjustment to changes in the home. Consulting with the client's family, friends, caregivers, or other relevant stakeholders can also optimize collaboration, agreement with recommendations, and satisfaction and improve overall client outcomes (Law, 1998).

To ensure that home modifications are tailored to the specific needs of each client, the occupational therapy evaluation is undertaken in the home where the activities are customarily performed (Corcoran, 2005; Law, King, & Russell, 2005; Siebert, 2005). Interviewing and observing people in their home environment provides occupational therapists with an opportunity to observe activities and interactions as they occur in that setting rather than relying on reports about the situation (Corcoran) or on evaluations undertaken in an unfamiliar environment. Interviewing the client in his or her own home also enhances the occupational therapist's understanding of the environmental context in which the client operates (Corcoran).

INFLUENCES ON OCCUPATIONAL THERAPY PRACTICE

Home modification practice varies across the world in terms of the extent and types of services provided. Differing funding and service priorities mean that some communities have well-developed home modification services while others rely on a patchwork of local resources to attend to people's specific needs. The legislative context and building regulations in different jurisdictions can also affect which services are provided and how they are delivered. In some regions, home modifications are provided within health and home care services; in other locations, these services are provided within the housing and building sector.

Within services, the types and levels of occupational therapy services provided for people requiring home modifications depend on the following:

+ The service delivery requirements of the programs
+ The source and level of funding available

+ The range of intervention options supported by the service

Further, occupational therapists working in a private practice might provide a specific range of home modification services, depending on reimbursement schedules or the level of funding available for their time. Occupational therapists' experience in home modification practice varies greatly because of different types and levels of experience and the availability and quality of home modification training and building advice.

Although occupational therapists might not be involved in the whole home modification process, they could still be required to provide the client with assistance and advice at any stage. For example, occupational therapists may be contacted to undertake the whole home modification process; they may be required to work with the client up to the point of identifying interventions; they may need to check modifications proposed by alternative parties to provide advice on their suitability or whether changes are required; or they may need to visit the client to train him or her in the use of the home modification after it has been installed. At times, the therapist might be required to visit a person's home to examine a modification that is not achieving the desired outcome to suggest alternative interventions. The timing and extent of occupational therapists' involvement during the home modification process depends on whether the referrer and other stakeholders understand the role or contribution of occupational therapists in the home modification process and whether occupational therapists have sufficient expertise in the area. With a good understanding of the role of occupational therapists, other parties concerned—such as clients, health and community care professionals, program administrators, insurance companies, lawyers, and design and construction professionals—can involve therapists constructively throughout the process.

Occupational therapists with appropriate knowledge and experience are able to demonstrate the benefits of their involvement at various stages and be called on repeatedly to contribute their expertise.

STAGES OF THE HOME MODIFICATION PROCESS

There are a number of stages in the home modification process, from the initial referral to the final evaluation of the home modification after installation. The specific stages of the home modification process include the following:

+ Receiving and analyzing the referral information
+ Prioritizing referrals
+ Arranging the home visit with the client
+ Preparing for the home visit
+ Traveling to the home and meeting the client
+ Entering the property
+ Interviewing the client
+ Inspecting the home
+ Measuring the client and his or her equipment and/or caregiver
+ Photographing, measuring, and drawing the built environment
+ Planning, selecting, and negotiating a range of interventions
+ Concluding the home visit
+ Seeking technical advice
+ Writing the report and completing drawings
+ Submitting the report to the referrer
+ Educating and training the client in the use of the home modifications
+ Evaluating the home modifications after installation

Occupational therapists can enter and exit at various points of the home modification service delivery, depending on the type and level of service required by the referrer, their level of expertise, and the expertise of other stakeholders involved in the process.

Receiving and Analyzing the Referral Information

The home modification process begins with the occupational therapist receiving and analyzing the referral information (Figure 6-1).

There are a range of reasons for seeking home modification advice from occupational therapists. Clients might have a newly diagnosed health condition, or they might have experienced a recent injury that requires changes to their existing environment before they can be discharged from care. Individuals might be aging and experiencing increasing difficulty coping in their current home situation. Home modifications might also be sought when people move to a new environment that does not adequately support their occupational performance. Alternatively, there might be changes to someone's social context or roles that impact on the fit between their performance skills and patterns, activity demands, and the environment (Siebert, 2005).

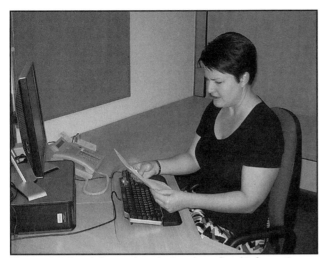

Figure 6-1. Receiving and analyzing the referral information.

Requests for a home modification evaluation are generally received from health practitioners and community and home care service providers; however, increasingly, informed clients and caregivers are contacting occupational therapists for home modification services. Referrals can arrive by phone, e-mail, fax, or letter and can contain variable amounts of information. Most contain a general request for a home evaluation because of an individual's health condition, injury, or increasing frailty. Some referrals seek a specific environmental intervention—for example, grab bars beside the toilet.

The referral stage signals the start of information gathering. As therapists review referrals, they note essential information, such as the client's name, address, and age. This background information and other details, such as the person's disability, health condition, or age-related changes, are entered into the service database often to assist with recording and tracking service requests and events. Existing records can be reviewed to determine whether clients have been seen previously and the nature of services they have accessed. Prior to the visit, therapists might need to carry out research on specific disabilities or health conditions to understand them more fully, their presentation and functional implications, in order to develop hypotheses about their likely impact on occupational performance and potential environmental barriers. Such information can help therapists think through the range of suitable interventions in advance of the home visit. Further, an understanding of prognoses alerts therapists to future equipment and support requirements that might need to be considered when planning interventions.

Other referral information of interest is whether the person is currently using equipment or receiving assistance in the home. If occupational therapists are not familiar with the equipment listed, they might have to undertake background research to ensure that they are well informed about the specifications of the equipment and how such devices can be used. Caregiver or family support information provides a prompt for the occupational therapist to ensure that these people are present at the time of the home visit and to engage them in the home-visit process (Klein, Rosage, & Shaw, 1999). It is also important to note who lives at home with the client and whether there are any regular visitors or guests. People who use the home environment regularly will also need to be consulted when devising environmental interventions, especially if substantial changes are to be made to the home.

Information about the treating doctor, therapist, nurse, or other service providers is also required to ensure that relevant providers can be contacted for further information or to discuss the suitability of interventions. It should be noted, however, that informed consent should be obtained from the client before making contact with these providers.

The referral might include information about the style of home or any environmental barriers being experienced in the home. The details about the style of home can provide an indication of any other environmental barriers in addition to those already documented. For example, knowing that a person with mobility impairment is living in an older, two-story house alerts the therapist to examine the condition of the stairs, stair usage, and the range of activities undertaken on the upper level.

Some specialist home modification providers and private therapists have developed a dedicated home modification referral information form to gather referral information and document other background information essential to providing a timely and appropriate service. The quality of referral information varies greatly in detail and quality. Referrers generally provide information on client demographics, background information on the person's disability and/or health condition, and a general statement of need. However, in order to prepare effectively for the visit, therapists require additional detail including the following:

+ The referrer and accompanying documentation
+ The current use of equipment and health and community services
+ The style of the home and existing environmental barriers
+ The type of modification/service required
+ The ownership of the home

+ The need for an interpreter or formal or informal decision maker

+ Other household members

In addition, to assist therapists in establishing timelines for service provision, they:

+ Require critical timeframes—for example, the client's expected discharge or court date

+ Need to know the level of risk to the client in his or her current situation—for example, the prevalence or likelihood of accident or injury, restricted activity, or unwanted dependence

Figure 6-2 is a sample home modification referral information form. When therapists make their initial phone calls to clients to set up a time for their home visit, this is a good opportunity to discuss occupational performance issues experienced in the home and to explain the role of the occupational therapist. Clients' expectations can be clarified in relation to the home modification and the timing, duration, and process of the home visit. Information gathered during these calls might also highlight additional issues—for example, that the client is not eligible for a particular service and might require a referral to an alternative.

Prioritizing Referrals

Occupational therapists often have to prioritize their work and allocate their time judiciously, especially if their services are in demand. Referrals are generally prioritized in light of the urgency of each individual client's need as well as the relative importance with respect to other referrals (Bradford, 1998). Factors to consider when prioritizing referrals are listed in Table 6-1.

When considering the urgency of referrals, therapists consider whether clients are at risk of being involved in an adverse event resulting in reduced activity, injury, institutionalization, or premature death if they are not visited immediately. Those who are at high risk are prioritized as being urgent. For example, an urgent home visit may be required if a referral indicates that the client has had falls in the home, has been hospitalized, and is not able to return home without adequate services and modifications. Alternatively, a visit may be considered non-urgent if the client has activity limitations that can be improved in the short-term with the use of equipment that can be purchased or borrowed or if they have care support in the home. Once the urgency of each client is determined, clients are then prioritized based on the degree of risk in relation to other people on the waiting list.

When determining the level of urgency, therapists need to determine and record the likelihood of an adverse event occurring and the consequences of an event.

For example, in the urgent case described above, the therapist would record that the client was highly likely to receive an injury resulting in further hospitalization should he or she return home without appropriate interventions. The non-urgent case would be recorded as being unlikely to result in an adverse event in the form of an injury and that any activity restrictions could be mitigated by the use of equipment while awaiting a home modification assessment (Table 6-2).

Where cases are not easily assessed as being high or low risk, various resources and tools are available to assist with decision making. For example, as illustrated in Figure 6-3, any event that is considered highly likely and with a high or moderate level of consequences would be considered high risk and therefore classified as urgent. Equally, any event that results in a high level of consequences and is highly or moderately likely is also considered to be high risk and therefore urgent. When events are unlikely to occur and have a low to moderate level of consequences, they are considered a low risk and priority. Similarly, events that have no or low consequences and have a low to moderate likelihood of occurring are low risk and priority; and events that have low likelihood with high consequence, moderate likelihood with moderate consequence, or high likelihood with low consequence would be considered as moderately risky and therefore prioritized over the low-risk cases (Pybus, 1996).

Arranging the Home Visit With the Client

Once the priority of the referral has been determined, the occupational therapist contacts the client by phone or letter within the recommended timeframe to arrange the home visit (Figure 6-4). Alternatively, the client may be advised that he or she has been placed on a waiting list and will be contacted in the future to arrange an appointment, assuming personal needs do not change. If clients are on a waiting list, they should be advised to contact the home modification program and the occupational therapist should their situation change. Clients might need to be reprioritized if their need for a visit becomes urgent or if their risk of accident, injury, or institutionalization increases.

Occupational Therapy Home Modification Referral Information Form

Demographic Information:

Client name:

Address:

Phone number:

Date of birth:

Gender:

ID number:

Referral Information:

Date of referral:

Referral source (including contact details):

Client's advocate or spokesperson (including contact details):

Does the client require an interpreter?

Does the client wish to have a particular person at the interview? If so, please provide the person's name and contact details.

Type of Referral:

Home modification:

Post modification evaluation:

Other:

List of Documentation Received

Confidential medical report from a doctor or other medical personnel:

Authority to request or disclose client information:

Other:

Health Condition or Disability Information

List client's health condition or disability, or details about any age related changes:

Is the client's condition permanent, improving, deteriorating, temporary or stable?

Has the client experienced a recent significant change in function or mobility? Describe.

Has there been a recent significant change in function or mobility?

What medication is the client taking for their conditions?

How many times has the client been hospitalized in the last 12 months?

What were the reasons for the client's hospitalization?

Is the client receiving family or informal caregiver assistance or community services to assist with self-care or home-maker tasks, or access within the community?

What community services or informal support services are being received by the client (include information on the treating doctor, therapist, nurse, or other service providers)?

Does the client live: alone, with a caregiver who is well, or with a caregiver who is aging or has a health or medical condition?

Figure 6-2. Sample Occupational Therapy Home Modification Referral Information Form (continued).

Description of the Client's Equipment

List the items of equipment that the client is currently using in the home and community to assist with mobility and day-to-day activities:

Description of the Home Environment

Describe the style of the client's home:

Is home owned or rented? If rented, state length of lease.

Description of the Environmental Barriers

Describe the environmental barriers being encountered by the client.

Describe the impact these barriers have on client or caregiver functioning.

Description of the Client's Home Modification Request:

Urgency of Home Visit

Provide an opinion on home modifications requirements:

Describe urgency of need for home modifications:

Occupational Therapist's Comments:

Signature Block

Staff Person Receiving Referral

 Name:

 Position Title:

 Signature:

 Date:

 Facility or Agency:

 Program:

Occupational Therapist Receiving or Reviewing Referral

 Name:

 Signature:

 Date:

 Facility or Agency:

 Program:

Figure 6-2 (continued). Sample Occupational Therapy Home Modification Referral Information Form.

Table 6-1. Considerations When Prioritizing Referrals

PRIORITY	High	Moderate	Moderate to low	Low
RESPONSE	See within the week	See within few weeks	See within 2 months	See within 6 months
CONSEQUENCE	Event likely to result in death or hospitalization	Event likely to result in compromised health or performance	Event likely to compromise independence	Event likely to impact on quality of life and participation
LIKELIHOOD	High likelihood of adverse event	Moderate likelihood of adverse event	Low likelihood of adverse event	Adverse event unlikely
TYPE OF LIMITATION	Transfers, mobility, and hygiene activities such as toileting and bathing	Other self-care activities such as eating and dressing	Cleaning, shopping, cooking, laundry	Leisure and community participation
ABILITY TO FUNCTION	Unable to perform essential elements of the activity	Difficulty performing essential elements of the activity	Difficulty performing some essential elements of the activity	Little difficulty performing essential elements of the activity
ALTERNATIVES	No viable alternative possible	Alternative method or equipment option possible but does not address issue fully	Alternative method or equipment option can temporarily address issue	Alternative method or equipment option possible
AVAILABLE SUPPORT	No alternative support available	No alternative support available onsite but can be purchased	No alternative support available onsite but can be accessed at no cost	Alternative support available onsite
TIMING	Palliative condition	Chronic/lifelong condition	Fluctuating condition	Acute, short-term condition

Table 6-2. Prioritization Table

NAME	SUSPECTED ENVIRONMENTAL HAZARD/BARRIER	CONSEQUENCE	LIKELIHOOD	URGENCY OF HOME VISIT
Mrs. Jones	Slippery bathroom floor	Injury—fall	High—already been hospitalized	High
Mrs. Smith	Low toilet	Reduced activity performance	Low—can be managed with additional equipment or caregiver support in interim	Low

The Timing and Duration of the Home Visit

The timing of the home visit is generally determined by the urgency of the client's situation and the availability of the client and other members of the household. Clients at high risk of injury will need to be seen urgently, whereas others can be scheduled routinely. The timing of the home visit might also need to be planned around the expected date of discharge from the hospital. If the client requires urgent home modifications to ensure his or her safety, the occupational therapist might undertake a home visit before or immediately after discharge. If it is not possible to complete all of the required work in time, the therapist might recommend basic modifications and plan a second visit to discuss other interventions after the client has returned home. In some instances, when the person has recently acquired a disabling condition, the occupational therapist might delay the visit until after the person has been living in the home for a short period and has had time to settle into his or her new routine and identify the environmental barriers. This can help

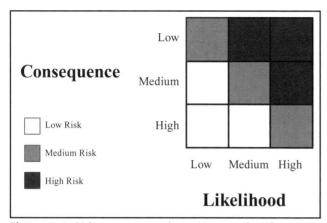

Figure 6-3. Risk assessment chart. (Reprinted with permission from *Safety Management: Strategy and Practice*, Pybus, R. Copyright © Elsevier 1996.)

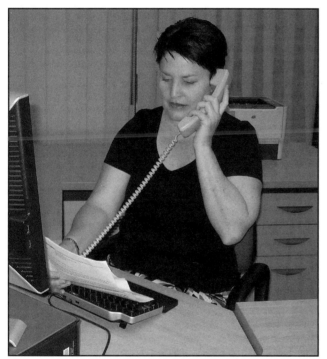

Figure 6-4. Contacting the client to arrange a home visit.

the service or reimbursement system may allocate a specific amount of time for home visits as defined by the client's health condition or the identified need. However, sometimes the complexity of the situation might only become evident during the visit.

There are a range of issues that can affect the timing and duration of the home visit. These include the following:

+ The energy levels of the client: The client might have limited physical, cognitive, or psychological capacity, which means that he or she can only manage short visits or visits conducted at particular times during the day or week.

+ The number of people in attendance to contribute to the decision-making process: The occupational therapist might need to negotiate an appointment time to suit a number of people and spend considerable time listening to the views of the client and others when gathering information and negotiating a range of intervention options.

+ The amount of equipment used: The occupational therapist might need time to undertake extensive measurement of the client, his or her equipment, and the home environment to determine the person's body dimensions, reach range, circulation, and storage space and dimensions and location of fittings and fixtures in the environment.

+ The number and nature of occupational performance difficulties being experienced: If the person is having trouble with a number of activities, the occupational therapist will need to allocate a reasonable timeframe to ensure that performance in each activity is adequately evaluated.

+ The number and type of barriers in the home environment: Some houses present numerous barriers to performance; others present challenges to being modified. The occupational therapist might need to take numerous photos and approximate measurements and seek technical advice from design or building professionals before the design of the modification. The greater the number and extent of environmental and construction barriers, the more time required.

If considerable time is required to evaluate the person, his or her occupational performance, and the home environment, the visit time may need to be extended or additional visits booked (Silverstein & Hyde, 1997). If the occupational therapist has been allocated only a limited time for the home visit, he or she will need to negotiate with the client and formulate a mutually agreeable structure for the interview,

the client make well-informed decisions about the issues and interventions required. When arranging home visits around the availability of the client, it is important to be aware that clients are often reliant on others for help with bathing, shopping, and medical appointments. Therefore, occupational therapists may need to arrange the visit around other scheduled activities.

The duration of home visits varies and should be negotiated with the client when making the appointment. Generally, occupational therapists are able to anticipate the time required for the visit, based on the referral or the initial conversation. Alternatively, allocating a specific time period for each stage of the visit, including the interview, observation, measurement, walk-through of the home, and discussion of intervention options.

Clients should be advised to have all concerned parties present at the visit. Involving the various stakeholders in the home modification process ensures that all relevant issues are discussed and carefully considered and that intervention options developed are acceptable and useful to everyone affected by them (Klein et al., 1999). Further, involving stakeholders at the time of the visit is likely to reduce the number of discussions and meetings, phone calls, and/or subsequent visits required to consult with various parties.

If clients rely on equipment to undertake different activities in the home, they need to be advised to have devices available at the time of the home visit. This allows the occupational therapist to measure them and observe their use in the home. Further home visits might be required if the client does not have his or her equipment available at the time of the initial home visit, particularly if the equipment dimensions and space requirements (with or without a caregiver using the equipment) are likely to impact on the design of the home modification.

Preparing for the Home Visit

Being well prepared ensures that the home visit is productive and efficient. Occupational therapists prepare for home visits by doing the following:

+ Filling in interview forms with relevant referral information in advance of the visit

+ Gathering required home visiting resources

+ Compiling appropriate forms and evaluation tools for information gathering

+ Collecting evaluation and environmental measurement tools

+ Collating information on various intervention options

Prior to the visit, therapists should read the referral information and any other background information on record and transfer relevant information onto forms to be used during the visit. It is also useful to take the referral documentation on the visit to confirm and clarify information with the client.

Therapists should ensure that they gather a range of resources that can be used during a home visit, including the following:

+ Personal identification information

+ A clipboard and pens or computer technology, such as a laptop or pocket PC

+ Occupational therapy evaluation tools, including interview guides, checklists, and report forms (if they are not on the laptop)

+ Extra paper and pencils for drawing diagrams

+ A cell phone

+ A street directory or satellite-navigation system for directions to the property

+ Water

+ Written information on whom to contact in the event of an emergency, such as a car breakdown

+ A first-aid kit in the vehicle

The forms that need to be taken on home visits can include an interview form with prompts, a home visit checklist listing specific features in different areas of the home, and privacy or consent forms—for use when information needs to be sought from other service providers, such as the doctor, hospital therapists, or home and community care nurses. Occupational therapists may need to take photos of the person and/or areas of the home, which might require the client's verbal and/or written permission.

Evaluation tools such as the Canadian Occupational Performance Measure (COPM; Law et al., 1998), the Performance Assessment of Self-Care Skills (PASS-Home; Rogers & Holm, 2007), the Safer-Home (Chiu & Oliver, 2006), the Housing Enabler (Iwarsson & Slaugh, 2001), and other standardized tools can be used to establish a picture of the person-environment-occupation transaction and provide a base measure of performance for comparison with outcomes measures (Law & Baum, 2005).

The choice of environmental measurement tools depends on the environmental barriers highlighted in the referral information. It is useful to have a kit that holds the following tools—with appropriate instruction sheets and forms—on all home visits:

+ 18-foot tape measure (5 meters) to measure dimensions

+ Distance meter to measure long distances

+ Camera (and spare batteries) for photos of the environmental barriers and the client's equipment to keep as a record from the visit and to incorporate into the home modification report

+ Light meter to measure lighting levels

+ Force measure

+ Electronic clinometer to measure the horizontal gradients of landings, paths, ramps, floors

+ String line and spirit level for setting out the proposed configuration of an outdoor ramp

Prior to the visit, therapists also need to research and collate resource information to take with them to assist with intervention planning. The resource information might include the following:

+ Drawings (site and floor plans or elevations) or photos of modified environments to show the client examples of completed work

+ Access standards or guidelines and/or local building codes relevant to the type of home being visited (to discuss specific design requirements with the client)

+ Photos and product information (for example, brochures or information from the Internet) to show the client illustrations of home modification designs and products and equipment solutions

Equipment such as an over-toilet frame or a bath board can serve as a less costly alternative to a home modification, and these may be taken on the home visit to try and evaluate suitability.

Safety Considerations

Prior to the visit, it is important that occupational therapists evaluate potential risks to themselves and the client during the home visit and ensure that safety measures are put in place.

Communicating the Home Visit Schedule

As a safety precaution, occupational therapists should advise their fellow workers of their schedule, the addresses and phone numbers of the clients they will be visiting, the expected duration of these visits, and their cell phone number. Staff working in private practice might need to identify a suitable contact and advise this person of their whereabouts, especially if they work on their own, outside of business hours, or in isolated locations.

Identification and Clothing

Occupational therapists should have personal identification on them at all times. They should also ensure that their appearance and clothing are appropriate and reflect community standards, in particular those that meet the expectations of the older generation. For example, when visiting older people, it is advisable for female occupational therapists to wear trousers rather than skirts to enable them to maintain their modesty while moving into various positions during measuring. It is also preferable that occupational therapists not wear shirts with plunging necklines or shorts or jeans that are low cut. Therapists should also wear enclosed shoes with low heels because they are likely to be walking on a variety of surfaces, both within and outside of the home. Shoes that can be slipped on and off easily allow occupational therapists to remove shoes before entering the house. When visiting construction sites, clothing and shoes should comply with workplace health and safety requirements. In such situations, occupational therapists may need hard hats and steel-tip boots.

Personal Safety, Training, and Support

Therapists need to be conscious of the environments they are entering and the background of the people they are visiting. They need to have plans in place to ensure their safety.

It is always advisable for occupational therapists to carry a cell phone at the time of the home visit. On arrival, they need to ensure that their vehicle is located in a safe, well-lit, easy-to-access location near the premises. The car should be parked on the street or in a designated parking area and should not block residents or caregivers needing access to and from the home.

A visual check of the property on entry can also provide information as to whether there are pets that might pose a safety risk to visitors. Discussion might be needed about restraining pets if the therapist is concerned about the animal or feels that it might disrupt the home visit.

Inside the premises, therapists should ensure that they position themselves between the client and the exit to ensure obstacle-free egress in the event of an adverse event. If the client or other householders exhibit any unusual behavior, it is advisable to record this information on file or report it to a supervisor on returning to the office. Similarly, if an adverse incident occurs at the time of the home visit, the therapist must advise a supervisor as soon as the home visit is completed and make a record of the incident on file.

Where therapists are dealing with remote, complex, or challenging clients, it is advisable for them to undergo safety training. At times, it might be necessary to take another person along on a visit. For example, if a client lives in a remote region that requires hours of driving, a second person might be required to share the driving and ensure safety in a remote location. When clients are frail, unwell, or live alone, the occupational therapist might require assistance to assess the person's safety in performing a range of activities in an unsupportive environment. If an occupational therapist is visiting a client who has just left a mental health facility or prison, he or she might need another staff member for support.

Traveling to the Home and Meeting the Client

The home visit process begins well before the therapist reaches the front door of the client's home (Figure 6-5). Occupational therapists survey the community and gather information en route to the person's home (Klein et al., 1999). They observe the location of local facilities in relation to the client's premises; the type and location of public transport; the general topography of the district; the presence and condition of footpaths, curbs, and roads in the surrounding area; and the style and condition of housing in the neighborhood. By observing the client's surroundings, therapists can gain an understanding of the potential environmental barriers to participation in the community. It also enables them to ensure that modifications to the exterior of the home will fit with the look of the rest of the street and neighborhood.

Entering the Property

Occupational therapists, prior to the visit, should ensure that they have the client's permission to enter the property (Figure 6-6). On walking to the front door, the therapist may notice aspects of the external layout of the home that might affect the client's occupational performance. For example, the therapist might note the slope of the land just outside of the boundary for street access to the site, the height and style of fencing for privacy, the slope of the land within the boundary, and the presence of any steps. It can also be noted whether paths are free of hazards and obstacles, the number of risers on the stairs, the condition of the steps and handrails, the presence of light fittings, and the age and style of home. These observations alert the therapist to potential barriers to occupational performance that may require further discussion and consideration (Figure 6-7).

When meeting the client at the front entry, the therapist should introduce him- or herself, show identification, and confirm that the client is available to begin the home visit and is comfortable with the therapist entering the home. As a courtesy, it is suggested to ask whether shoes need to be removed before entering.

On entry, the therapist should observe the environment to ascertain his or her level of personal safety. If there is any feeling of unease for any reason during the home visit, the therapist needs to discontinue the visit and exit the premises. If there are no perceived threats, the visit can proceed, and the therapist can establish a presence in the home.

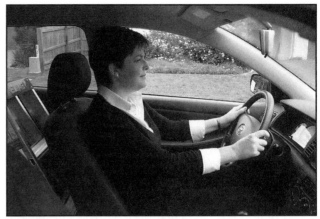

Figure 6-5. Driving to the client's home.

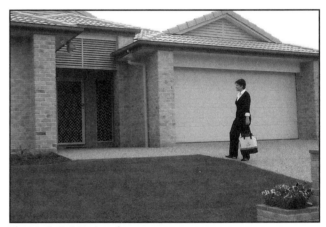

Figure 6-6. Entering the property.

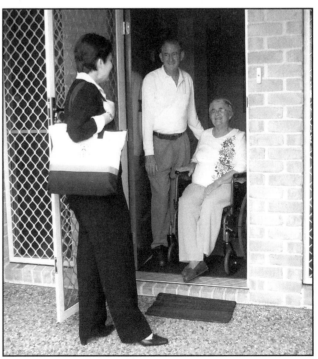

Figure 6-7. Observing the property features and the client.

The occupational therapist should ask the client and other householders where they would be most comfortably seated and ensure that this location is well-suited to conducting an interview and viewing resource materials. The occupational therapist then takes the seat suggested by the client. The therapist may politely request that seating be rearranged, the radio or television be turned off, or lights be turned on to create a more conducive interview environment.

If the client offers a drink, the therapist can accept it and use this time to establish a rapport. It is also an opportunity to become familiar with the home environment, commenting, for example, on the view; the décor; or the prints, objects, or photos on display. The therapist might note the layout and condition of the home, existing obstacles, and lighting and discuss issues of concern with the client as they become relevant during the interview.

The therapist might also use this opportunity to observe the client as he or she prepares the refreshments, noting any concerns about mobility, ability to structure and complete the task, as well as concentration and communication during the activity. The therapist should be aware that performance during this activity may not be representative of the person's usual performance and that hypotheses formulated at this time need to be confirmed through further evaluation.

When the client is finally seated, the therapist makes a full introduction, providing information about the home modification program, his or her role, and the purpose of the visit. The therapist should introduce him- or herself to everyone present and develop an understanding of each person's relationship with the client and his or her place in the home and its routines. The therapist may also need to clarify each person's role in any decision making to do with modification of the home environment. For example, the client's husband might have been involved in building and maintaining the home and would therefore need to be consulted about changes; a community care nurse might provide assistance during bathing and would therefore need to be consulted about modifications to the bathroom; the client's daughter might be concerned about disruptions to the household that would necessitate her accommodating her parents if major modifications are undertaken.

In different situations, the occupational therapist might have to vary the way the visit is conducted. For example, the therapist might sit and complete the interview first before asking the client to show how he or she currently undertakes activities in various areas of the home. Alternatively, the client may be anxious to discuss his or her concerns and

show the problem areas in the home first to ensure that the occupational therapist is clear about the issues. The therapist might also decide that viewing the home is important before the interview because it could provide important information on the layout of the home and specific fixtures and fittings. Regardless of the order of events, it is essential that the therapist gains all of the information required before discussing interventions.

Interviewing the Client

At the start of the interview process, the occupational therapist confirms the referral information and the background details with the client to ensure these are accurate (Figure 6-8). During the interview, the therapist listens to the person's story to understand the following:

+ The person's health condition and concerns
+ Activities, routines, and roles within the home and community
+ Use of the various areas of the home
+ The personal meaning of the home, including the objects, spaces, and features within the home
+ The history of the home
+ The person's future hopes and dreams in relation to his or her home (Siebert, 2005)

The occupational therapist can use a series of open and closed questions to develop a deeper understanding of the person, his or her occupations, and occupational performance concerns and barriers in the home environment. This questioning process involves identifying and defining issues of importance to the client and understanding the history and routines within the household and how these may influence the nature, feasibility, and appropriateness of interventions (Siebert, 2005). The client's wants, needs, occupational risks, and problems are evaluated, and information is gathered, synthesized, and framed from an occupational perspective (AOTA, 2008). This information is then considered as the occupational therapist observes the client undertaking various activities in the home at a later stage in the visit.

Information gathered at the time of the interview is documented to ensure a record of the detail is retained (Stark, 2003). Occupational therapists may use one or more of the following to document information:

+ A notebook for handwritten interview notes or drawings
+ Paper forms with key headings or checklists to guide the interview process

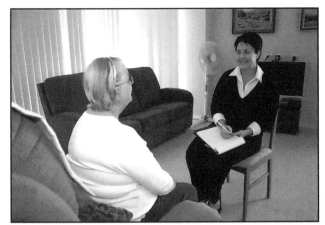

Figure 6-8. Interviewing the client.

+ Personal computers (handheld or laptop or tablet) that contain documents with key headings or checklists. This technology may be used to type in responses directly or convert handwriting to text and upload photos so that changes can be drawn on the photo directly.

+ Digital pens and dedicated documents with key headings or checklists. The digital pens can record handwriting and drawings or convert these to text and electronic diagrams.

The type of technology used depends on a range of factors, including the therapist's experience with, and confidence in, using technology; the cost, availability, and reliability of the technology; and access to technical support.

Inspecting the Home

During the visit, the therapist examines the environment carefully to develop a full understanding of its layout, structure, fixtures and fittings, and the barriers to occupational performance (Figures 6-9 through 6-11). Of particular interest will be:

+ External access around the home—for example, access to the mailbox, trash cans, clothesline, pool, greenhouse, front and back yards, and to the front gate; the quality and type of paths, stairs, ramps, and driveway areas

+ Internal access within the home—for example, the layout of the home (open plan or with corridors); the location and number of internal stairs; the number of bedrooms and route of access to the various areas of the home; changes in floor levels and the types of floor finishes

+ Kitchen, bathroom, laundry, and bedrooms—for example, layout and the types of fittings and fixtures

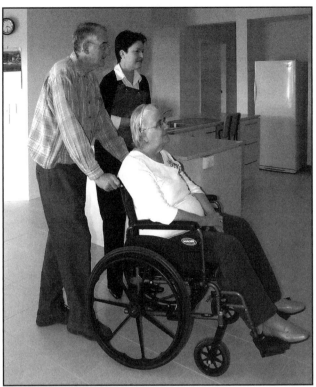

Figure 6-9. Inspecting the home with the client.

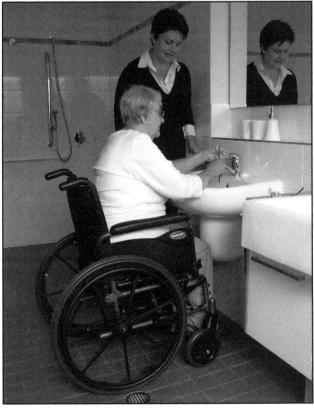

Figure 6-10. Observing the client.

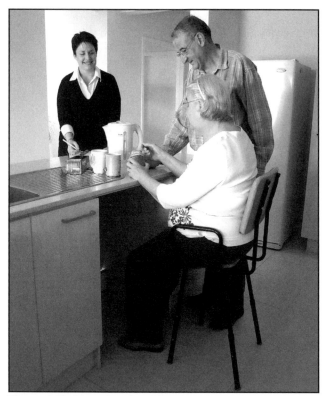

Figure 6-11. Observing the client.

+ Car-parking facilities—for example, space, lighting, and access

+ Access to the vehicle or public transport—for example, access from the car parking facility to the home, the distance to public transport facilities

A walk-through of the different areas with the client will enable the occupational therapist to analyze the physical environment and its potential to enhance or constrain occupational performance (Siebert, 2005). It will also afford the client an opportunity to show where occupational performance difficulties occur. The occupational therapist then uses skilled observation and occupational analysis to analyze the client's occupational performance as he or she demonstrates activities of concern or simulates elements of activities, such as transfers, bending, and reaching (Klein et al., 1999). The therapist listens to the client's concerns and then observes his or her performance, analyzing the sequence of activities and discussing how, when, where, and why the difficulties occur with the client (Ohta & Ohta, 1997). This ensures that the hypotheses formulated by the therapist about the person's capacity at the time of referral and interview are fully explored and validated or refuted as appropriate. Examining occupational performance in different areas of the home with the client ensures that he or she understands how the current design and layout of the home, or the existing fittings and fixtures, might hamper occupational performance and allows the therapist to discuss potential environmental modifications.

Measuring the Client, Equipment, and Caregiver

The occupational therapist might need to measure the client, his or her equipment, and the caregiver to determine the required size of openings and circulation spaces and the location of fittings and fixtures (Figures 6-12 through 6-14).

When the client's dimensions are required, the therapist measures the following:

+ Height, width, and length of various body parts

+ Reach range in seated and/or standing positions

+ Eye height and examines his or her visual fields

In addition, the therapist measures the height, length, width, and circulation space of the equipment and caregivers. The therapist also checks the positioning and movement of the client with the equipment and caregivers in relation to managing the spaces, fittings, and fixtures. This information ensures that spaces can be designed to optimize the ease of approach and use and that fixtures and fittings are within reach.

If there are going to be multiple users of a specific area, the anthropometrics of all users will need to be considered in the redesign of space and placement of fittings and fixtures, with adjustable options being integrated into the design if necessary.

Photographing, Measuring, and Drawing the Environment

Drawings and photographs can become a valuable record of the home visit and can be used to complement the written detail in the report. Therapists are reminded to seek permission from clients to photograph, measure, and draw areas of the home.

Photographs

Therapists may take photos of key areas and features in the home from various angles to ensure that comprehensive information is collected. Photographs can be useful in reports because they add visual detail about the home and environmental barriers. Digital photographs can be easily inserted into a Word document and can be annotated by hand or electronically to highlight barriers and illustrate where the modifications are to be installed.

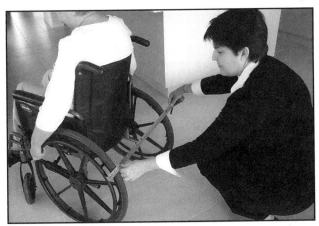

Figure 6-12. Measuring the client's equipment.

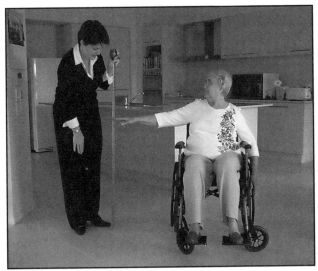

Figure 6-13. Measuring the client's reach range.

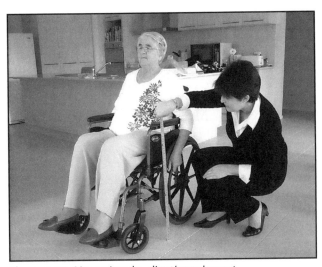

Figure 6-14. Measuring the client's equipment.

A digital photo might also be useful for the therapist to discuss the environmental barriers and range of solutions with the client if he or she is not able to access an area of the home. Printouts can be drawn on to illustrate the location of the proposed modifications. Photos can also serve as a record of the environment before, during, and after the home modification and can be a visual aid for informing other clients, their families, and caregivers about alternative environmental interventions.

Measurements

The occupational therapist needs to collect a comprehensive set of measurements of the problem areas in the home environment (Figures 6-15 and 6-16). Measurements of features that are working well for the client should also be taken so that these dimensions can be incorporated in any redesign.

The type of measurements taken will depend on the environmental barriers or enablers identified. Measurements can include lengths, widths, depths, and heights of fittings, fixtures, and the circulation spaces in problem areas of the home. It might also be necessary to measure the spaces adjacent to or along a path of travel to these areas as these areas might need to be incorporated in the final redesign. It is advisable to collect any additional measurements that might be useful if alternative solutions need to be explored at a later stage.

All relevant measurement information, including drawings of the layout of specific areas in floor plan and elevation views, is recorded at the time of the visit and is incorporated in the design of the modification.

Chapter 8 provides further information about measuring the person and the environment.

Drawings

Measurements of the environment are recorded on a concept drawing, which can be used when communicating design requirements to various stakeholders.

Therapists employ various drawing methods, depending on their expertise and the type of work they do. They may choose to take only approximate measurements and create concept sketches to send on to a skilled contractor or building design professional to refine and develop into scale drawings. Alternatively, they may develop simple concept drawings, drawn to scale, to ensure that there is adequate space for circulation and fixtures and fittings in the proposed design before passing it on to building and design professionals for detailed drawings. Therapists should check the level of service they are required to provide with their licensing

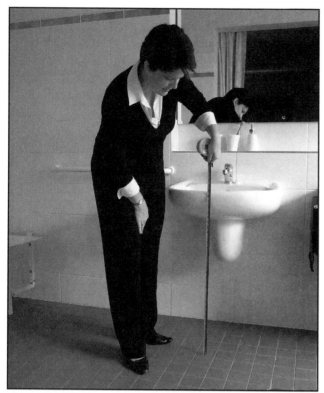

Figure 6-15. Measuring the environment.

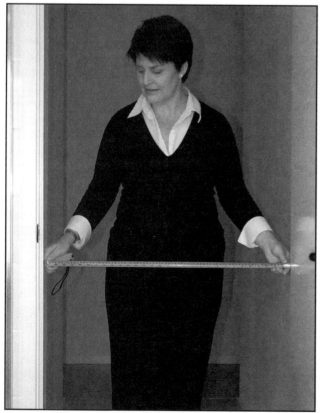

Figure 6-16. Measuring the environment.

boards to ensure that they do not work outside of their scope of practice.

Once a draftsperson or builder has developed a scale drawing, the therapist needs to review the drawing and evaluate the usefulness of the design for each individual. A scale ruler is used at this point to confirm that required clearances and circulation spaces have been included in the design.

Chapter 9 provides information on drawing the built environment.

Planning, Selecting, and Negotiating Interventions

An individual's occupational performance can be enhanced through a range of interventions, such as seeking alternative ways to undertake activities, providing assistive devices and social supports, and/or modifying the home environment (Figure 6-17). Once therapists have a clear understanding of the client's occupational profile and his or her key occupational performance issues, they can select, review, negotiate, plan, and implement a range of suitable interventions. When designing interventions, therapists draw on theory, practice models, and research evidence and use professional reasoning to choose the best solution for each situation (AOTA, 2008; Boyt Schell, 2003; Fisher, 1998).

Occupational therapists collaborate with clients to establish short- and long-term goals related to occupational performance in the home and community (Grayson, 1997). Short-term goals might include addressing problems associated with performance components or environmental issues; long-term goals might be to maintain or enhance the performance of daily occupations related to performing different roles in the home and community (Law & Baum, 2005). Once the client's goals are identified and prioritized, the therapist works with him or her to identify the interventions to address these goals (AOTA, 2008).

When an extensive number of changes is required, staff may need to discuss the list of recommendations with clients and, if relevant, caregivers, so that items can be prioritized (Connell & Sanford, 1997; Silverstein & Hyde, 1997). Prioritizing home modifications is especially important if there are issues relating to the funding and timing of the work.

Factors Influencing Intervention Options

The process of planning and discussing intervention options with the client can be a complex undertaking influenced by a range of factors: client related, therapist related, and environment related.

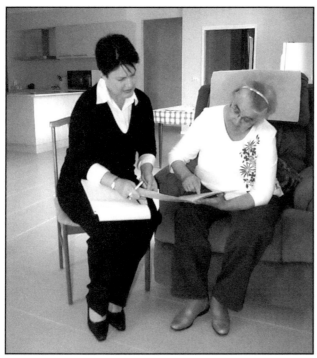

Figure 6-17. Planning, selecting, and negotiating interventions.

Client-Related Factors

Occupational therapists should consider various areas of the home as they talk through the range of intervention options. Clients may be unable to change when and how specific activities are undertaken and therefore may be reluctant to consider some intervention options. However, they can also grow accustomed to reduced levels of performance and underestimate the barriers in the home environment (Pynoos, Sanford, & Rosenfelt, 2002; Wylde, 1998). Interventions can also have an impact on the physical, social, cultural, personal, spiritual, and temporal elements of the home environment, which should be considered carefully when selecting and negotiating modifications (Hawkins & Stewart, 2002).

Other factors that can affect the selection, negotiation, and acceptance of home modifications include the following:

+ The cost of the modification: Clients might not have the funds to make changes to their home, especially if most of the home modifications are to be self-funded, as they generally are (American Association of Retired Persons [AARP], 2000). In addition, some modifications require additional structural or maintenance work to be undertaken before the modification is completed, which is often at a cost clients can ill-afford (Jones, de Jonge, & Phillips, 2008).

+ The person's knowledge of the range of possible intervention options: Without a clear understanding of what is possible, clients are often not able to envision how their situation can be improved (Jones et al., 2008).

+ The person's perception of the need, usefulness, and acceptability of the intervention: Clients are more likely to accept an intervention if they believe it supports their sense of personal identity. Conversely, interventions that undermine their sense of identity are unlikely to be welcomed (McCreadie & Tinker, 2005).

+ The availability of information about arranging the work: Clients are better able to undertake a modification if they understand the building process: how to choose and engage a contractor, how the work would be done, how to manage in the home while the work is underway, and how to cope with any mess caused by contractors (AARP, 2000; Duncan, 1998; Pynoos & Nishita, 2003).

+ The amount of disruption the intervention is likely to cause: Clients are sometimes reluctant to undertake extensive work in areas such as the bathroom if it will be out of commission for a period.

Therapist-Related Factors

Interventions recommended by occupational therapists are likely to be influenced by their own level of expertise and experience in the home modification field as well as their model of practice. For example, occupational therapists with a wide-ranging knowledge of domestic products, design standards or guidelines, and resources and who undertake post-modification evaluation of previous work are likely to have a wealth of valuable information and experience that they can draw on. Therapists who use an ecological or transactive model of practice are also more likely to address occupational performance difficulties using environmental interventions than therapists who use models focused on remediating performance components.

Environment-Related Factors

When considering modifications for the home, the team and the client need to consider a range of factors relating to the suitability of the dwelling for alteration, including the following:

+ The cost-effectiveness of any changes, given the size, value, age, and structural suitability of the home (Connell & Sanford, 1997; Silverstein & Hyde, 1997)

+ Building rules and regulations relevant to the redesign of the area to ensure compliance with the law

+ The fit of any modification with the style and design of the dwelling and existing streetscape, if the work is located outside of the home

+ The long-term viability of the design and suitability to current and future householders. Current design trends, such as universal design, aim to ensure that products and designs are "useable by all" (Center for Universal Design, 1997) and reduce the likelihood that the modification needs to be altered or removed later as the needs change (Ringaert, 2003).

Other Factors

In most services, there are policies and procedures relating to home modification recommendations and a specific range of resources available to assist in the planning of interventions. Legislation, industry standards, and design guidelines might also guide the design and implementation of environmental interventions (Ringaert, 2003).

Chapter 4 provides information on legislation influencing home modification practice, and Chapter 12 provides details about design standards and their role in guiding interventions.

Educating Clients About Proposed Interventions and the Modification Process

Throughout the process of selecting and negotiating interventions, the therapist has a responsibility to inform the client about the extent of change to an area required, the range of people to be involved in the process and their respective responsibilities, and the expected timeframe for the modification work. In addition, the therapist should discuss the expected impact of the home modification on the way activities would be undertaken and the expected appearance of the final modification. The therapist might show the client photos and diagrams of the layout of a room to help him or her better understand how it will look and how he or she might be able to move through or use the area.

Some occupational therapists find it useful to take clients to facilities that have already been modified to allow them to move around in the space and try the fittings and fixtures. This may include visiting:

+ A demonstration home or display center to view and try accessible design features

+ A hydrotherapy center to try an accessible toilet, vanity unit, and shower recess

+ A shopping center to try the gradients of accessible ramps

Information gleaned from these trials can be used to confirm or guide the redesign of proposed home modifications.

Chapter 10 provides information on identifying suitable interventions, and Chapter 11 provides detail about sourcing and evaluating products and designs.

Concluding the Home Visit

At the conclusion of the home visit, the therapist should provide the client with a brief verbal summary of the outcomes from the visit and confirm the full range of issues and options to be included in the home modification report (Figure 6-18). It is also beneficial to leave a brief written summary of the proposed interventions and an action plan stating who is responsible for each step of the plan. At this time, it is important to ensure that the client agrees with the recommendations. If the client does not agree, the therapist should extend the visit or make another time for further discussion and negotiation with the client and other stakeholders. If technical advice is required on the proposed modification, the therapist might also arrange to visit with a designer or builder before the home modification report is written and finalized.

Seeking Technical Advice

Technical building advice is sometimes required, particularly where home modification work is expected to be extensive. Because occupational therapists do not receive training in construction and renovation, they consult with experts, such as design or building professionals, when they require expertise on design and building matters. For example, a therapist might need to know whether:

+ A wall can support a grab bar

+ A wall can be removed to allow more circulation space without compromising the integrity of the roof

+ Light fittings and power points can be of a particular type and positioned in specific locations in a bathroom

+ A garage can be converted into an extra bedroom

+ A ramp can be designed with an appropriate gradient to suit an area with limited space or if the yard has a slope

+ A proposed extension of a home is possible under local building regulations

+ A stair lift can be installed on stairs leading to several units under local building regulations

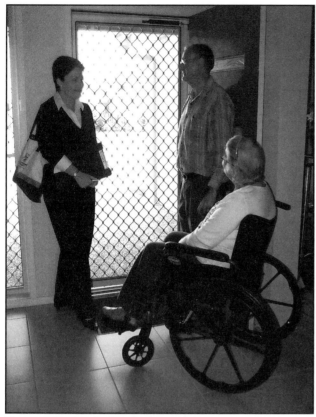

Figure 6-18. Concluding the home visit.

Design or building professionals generally contribute to the design and construction of modifications by:

+ Noting environmental barriers and constraints, including property boundaries, immovable structures, or items that will affect the design—for example, protected trees and fire-rated or load-bearing walls

+ Systematically measuring relevant areas and noting the position of services and other permanent fittings and fixtures, such as windows and doors

+ Deciding on the structural work required, such as modifying the levels or finishes of the floor and removing, moving, or installing new walls, doorways, or windows

+ Deciding on the changes required to services, such as the location of electrical points, water pipes, or drains

+ Planning the location of fittings and fixtures

+ Drawing the redesigned area to scale

+ Finalizing product finishes, such as flooring and surfaces, lighting, and color options

Issues discussed among the occupational therapist, the design or building professional, and the client might include the following:

+ The feasibility of the proposed environmental modification, that is, whether the home modification is reasonable given the age and type of construction of the home or whether the changes can be easily and stylishly included in the existing layout of the home

+ The existing dimensions and space for the home modifications, such as adequate floor area to incorporate the home modification

+ The required dimensions of the modifications, such as length, height, width, or depth of spaces, fixtures, and fittings

+ The range of products and features to be incorporated into the alterations, with due consideration given to the specific needs of the client as well as other people in the household

+ The cost and design of the proposed work in relation to the household budget and the degree of design elegance associated with the cost of the proposed modification

The information gathered from discussions with the design and building professional might be included in the therapist's report, or the design and building professional might provide a written technical specification report with accompanying drawings and photos. If the technical specification report and drawings have more technical detail than the therapist's home modification report, they should be used by the contractor for quoting and completing the work.

Reviewing Professional Drawings

To ensure that the developed drawings are consistent with those agreed to by the therapist in collaboration with the client, the therapist compares them with those created by the design or building professional (Figure 6-19). The therapist ensures that all relevant information is included and that there are no discrepancies, omissions, or inadequate adherence to recommendations or design guidelines or standards. Once the plans are reviewed, the therapist provides a report on how the proposed design will or will not meet the client's needs and either endorses the drawings or provides a report about the discrepancies noted on the plans. This report provides feedback to the design or building professional and ensures the drawings are revised to suit the client's specific requirements.

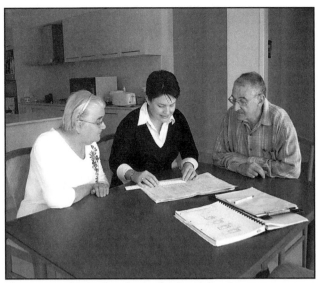

Figure 6-19. Reviewing the professional drawings.

Role Differences

It is important to note that design or building professionals are not trained to have an understanding of a client's health conditions and disabilities and the associated impact on occupational performance; hence, they have no expertise in evaluating the specific needs of clients. They are not trained to analyze the person-environment-occupation transaction, to identify a specific cause of performance difficulties, or to determine how occupational performance can be further enabled using a range of interventions. However, building and design professionals do possess important technical expertise on the design and construction of buildings and surrounding environments, which can assist in the planning of environmental interventions. Consequently, it is imperative that a team approach is used in home modification practice so that various professionals can contribute their unique expertise to the home modification process and the design of environmental interventions (Pynoos et al., 2002).

Writing the Report and Completing the Drawings

Therapists should document the findings and recommendations as soon as possible after the home visit. This will ensure that the details of the visit are captured accurately in the report. Notes and photos taken at the time of the visit can also assist with recall.

The occupational therapy report should summarize information gathered at the time of the home visit. It is also important that the therapist contacts the client, family or people assisting the client to make decisions, or other service providers after the visit to seek further information about the client's health condition or disability and their functional capacity. As stated earlier, permission should be sought from the client prior to making contact with relevant stakeholders. Some services require that client permission be recorded in writing and placed on file for future reference.

It is important that therapists are clear about the documentation requirements of the original referrer—the program or individual who will receive the report—because each might have their own reporting expectations. The report should be in politically correct language and worded simply so that it can be clearly understood by the intended reader. Details about whether information has been reported by the client, family, caregivers, or others or observed by the occupational therapist should be included. More essentially, the report should provide a record of the professional and clinical reasoning and decision-making process and not just the outcomes of the home visit. If required, photos and drawings should be incorporated into the report to provide a detailed picture of the client's circumstances and the areas of the home environment requiring alteration. Finally, the report should provide the client with a record of the visit—the issues and solutions discussed and the final recommendations.

The Structure of a Home Modification Report

Not all occupational therapists or home modification services stipulate a structure for home modification reports; however, it is recommended that they establish a structure for these documents. For example, some services might choose to document the occupational therapy report in two sections as follows.

The first section of the report should provide background information about the client, their disability or medical condition, and any personal or environmental impacts on their occupational performance, valued roles, and day-to-day activities. Other background information can include details of the equipment being used by the client in the home and, where appropriate, the dimensions of these items with and without the client. Information on the client's current living situation and use of support services should also be included in this first section.

The second section of the report should detail the issues identified and discussed during the interview as well as the options explored. Justification for the final option should also be provided, explaining why this is the best option for the client and his or her situation. This section should detail the specific needs of the client and the physical, social, cultural, personal, and temporal aspects of the home that impact on decision making.

The third section of the report is a guide for the building professional when undertaking the home modification work. This section should incorporate a general list of the modifications required, including the location and dimensions of features, the circulation spaces and clearances, and the performance requirements of products and finishes (Bradford, 1998). The building professional does not need to read the confidential information about the client contained in the first section; he or she requires only the technical information to undertake the home modification work. It is therefore necessary that the third section provides sufficient detail for the modification work to be undertaken successfully and, where appropriate, include the detailed specification and plans provided by the builder or architect. This section of the report should be able to stand alone in its own right and have sufficient detail to guide a builder, particularly if the building professional's drawings and specifications become detached from the occupational therapy report. It is not satisfactory for the therapist to refer the reader to the builder or architect's report and not include a detailed summary of the home modification requirements in that report.

When making recommendations, it is preferable that therapists indicate only the performance requirements of products rather than specify particular brands. This practice ensures that a range of products are considered. There might be specific occasions when the client requires a particular product to suit his or her needs. In such situations, occupational therapists might have to provide product information in their report to ensure that the client's needs are met (Bradford, 1998).

It is important that therapists develop an intimate knowledge of the wide range of products suitable for use in home modifications. In particular, they should be familiar with industry standards: how the product should be manufactured, tested for safety, and labeled for correct use.

Therapists can provide each client with a copy of the report and its recommendations to ensure he or she has a record to refer to while the work is being undertaken. The therapist should be mindful that the report, and any other associated documentation relating to the client on file, is a legal document and might one day be used in court. It is therefore important to consider the extent and type of information to be kept on file and included in reports.

Submitting the Report

In the next step of the home modification process, the therapists submit the report for approval and action. Some services require information only for the builder and do not need the client's background information. In this instance, therapists can keep notes on file for future reference and to comply with the legislative requirements for storage of client records.

If therapists have provided sufficient justification for the recommendations and details of the modification in the report, the work can be approved and started. On occasion, the person or program providing the funding for the home modification might not approve the modification: the alterations might be considered too costly, too invasive, an inappropriate intervention given the client's requirements, or outside of the scope of the provision of the program. There might be requested changes to the recommendations, which would require another home visit to renegotiate the interventions with the client. It is important that therapists be clear about the parameters of the program before making recommendations because this will inevitably save time. However, they should always ensure that their recommendations are in the best interests of their clients and provide them with sufficient information to make informed choices. Clients might decide to fund their preferred option themselves. Alternatively, therapists might refer clients to another service should their needs fall outside the scope of the existing service or funding.

If therapists are in doubt about what might be approved, they might propose a range of options in the home modification report—from the least costly and least invasive option through to the ideal solution that may be more expensive. It is important that therapists clearly document their clinical reasoning in relation to the proposed interventions, the level of importance or priority assigned to these interventions, and the consequence of each for the client. This information will provide helpful detail for the decision maker as he or she reads the report.

Further information about ethical, legal, and reporting issues can be found in Chapter 13.

Educating and Training Clients in the Use of Home Modifications

Occupational therapists have a role in educating and training clients in the use of modifications once they have been installed. This training is particularly relevant in situations where:

+ The modifications have been extensive

+ The person's impairments are newly acquired

+ The person's occupational performance has declined over time

+ A range of equipment has been considered in the planning of the modification

+ Caregivers need to use the modification when providing assistance to the client (Siebert, 2005)

Further, education and training in the use of modifications may be required if the client has demonstrated difficulty managing alternative interventions.

Therapists might also provide contact information for repair or maintenance (Bradford, 1998) so that the client can contact the supplier or builder for assistance if problems arise during the warranty period.

Evaluating Home Modifications After Installation

The home modification process concludes with the occupational therapist inspecting the modification and other interventions to determine whether they have achieved the desired outcomes and have not presented any unexpected difficulties (Figures 6-20 through 6-22). The therapist also confirms that the modifications and interventions have met client expectations and fit in with the look and feel of the home and household routines. In addition, they discuss whether the client's occupational performance has been supported or enhanced through the new interventions. Further changes might have to be made if the modification has not helped the person's occupational performance or if it has created further environmental barriers.

The postmodification inspection can take one of two forms: it can involve therapists taking a walk-through of the property with clients to examine the effectiveness of the modifications, or it can comprise a formal evaluation of the outcomes of the modification using a standardized evaluation tool. In the first instance, occupational therapists might complete a detailed review of the products and finishes installed and check the specific measurements to ensure that the home modification has been completed as per the therapist's documented recommendations and drawings or as per the design or building professional's specification and drawings.

Therapists should inform clients (or advocates) if they identify problems resulting from poor workmanship, incorrect installation of fittings and

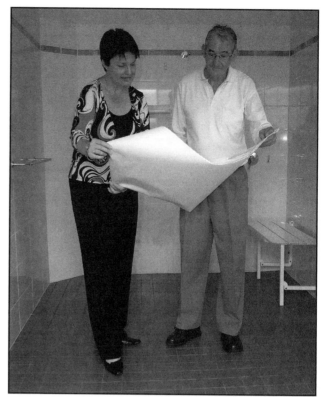

Figure 6-20. Checking the built environment against the plans.

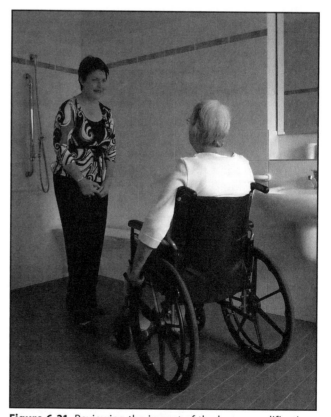

Figure 6-21. Reviewing the impact of the home modifications on the client's occupational performance.

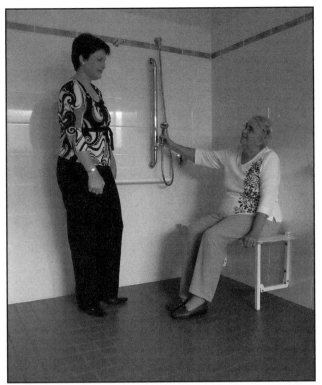

Figure 6-22. Observing the client using the home modifications.

fixtures, or delays with work completion by tradesmen. To act in this capacity, they will need to have an understanding of the relevant legislation, such as building or human rights legislation, to help resolve issues. They will also need some knowledge of advocacy and building service organizations that can assist in the resolution of disputes.

Improved occupational performance is the expected outcome of occupational therapy interventions (Backman, 2005). Performance outcomes discussed during the initial evaluation process (at the time of interviewing and observing the client) can be revisited after the modification to note any change in that performance. By using standardized tools to identify goals and evaluate performance, therapists can assess the extent of change following the modification. This information is invaluable in informing practice and demonstrating the effectiveness of home modification practice.

Further information about evaluating client outcomes can be found in Chapter 14.

CONCLUSION

This chapter described how occupational therapists receive and analyze referral information with a view to prioritizing their visit in relation to other referrals. After contacting clients to arrange a suitable time and preparing and collating required resources in advance of the visit, therapists travel to the clients' homes where they complete interviews, inspect the homes, measure the clients and their equipment and/or caregivers, and photograph, measure, and draw the built environment. They sit with the clients to plan, select, and negotiate a range of interventions before concluding the visit. This chapter has also discussed how technical advice may be required from professionals with design or construction expertise, before the report and drawings are finalized and submitted to the referrer. Information has been provided on the valuable role of occupational therapists in educating and training the client in the use of the home modification and evaluating its effectiveness after installation.

REFERENCES

American Association of Retired Persons. (2000). *Fixing to stay: A national survey on housing and home modification issues.* Washington, DC: Author.

American Occupational Therapy Association. (2008). Occupational therapy practice framework: Domain and process. *American Journal of Occupational Therapy, 62,* 625-683.

Backman, C. L. (2005). Outcomes and outcome measures: Measuring what matters is in the eye of the beholder. *Canadian Journal of Occupational Therapy, 72*(5), 259-261.

Boyt Schell, B. A. (2003). Clinical reasoning: The basis of practice. In E. B. Crepeau, E. S. Cohn, & B. A. Boyt Schell (Eds.), *Willard and Spackman's occupational therapy* (11th ed., pp. 131-139). Philadelphia: Lippincott, Williams & Wilkins.

Boyt Schell, B. A., & Schell, J. W. (2008). Professional reasoning as the basis for practice. In B. A. Boyt Schell & J. W. Schell (Eds.), *Clinical and professional reasoning in occupational therapy* (pp. 3-12). Philadelphia, PA: Lippincott, Williams & Wilkins.

Bradford, I. (1998). The adaptation process. In R. Bull (Ed.), *Housing options for disabled people* (pp. 78-113). Cambridge, MA: Athenaeum Press.

Brown, C. E. (2009). Ecological models in occupational therapy. In E. B. Crepeau, E. S. Cohn, & B. A. Boyt Schell (Eds.), *Willard and Spackman's occupational therapy* (11th ed., pp. 435-445). Philadelphia, PA: Wolters Kluwer Lippincott, Williams & Wilkins.

Center for Universal Design. (1997). *The Principles of Universal Design, Version 2.0.* Raleigh, NC: North Carolina State University. Retrieved from http://www.design.ncsu.edu/cud/about_ud/udprinciplestext.htm

Chiu, T., & Oliver, R. (2006). Factor analysis and construct validity of the SAFER-HOME. *Occupational Therapy Journal of Research: Occupation, Participation and Health, 26*(4), 132-142.

Connell, B. R., & Sanford, J. A. (1997). Individualizing home modification recommendations to facilitate performance of routine activities. In S. Lanspery & J. Hyde (Eds.), *Staying put: Adapting the places instead of the people* (pp. 113-148). Amityville, NY: Baywood Publishing Company Incorporated.

Corcoran, M. (2005). Using qualitative measurement methods to understand occupational performance. In M. Law, C. Baum, & W. Dunn (Eds.), *Measuring occupational performance: Supporting best practice in occupational therapy* (pp. 65-78). Thorofare, NJ: SLACK Incorporated.

Crabtree, M. (1998). Images of reasoning: A literature review. *Australian Occupational Therapy Journal, 45*, 113-123.

Duncan, R. (1998). Funding, financing and other resources for home modifications. *Technology and Disability, 8*, 37-50.

Fisher, A. G. (1998). Uniting practice and theory in an occupational framework. *American Journal of Occupational Therapy, 52*(7), 509-520.

Gitlin, L. N. (2009). Environmental adaptations for older adults and their families in the home and community. In I. Soderback (Ed.), *International handbook of occupational therapy interventions* (pp. 52-62). New York, NY: Springer Publishing Company.

Grayson, P. J. (1997). Technology and home adaptations. In S. Lanspery & J. Hyde (Eds.), *Staying put: Adapting the places instead of the people* (pp. 55-74). Amityville, NY: Baywood Publishing Company Incorporated.

Hawkins, R., & Stewart, S. (2002). Changing rooms: The impact of adaptations on the meaning of home for a disabled person and the role of the occupational therapist in the process. *British Journal of Occupational Therapy, 65*(2), 81-87.

Iwarsson, S., & Slaugh, B. (2001). *The housing enabler: An instrument for assessing and analyzing accessibility problems in housing.* Navlinge och Staffanstorp, Sweden: Veten & Stapen HB & Slaug Data Management.

Jones, A., de Jonge, D., & Phillips, R. (2008). *The impact of home maintenance and modification services on health, community care and housing outcomes in later life.* Melbourne, Australia: Australian Housing and Urban Research Institute.

Klein, S. K., Rosage, L., & Shaw, G. (1999). The role of occupational therapists in home modification programs at an area agency on aging. In E. D. Taira & J. L. Carlson (Eds.), *Aging in place: Designing, adapting, and enhancing the home environment* (pp. 19-38). Binghamton, NY: The Haworth Press.

Law, M. (1998). *Client-centered occupational therapy.* Thorofare, NJ: SLACK Incorporated.

Law, M., Baptiste, S., Carswell, A., McColl, M., Polatajko, H., & Pollock, N. (1998). *Canadian occupational performance measure* (3rd ed.). Toronto, Ontario: Canadian Association of Occupational Therapists.

Law, M., Baptiste, S., & Mills, J. (1995). Client-centered practice: What does it mean and does it make a difference. *Canadian Journal of Occupational Therapy, 62*, 250-257.

Law, M., & Baum, C. (2005). Measurement in occupational therapy. In M. Law, C. Baum, & W. Dunn (Eds.), *Measuring occupational performance: Supporting best practice in occupational therapy* (pp. 3-20). Thorofare, NJ: SLACK Incorporated.

Law, M., King, G., & Russell, D. (2005). Guiding therapist decisions about measuring outcomes in occupational therapy. In M. Law, C. Baum, & W. Dunn (Eds.), *Measuring occupational performance: Supporting best practice in occupational therapy* (pp. 33-44). Thorofare, NJ: SLACK Incorporated.

McCreadie, C., & Tinker, A. (2005). The acceptability of assistance technology to older people. *Ageing and Society, 25*(1), 91-110.

Ohta, R. J., & Ohta, B. M. (1997). The elderly consumer's decision to accept or reject home adaptations: Issues and perspectives. In S. Lanspery & J. Hyde (Eds.), *Staying put: Adapting the places instead of the people* (pp. 79-89). Amityville, NY: Baywood Publishing Company Incorporated.

Pybus, R. (1996). *Safety management: Strategy and practice.* Boston, MA: Butterworth-Heinemann.

Pynoos, J., & Nishita, C. J. (2003). The cost and financing of home modifications in the United States. *Journal of Disability Policy Studies, 14*(2), 68-73.

Pynoos, J., Sanford, J., & Rosenfelt, T. (2002). A team approach to home modifications. *OT Practice, 7*(7), 15-19.

Ringaert, L. (2003). Universal design of the built environment to enable occupational performance. In L. Letts, P. Rigby, & D. Stewart (Eds.), *Using environments to enable occupational performance* (pp. 97-115). Thorofare, NJ: SLACK Incorporated.

Rogers, J. C., & Holm, M. B. (2007). The performance assessment of self-care skills (PASS). In I. E. Asher (Ed.), *An annotated index of occupational therapy evaluation tools* (3rd ed., pp. 102-110). Bethesda, MD: American Occupational Therapy Association.

Siebert, C. (2005). *Occupational therapy practice guidelines for home modifications.* Bethesda, MD: American Occupational Therapy Association.

Silverstein, N. M., & Hyde, J. (1997). The importance of a consumer perspective in home adaptation of Alzheimer's households. In S. Lanspery & J. Hyde (Eds.), *Staying put: Adapting the places instead of the people* (pp. 91-111). Amityville, NY: Baywood Publishing Company.

Stark, S. (2003). Home modifications that enable occupational performance. In L. Letts, R. Rigby, & P. Stewart (Eds.), *Using environments to enable occupational performance* (pp. 219-234). Thorofare, NJ: SLACK Incorporated.

Wylde, M. A. (1998). Consumer knowledge of home modifications. *Technology and Disability, 8*, 51-68.

7

Evaluating Clients' Home Modification Needs and Priorities

*Desleigh de Jonge, MPhil (OccThy), Grad Cert Soc Sci
and Ruth Cordiner, DipCOT, Grad Cert OccThy*

In occupational therapy, evaluation is viewed as a collaborative process that aims to understand people as occupational beings and how they create meaning in their lives through occupation (Cohn, Schell, & Neistadt, 2003). A home evaluation seeks to understand and analyze the dynamic transaction between people, their occupational patterns, and the home environment. Using a top-down approach and an occupation-based framework, occupational therapists analyze occupational performance by first seeking to understand the roles and occupations of importance to the person and the impact of the injury, impairment, or health condition on the person's life. The therapist then observes and examines the person's performance, the home environment, and occupational elements (activities, tasks, and sequences) to identify barriers and facilitators to performance. Clients are considered to be central to the evaluation process, actively contributing to the therapist's understanding of their experience and capacities, the value of the activities they engage in, and the intricacies of the home environment.

Given the unique and complex nature of occupational performance in the home, therapists rely heavily on professional reasoning to deal with the diversity of information they gather during the evaluation process. This chapter describes the range of reasoning styles therapists use and how they are used throughout the process to develop and test hypotheses, understand the client's perspective, and determine what is achievable to ensure the best possible outcomes. The chapter also details the variety of evaluation strategies therapists use to understand and interpret occupational performance in the home—including informal and structured interviews, skilled observation, and standardized assessment tools—and discusses what each strategy contributes to the home modification process. Criteria are also provided to guide therapists when they are selecting and evaluating standardized assessment tools.

CHAPTER OBJECTIVES

By the end of this chapter, the reader will be able to:

+ Describe the purpose of a home evaluation

+ Explain the framework therapists use for evaluating occupational performance in the home

+ Describe how professional reasoning is used throughout a home evaluation

+ Identify the types of evaluation strategies occupational therapists use during a home visit and what each contributes to the evaluation process

+ Identify important considerations in choosing standardized assessment tools for home modifications

Ainsworth, E., & de Jonge, D.
An Occupational Therapist's Guide to Home Modification Practice (pp. 113-138)
© 2011 SLACK Incorporated

Purpose of Evaluation

When providing a home modification service, the purpose of an occupational therapy evaluation is to gain an understanding of the clients' abilities and the barriers that prevent them from successfully completing the necessary and valued activities in their home. The home is a natural environment in which the therapist and client can develop a shared understanding of occupational performance issues. It is here that therapists can observe their clients undertaking everyday activities and see how and where they are usually done. By using a range of evaluation strategies, the therapist identifies "misfits" involving the person, occupations, and the environment. Throughout the visit, the therapist monitors the environment and talks with people who live in the home to understand the dimensions of the home environment that influence occupational performance and are likely to impact on decision making.

Therapists undertake evaluations in the home to:

+ Ensure that clients being discharged from a hospital or institution are safe and able to undertake basic self care activities independently (Rigby, Stark, Letts, & Ringaert, 2009)

+ Identify fall risks, especially in the homes of older people and people with a history of falling

+ Ensure that people with congenital and acquired impairments (e.g., cerebral palsy, stroke, spinal or head injury, Parkinsonism) are able to mobilize safely and function effectively in their home environments (Rigby et al., 2009)

+ Ensure that older people, including those with and without an identified health condition, are able to remain living in their homes for as long as possible

+ Assist families to care for children or older people with impairments

Home is where many and varied occupations are undertaken (Rigby et al., 2009). It is where people commonly eat; rest; look after themselves and others; and manage their finances, goods, and resources. It is where they develop and maintain relationships or refresh and replenish their energies through a range of restful and active leisure activities. It is the base from which they engage in the community and explore the world. Some activities happen routinely on a daily or weekly basis while others happen seasonally or periodically. Home evaluations generally involve an assessment of the person's ability to perform valued and important occupations in the home. Depending on the person's roles and priorities, an evaluation would generally include an assessment of self-care and household activities as well as those to do with leisure and community participation. Some evaluations focus primarily on the accessibility or safety of the home and community.

Evaluations generally take a number of forms. First, they are used as a means of screening—that is, determining whether a person requires occupational therapy services and how urgently. Evaluations also assist therapists to analyze and diagnose the nature and, in some cases, the extent of the occupational performance issue. Finally, evaluation allows therapists to determine whether there has been a change in occupational performance as a result of occupational therapy intervention, commonly referred to as outcome measurement. Each of these evaluation approaches uses different strategies, although some traverse a number of purposes.

Screening

Screening involves a cursory evaluation of the person's occupational performance to determine whether a more thorough evaluation is required (Rogers & Holm, 2003). This can take the form of a brief, informal interview with the person (or the referrer) to determine whether he or she has any specific occupational performance concerns or is at risk of developing associated problems. Therapists commonly use structured questioning to understand the nature of the person's impairment or health condition and its current and future impact on occupational performance. Therapists also briefly explore the demands of various roles and activities and the nature of the home environment and potential impacts on occupational performance (Law, Baum, & Dunn, 2005a). Alternatively, they use standardized tools to evaluate the person's capacity to perform a range of activities or identify environmental hazards that may place the person at risk of occupational performance difficulties in the home. Both informal and structured questioning rely on the therapist's experience and professional judgment to decide whether the client requires a service and how urgently it should be delivered. The information gathered using standardized assessments provides a mechanism for determining the extent of a performance problem, which can be used to justify and prioritize service provision. In addition, information gained from screening all referrals can assist in determining the extent of need, generally, in the community.

Analyzing and Diagnosing Occupational Performance

Therapists are familiar, primarily, with using evaluations to analyze and diagnose occupational performance difficulties. These evaluations require a thorough approach to information gathering and analysis and are essential to designing effective interventions. Therapists generally use a range of evaluation strategies to understand the precise nature of the occupational performance difficulties being experienced and to identify aspects of the person-environment-occupation transaction that are contributing factors.

There is a range of evaluation strategies therapists use to identify and analyze occupational performance issues. Informal and structured interviews provide background information on clients and their living environment and help therapists develop an understanding of client concerns and their perspective on the nature and impact of occupational performance problems. Therapists also use skilled observation to closely examine occupational performance, identify where performance is ineffective or hazardous, and investigate factors contributing to inadequate performance. These observations are often undertaken in a semi-structured way with performance described qualitatively, which relies heavily on the professional experience and judgment of the therapist. Therapists also use standardized assessment tools to measure the extent of the performance problem and diagnose the cause of the presenting problem.

Evaluation of Outcomes

Outcome evaluation assists therapists to determine the effectiveness of home modification interventions. These evaluations are undertaken to confirm that the changes have produced the desired improvements in occupational performance and to ensure there are no adverse consequences resulting from the introduced changes. The consistent use of outcome measures is also fundamental to evidence-based practice (Law, Baum, & Dunn, 2005b). These evaluations inform therapists about the most effective interventions in a range of situations and build a body of evidence of their effectiveness. This information is being used increasingly by policymakers and management to make decisions about policy directions and the future funding of various service programs (Law et al.). Outcomes can be evaluated qualitatively and quantitatively. Qualitative evaluation provides an opportunity to record the client's and the therapist's perception of the impact of the

intervention. Quantitative evaluation can demonstrate the extent of impact and establish whether there have been any measurable changes as a result of the intervention, especially if standardized measures are used before and after the event.

FRAMEWORK FOR EVALUATION

In home modification practice, it is important that the evaluation strategies chosen reflect client-centered practice so that consumers are empowered by the process and have a sense of ownership of the modifications undertaken in their home. Evaluation methods should allow consumers to identify their specific concerns about valued occupations, record their unique occupational performance requirements, and document the impact of interventions on their lives (Law et al., 2005b). This requires that evaluation strategies do the following:

+ Allow occupational performance issues or problems to be identified by the client and household members and not solely by the therapist and team

+ Permit the unique nature of each person's participation in occupations to be recognized

+ Provide opportunities for both the subjective experience and the observable qualities of occupational performance to be recorded

+ Afford the client (and relevant others) to have a say in evaluating the outcomes of the interventions

+ Recognize the unique qualities of the home environment

+ Assist clients and household members to develop a mutual understanding of therapists' safety, prevention, or health maintenance concerns (Law & Baum, 2005)

Client-centered evaluation requires that evaluation strategies extend beyond the measurement of performance components. Evaluation strategies need to be able to measure the extent of occupational engagement, giving due recognition to the uniqueness of each person's valued roles and occupations. They should also allow the client and therapist to jointly plan interventions (Law & Baum, 2005) and to determine the effectiveness and value of these to the consumer in the short and long term.

Evaluation should also accurately reflect the scope and focus of the profession and its practice frameworks. When using the occupational therapy practice framework, evaluation focuses on understanding the person's occupational history and experiences and his or her patterns of daily living, interests, values, and needs as well as his or her priorities and concerns about occupational performance (American Occupational Therapy Association [AOTA], 2008). Occupational performance is observed in context in order to determine supports or barriers to performance, giving due consideration to body structures and function, performance skills and patterns, and activity demands as well as the environment. The therapist, in collaboration with the client, then determines concerns and risks and identifies problems and the probable causes.

When using an ecological approach, evaluation should focus on the quantity and quality of occupational performance using both objective and subjective methods. It examines the "fit" of the person, environment, and occupations, acknowledging that these are constantly changing and evolving. These models recognize the unique personal attributes, capacities, and life experiences each individual brings to the collaboration. Evaluations need to examine the physical, sociocultural, personal, and temporal elements of the environment and the potential impact of these on occupational performance. It would also consider these environmental domains from an individual, household, neighborhood, and community perspective.

PROFESSIONAL REASONING

As a result of the individual and complex nature of home modification practice, therapists rely heavily on professional reasoning throughout the evaluation and intervention process. This section focuses on the use of professional reasoning during evaluation. The role of professional reasoning in designing acceptable, effective, and workable home modification interventions will be discussed further in Chapter 10; however, good reasoning in the evaluation process is critical to developing a thorough understanding of the issues, which then contributes to developing effective interventions and achieving good outcomes.

Therapists use a "whole body" process (Schell, 2009) to understand occupational performance in the home, identify factors that constrain performance, and create a home environment that enables occupational engagement. Using a combination of theoretical knowledge and personal and professional experience, therapists analyze copious amounts of diverse information to fully understand each person and his or her occupational performance issues. They can then recommend interventions that will fit well with each unique person-environment-occupation transaction.

There is a combination of thinking approaches that therapists use to understand occupational performance issues in the home environment: scientific, narrative, pragmatic, and ethical reasoning (Schell, 2009). For example, from the moment therapists receive a referral, they begin to gather information and use scientific reasoning to anticipate occupational performance difficulties or generate hypotheses from their bank of theoretical knowledge of impairments and health conditions and the role the environment plays in creating disability. Therapists continue to use scientific reasoning throughout the evaluation process when choosing appropriate evaluation methods and analyzing and interpreting behavior. When talking with their clients and listening to their stories, therapists use narrative reasoning to develop a deeper understanding of people's lifestyles, aspirations, concerns, and valued occupations. They then work with their clients throughout the visit to develop a rich understanding of their experiences and environments and to explore and create a new future. Pragmatic reasoning assists therapists to use their personal resources to their best advantage, understand the service delivery context, and work sensibly and effectively within the policy framework and available resources. Finally, ethical reasoning ensures that the therapist maintains respect for the values and rights of all clients and provides the best possible service in every situation. Professional reasoning has been described as "a dynamic process simultaneously influenced by the client and therapist's characteristics, experience, and background" (Radomski, 2008, p. 41). The dynamic nature of professional reasoning is particularly evident when therapists use a client-centered approach, where they need to be flexible and responsive to the uniqueness of each person and his or her home environment.

Scientific Reasoning

What Is Scientific Reasoning?

Scientific reasoning is described as "a logical process that parallels scientific inquiry" (Schell, 2009, p. 318). There are two forms of scientific reasoning described in the literature: diagnostic reasoning and procedural reasoning (Schell). Diagnostic reasoning is concerned with sensing and defining professional problems (Rogers & Holm, 1991; Schell), and procedural reasoning is the thinking that comes from choosing suitable evaluation and intervention approaches (Fleming, 1991, 1994). In combination, these processes assist therapists to progress from defining to resolving occupational performance problems (Chapparo & Ranka, 2000). Drawing on relevant bodies of knowledge, the therapist seeks and interprets cues and then generates and tests hypotheses (Rogers & Holm) about the person's occupational performance difficulties and contributing factors.

How Is It Used?

The process begins with the therapist gleaning cues from the written referral, case file, preliminary conversation with the client, presentation of the neighborhood, appearance and design of the home, and initial encounter with the client. For example, Glenda, an older woman, is referred a home assessment following a fall. The therapist would initially determine her age, living situation, general health, and whether she sustained any injuries from the fall by reading the referral or file. He or she would ask Glenda about the circumstances of the fall to identify potential precipitating and contributing factors. During the visit, the therapist would note the age, design, and state of repair of the house, and he or she would scan the environment for known hazards. He or she would also observe the client as she walks through the house and note her agility and ability to negotiate obstacles and changes in light levels and flooring. These are the cues that provide therapists with initial information about clients, their occupations, and their home environments, which assist them to generate hypotheses about the person's occupational performance.

How Does It Influence the Evaluation Process?

The cues sought and noted by therapists are shaped by their knowledge, experiences, and models of practice. For example, a therapist's knowledge of factors that contribute to falls would direct him or her to collect information about a client's fall history, number of medications, and so forth. Knowing about the consequences of a fall for someone with osteoporosis also alerts the therapist to investigate this and other co-morbidities. Therapists with experience working with people with a history of falls would be alert to features in the environment that could be injurious during a fall. The various models to which therapists ascribe also define what they attend to and what they understand to have contributed to the observed problem. A rehabilitation therapist might focus primarily on measuring the extent of the person's functional impairment; therapists using an occupational performance model would focus on understanding how the person undertakes activities, while those using an ecological model would also examine the environment and how well it supports activity engagement.

When using diagnostic reasoning, therapists draw on existing knowledge to acquire and interpret cues and generate and test hypotheses. From a given diagnosis, therapists can anticipate functional difficulties and hypothesize about how these are likely to impact on occupational performance and progress in the long term. In addition, therapists analyze and interpret behavior in an effort to understand what is contributing to it. If Glenda were to trip when walking to the bathroom during the home visit, the therapist might attribute this to wearing poor footwear, being distracted, a developing dementia or neurological impairment, or an uneven carpet. These hypotheses would then be tested or adjusted as further cues are sought and interpreted. For example, the therapist might ask Glenda to demonstrate how she gets into the shower recess. By asking her to remove her shoes, the therapist can test whether the problem persists without footwear. Allowing her to concentrate on the task allows the therapist to observe her performance without distractions. Observing her capacity to notice and lift her feet over obstacles or level changes on the floor enables the therapist to test her concerns about her physical and cognitive function. Finally, her ability to negotiate changes in floor level allows the therapist to examine the impact of environmental barriers on Glenda's performance.

Procedural reasoning is used to choose appropriate evaluation strategies, including valid and reliable assessment tools (Radomski, 2008). Therapists select strategies and tools that allow them to gather information about the person, his or her occupations and the environment, and the transaction between them. A combination of observation, assessment, and discussion allows various hypotheses to be modified and tested until the therapist develops a clear understanding of occupational performance and the person-environment-occupation transaction.

What Does It Offer the Therapist and Client?

Scientific reasoning allows therapists to draw on their knowledge and experience to gather, analyze, and interpret vast amounts of information. When therapists are well informed and able to use this information to generate a number of hypotheses, they are well placed to observe and interpret the person-environment-occupation transaction and understand how and why occupational performance difficulties occur. This complex process is often easier for experienced therapists who have integrated their model of practice, have acquired a broad knowledge base through experience and reading, and have developed the capacity to attend to and process a diversity of information simultaneously. Less-experienced therapists often struggle to use their models of practice and limited knowledge effectively, to attend to a number of cues at the same time, and to generate multiple hypotheses. This can result in a tendency for them to jump to conclusions quickly if time is not taken to critically reflect on assumptions (Chapparo & Ranka, 2000). Experienced therapists are also at risk of contracting to routine practices if they over-rely on experience, do not keep their knowledge current, or actively reflect on their reasoning processes (Chapparo & Ranka).

Although scientific reasoning might appear to be the realm of the therapist, clients also benefit from this form of reasoning. When therapists are able to share their knowledge and articulate their reasoning, they can engage clients in a meaningful and informative discussion about risks and potentially contributing factors. This allows the client to be an active part of the diagnosis and decision-making process rather than feeling uninformed and disempowered by "expert" opinion.

Narrative and Conditional Reasoning

What Is Narrative Reasoning?

Occupational therapy has been described as both an art and a science (Peloquin, 1994). Narrative reasoning, which addresses the art of the profession, contrasts with and compliments scientific reasoning. Narrative reasoning is used to understand and describe a person's unique experience of his or her situation and to work with that person to create an impelling future. It assists therapists to make sense of each person's situation and imagine the impact of the illness, injury, or health condition on their lives (Schell, 2009).

How Is It Used?

Throughout the home visit, therapists engage in natural conversations with the householder, making comments about spaces in the house and asking questions such as, "Did you decorate this room yourself?" and "Are these photos of your family?" This generally elicits storytelling that assists in developing rapport and gaining a richer understanding of the home and the people living in it. Therapists also use structured interviews to gather information. These interviews can include open-ended questions that allow clients to describe their experience in the home. This allows therapists to draw information from these stories to enrich their understanding of the impact of the health condition or impairment on a client's engagement in activities in the home and gain information about his or her occupational history. It also provides the client with an opportunity to introduce new or unexpected elements to the story that might not have been uncovered through direct or closed questioning. Active and empathetic listening is also important in building rapport and encouraging clients to openly share their experiences and aspirations. Creating a safe space for disclosure might be as simple as having a cup of tea and saying nothing, instead allowing the client to discuss things that are important to him or her.

By taking the time to talk with Glenda, the older woman described previously in this chapter, the therapist developed a rich understanding of the impact of her condition and the significance of her home environment. She learned that Glenda was experiencing an increasing number of falls and that this was making her feel unsafe in her home and reluctant to go out without someone accompanying her. Consequently, she finds herself doing less and feeling even more uncertain. The therapist also learned that Glenda had lived in the house all 45 years of her married life and had raised five children there. Of significance is that she now lives alone in the home that her recently deceased husband built. Glenda is reluctant to make changes because the home provides her with a strong connection to him and their family. She also looks after two of her young grandchildren after school, bathing and feeding them before her daughter collects them after work.

Narrative reasoning is not only useful for developing a deeper understanding of each person and his or her personal preferences and priorities, it is also valuable in assisting clients to explore and create a new future for themselves. When discussing issues, the therapist has an opportunity to share stories with a client and create new possibilities and a future for him or her. For example, therapists can sometimes assist clients to articulate and analyze their concerns by sharing stories about other people's experiences. Stories also help clients envision possibilities and create goals that may have been long abandoned. For example, when discussing a recent experience with a client with similar reservations about going out into the community, the therapist shared a story about how a simple modification to the front entry of the house had provided the client with greater confidence and a sense of security when entering and exiting the house. This story allowed Glenda to contemplate developing a goal she might not otherwise have considered.

How Does It Influence the Evaluation Process?

Spending time developing a deeper understanding of each client and his or her home environments allows therapists to contextualize and make sense of information gathered during the evaluation. For example, understanding the value a client places on chairs and objects in the home assists the therapist to acknowledge that they are more than environmental hazards. It allows them to remain open and respectful and to anticipate issues where their evaluation of risk might differ from that of their client.

Narrative reasoning can often be automatic and unconscious even for novice therapists. For example, informally observing people in their homes can reveal a great deal about their life stories. A well-tended garden informs the therapist that the householder appreciates plants and that they spend a great deal of time either tending to the garden themselves or paying someone else to do it. Photographs on the wall reveal personal connections. Shelves and floor space cluttered with valued objects and trinkets alerts the therapist to the attachment that the person has to his or her belongings. These observations are different from the cues sought in scientific reasoning, where therapists seek cues to generate and test hypotheses and then filter information through their scientific knowledge to analyze or diagnose issues. In narrative reasoning, the therapist absorbs information from someone's stories and from the environment to build an understanding of his or her life experience and the personal and social culture of the home environment.

What Does It Offer the Client and Therapist?

Narrative reasoning allows clients to examine their issues and air their concerns in a safe environment. It also enables therapists to develop a deep understanding of each client's unique experience of his or her situation. The trust and rapport developed in this process makes it easier for the client to disclose personal information and have faith in the therapist's evaluation of the issues because it is founded on a deep understanding of the situation. This type of reasoning also allows therapists to explore the symbolic meaning of home with the consumer and to ensure that modifications are life enhancing, as well as rational and pragmatic. It shifts the focus from simply addressing issues of safety, function, and independence to developing a rich and deep understanding of the person, his or her valued occupations, and the home environment. It also affords clients the opportunity to be the authors of their own life story.

Pragmatic Reasoning

What Is Pragmatic Reasoning?

Pragmatic reasoning is the consideration given to the practical realities encountered in practice. It assists therapists to work sensibly and effectively within their personal resources as well as within the resources available in the practice context (Schell,

2009). Therapists bring personal experiences, professional competencies, and a level of commitment to professional practice that impact on their capacity to deliver a service. The demands on therapists' time within the service and outside work will also influence their availability. In addition, the practicalities and logistics of delivering services within a particular setting—in this case, the home—and the processes and resources within the service organization (Schell & Cervero, 1993) influence the type and level of service that can be delivered.

How Is It Used?

In daily practice, therapists use pragmatic reasoning to make the best use of their personal resources—such as knowledge, skills, time, and level of commitment—as well as service resources—such as evaluation resources, structures and processes, reimbursement schedules, and policy directives. For example, a therapist might have limited experience in dealing with people like Glenda who have an increased falls risk, so he or she would dedicate time prior to the visit to reading about and becoming familiar with known falls risks. This would ensure the most effective use of visit time. If a specific time was allocated for the visit by the service or reimbursement schedule, the therapist would try to structure it to ensure that all issues were addressed and prioritized efficiently. If the service did not have resources dedicated to assessing falls risk, the therapist might borrow them from another center to use in this instance with plans to order them for the service should more clients with falls risks be anticipated. The constraints placed on the evaluation by the client and the environment would also be considered to maximize the effectiveness of the visit— for example, advising Glenda of the time required for the visit so that she can make this time available. If the environment has many hazards, the therapist might need to spend more time at Glenda's house and postpone the next client visit.

How Does It Influence the Evaluation Process?

During the evaluation process, therapists use their knowledge of and experience with various evaluation strategies to identify and define occupational performance issues. The diversity of experience and competency among therapists leads to variability in the nature and quality of evaluation, especially in a new or developing area of practice such as home modification. It is therefore important that, as a profession, therapists develop and share practice knowledge and evaluation tools and protocols to ensure that service delivery is consistent and of a high quality. Therapists with limited experience should consult with more experienced colleagues to ensure that they have been effective in identifying all of the relevant issues in the complex practice environment.

Therapists need to be flexible and responsive to the specific needs and circumstances of each client and therefore use pragmatic reasoning to choose the most appropriate strategies for any given situation. The home setting presents particular challenges to traditional evaluation methods and assessment tools. Being a private space, the client or homeowner might have sensitivities or preferences that impact on which, and how, things can be evaluated. This requires therapists to search for new evaluation strategies that accommodate the diversity of issues and circumstances they encounter in this complex environment.

The time available for a home visit can also influence the nature of evaluation undertaken. Time-limited or one-off home visits can make it difficult for therapists to develop a deep understanding of the person-environment-occupation transaction and to be entrusted sufficiently to recommend changes to personal routines and spaces. Consequently, therapists use pragmatic reasoning to prioritize issues with clients to ensure that the most important issues are attended to in the time available.

Service organizations often have a particular focus and assessment protocols that might or might not align well with professional practice. In these situations, therapists fulfill their employment responsibilities by clarifying what they are able to offer the client within this service and referring him or her to other services that can address additional needs. Therapists then work with the organization to refine and develop procedures and protocols within the service so that they are more in line with current professional knowledge or best practice.

What Does It Offer the Therapist and Client?

Therapists are faced with a considerable number of pragmatic considerations when undertaking home modification evaluations. They are acutely aware of the many factors in the practice context that impinge on home modification practice and use pragmatic reasoning to manage the many competing demands on their time and resources. When managed well, therapists can optimize the use of their time and resources to address occupational performance issues in the home. However, sometimes pragmatic issues can significantly constrain practice. A focus on cost effectiveness and efficient use of resources, including therapists' time, can sometimes result in an emphasis on throughput and short-term outcomes. The home is a very personal and private environment and, as such, sufficient time is required

to allow the therapist to get to know the client and to allow him or her to focus and direct the evaluation process. The challenge for therapists is to achieve a balance between working within available resources and working long-term to maximize the resources available, which includes building the capacity of therapists and services to respond to people's diverse home modification needs. Pragmatic reasoning therefore necessarily requires therapists to provide ongoing input to facilitate the development of service policies, procedures, and resources to ensure that home modification services are as effective as they are efficient.

Ethical Reasoning

What Is Ethical Reasoning?

Ethical reasoning is the final and most critical type of reasoning. When the art and science of occupational therapy meet reality, therapists call on their personal and professional values to ensure that quality services are delivered to all clients. Ethical reasoning is the thinking that therapists undertake to synthesize knowledge and evidence, client values and goals, an appraisal of his or her competencies, and practical aspects of service delivery to provide the best possible care (Radomski, 2008). When dealing with the many competing forces that impact on their thinking and decision making, therapists filter decisions through the core values and attitudes of the profession and its code of ethics. The profession holds a number of enduring values, one of which is that all humans are unique. This value challenges therapists to appreciate each individual's experiences, values, and goals over theoretical understandings and routine procedures and implores them to make time and use evaluation strategies that recognize and understand each person's distinctive nature.

How Is It Used?

When considering scientific, narrative, and pragmatic aspects of practice, therapists are often confronted with conflicting information and demands. Ethical reasoning requires therapists to critically reflect on competing perspectives to ensure that their actions manifest ethical practice. The occupational therapy code of practice requires therapists to:

+ Demonstrate a concern for the well-being of the recipients of their services (beneficence)

+ Take reasonable precautions to avoid imposing or inflicting harm upon the recipient of services or to his or her property (non-maleficence)

+ Respect the recipient and/or his or her surrogate(s) as well as the recipient's rights (autonomy, privacy, confidentiality)

+ Achieve and continually maintain high standards of competence (duties)

+ Provide accurate information about occupational therapy services (veracity; AOTA, 2000).

When visiting clients' homes, therapists are privy to a great deal of information about their clients. For example, on entering Glenda's home, the therapist becomes aware of a number of hazards that put her at a high risk of falling. Ethical reasoning alerts the therapist to his or her responsibility to address each of these before leaving the home. The therapist is also aware that he or she should not introduce any additional risks by placing equipment in Glenda's path or asking her to perform an activity that would unnecessarily place her at risk. At the same time, the therapist has to respect Glenda's right to privacy and control in her own home and can therefore not enter rooms without permission or impose solutions that are not welcomed. Additionally, the therapist must not disclose information to others about Glenda and her living situation without her permission. Ethical reasoning also impels the therapist to provide a high quality of service to all clients, regardless of race, social circumstances, or attitude, and ensures that clients are well informed about what can and cannot be provided by the particular service. The therapist would also ensure that Glenda is referred to more appropriate services should her needs fall outside of his or her responsibilities.

How Does It Influence the Evaluation Process?

It is not uncommon that the values of therapists or service organizations sometimes differ from those of clients. These conflicts are inevitable and require the therapist to use sound reasoning to resolve differences of opinion. Respectful and open discussion with the client ensures that the therapist understands his or her perspective and collaborates to achieve a mutually satisfying outcome. Therapists also need to critically reflect on their personal and professional values in order to "confront, understand and work towards resolving the contradictions within his/her practice between what is desirable and actual practice" (Johns, 2000, p. 34). An evaluation with sound ethical reasoning ensures that the therapist evaluates the right things using the best possible approach for the particular situation, regardless of the challenges presented.

What Does It Offer the Therapist and Client?

Ethical reasoning provides the therapist with a systematic way of addressing conflicts between what

should be done and what can be done (Doherty, 2009). It also ensures that that all clients are treated respectfully and receive a high-quality service regardless of the situation. Within the evaluation process, ethical reasoning allows the therapist to fully explore the client's perspective and work collaboratively with them to define and prioritize issues.

TYPES OF EVALUATION STRATEGIES

Therapists use a range of evaluation strategies, such as informal and structured interviews, skilled observation, and standardized assessments, to gather information about the client and his or her home and to test hypotheses.

Informal Interview

Home modification evaluations generally begin with the therapist engaging in an informal discussion with the client about the home, the reason for referral, or concerns the client has about his or her occupational performance. Interviewing is an essential step in the evaluation process and generally serves a dual purpose. First, interviews allow therapists to gather information, hear clients' stories, and understand their experiences, concerns, goals, and aspirations (Henry & Kramer, 2009). Second, interviews afford therapists an opportunity to build collaborative relationships with their clients and gain their trust (Henry & Kramer). Interviewing is used by therapists to create a shared understanding of each client's situation, so that the home modification process can address his or her individual concerns and priorities.

Informal interviews are useful in gathering qualitative information about the client and the home, which is essential in providing a client-focused service. These interviews can be semi-structured and unstructured but generally take the form of a conversation, where questions are asked and information is provided without using a predetermined format. This two-way communication is commonly guided by broad goals or, at most, a set of prompts that direct therapists through a range of topics. However, to explore issues further, therapists often develop additional questions in response to the client's comments or responses. This style of questioning is used at the start of the visit to explore clients' priorities and aspirations and then throughout the visit, as they move through the home and demonstrate performance in specific areas, to gather further insights into clients' concerns and experiences.

Although individual therapists are likely to have their own personal style of communication, there are a range of strategies that can be used to increase the effectiveness of informal interviews. At the outset, it is essential to create a safe and accepting interpersonal climate for the interview. Finding a quiet, comfortable place in the house where the client and therapist can sit close to each other (3 to 4 feet apart and at right angles) is an important first step. It is equally important, however, that the therapist allows the initial conversation to flow freely while both parties are settling into the interview and becoming comfortable with each other. It can be valuable to let the client raise the topic of conversation, because the therapist can learn more about the client and what he or she feels is important. This also provides the therapist with an opportunity to demonstrate genuine interest in the client's concerns and value his or her perspective.

Once the interview climate has been established, the therapist uses a range of questioning techniques, such as open and closed questions and probing, to encourage discussion and to explore occupational performance issues in greater depth. Regardless of the quality of the interview questions, therapists need to constantly monitor the effectiveness of each interview and the quality of the information acquired. Informal interviews are difficult to conduct without a lot of experience; however, they are likely to be most effective when the interviewer:

+ Is knowledgeable about the content of the interview

+ Structures a purposeful and well-rounded interview

+ Is open and responsive to topics introduced by the interviewee

+ Uses clear communication that can be understood by everyone involved in the interview

+ Employs a gentle approach that allows the interviewees sufficient time to consider their responses and reply

+ Is empathetic and listens attentively to what is being said, how it is said, and what is not said

+ Has sensitive responses to the interviewees' expressed opinions and concerns

+ Is able to take positive control of the direction of the interview, or steer the interview, based on agreed goals for the interaction

+ Is able to critique or challenge what is said if inconsistencies occur or issues require closer examination

+ Remembers what has been said previously and relates back to information obtained at different parts of the interview

+ Clarifies information gained and explores the client's perceptions of events without imposing meaning or over-interpreting information (Kvale, 1996)

Informal interviews allow clients to provide therapists with a wealth of information at their own pace; however, this information can be easily overlooked or lost if it is not adequately managed or recorded. Therapists use structured interviews to screen whether clients have occupational performance issues and to establish the extent and urgency of the concerns; they use semi-structured interviews to explore, probe, and analyze the nature of difficulties they are experiencing. It takes time and experience to learn to use informal interviewing well because it can be difficult to obtain the right information and integrate the information provided, especially when clients are eager to talk about a broad range of topics. Equally, it can take a great deal of skill to coax reserved clients to disclose personal information, which is often required in home modification practice. Experienced therapists, who have developed an internalized framework and procedure for interviewing, are comfortably placed to use informal interviewing well. However, without a systematic approach and regular review, informal interviewing can result in some issues being explored haphazardly or being neglected altogether.

Informal interviewing generally allows therapists to learn a great deal about clients' particular concerns and requirements and the impact of occupational performance difficulties. Although this information is invaluable in shaping decision making and negotiations with clients, it is often not recorded formally. This lack of documentation results in "underground practice" (Mattingly & Fleming, 1994; Pierre, 2001), where discrepancies occur between what therapists do and what they record. Consequently, the complexity of issues considered when making home modification decisions is often not acknowledged and documented by therapists or recognized within services. Even if this qualitative information was effectively recorded, it is not in a form that readily allows the outcomes of home modification interventions to be measured. With the growing focus on evidence-based practice, therapists need to ensure that the client's perspective, which occupational therapy claims to be vital, is recorded. It is crucial that this perspective is not lost in the search for standardized evaluation tools in determining the nature and extent of need and quantifying the effectiveness of interventions.

Structured Interviews and Checklists

Many occupational therapy services develop structured forms and checklists that are targeted at identifying occupational performance issues in the home for a particular client group. These forms provide therapists with a structure for collecting demographic information, medical history, and self-reported ability to undertake activities of daily living. In services that offer home modification services, information is also gathered on the age, design, and features of the house. There are also a number of environmental checklists that assist therapists to identify environmental features that are potential hazards or barriers to people with specific impairments or health conditions. These tools are a useful guide for therapists who are new to the service or area of practice because they help them to collect all information relevant to the particular service. With the many distractions that can occur in a home environment, these tools can ensure that therapists address everything on the form during the interview or environmental inspection. The structure of these tools ensures some consistency in the information gathered and makes it easier when clients are transferred to other therapists within the service or revisit the service at a later date. Although these tools are not standardized and don't often provide the quantitative information required for evaluating the effectiveness of an intervention, they do provide information on the preintervention situation. When clients or other staff view the information collected using these tools, the domain of concern of occupational therapy becomes immediately apparent.

Although structured forms and checklists are useful, they do have a number of limitations. It has been said that "what occupational therapists do looks simple, what they know is quite complex" (Mattingly & Fleming, 1994, p. 24). The use of set forms to ensure consistent information gathering often oversimplifies what occupational therapists really do. Two-dimensional information about the person, activity performance, or the environment belies the complexity of the person-environment-occupation transaction. Often, these forms and checklists do not reflect the breadth and depth of information that therapists gain when interviewing clients, which misrepresents the nature of information therapists operate from. Second, once a form has been developed, it is often assumed that anyone could collect the information, which leads to services sometimes questioning why other staff could not be trained to do a home assessment. Third, in the interest of comprehensiveness, these forms frequently require therapists to collect additional nonspecified information to address the specific concerns of the client at the time of the interview. This may result in an unnecessary invasion of the person's privacy, especially when information about irrelevant medical conditions is collected or spaces in the house are inspected unnecessarily. Finally, these tools are often not reviewed regularly enough in light of new evidence, theoretical knowledge, or changes in service practice, which results in traditional practices often persisting well beyond their use-by date.

Skilled Observations and Occupational Analysis

Observing clients in their homes, where they perform their usual daily activities, provides a wealth of valuable information more comprehensive and detailed than can be gained from interviewing alone. During the course of the home visit, occupational therapists observe clients as they move and perform various activities around the home—for example, answering the door, moving through the home, and possibly making refreshments. These general observations, often automatic to experienced clinicians, provide a basis for discussing the impact of the health condition or impairment on life within the home. However, therapists also ask clients to perform specific occupations, in particular those identified as problematic, during the initial interview. By skillfully observing occupational performance, therapists can observe behavior in its natural environment and identify factors that are contributing to, or interfering with, performance (Dunn, 2000).

Occupational therapists have specialized knowledge and skills that allow them to analyze and evaluate occupational performance (Dunn, 2000) and they use different theoretical lenses to understand occupational performance and factors that contribute to performance difficulties (Crepeau & Schell, 2009). For example, when using an ecological model such as person-environment-occupation or person-environment-occupation-performance model, therapists focus on analyzing the fit between the person, the occupation, and the environment. Occupational therapists also use their skills in occupational and activity analysis to identify the important elements of various occupations in the home and where and how breakdowns in performance occur.

Occupational Analysis

Occupational analysis is core to occupational therapy practice. It allows therapists to analyze occupations of value and concern to clients in the actual context in which they are performed and to gain an understanding of their possible meaning, component tasks, specific performance requirements, and potential facilitators and barriers to performance (Crepeau & Schell, 2009). This qualitative information allows therapists to identify the particular aspects of the task that result in difficulties or compromise. Using whole body reasoning, therapists then examine aspects of the individual's performance and occupational or environmental demands that are impinging on successful completion. This type of analysis acknowledges the unique meaning and purpose of the activity for the individual and recognizes the distinctive way tasks are performed, depending on the purpose of the task, the experience and preferences of the person, and the demands and structure of the occupation and environment.

Activity analysis, on the other hand, analyzes activities in a more abstract sense so as to assist therapists in anticipating potential difficulties in performance (Crepeau & Schell, 2009). When undertaking an activity analysis, therapists tend to identify common components of the task and capacities and environmental elements required for successful completion. This alerts therapists to the specific aspects of the task where breakdowns in performance are likely and helps them to understand possible contributions to difficulties and errors. For example, a simple activity such as going to the toilet incorporates a number of tasks, and there can be a breakdown at any stage of this activity if there is a poor person-environment-occupation fit. Table 7-1 details the procedural component tasks of going to the toilet.

Task breakdown can occur if the person has specific impairments that make it difficult to anticipate a toileting need, mobilize to the toilet, locate the toilet, or see various fixtures and fittings. In addition, there may be aspects of the environment that make it difficult for the person to carry out the activity—for example, too great a distance, convoluted or obstructed pathways, unfamiliar presentation, high door furniture, unfamiliar or inaccessible positioning of light fittings, low toilet pan, inoperable flush button, poorly located or difficult-to-tear toilet paper, or tight space between door and toilet pan. Therapists commonly observe people performing various aspects of activities and analyze performance difficulties as they occur. This is not a formalized process but rather one where each therapist uses an individual approach to analyzing tasks and interpreting problems.

Some standardized tools, such as the Performance Assessment of Self-Care Skills (PASS-Home; Rogers

Table 7-1. Activity Analysis of Going to the Toilet

Register need to go to the toilet

Locate and find way to toilet

Open the door

Enter the room

Turn on the light

Close the door

Travel, turn, and position at front of pedestal

Undress

Sit down onto toilet

Reach for toilet paper/release sheet

Transfer weight for wiping

Attend to personal hygiene

Move from sitting to standing

Don and adjust clothing

Clean toilet bowl

Turn and flush toilet

Open door

Negotiate doorway

Find way to sink to wash hands

Turn on taps

Wet hands

Soap hands

Rub hands together

Rinse hands

Dry hands

NB collapse or need assistance

& Holm, 1994) and Comprehensive Assessment and Solution Process for Aging Residents (CASPAR; Sanford, Pynoos, Tejral, & Browne, 2002), provide a framework for analyzing and evaluating various household activities. These tools present essential task elements and a structure for examining and recording difficulties experienced and assistance required for successful completion. Although this type of analysis provides a foundation for identifying potential performance breakdowns and contributing factors, these and other activity analysis frameworks tend to focus on the physical and immediately observable aspects of activities. Less attention is paid to the sensory, cognitive, and emotional demands of activities: preparing for, initiating, and terminating activities and the routines and habits required when undertaking daily tasks in the home. There needs to be further evaluation to determine when, where, and how people undertake tasks, their experience of the performance, and the specific qualities of performance that are important to them.

Therapists generally use a combination of activity and occupational analysis when observing occupational performance in the home (Crepeau & Schell, 2009). Using a blended approach to analysis allows therapists to understand the particular importance and issues for specific clients as well as the factors contributing to performance difficulties and how these can be addressed (Crepeau & Schell). Because skilled observation is generally undertaken qualitatively, it can be difficult to measure changes in performance objectively. The nature and quality of analysis is also dependent on the therapist's clinical experience. Furthermore, it is important to be aware that an individual's performance is likely to vary throughout the day as his or her capacities and environmental conditions change, and therapists need to account for this variability when evaluating an individual's performance in various household activities.

Rogers and Holm (2009) have identified a number of parameters that therapists examine when analyzing occupational performance: value, independence, adequacy, and safety.

Value

Value is the importance or significance of the occupation to the individual. When resources are limited, people generally establish priorities and reserve their energies for highly valued occupations (Rogers & Holm, 2009). The relative value of tasks is often addressed in the interview or other assessment processes and assists in identifying consumer goals and priorities. However, the therapist may review and revise these priorities in collaboration with the consumer if further performance concerns become evident while activities are being performed.

Independence

Independence generally refers to a person's ability to complete activities without assistance. A person's level of dependence is measured in terms of the type of assistance he or she requires to complete an activity. Assistance is commonly assessed as progressing from low levels of support, in the form of using assistive devices and the need for supervision or task setup, to high levels of support, such as another person providing verbal or physical prompting or physical assistance. People's confidence in their ability to perform activities in the home is another facet of independence (Rogers & Holm, 2009). If they believe they cannot perform a task, it is likely that their performance will be compromised. Though

independence is the primary goal of many services and therapists, it may not be important to the client. There are people with a disability who prefer to receive assistance with routine daily living tasks to allow time and energy for activities they prefer, such as working or spending quality time with loved ones (Baum, Bass-Haugen, & Christiansen, 2005). Sacrificing independence in one activity can result in more autonomy in overall lifestyle and a greater quality of life.

Adequacy

Adequacy refers to the efficiency and acceptability of the process and outcome of the activity (Rogers & Holm, 2009). Efficiency refers to minimizing the amount of effort required to achieve a given outcome. Rogers and Holm evaluate efficiency by examining the degree of difficulty, pain, fatigue, and dyspnea exhibited or experienced during the task as well as the amount of time taken. Acceptability of the outcome is evaluated in terms of social standards, personal satisfaction, and presence of aberrant behaviors (Rogers & Holm).

The ease and comfort with which an individual undertakes activities are important considerations when analyzing occupational performance because they impact on his or her personal experience of daily life within the home, which can subsequently influence overall quality of life. Therapists generally gather information about the experience of the performance from clients, informally asking whether they experience any difficulty, pain, fatigue, and dyspnea during performance. Therapists can also obtain information on the level of difficulty or discomfort experienced by using standardized tools such as the following:

+ The Usability Rating Scale (URS; Pitrella & Kappler, 1988; Steinfeld & Danford, 1997)—a 7-point bipolar measure of difficulty ranging from –3 (very difficult) to +3 (very easy), with 0 providing a neutral point at the center of the scale

+ The Brief Pain Inventory (Cleeland & Ryan, 1994)—a measure of the intensity and interference of pain

+ The Faces Pain Scale (Bieri, Reeve, Champion, Addicoat, & Ziegler, 1990)—a picture scale of pain intensity

Alternatively, therapists can use customized scales in the form of Likert scales and semantic differentials or picture scales. Although customized scales might not be standardized, they provide therapists with a mechanism for identifying and discussing clients' experiences of performance and perceptions of difficulty or discomfort.

A typical 5-level Likert scale is set out as follows: How difficult is your current showering routine?

1. Very difficult

2. Difficult

3. Neither easy nor difficult

4. Easy

5. Very easy

Semantic differential scales usually feature descriptive adjectives with opposite meanings at either end of a scale. For example:

No pain |___|____|____|___| Worst pain imaginable
No difficulty |___|____|____|___| Severe difficulty

Therapists also monitor clients for clinical signs of exertion—for example, increased effort, pallor, sweating, or labored breathing. Tools such as wrist-pulse monitors can also be useful in gauging increased effort. The duration of activities can be measured using a stopwatch; however, the ideal time required for various household tasks is yet to be calculated and is likely to vary from one person to another (Rogers & Holm, 2009). It is likely that clients and their significant others will report whether the time taken for the activity is acceptable or manageable.

The acceptability of the outcome is determined by establishing the person's level of satisfaction with the end product and comparing the result with social expectations (Rogers & Holm, 2009). Overall satisfaction can be evaluated using qualitative comments, customized scales, or a standardized measure such as the Canadian Occupational Performance Measure (COPM; Law et al., 1998), which measures the client's perception of performance and satisfaction with performance. It is difficult to clearly define socially acceptable performance. Therapists generally rely on the client's level of satisfaction but would be concerned when outcomes vary significantly from social standards and place an individual at risk of social alienation from his or her family, friends, and peer group. The therapist would then discuss with the person his or her perception of performance to confirm whether the outcome required improvement. Therapists also use skilled observation to note behaviors that interfere with the process or outcome and vary greatly from the way tasks are typically performed, such as confusion in the order of the procedure, repetitive checking, inappropriate use of fixtures and fittings, and impulsive or disruptive behavior. These are then discussed with the client and significant others.

Safety

In home modification practice, therapists are routinely required to assess the safety of individuals in their homes. Safety is defined as the level of risk that individuals are exposed to when they are performing specific tasks and is a product of the interaction between the capacity of the individual at any given moment, the nature of the task he or she is performing, and the challenges presented by the environment (Rogers & Holm, 2009). While safety is a complex parameter to measure and control for, it is also critical to the success of the home modification process. If it is not addressed adequately, there could be potentially catastrophic consequences for the consumer.

A risk management framework is a useful structure for evaluating and managing risks in the home in a logical and systematic manner. Risk management involves developing processes, structures, and a culture to manage adverse events and optimize opportunities for safety (Standards Association of Australia, 2004). It is a recognized process within a range of settings and is used by a variety of organizations. Risk management is a consultative process that involves all stakeholders—in particular, the person exposed to the risk. This ensures that all views are considered in identifying and evaluating risk and that everyone involved has ownership of the measure to be undertaken to manage the risk. Risk management in the home is likely to include consultation with the client and, in many cases, to extend to the people he or she lives with, family, health providers, personal assistance providers, and advocates.

When undertaking a risk management process, it is important to define the context and determine the purpose of the risk management activity. The context refers to the internal and external environment and, in home modification practice, involves understanding the goals and priorities of clients, their capacities, their social resources, and the physical environments in which they live. The purpose of the risk management activity in this setting is to minimize risk of injury and maximize opportunities for meaningful activity in the home—two purposes that sometimes conflict. Negotiations may need to be undertaken to achieve a balanced plan that meets the needs and wants of the client. For example, a client may wish to soak in a bath regularly to relieve joint pain but may be exposed to a number of risks getting in and out of the bath. The occupational therapist or the organization for which he or she works might also be concerned about their duty of care and potential litigation in relation to the recommendations made. This may lead to risk minimization at the expense of the client's quality of life. Therapists can use a systematic and inclusive approach of risk management to meet their duty of care while still allowing clients to take responsibility for the levels of risk they wish to include in their daily lives. This process involves identifying, analyzing, evaluating, managing, monitoring, and reviewing risks.

Identifying Risks

Identifying risks involves establishing which events are likely to have adverse or uncertain outcomes. When identifying risk in the home environment, it is necessary to observe the person performing the relevant tasks in his or her home. Self-report is not an adequate method of determining risk because people might not always be aware of potential risks in their home. Neither is a simple audit of the physical environment sufficient because, although an audit might identify hazards—events or situations that are the source of danger with the potential to cause harm or injury—it does not determine the degree of risk involved with the hazard. Risk is the likelihood of harm resulting from exposure to a hazard. Simply auditing the physical environment for hazards does not take into account the likelihood of exposure to the hazard and the capacities, vulnerabilities, and experience of the person and how these interact with the environment.

Analyzing Risks

Once the potential hazards have been identified, it is necessary to develop an understanding of the level of risk. Analyzing each risk involves all of the stakeholders making a judgment about the likelihood of an adverse event occurring and the consequences of such an event. When determining the level of risk, the therapist, client, and other relevant stakeholders need to consider the following:

1. *Frequency*: How often the person is exposed to the hazard

2. *Probability*: The probability of an adverse event occurring

3. *Consequences*: The likely consequences of an adverse event

4. *History*: Previous experience of an adverse event (Pybus, 1996)

In a home evaluation, a qualitative analysis of risk is undertaken in consultation with the client and other household members. For example, if we were to analyze the risk of falling or tripping on the front stairs, the client and the therapist would need to determine how often the stairs are used, the chances of the person tripping or falling, the consequences of an incident, and whether an incident has occurred in the past and how often. Levels of risk vary from one situation to another. For example, the risk would be low where a fit and agile older person lived in a dwelling in good repair, rarely used the front stairs, and had no history of tripping on the stairs. In another situation, where an older person with osteoporosis lived in a house in poor repair, used the stairs frequently, and had tripped on the stairs previously, the risk would be high. Even if this person used the stairs only intermittently—for example, to collect the mail—the potential consequences of a fall would warrant management of the risk. The process of identifying and discussing the frequency of exposure, the probability of an event, the likely consequences, and the history of incidents provides a useful structure for therapists to discuss their concerns and understand the client's perception of the risk. By affording clients an opportunity to discuss the frequency of exposure and history of adverse events, therapists can gain a deeper understanding of the potential risk.

Evaluating Risks

Once a judgment has been made about the level of each identified risk, it is then possible to decide which risks need to be addressed and their order of priority. In home modifications, the decisions will need to take into account the level of risk, the personal priorities of the consumer, the role of the organization providing the service, and the resources available for managing the risk.

Managing Risks

In selecting the most appropriate risk management option, therapists generate a range of options and collaborate with clients and other stakeholders to agree on the most effective and acceptable solutions. There are several risk management strategies employed:

+ *Avoiding the risk*: In the home, one option for managing a risk is to avoid that area of the home or the activity completely. For example, a person might choose to use another entry to the house exclusively and avoid the flight of stairs in need of repair.

+ *Reducing the likelihood of the risk*: Possibly the most common is to reduce the likelihood of an accident by providing modifications, assistive equipment, alternative ways of performing tasks, or any combination of these strategies. However, an additional evaluation will then be required to ensure that additional or different risks are not being introduced.

+ *Changing the consequences*: Changing the consequences to reduce the extent of injury is another approach. For example, the person might take medication, wear protective equipment to reduce the risk of fracture, or wear a personal alarm to call for help.

+ *Sharing the risk*: The risk could be shared—for example, by getting someone else to collect the mail or enlisting some help in using the stairs.

+ *Retaining the risk*: This is a valid choice where the activity is highly valued by the individual and other risk management strategies are neither feasible nor acceptable to the client. For example, people may choose to continue to use the stairs to collect mail, regardless of falls risks, because they have done so all their lives and would not entertain having someone else do it for them (Standards Association of Australia, 2004).

Therapists, and the organizations they work for, might be averse to this last option because of concerns about meeting their duty of care and possible litigation. However, imposing unacceptable risk-management strategies on the consumer is counter-productive because they are likely to cause distress or not be used. In these situations, it is imperative that the therapist work with the client to ensure he or she fully understands the probability of an event occurring and the consequences involved. It is also important that the client is fully informed on how to manage the risk and knows where to seek further assistance if required.

Monitoring and Reviewing Risks

It is essential that therapists maintain an ongoing review of risk management strategies to ensure that the management plan is sustainable and remains effective. Factors that affect the probability and consequences of an outcome will inevitably change over time and impact on the suitability of a strategy. Therefore, it is important to follow up once a management strategy has been put in place and then again at regular intervals to ensure it continues to manage the risk. Alternatively, clients should be encouraged to contact the service should they feel that the probability or consequences of a risk have changed. Outcome measures can be used to monitor and review the effectiveness of risk management strategies.

Skilled observation allows therapists to analyze the person-environment-occupation fit and to identify where and how breakdowns are occurring, which then provides the foundation for developing successful interventions. This form of evaluation requires highly developed skills in observation, occupational analysis, and risk management and is often difficult for students and inexperienced clinicians to use effectively. Because of the complexity of the information gathered and the qualitative nature of it, it is difficult to assess the quality of evaluations undertaken by various therapists and quantify the effectiveness of interventions. Once again, without clear documentation of the evaluation undertaken, the profession is not able to articulate its unique approach and contribution to service delivery.

Standardized Assessment

The Nature of Standardized Assessment

Standardized assessments, whether qualitative or quantitative in nature, are developed and tested to ensure that the information collected is comprehensive, trustworthy or valid, and consistent or reliable. *Trustworthiness* is a term used to refer to ensuring the credibility and quality of qualitative data. For quantitative measures, validity ensures that the tool measures what it is intended to and that there is agreement about what it is measuring; reliability ensures that the measures are consistent (Dunn, 2005). Standardized assessments ensure effective, systematic, and consistent information gathering (Law & Baum, 2005). They provide therapists with a mechanism for appraising or calculating the magnitude, quantity, or quality of a particular characteristic or attribute (Law & Baum). These tools provide a uniform procedure for administering the assessment by specifying the conditions, tools, instructions, and questions. Some standardized assessments are norm referenced while others are criterion referenced (Dunn). Norm-referenced tools compare individual test scores with those of a general or specific sample or an ideal. These tools are useful for diagnosis or screening because they assist the therapist in determining the extent of impairment or difficulty and whether performance warrants further investigation. Criterion-referenced assessments are especially useful for occupational therapists because they measure performance against an identified standard rather than an "ideal." These tools can be used to identify and specify the goals and needs of individuals and allow therapists to evaluate the effectiveness of an intervention. When using standardized tools, it is imperative that therapists understand the focus and purpose of the tool and "choose the most appropriate measure with the best psychometric properties" (Cooper, Letts, Rigby, Stewart, & Strong, 2005, p. 316). In home modification practice, assessment tools need to be sensitive to changes in occupational performance and ensure that the environment is adequately acknowledged.

Traditional Assessment Tools

The use of standardized assessments can result in therapists measuring "variables that can be measured rather than what should be measured" (Corcoran, 2005, p. 65). Traditionally, occupational therapists have used a range of standardized tools to assess clients' functional capacities, independence in activities of daily living, or accessibility or safety of the environment (Table 7-2). Assessing the functional capacities of an individual, such as motor (sensorimotor), process or cognitive, communication and interaction or social capacities in a standardized environment assists therapists in anticipating performance issues or understanding aspects of the person that are likely to constrain occupational performance. Establishing the person's level of dependence in a range of activities of daily living also alerts the therapist to potential occupational performance concerns in the home environment. Therapists can develop an awareness of challenges to occupational performance in the home by using standardized tools to identify barriers and hazards in the home environment. Table 7-2 provides an overview of the range of standardized assessments available to therapists.

Historically, the person, occupation, and environment have been viewed as discrete elements that could be assessed independently (Cooper et al., 2005). However, the interdependent relationship between these elements is increasingly being acknowledged. Occupational performance is considered to be the result of all three elements working together and impacting on each other. These traditional assessments tell us little about the person-environment-occupation transaction in the home and how this impacts on occupational performance, something that is considered critical in assessing occupational performance in this natural environment (Law et al., 2005a). They often have a specific purpose and focus, which makes it difficult to address the unique needs of individual clients, the person's occupational experience and interests, the specific demands of the activity, the fit between the person and the environment, or the capacity of the environment to support specific occupations (Law et al.).

Measures of Occupational Performance

There are few standardized assessment tools that quickly and accurately assess many of the parameters of interest for occupational therapists and their clients (Corcoran, 2005), in particular, occupational performance and the person-environment-occupation transaction. When measuring occupational performance, occupational therapists need to capture both the subjective experience and the objective performance (McColl & Pollock, 2005). They require tools that allow them to understand the specific needs of the individual and assist them to explain behavior. A number of structured and semi-structured interview schedules have been developed that guide

therapists to systematically examine the individual's experience of occupation—for example, Canadian Occupational Performance Measure (COPM; Law et al., 1998), Occupational Self-Assessment (OSA; Baron, Kielhofner, Ienger, Goldhammer, & Wolenski, 2002), and the Occupational Performance History Interview-II (OPHI-II; Kielhofner et al., 1998). While the OPHI-II and the OSA both examine the impact of the environment on occupational performance, the COPM focuses primarily on defining occupational performance issues and relies on the client and therapist exploring the impact of the environment on performance through informal discussion and observation. A detailed description and review of these tools is available in McColl and Pollock. These standardized tools allow therapists to develop an understanding of clients' past and present experiences and perceptions of their occupational performance and assist in the development of occupation-focused goals (Fasoli, 2008). The client-centered nature of these tools engages the client in identifying occupational performance issues, thus increasing his or her involvement in the evaluation process and the therapist's understanding from the client's perspective. These tools also allow individualized intervention plans to be developed and the impact of these to be evaluated.

Occupational therapists frequently use standardized assessments to assess occupational performance in relation to basic and instrumental activities of daily living and community participation. Assessments of activities of daily living (ADL) usually focus on determining the level of independence across a range of tasks for the purposes of screening or measuring outcomes—for example, Barthel (Mahoney & Barthel, 1965), Functional Independence Measure (FIM; Uniform Data System for Medical Rehabilitation [UDS], 1997), and Katz Index of Activities of Daily Living (Katz, Ford, Moskowitz, Jackson, & Jaffe, 1963). Generally, these global measures of independence do not provide information on the quality of performance or problematic aspects of the tasks (Gitlin, 2005). Though they may be a useful screening tool, they are not useful in analyzing or diagnosing occupational performance issues or evaluating home modification outcomes.

Recently, a number of performance-based assessments have been designed to assist therapists to objectively analyze the quality of performance and identify barriers to valued occupations. A detailed description of assessments of basic and instrumental activities of daily living and community participation is available in Law et al. (2005a). Some of these tools rely on self, or proxy, report.

Table 7-2. Standardized Measures of Functional Capacity, Independence, the Environment, and Occupational Performance

OCCUPATIONAL PERFORMANCE	REFERENCE
Canadian Occupational Performance Measure (COPM)	Law, M., Baptiste, S., Carswell, A., McColl, M., Polatajko, H., & Pollock, N. (1998). *The Canadian Occupational Performance Measure* (3rd ed.). Toronto, Ontario: Canadian Association of Occupational Therapists.
Occupational Circumstances Assessment—Interview and Rating Scale (OCAIRS)	Deshpande, S., Kielhophner, G., Henricksson, C., Haglund, L., Olson, L., Forsyth, K., & Kulkarni, S. (2002). *Model of Human Occupation*. Chicago, IL: Model of Human Occupation Clearinghouse.
Occupational Self-Assessment (OSA)	Baron, K., Kielhofner, G., Ienger, A., Goldhammer, V., & Wolenski, J. (2002). *Occupational Self-Assessment Version 2.1*. Chicago, IL: Model of Human Occupation Clearinghouse.
Occupational Performance History Interview II (OPHI II)	Kielhofner, G., Mallison, T., Crawford, D., Nowak, M., Rigby, M., & Henry, A. (1998). *The Occupational Performance History Interview (Version 2.0) OPHI-11*. Chicago, IL: Model of Human Occupation Clearinghouse.
FUNCTIONAL CAPACITIES	REFERENCE
Lighthouse Near Acuity Card	Ferris, F. L., Kassoff, A., Bresnick, G. H., & Bailey, I. (1982). New visual acuity charts for clinical research. *American Journal of Ophthalmology, 94*, 91-96.
Lighthouse International Functional Vision Screening Questionnaire	Lighthouse International, 111 East 59th Street, New York, NY, 10022. Tel: (212) 821-9525, Fax: (212) 821-9706
Audition Screening Tool	Popelka, G. R. (1997). *High and low pitch sounds: A screening tool*. Unpublished manuscript.
Timed Up-and-Go Test	Podsiadlo, D., & Richardson, S. (1991). The timed "up-and-go": A test of basic mobility for frail elderly persons. *Journal of the American Geriatrics Society, 39*, 142-148.
Functional Reach Test	Duncan, P. W., Weiner, D. K., Chandler, J., & Studenski, S. (1990). Functional reach: A new clinical measure of balance. *Journal of Gerontology: Medical Sciences, 45*, M192-M195.
Short Blessed	Katzman, R., Brown, T., Fuld, P., Peck, A., Schechter, R., & Schimmell, H. (1983). Validation of a short orientation-memory-concentration test of cognitive impairment. *American Journal of Psychiatry, 140*(5), 734-739.
Mini-Mental State Examination (MMSE)	Folstein, M. F., Folstein, S. E., & McHugh, P. R. (1975). "Mini-Mental State": A practical method for grading cognitive state if patients for the clinician. *Journal of Psychiatric Research, 12*, 189-198.
Geriatric Depression Scale	Alden, D., Austin, C., & Sturgeon, R. (1989). A correlation between the geriatric depression scale long and short forms. *Journal of Gerontology, 44*, 124-125.
Caregiver Strain Index	Robinson, B. C. (1983). Validation of a caregiver strain index. *Journal of Gerontology, 38*, 344-348.
Zarit Burden Interview	Zarit, S. H., Reever, K. E., & Bach-Peterson, J. (1980). Relatives of the impaired elderly, correlates of feeling of burden. *Gerontologist, 20*(6), 649-655.

(continued)

Table 7-2. Standardized Measures of Functional Capacity, Independence, the Environment, and Occupational Performance (continued)

LEVEL OF INDEPENDENCE	REFERENCE
Barthel	Mahoney, S. I., & Barthel, D. W. (1965). Functional evaluation: The Barthel index. *Maryland State Medical Journal, 14*, 61-65.
Functional Independence Measure (FIM)	Uniform Data System for Medical Rehabilitation. (1997). *Functional Independence Measure (Version 5.1)*. Buffalo, NY: Buffalo General Hospital, State University of New York.
Katz Index of Activities of Daily Living	Katz, S., Ford, A. B., Moskowitz, R. W., Jackson, B. A., & Jaffe, M. W. (1963). Studies of illness in the aged: The index of ADL: A standardized measure of biological and psychosocial function. *Journal of the American Medical Association, 185*(12), 94-99.
ACCESSIBILITY AND SAFETY OF THE ENVIRONMENT	REFERENCE
Comprehensive Assessment and Solutions Process for Aging Residents (CASPAR) www.ecaspar.com/ec/	Sanford, J. A., Pynoos, J., Tejral, A., & Browne, A. (2002). Development of a comprehensive assessment for delivery of home modifications. *Physical & Occupational Therapy in Geriatrics, 20*(2), 43-55.
The Home Environmental Assessment Protocol (HEAP)	Gitlin, L. N., Schinfeld, S., Winter, L., Corcoran, M., Boyce, A., & Hauck, W. (2002). Evaluating home environments of persons with dementia: inter-rater reliability and validity of the home environmental assessment protocol (HEAP). *Disability and Rehabilitation, 24*(1), 59-71.
HOME FAST	Mackenzie, L., Byles, J., & Higginbotham, N. (2000). Designing the Home Falls and Accidents Screening Tool (HOME FAST): Selecting the items. *British Journal of Occupational Therapy, 63*(6), 260-269.
Housing Enabler www.enabler.nu	Iwarsson, S., & Slaug, B. (2001). *The Housing Enabler: An instrument for assessing and analyzing accessibility problems in housing.* Navlinge och Staffanstorp, Sweden: Veten & Stapen HB & Slaug Data Management.
Usability in My Home (UIMH)	Fange, A. (2002). *Usability in My Home, manual.* Lund, Sweden: Lund University, Division of Occupational Therapy.
SAFER	Oliver, R., Blathwayt, J., Brackley, C., & Tamaki, T. (1993). Development of the Safety Assessment of Function and the Environment for Rehabilitation (SAFER) tool. *Canadian Journal of Occupational Therapy, 60*(2), 78-82.
SAFER-HOME v.2	Chiu, T., & Oliver, R. (2006). Factor analysis and construct validity of the SAFER-HOME. *OTJR: Occupation, Participation and Health, 26*(4), 132-142.
The Home Occupational Environment Assessment (HOEA)	Baum, C. M., & Edwards, D. F. (1998). *Guide for the Home Occupational-Environmental Assessment.* St. Louis, MO: Washington University Program of Occupational Therapy.
Wesha	Clemson, L. (1997). *Home fall hazards. A guide to identifying fall hazards in the homes of elderly people and an accompaniment to the assessment tool the Westmead Home Safety Assessment.* Victoria, Australia: Co-ordinates Publications.

However, tools that use performance observation are of particular interest to home modification therapists because they allow them to evaluate the quality of occupational performance in daily activities and the factors that contribute to this. Tools of particular interest are the Assessment of Motor and Process Skills (AMPS; Fisher, 1995) and the Performance Assessment of Self-Care Skills (PASS; Rogers & Holm, 1994). Therapists using these tools can select tasks relevant to the client in his or her own environment and to diagnose the precise moment and nature of performance breakdown. They examine the quality of performance rather than focusing solely on the outcome of performance. The AMPS is used by therapists who undergo extensive training to examine an individual's ability to perform specific motor and process skills within two or three meaningful instrumental activities of daily living (IADL) tasks selected from a bank of 56 tasks (Gitlin, 2005). This tool allows therapists to diagnose specific performance difficulties that clients experience when undertaking activities but does not measure the impact of the environment or environmental interventions on performance.

The PASS is one of the few tools that examines safety and adequacy of performance in addition to level of independence on a 4-point scale (Gitlin, 2005). The PASS is available in a clinic and home version, and both include 26 core tasks related to functional mobility (5), personal self-care (3), instrumental activities of daily living with cognitive emphasis (14), and instrumental activities of daily living with physical emphasis (4) (Rogers & Holm, 2007). Each task is criterion referenced, detailing the subtasks required for successful completion (Figure 7-1). Practitioners can select specific tasks depending on the client's priorities or lifestyle or use the task development template to develop a new task. The tool allows therapists to identify the precise point of task breakdown and to provide verbal support, nondirective or directive verbal support, gestures, task and environmental modification, demonstration, physical guidance, physical support, or total assistance to support task completion.

Environmental Assessments

With the growing recognition of the role of the environment in disablement, a number of assessments have been developed to examine the environment in relation to the person and his or her ability to operate effectively in that environment. For a comprehensive review of quality environmental measures, refer to Cooper et al. (2005). Cooper et al. note it is difficult for any one tool to assess this multifaceted and complex entity comprehensively.

Consequently, it is important to be clear about the purpose and focus of the tools available and what each can contribute to an understanding of the impact of the environment on occupational performance. There are two tools designed specifically to analyze the home environment: the Housing Enabler (Iwarsson & Slaug, 2010) and the CASPAR (Sanford et al., 2002).

The Housing Enabler (HE) is based on the Enabler developed by Steinfeld in the 1980s (Fange, Risser, & Iwarsson, 2007) and is particularly useful for examining the congruence between the person's functional capacities and his or her physical environment. There is a particular focus on assessing the accessibility of the home environment for people with a range of functional and mobility impairments, such as difficulty interpreting information, severe loss of sight, complete loss of sight, severe loss of hearing, prevalence of poor balance, incoordination, limitations of stamina, difficulty in moving head, difficulty in reaching with arms, difficulty in handling and fingering, loss of upper extremity skills, difficulty bending or kneeling, reliance on walking aids, reliance on wheelchair, and extremes of size and weight (Figure 7-2). This tool (demonstration version available at www.enabler.nu) allows therapists to identify potential accessibility barriers in the home, which can then be examined further through additional performance testing (Cooper et al., 2005).

The Housing Enabler is administered in three steps:

1. Using a combination of interview and observation, the functional limitations (13 items) and dependence in mobility (2 items) are identified.

2. The physical barriers in the home and immediate outdoor environment (188 items) are noted.

3. The accessibility score is calculated using a complex matrix and specialized software to examine the profile of functional limitations and mobility dependence against the accessibility barriers in the environment where a predefined severity score has been provided for each barrier. The severity of accessibility barrier is rated 1 through 4, with higher points awarded to items that are likely to present more severe problems to people with that limitation (Figure 7-3). The final score indicates the magnitude of accessibility problems in the environment. Scores higher than zero indicated the presence of accessibility problems (Iwarsson & Slaug, 2010).

Task #H3: Functional Mobility: Toilet Transfers

HOME CONDITIONS: Bathroom area and
1. Toilet "as is"
2. Ct positioned facing the toilet

HOME INSTRUCTIONS

"Now let's go into the bathroom to assess morning care activities." [Wait for Ct to locate bathroom]

[As Ct enters the bathroom] "First I'd like you to show me how you sit down on the toilet, and how you reach for and gather toilet paper. You do not need to remove your clothing. Put the toilet paper into the toilet as you normally would. Do you know what you are to do? [Wait for response]

"Now show me how you get up from the toilet." [Wait for response]

SCORE	INDEPENDENCE	SAFETY	ADEQUACY	
			QUALITY	PROCESS
3	No assists given for task initiation, continuation, or completion	Safe practices were observed	Acceptable (Standards met)	Subtasks performed with precision & economy of effort & action
2	No Level 7-9 assists given, but occasional Level 1-6 assists given	Minor risks were evident but no assistance provided	Acceptable (Standards met, but improvement possible)	Subtasks generally performed with precision & economy of effort & action; occasional lack of efficiency, redundant or extraneous actions; no missing steps
1	No Level 9 assists given; or occasional Level 7 or 8 assists given; or continuous Level 1-6 assists given	Risks to safety were observed and assistance given to prevent potential harm	Marginal (Standards partially met)	Subtasks generally performed with lack of precision and/or economy of effort & action; consistent extraneous or redundant actions; steps may be missing
0	Level 9 assists given; or continuous Level 7 or 8 assists given; or unable to initiate, continue, or complete subtask or task	Risks to safety of such severity were observed that task was stopped or taken over by assessor to prevent harm	Unacceptable (Standards not met)	Subtasks are consistently performed with lack of precision and/or economy of effort & action so that task progress is unattainable

---

Task #H3: Functional Mobility: Toilet Transfers

Assistive Technology Devices (ATDs) used during task:
1.
2.
3.
Total # of ATDs used: ___

Subtasks	MOBILITY/ADL/IADL SUBTASKS	Verbal Supportive (Encouragement)	Verbal Non-Directive	Verbal Directive	Gestures	Task of Environment Rearrangement	Demonstration	Physical Guidance	Physical Support	Total Assist	Unsafe Observations	QUALITY: Standards not met; improvement needed	PROCESS: Imprecision, lack of economy, missing steps	INDEPENDENCE	SAFETY	ADEQUACY
Assist Level →		1	2	3	4	5	6	7	8	9						
1	Locates bathroom efficiently (goes directly to bathroom)															
2	Turns to position self in front of toilet and maintains balance (does not grab sink for support; does not grab towel rack for support)															
3	Lowers self onto toilet in a controlled manner (does not "pop" down; buttocks are centered on and touching seat)															
4	Reaches for and gathers (grasps and folds) toilet paper and maintains balance (does not fall forward or sideways)															
5	Places toilet paper into toilet and maintains balance (does not fall forward or sideways)															
6	Raises self from toilet in a controlled manner (does not "rock" down to gain momentum; no loss of balance) and achieves and maintains standing balance (does not sway or "catch" self on sink or other object)															

Column groupings: INDEPENDENCE DATA (Assist Levels 1–9); SAFETY DATA (Unsafe Observations); ADEQUACY DATA (Quality, Process); SUMMARY SCORED (Independence, Safety, Adequacy).

Figure 7-1. Extract from PASS—functional mobility: toilet transfers. (Reprinted with permission from J. C. Rogers and M. B. Holm, University of Pittsburgh, Pittsburgh, PA.)

Currently, this tool is used to evaluate the suitability of accommodation for people with a range of functional and mobility impairments to assist in municipal planning (Fange et al., 2007) and in research to identify the number and magnitude of accessibility problems in housing for older people and its relationship to healthy aging outcomes (Fange & Iwarsson, 2005; Iwarsson, 2005; Iwarsson, Horstmann, & Slaug, 2007). Although the accessibility measures in this tool are based on the Scandinavian accessibility standards, this tool directs therapists to environmental features that are potential accessibility barriers to people with a range of mobility and functional impairments.

FUNCTIONAL LIMITATIONS AND DEPENDENCE ON MOBILITY DEVICES

Yes No

☐	☐	A. Difficulty interpreting information	A
☐	☐	B1. Visual impairment	B1
☐	☐	B2. Blindness	B2
☐	☐	C. Loss of hearing	C
☐	☐	D. Poor balance	D
☐	☐	E. Incoordination	E
☐	☐	F. Limitations of stamina	F
☐	☐	G. Difficulty in moving head	G
☐	☐	H. Reduced upper extremity function	H
☐	☐	I. Reduced fine motor skill	I
☐	☐	J. Loss of upper extremity function	J
☐	☐	K. Reduced spine and/or lower extremity function	K
☐	☐	L. Dependence on walking aid(s) **A B C*** ☐☐☐	L
☐	☐	M. Dependence on wheelchair ☐☐☐	M

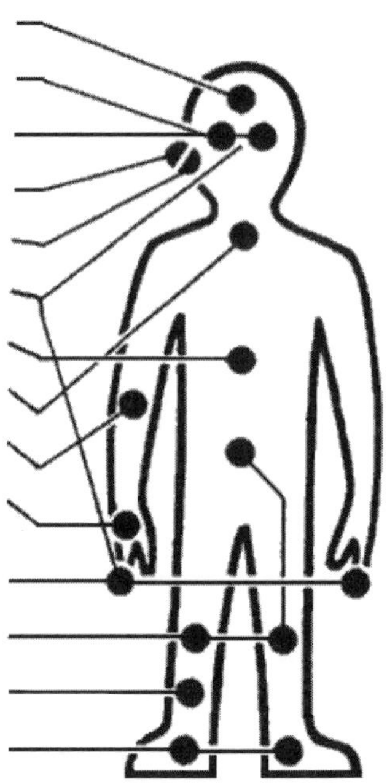

*Section in the environmental component: A. Exterior surroundings. B. Entrance. C. Indoor environment

Figure 7-2. Housing Enabler—functional limitations form. (Reprinted with permission from Iwarsson, S., & Slaug, B. (2010). *The Housing Enabler: A method for rating/screening and analysing accessibility problems in housing* (2nd ed.). Lund & Staffanstorp, Sweden: Veten & Skapen HB and Slaug Enabling Development.)

Personal component / functional profile	Yes / No / Bygg ikapp, page ref.	A	B1	B2	C	D	E	F	G	H	I	J	K	L	M	RATING
A. Exterior surroundings																
General **A1.** Paths narrower than 1.5 m. *A width of 1.0 m is acceptable provided there are 1.5 m turning zones at least every 10 m.*	p. 304					3	3							3	3	☐ Yes ☐ No ☐ Not rated
A2. Irregular/uneven surface. *(irregular surfacing, joins, sloping sections cracks, holes; 5 mm or more).*	p. 305		2	3		1	1		3				1	3	3	☐ Yes ☐ No ☐ Not rated
A3. Unstable surface (loose gravel, sand, clay, etc). *Mark if it causes difficulties e.g. when using a wheelchair or rollator.*			2	3		3	3	2					1	3	4	☐ Yes ☐ No ☐ Not rated

Figure 7-3. Housing Enabler—environmental assessment form. (Reprinted with permission from Iwarsson, S., & Slaug, B. (2010). *The Housing Enabler: A method for rating/screening and analysing accessibility problems in housing* (2nd ed.). Lund & Staffanstorp, Sweden: Veten & Skapen HB and Slaug Enabling Development.)

The CASPAR (Sanford et al., 2002) is a consumer-directed assessment that enables an older adult, family, or nonspecialist therapist to identify problems in undertaking tasks in the home (Sanford et al.). This tool examines the person's interaction with the specific elements in the built environment when accessing the house, mobilizing throughout the house, managing controls such as lighting and temperature controls, getting in and out of bed, and undertaking daily living tasks such as toileting, bathing, grooming, cooking, and washing. Figure 7-4 provides an excerpt from the CASPAR, which examines the use of the bathroom.

The CASPAR allows therapists to record instances where the client experiences a problem with specific task elements, receives help, or uses a device for assistance. This tool provides a useful structure for documenting problems and prioritizing person-environment issues but does not allow therapists to document or record changes in the quality of performance. It does, however, provide detailed diagrams to guide therapists in measuring specific aspects of the built environment related to common problems and modifications.

Selecting and Evaluating Standardized Assessment Tools

When choosing an assessment tool, it is critical to understand the purpose and focus of the tool and to ensure that these align with the intended application (Cooper et al., 2005). Unfortunately, there are few tools that address the issues of concern of occupational therapists and their clients and assess them in the way they need to be assessed. Once a suitable standardized tool has been identified, therapists investigate the psychometric properties of the tool to ensure that it has adequate validity, reliability, and sensitivity for its purpose. Using valid and reliable measures allows therapists to determine the extent of the problem and evaluate the effectiveness of interventions in addressing them. Standardized evaluation tools ensure consistency and assist those therapists with limited experience to identify and address issues systematically. However, standardized tools may have limited flexibility when used to address clients' specific concerns; the complex interaction between the person, environment, and occupations; and the unique situations encountered in home environments. It is often challenging to use standardized tools effectively in the home because time is often limited and it is difficult to follow instructions rigidly in an unfamiliar and unstructured environment (Gitlin, 2005). Some tools require specialist training and have specific setup requirements. Many standardized measures are not sensitive to the changes that can result from

interventions, such as decrease in time taken and making the client feel safer, and can penalize the use of standard interventions, such as the use of an assistive device. These limit their usefulness in evaluating outcomes. For example, the FIM (UDS, 1997) is considered a gold standard in terms of its psychometric properties. While it may be a useful tool for screening level of independence, it does not provide therapists with useful information about the adequacy and safety of performance or the person-environment-occupation transaction, and it is not responsive to changes resulting from typical occupational therapy interventions, such as assistive devices (Johansson, Lilja, Petersson, & Borell, 2007). Regardless of its psychometric properties, the FIM is useful only in specific circumstances—for example, screening and measuring the outcomes of remediation interventions—and is potentially detrimental in demonstrating the efficacy of adaptive interventions. When standardized tools are not available or not appropriate, therapists should use qualitative evaluation strategies, such as interviews and skilled observations, that are trustworthy and consistent (Law et al., 2005a) and ensure that information gathered using these invaluable strategies is adequately documented.

CONCLUSION

Evaluation serves a number of purposes. Primarily, therapists use evaluation to examine and identify misfits between the person, occupations, and the environment. However, it is also valuable in screening referrals to identify people with potential occupational performance issues and to measure the magnitude of change in occupational performance resulting from home modification interventions. Professional reasoning is used throughout the evaluation process. Drawing on relevant practice frameworks and existing bodies of knowledge, therapists seek and interpret cues and generate and test hypotheses about the person's occupational performance difficulties and contributing factors. They use narrative reasoning to understand and describe each client's unique experience of his or her situation and to work with him or her to create an impelling future. Pragmatic reasoning assists therapists to work sensibly and effectively within their personal resources as well as the resources available in the practice contex and ethical reasoning requires therapists to reflect on their personal and professional values when dealing with the many competing forces that impact on their thinking and decision making.

3.4 Using the Bathroom				
Tasks	**Problem**	**Help**	**Device**	**Comments**
Toileting				
Getting close enough to any toilet.	☐	☐		
Getting on/off any toilet.	☐	☐		
Reaching the toilet paper at any toilet.	☐	☐		
Flushing any toilet.	☐	☐		
Other (specify):	☐	☐		
	☐	☐		
	☐	☐		
Bathing/Showering				
Getting close enough to any bathtub/shower.	☐	☐		
Getting in/out of any bathtub/shower.	☐	☐		
Lowering down to/rising up from the bottom of any bathtub.	☐	☐		
Standing while showering in any shower.	☐	☐		
Reaching the faucet and turning the water on/off in any bathtub/shower.	☐	☐		
	☐	☐		
Reaching the water, soap, shampoo, etc. in any bathtub/shower.	☐	☐		
Other (specify):	☐	☐		
	☐	☐		

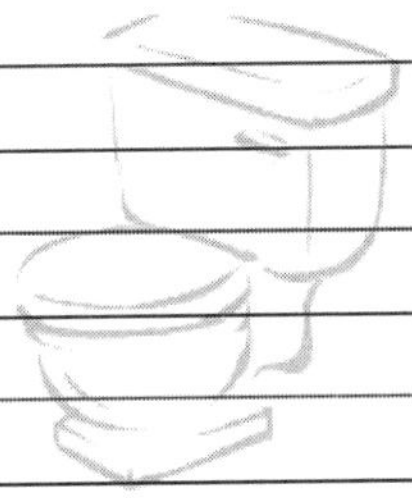

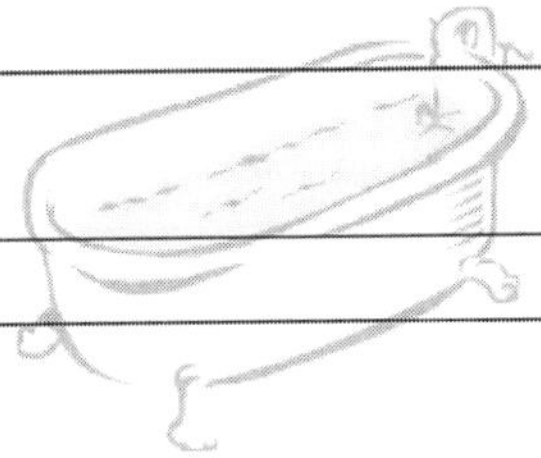

Figure 7-4. Example of CASPAR item. Permission to reproduce CASPAR item provided by Extended Home Living Services, Wheeling, IL.

Therapists use a range of evaluation strategies to gather information about the client, his or her occupational performance, and his or her home. Informal interviewing is used to develop two-way communication between the therapist and the client, allowing therapists to build collaborative partnerships, earn clients' trust and confidence, gather information, hear stories, and understand clients' experiences, concerns, goals, and aspirations. Structured interviews provide therapists with a framework for collecting demographic information, medical history, and self-reported ability to undertake activities of daily living as well as information on the age, design, and features of the house. Dedicated checklists prompt therapists to identify potential hazards or barriers to people with specific impairments or health conditions.

Skilled observation allows therapists to observe occupational performance in the client's natural environment and identify factors that are contributing to, or interfering with, performance. General observations provide a basis for discussing the impact of the health condition or impairment on life within the home, while analysis of specific occupations, in particular those identified as problematic during the initial interview, allows therapists to examine the value, independence, adequacy, and safety of performance. A growing number of standardized assessments are available to therapists to ensure that the information collected is comprehensive, trustworthy or valid, and consistent or reliable. Using valid and reliable measures allows therapists to determine the extent of the problem and evaluate the effectiveness of interventions in addressing the identified problem or concern.

REFERENCES

American Occupational Therapy Association. (2000). Occupational therapy code of ethics. *American Journal of Occupational Therapy, 54*, 614-616.

American Occupational Therapy Association. (2008). Occupational therapy practice framework: Domain and process (2nd ed.). *American Journal of Occupational Therapy, 62*, 625-683.

Baron, K., Kielhofner, G., Ienger, A., Goldhammer, V., & Wolenski, J. (2002). *Occupational Self-Assessment Version 2.1.* Chicago, IL: Model of Human Occupation Clearinghouse.

Baum, C. M., Bass-Haugen, J., & Christiansen, C. H. (2005). Person-environment-occupational-performance: A model for planning interventions for individuals and organizations. In C. H. Christiansen, C. M. Baum, & J. Bass-Haugen (Eds.), *Occupational therapy: Performance, participation and well-being* (3rd ed., pp. 373-392). Thorofare, NJ: SLACK Incorporated.

Bieri, D., Reeve, R. A., Champion, G. D., Addicoat, L., & Ziegler, J. B. (1990). The Faces Pain Scale for the self-assessment of the severity of pain experienced by children: Development, initial validation, and preliminary investigation for ratio scale properties. *Pain, 41*, 139-150.

Chapparo, C., & Ranka, J. (2000). Clinical reasoning in occupational therapy. In J. Higgs & M. Jones (Eds.), *Clinical reasoning in the health professions* (pp. 128-137). Oxford, UK: Butterworth-Heinemann.

Cleeland, C. S., & Ryan, K. M. (1994) Pain assessment: Global use of the Brief Pain Inventory. *Annuals of the Academy of Medicine Singapore, 23*(2), 129-138.

Cohn, E. S., Schell, B. A., & Neistadt, M. E. (2003). Introduction to evaluation and interviewing. In E. B. Crepeau, E. S. Cohn, & B. A. Boyt Schell (Eds.), *Willard & Spackman's occupational therapy* (10th ed., pp. 279-285). Philadelphia, PA: Lippincott, Williams & Wilkins.

Cooper, B., Letts, L., Rigby, P., Stewart, D., & Strong, S. (2005). Measuring environmental factors. In M. Law, C. Baum, & W. Dunn (Eds.), *Measuring occupational performance: Supporting best practice in occupational therapy* (pp. 316-344). Thorofare, NJ: SLACK Incorporated.

Corcoran, M. (2005). Using qualitative measurement methods to understand occupational performance. In M. Law, C. Baum, & W. Dunn (Eds.), *Measuring occupational performance: Supporting best practice in occupational therapy* (pp. 65-78). Thorofare, NJ: SLACK Incorporated.

Crepeau, E. B., & Schell, B. A. B. (2009). Analyzing occupations and activity. In E. B. Crepeau, E. S. Cohn, & B. A. Boyt Schell (Eds.), *Willard & Spackman's occupational therapy* (11th ed., pp. 359-374). Philadelphia, PA: Wolters Kluwer Lippincott Williams & Wilkins.

Doherty, R. F. (2009). Ethical decision making in occupational therapy practice. In E. B. Crepeau, E. S. Cohn, & B. A. Boyt Schell (Eds.), *Willard & Spackman's occupational therapy* (11th ed., pp. 274-285). Philadelphia, PA: Wolters Kluwer Lippincott Williams & Wilkins.

Dunn, W. (2000). Best practice occupational therapy assessment. In W. Dunn (Ed.), *Best practice occupational therapy: In community services with children and families* (pp. 79-108). Thorofare, NJ: SLACK Incorporated.

Dunn, W. (2005). Measurement issues and practices. In M. Law, C. Baum, & W. Dunn (Eds.), *Measuring occupational performance: Supporting best practice in occupational therapy* (pp. 21-32). Thorofare, NJ: SLACK Incorporated.

Extended Home Living Services. (n.d). *CASPAR: Comprehensive assessment and solution process for aging residents.* Retrieved from http://www.ehls.com/CASPAROverview.pdf

Fange, A., & Iwarsson, S. (2005). Changes in ADL dependence and aspects of usability following housing adaptation: A longitudinal perspective. *American Journal of Occupational Therapy, 59*, 296-304.

Fange, A., Risser, R., & Iwarsson, S. (2007). Challenges in implementation of research methodology in community-based occupational therapy: The Housing Enabler example. *Scandinavian Journal of Occupational Therapy, 14*, 54-62.

Fasoli, S. E. (2008). Assessing roles and competence. In M. V. Radomski & C. A. Trombly Latham (Eds.), *Occupational therapy for physical dysfunction* (6th ed., pp. 65-90). Philadelphia, PA: Wolters Kluwer/Lippincott, Williams & Wilkins.

Fisher, A. (1995). *Assessment of motor and process skills.* Fort Collins, CO: Three Star Press.

Fleming, M. H. (1991). The therapists with a three track mind. *American Journal of Occupational Therapy, 45*(11), 1007-1014.

Fleming, M. H. (1994). Procedural reasoning: Addressing functional limitations. In C. Mattingly & M. H. Fleming (Eds.), *Clinical reasoning: Forms of inquiry in a therapeutic practice* (pp. 137-177). Philadelphia, PA: Davis.

Gitlin, L. (2005). Measuring performance in instrumental activities of daily living. In M. Law, C. Baum, & W. Dunn (Eds.), *Measuring occupational performance: Supporting best practice in occupational therapy* (pp. 227-247). Thorofare, NJ: SLACK Incorporated.

Henry, A. D., & Kramer, J. M. (2009). The interview process in occupational therapy. In E. B. Crepeau, E. S. Cohn, & B. A. Boyt Schell (Eds.), *Willard & Spackman's occupational therapy* (11th ed., pp. 342-358). Philadelphia, PA: Wolters Kluwer Lippincott Williams & Wilkins.

Iwarsson, S. (2005). A long-term perspective on person-environment fit and ADL dependence among older Swedish adults. *Gerontologist, 45*, 327-336.

Iwarsson, S., Horstmann, V., & Slaug, B. (2007). Housing matters in very old age—Yet differently due to ADL dependence level differences. *Scandinavian Journal of Occupational Therapy, 14*, 3-15.

Iwarsson, S., & Slaug, B. (2010). *The Housing Enabler: A method for rating/screening and analysing accessibility problems in housing* (2nd ed.). Lund & Staffanstorp, Sweden: Veten & Skapen HB and Slaug Enabling Development.

Johansson, K., Lilja, M., Petersson, I., & Borell, L. (2007). Performance of activities of daily living in a sample of applicants for home modification services. *Scandinavian Journal of Occupational Therapy, 14*(1), 44-53.

Johns, C. (2000). *Becoming a reflective practitioner.* Oxford, UK: Blackwell Science.

Katz, S., Ford, A. B., Moskowitz, R. W., Jackson, B. A., & Jaffe, M. W. (1963). Studies of illness in the aged. The index of ADL, a standardized measure of biological and psychological function. *Journal of the American Medical Association, 185*, 914-919.

Kielhofner, G., Mallinson, T., Crawford, D., Nowak, M., Rigby, M., & Henry, A. (1998). *User's manual for the OPHI-II.* Chicago, IL: Model of Human Occupation Clearing House, University of Illinois at Chicago, Department of Occupational Therapy.

Kvale, S. (1996). *Interviews: An introduction to qualitative research interviewing.* Thousand Oaks, CA: Sage Publications.

Law, M., Baptiste, S., Carswell, A., McColl, M., Polatajko, H., & Pollock, N. (1998). *Canadian Occupational Performance Measure* (3rd ed.). Toronto, Ontario: Canadian Association of Occupational Therapists.

Law, M., & Baum, C. (2005). Measurement in occupational therapy. In M. Law, C. Baum, & W. Dunn (Eds.), *Measuring occupational performance: Supporting best practice in occupational therapy* (pp. 1-20). Thorofare, NJ: SLACK Incorporated.

Law, M., Baum, C., & Dunn, W. (2005a). Occupational performance assessment. In C. H. Christiansen, C. M. Baum, & J. Bass-Haugen (Eds.), *Occupational therapy: Performance, participation, and well-being* (pp. 339-360). Thorofare, NJ: SLACK Incorporated.

Law, M., Baum, C., & Dunn, W. (2005b). *Measuring occupational performance: Supporting best practice in occupational therapy.* Thorofare, NJ: SLACK Incorporated.

Mahoney, F. I., & Barthel, D. W. (1965). Functional evaluation: The Barthel Index. *Maryland State Medical Journal, 14,* 61-65.

Mattingly, C., & Fleming, M. (1994). *Clinical reasoning: Forms of inquiry in a therapeutic practice.* Philadelphia, PA: Davis Company.

McColl, M. A., & Pollock, N. (2005). Measuring occupational performance using a client-centered perspective. In M. Law, C. Baum, & W. Dunn (Eds.), *Measuring occupational performance: Supporting best practice in occupational therapy* (pp. 81-91). Thorofare, NJ: SLACK Incorporated.

Peloquin, S. M. (1994). Occupational therapy as art and science: should the older definition be reclaimed? *America Journal of Occupational Therapy, 48*(11), 1093-1096.

Pierre, B. L. (2001). Occupational therapy as documented in patients' records--Part III. Valued but not documented. Underground practice in the context of professional written communication. *Scandinavian Journal of Occupational Therapy, 8,* 174-183.

Pitrella, F., & Kappler, W. (1988). *Identification and evaluation of scale design principles in the development of the Extended Range Sequential Judgement Scale.* Wachtberg, Germany: Research Institute for Human Engineering.

Pybus, R. (1996). *Safety management: Strategy and practice.* Oxford, UK: Butterworth-Heinemann.

Radomski, M. V. (2008). Planning, guiding and documenting practice. In M. V. Radomski & C. A. Trombly Latham (Eds.), *Occupational therapy for physical dysfunction* (6th ed., pp. 41-64). Philadelphia, PA: Wolters Kluwer/Lippincott, Williams & Wilkins.

Rigby, P., Stark, S., Letts, L., & Ringaert, L. (2009). Physical environments. In E. B. Crepeau, E. S. Cohn, & B. A. Boyt Schell (Eds.), *Willard & Spackman's occupational therapy* (11th ed., pp. 820-849). Philadelphia, PA: Wolters Kluwer Lippincott Williams & Wilkins.

Rogers, J. C., & Holm, M. B. (1991). Occupational therapy diagnostic reasoning: A component of clinical reasoning. *American Journal of Occupational Therapy, 45,* 1045-1053.

Rogers, J. C., & Holm, M. B. (1994). *The Performance Assessment of Self-Care Skills (PASS), Version 3.1.* Pittsburgh, PA: University of Pittsburgh.

Rogers, J. C., & Holm, M. B. (2003). Activities of daily living and instrumental activities of daily living. In E. B. Crepeau, E. S. Cohn, & B. A. Boyt Schell (Eds.), *Willard & Spackman's occupational therapy* (10th ed., pp. 315-339). Philadelphia, PA: Lippincott, Williams & Wilkins.

Rogers, J. C., & Holm, M. B. (2007). The Performance Assessment of Self-Care Skills (PASS). In I. E. Asher (Ed.), *An annotated index of occupational therapy evaluation tools* (3rd ed., pp. 102-110). Bethesda, MD: American Occupational Therapy Association.

Rogers, J. C., & Holm, M. B. (2009). The occupational therapy process. In E. B. Crepeau, E. S. Cohn, & B. A. Boyt Schell (Eds.), *Willard & Spackman's occupational therapy* (11th ed., pp. 478-518). Philadelphia, PA: Wolters Kluwer Lippincott Williams & Wilkins.

Sanford, J. A., Pynoos, J., Tejral, A., & Browne, A. (2002). Development of a comprehensive assessment for delivery of home modifications. *Physical & Occupational Therapy in Geriatrics, 20*(2), 43-55.

Schell, B. A. (2009). Professional reasoning in practice. In E. B. Crepeau, E. S. Cohn, & B. A. Boyt Schell (Eds.), *Willard & Spackman's occupational therapy* (11th ed., pp. 314-327). Philadelphia, PA: Wolters Kluwer Lippincott Williams & Wilkins.

Schell, B. A., & Cervero, R. M. (1993). Clinical reasoning in occupational therapy: An integrative review. *American Journal of Occupational Therapy, 47,* 605-610.

Standards Association of Australia. (2004). Australian New Zealand Risk Management Standard (AS/NZ 4360:2004).

Standards Association of Australia (2004). *Australian New Zealand Risk Management Standard* (AS/NZ 4360:2004), Sydney, Australia: Author.

Steinfeld, E. H., & Danford, G. S. (1997). Environment as mediating factor in functional assessment. In S. S. Dittmar & G. E. Gresham (Eds.), *Functional assessment and outcome measures for the rehabilitation health professional* (pp. 37-57). Gaithersburg, MD: Aspen Publishers.

Uniform Data System for Medical Rehabilitation. (1997). *Functional Independence Measure (Version 5.1).* Buffalo, NY: Buffalo General Hospital, State University of New York.

Measuring the Person and the Home Environment

Elizabeth Ainsworth, MOccThy, Grad Cert Health Sci
and Desleigh de Jonge, MPhil (OccThy), Grad Cert Soc Sci

Having a health condition or impairment can be disabling, limiting a person's capacity to manage everyday tasks in the home or community. A home environment that is not designed for a person's specific needs is more handicapping than one whose design is well suited to the occupant.

This chapter describes the information that needs to be obtained to facilitate goodness of fit of the person with his or her home and discusses the contribution to this of an understanding of anthropometrics, ergonomics, and biomechanics. The chapter describes the characteristics of the home environment, such as the size of spaces, gradients, illuminance, force, and sound, that affect occupational performance and identifies tools for measuring these characteristics. The chapter concludes with information about factors that may influence measurement practice in the home.

CHAPTER OBJECTIVES

By the end of this chapter, the reader will be able to:

+ Describe measurement and the types needed for home modification

+ Explain the relevance and limitations of anthropometrics, ergonomics, and biomechanics

+ Describe methods for measuring people, equipment, and the home environment

+ Discuss various measures that relate to home design

+ Describe measuring tools and resources

+ Describe factors influencing measuring practice

+ Explain the consequences of not using reliable measuring techniques

THE IMPORTANCE OF MEASUREMENT

Increasingly, occupational therapists are recognizing the importance of measurement in detailing the attributes of clients, their equipment, and caregivers so that they can be incorporated in the redesign of the home environment. The following discussion provides a general overview of measurement and its importance, the types of measurements required for home modification practice, and the consequences of not using sound measurement techniques.

During the home modification process, therapists gather information about the person-occupation-environment fit by taking systematic and accurate measurements of that person's physical characteristics and features in the home environment that impact occupational performance. Measurements are taken of the person, the equipment he or she uses, and the caregiver to determine the environmental characteristics required to support successful

Ainsworth, E., & de Jonge, D.
An Occupational Therapists's Guide to Home Modification Practice (pp. 139-170)

completion of a range of occupations in and around the home. The person's height, weight, width, and depth—and those of his or her equipment and caregiver—and the person's visual capacity are examined to determine the space, load capacity, clearance, size, and placement of features and illumination requirements in the environment. For example, when designing a shower area for a tall, heavy client who uses a customized wheelchair, the therapist takes measurements of the person in his or her wheelchair and observes transfers and movement within the bathroom to determine the circulation spaces required and the load capacity, size, and placement of the drop-down shower seat. A broad range of activities may occur within the different areas of the home, so it is important that therapists talk with the residents to understand how each area of the home is used and how various activities are undertaken in each area.

Therapists also measure aspects of the environment and their impact on occupational performance or the health, safety, independence, quality of life, and participation of people within the home. The features that are commonly examined include lighting, color, space, heights, widths, distances, gradients, force, and sound (Bridge, 2005). For example, a person with age-related vision changes who is experiencing difficulty mobilizing at night and in transition zones—that is, between the outside and inside of the home—may need lighting levels measured to determine the need for enhanced lighting.

Good measurement practice is critical to good design. Measurement, rather than assumption or guesswork, enables modifications to be tailored to clients' requirements. Occupational therapists can use these measurements to inform clients and other stakeholders about the functional implications of the various aspects of the design and location of features in the environment. Measurements can be used as a foundation for discussing the limitations of the current situation and how activities or the environment can be changed to support occupational performance. These measurements are especially useful for highlighting the extent to which clients' requirements fall outside of the design and performance criteria in the existing access and design standards.

There are several problems that can arise when clients and their environment are inaccurately measured. Clients can be unwilling to accept recommended changes if they perceive that these have not been tailored to suit their specific requirements. Inadequate measurement can also result in solutions being poorly designed, which can cause delays, disruption, and extra expense for the service

or client as he or she navigates problems and renegotiates alternative options with the client. Further, interventions that have not been adequately tailored to the individual's needs are likely to fail, resulting in an accident or injury, poor health, premature or unnecessary institutionalization, increased reliance on others, and a reduced quality of life.

Effective measurement is informed by an understanding of the relevance and application of anthropometrics, ergonomics, and biomechanics. Each of these fields can contribute to an understanding of the person-environment-occupation fit. Anthropometrics can assist in understanding the dimensions of static postures and dynamic movement and how population data are used to inform design. This field of study informs therapists about the diversity of human body characteristics and the importance of providing individualized measures of people who fall outside of the typical population design range. It has also established standardized methods of measurement, which can be used by therapists when gathering individualized measurement information. Ergonomics provides therapists with an understanding of human task demands, the usability of environments, and the person-environment transaction. Biomechanics enables occupational therapists to appreciate the structural basis for human performance, the strength or power capabilities of the human body, and the forces generated by the body as people undertake activities (Standards Australia, 1994).

ANTHROPOMETRY AND ANTHROPOMETRIC MEASUREMENT

Anthropometry is the study of the shape, size, and proportion of the human body, the strength and working capacity or abilities, and the variation of these characteristics in populations (Ching, 1995; Paquet & Feathers, 2004; Pheasant, 1996; Pheasant & Haslegrave, 2006; Steinfeld, Lenker, & Paquet, 2002). Anthropometric data arising from the static and dynamic measurements of the human body (Australian Safety and Compensation Council, 2009) are collected on various populations and are used to guide the design of products, spaces, environments, and systems (Australian Safety and Compensation Council; Baker, 2008; Connell & Sanford, 1999; Cooper, 1998; Pheasant & Haslegrave; Steinfeld et al.).

Large anthropometric data sets, some of which have been derived from people in the armed forces in various countries, have been compiled and presented in multiple tables with detailed measures for

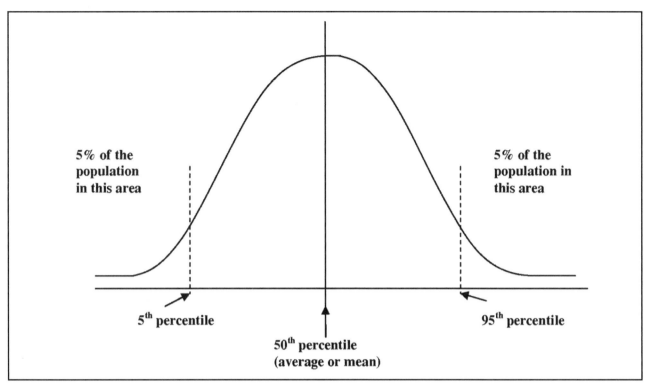

Figure 8-1. The normal distribution represented by the bell-shaped curve.

different subgroups—for example, age and gender (Conway, 2008). When measures of individuals within populations are graphed, they commonly form a normal or bell-shaped curve, with an increasing proportion of the population tending toward the mean near the middle of the curve and a decreasing proportion tending toward the tails of the curve (Diffrient, Tilley, & Bardagjy, 1974), although not all anthropometric measures are symmetrically distributed. It is important that designs sufficiently accommodate anthropometric variability (Pheasant & Haslegrave, 2006). Customarily, the proportion of the population that is used for designs is 90%; that is, anthropometric dimensions occurring at either of or between the 5th and 95th percentiles (Goldsmith, 2000; Pheasant & Haslegrave) or at or below the 90th percentile (Figure 8-1). Expressing population proportions in terms of percentiles is a simple way of indicating the degree of inclusion or exclusion of members of a population (Goldsmith, 1976).

Published anthropometric data may be relevant to the majority of people within populations but not to a sufficient majority because the data have historically tended to exclude people with disabilities. Published anthropometric data might therefore provide little information about the characteristics of people with disabilities (Steinfeld, 2004). A small number of studies, undertaken in the late 1970s and early 1980s, have provided limited data on the anthropometrics of people with disabilities. Many studies on people with disabilities are limited in their usefulness because they have tended to focus on specific disability groups rather than the full range of people with disabilities, lack standardized dimensional definitions and measurement methods (Bridge, 2005; Paquet & Feathers, 2004), and do not include or acknowledge the specific requirements of people with more than one disability (Bridge). Further, the data do not consider the various types of assistive devices used by a range of people with disabilities and how and when they are used (Steinfeld).

Despite the difficulties associated with applying anthropometric data to people with disabilities and across subgroups of them, the available data can assist therapists in understanding the complexities of the human form and how it interfaces with the environment (Baker, 2008). Anthropometric data are necessary when the characteristics of individuals are unknown or when establishing initial estimates of measures of the characteristics where the individual is known. Whatever the case, therapists should understand that when designing for a particular person, it is important that individualized measuring occurs. Without individualized measurements, the suitability of the home modification for the client might be compromised.

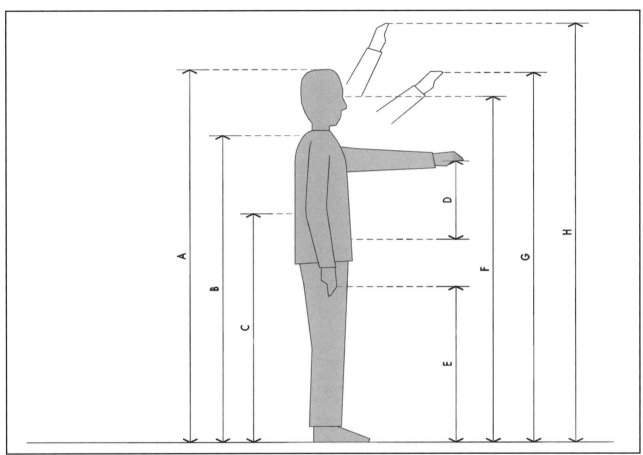

Figure 8-2. Standing anthropometrics. (Adapted from Goldsmith, S. (2000). *Universal design: A manual of practical guidance for architects.* London, UK: Elsevier.)

Types of Anthropometry and Their Application

Two types of anthropometry are used to guide design: structural, or static, anthropometry, and functional, or dynamic, anthropometry.

Structural, or Static, Anthropometry

This form of anthropometry "is the science of measuring length, breadth, and the width of the human population" (Baker, 2008, p. 75). Static measurements are usually taken with the person in the standing and/or seated position. Human dimensions are always considered in the sagittal plane—the vertical plane through the longitudinal axis that divides the body into left and right sections—or the coronal plane—the vertical plane through the longitudinal axis that divides the body into front and back sections (Baker).

The standing posture involves the subjects standing erect and looking straight ahead, with their arms in a relaxed position by their side (Baker, 2008). The seated posture involves the subjects sitting erect and looking straight ahead. Their thighs should be parallel to the floor and their knees bent at a 90 degree angle with feet flat on the floor; the upper arms are to be relaxed and perpendicular to the horizontal plane with the forearm at right angles to the upper arm and parallel to the floor (Baker). Measurements are taken along imaginary horizontal or vertical lines using specific anatomical landmarks, such as popliteal crease at the back of the knee, greater trochanter of the femur, and parts of the body, as reference points. For example, a person's stature is determined by measuring the vertical distance from the floor to the vertex (the crown of the head). This measurement is then used to define the vertical clearance required when standing, walking, or wheeling in an area of the minimum acceptable space or with overhead obstructions. The most common static body dimensions to obtain in relation to the design of home interiors include height, weight, sitting height, eye height, buttock-knee and buttock-popliteal lengths, breadths across elbows and hips, seated knee and popliteal heights, and thigh clearance height (Panero & Zelnik, 1979; Figures 8-2 and 8-3).

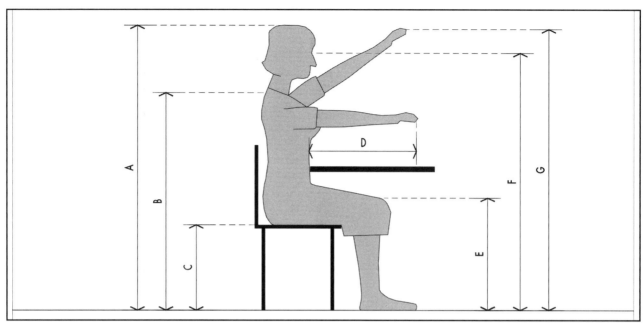

Figure 8-3. Seated anthropometrics. (Adapted from Goldsmith, S. (2000). *Universal design: A manual of practical guidance for architects*. London, UK: Elsevier.)

Measurements to note in Figure 8-2:

+ A = Floor to top of head
+ B = Floor to shoulder
+ C = Floor to elbow
+ D = Waist to hand
+ E = Floor to wrist
+ F = Floor to eye level
+ G = Diagonal reach range—floor to hand
+ H = Diagonal reach range—floor to hand

Measurements to note in Figure 8-3:

+ A = Floor to top of head
+ B = Floor to top of shoulder
+ C = Floor to popliteal area
+ D = Chest to end of hand
+ E = Floor to top of knee
+ F = Floor to eye level
+ G = Diagonal forward reach

Anthropometric data on people with disabilities also include dimensions of people occupying assistive devices. Dimensions of an occupied wheelchair are used to determine the floor space and vertical and horizontal clearance requirements of people using wheelchairs.

Functional, or Dynamic, Anthropometry

This form of anthropometry involves the measurement of a subject while in motion to help determine the properties of the body, such as range of motion or reach, and stride or clearance (Ching, 1995; Cooper, 1998). This can also include the measurement of the subject during movement associated with certain tasks, such as reaching, using an assistive device, or the measurement of the subject's strength (Steinfeld et al., 2002). These types of data are more difficult to reliably obtain because of the movement of the subject during the measurement process. However, functional or dynamic anthropometry provides more accurate information about the movement within spaces and during activities. For example, when considering the ability of the body to reach forward, the static measurement that would be used is "arm length" (Australian Safety and Compensation Council, 2009). However, dynamic analysis of a person reaching forward shows that the shoulder joint also moves forward with the arm, thus increasing the person's forward reach capacity beyond the static length of the arm (Australian Safety and Compensation Council, p. 42).

The size, shape, weight, and movement patterns of people with disabilities vary considerably, requiring the environment to be customized to their unique requirements. Occupational therapists use the principles of anthropometric measurement to position clients and locate anatomical landmarks and parts of the body when establishing clients' specific dimensions. Using an established and standardized approach to measurement, where possible, ensures that practice is accurately and consistently replicated by staff, particularly when there is a range of approaches. Individualizing the measurement process is particularly useful where usability and safety require a close fit between individuals, their equipment and caregivers, and their environment (Steinfeld et al., 1979; Steinfeld et al., 2002). For example, a bathroom needs to be designed to "fit" an individual's stature and functional reach range to ensure his or her safety and the usability of the fittings. Specifically measuring a person allows therapists to collect concrete and scientific information that can be used to analyze why a space is not working and design or redesign spaces to suit the needs of users with specific requirements (Goldsmith, 2000).

BIOMECHANICS

Biomechanics is the study of human movement using mechanical principles (Spaulding, 2008a). It examines movement and equilibrium using the principles of physics to investigate the influence of forces, levers, and torque on performance (Pedretti, 1996). Because the biomechanics of the human body are so complex, no single biomechanical model of the human body currently exists; rather, there are many models from various fields of use to explain movement of the human body (Kroemer, 1987).

Biomechanics can be used to analyze movement in everyday activities to understand the mechanical aspects of the movement. In a biomechanical analysis of the sit-to-stand transfer, Laporte, Chan, and Sveistrup (1999) highlight the role of displacement, momentum, velocity, and the relationship between the center of pressure and center of mass throughout the four phases of the sit-to-stand transfer. This type of analysis provides therapists with a detailed understanding of the elements of the movement and how variations in movement may result in performance difficulties.

Using biomechanical principles, therapists systematically observe performance in order to examine the quality of the movement, the effectiveness of performance, and the potential for injury (Kreighbaum & Barthels, 1996; Pheasant, 1987). By using a qualitative biomechanical analysis, therapists can identify ineffective or problematic aspects of movement. Considerations commonly include the following:

+ *Range of movement*: Working outside of safe ranges of motion and/or within extreme ranges

+ *Center of gravity*: Displacement of the person's center of gravity outside of the base of support

+ *Accuracy*: Imprecise or uncoordinated movements

+ *Speed and momentum*: Slow, hesitant, uncontrolled, or impulsive actions

+ *Strength*: Overexertion or ineffective positioning resulting in poor use of force, levers, and torque

+ *Endurance*: Limited activity tolerance or excessive energy expenditure (Steinfeld et al., 1979)

Occupational therapists also draw on biomechanical principles to improve movement and make it safer. They identify the most appropriate posture for the performance of a task with a view to maximizing the effect of forces and minimizing muscular effort (Pheasant, 1987). They also advise on strategies to improve the effectiveness and efficiency of movement and reduce the likelihood of injury. Based on their biomechanical analysis of the sit-to-stand transfer, Chan, Laporte, and Sveistrup (1999) identify a range of strategies to improve the effectiveness and safety of the movement—for example, the ideal initial body position and the proper use of body mechanics throughout the movement.

ERGONOMICS

Ergonomics is concerned with shaping environments and tasks to optimize the abilities of individuals to perform activities (Baker, 2008; Conway, 2008; Stein, Soderback, Cutler, & Larson, 2006). It involves measuring and using the dimensions of objects and spaces to examine the human task demands (Conway; Stein et al.). Though ergonomics emerged from the area of work performance, worker safety, and productivity, it is not solely confined to workplace environments (Berg Rice, 2008). The concepts and principles are derived from research in many fields, including industrial engineering, human factors psychology, occupational medicine, and nursing as well as occupational therapy (Stein et al.). Like occupational therapy, the field of ergonomics is concerned with the usability of environments and the person-environment transaction (Conway). The principles of ergonomics can be used to prevent musculoskeletal injures, conserve energy, and use the body in the most efficient way possible when engaging in activity or occupation (Stein et al.).

Two approaches are commonly used in an ergonomic evaluation—task analysis and user trial (Pheasant, 2006). Task analysis involves examining what the person is doing or needs to do and analyzing the physical movements and information processing involved and the actual or potential environmental barriers or constraints (Conway, 2008). An effective task analysis involves clarifying the person's goals, the intended outcome, and the potential areas of mismatch between the person, the activity, and the environment (Conway). A user trial involves the naturalistic trial of a product or environment to determine its usability (Conway) and to evaluate whether there is a satisfactory match with the user when considering its comfort, usability, and performance (Pheasant, 1987).

With its user-centered approach and person-environment transactive perspective (Pheasant & Haselgrave, 2006), ergonomics can assist occupational therapists to determine the adequacy of the person-environment fit (Conway, 2008; Stein et al., 2006). Ergonomic principles guide the analysis of the person's posture, movement, and performance and the impact of the environment (Berg Rice, 2008). An ergonomic approach provides therapists with a framework for evaluating and matching the design of the layout, fittings, and fixtures to suit the specific capabilities of the person; additionally, it assists in selecting products, equipment, and designs to improve client or caregiver efficiency, effectiveness, and safety (Berg Rice).

MEASURING THE CLIENT, EQUIPMENT, AND CAREGIVERS

People vary in terms of their body size and movement patterns, the equipment they use, and the assistance they receive; hence, therapists often need to take an individualized approach when measuring clients, their caregivers, and their equipment. Therapists gather this information to alert builders and designers to the specific requirements of clients whose dimensions or abilities fall outside of the population addressed by the standards. Individualized measurement is advisable, particularly, for people who vary substantially in terms of height, size, or weight and for those who use equipment other than a standard wheelchair; have impairments that affect their posture, movement, or balance; have limited use of their upper limbs; or require caregiver assistance for various activities.

The challenge for occupational therapists lies in knowing what to measure and how to measure it. By measuring people's size, shape, weight, space requirements (with consideration for their equipment and/or caregiver dimensions), reach, clearance, posture, and strength, the therapist can determine the space they require and the best location for fixtures and fittings.

Individuals' body dimensions might need to be measured in various static or dynamic postures, such as sitting, standing, bending, kneeling, or lying positions, depending on the nature of the activities they are involved in around the home. Posture relates to the orientation of body parts in space and depends on the dimensions of the body and their relationship with items in the environment. People with poor strength and endurance or visual difficulties might experience change in posture throughout the day or alter their posture for different activities. Posture might vary as a result of natural biological fluctuations. For example, a person's stature can vary approximately 15 mm over 24 hours, being the greatest first thing in the morning when the spine has been relieved of supporting body weight through lying down overnight (Pheasant & Haslegrave, 2006). Shrinkage of the spine tends to occur rapidly within the first 3 hours of rising (Pheasant & Haslegrave). It may not always be possible to measure clients in seated or standing positions. In these cases, therapists need to choose the posture that best suits the clients' disabilities, the activities they wish to complete, and the environment in which they will function in that position. For example, if a client needs to reach to operate an intercom while in bed, he or she will need to be measured lying down and reaching to the area on the wall that would best suit the person's capacity to operate the device.

The following diagrams and photos provide an illustration of typical body postures and the location of the body landmarks used as reference points during the measurement process. Pheasant and Haslegrave (2006) provide a detailed description of body dimensions and what these dimensions apply to in relation to the design of the built environment. The examples provided in the following discussion are the measures most commonly taken by occupational therapists.

The Height, Width, and Depth of Parts of the Body

The therapist uses a tape measure to determine height, width, and depth of parts of the person and the equipment above floor level (AFL). Pheasant and Haslegrave (2006) provide the following detail:

+ A person's stature is determined by measuring the vertical distance from the floor to the vertex (the crown of the head). This measurement defines the vertical clearance required when standing, walking, or wheeling in an area or the minimum acceptable space of overhead obstructions.

+ Shoulder height is measured from the floor to the acromion (the bony tip of the shoulder), and it is the reference point for the location of fittings, fixtures, and controls.

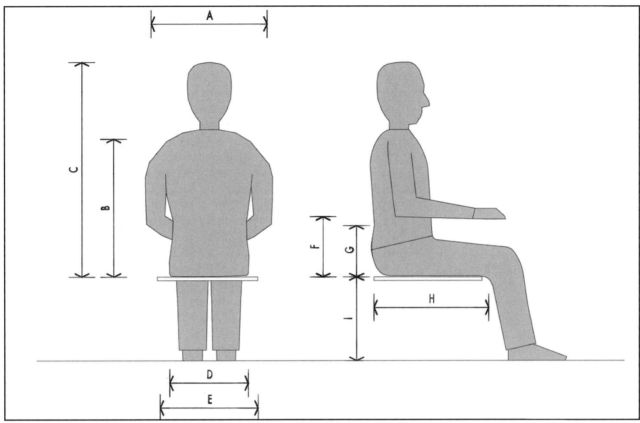

Figure 8-4. Rear and side views of a seated person. (Adapted from Pheasant, S. (1996). *Bodyspace: Anthropometry, ergonomics and the design of work.* London, UK: T.J. Press.)

+ Knee height includes the horizontal distance from the floor to the upper surface of the knee (measured to the quadriceps muscle and not the knee cap), and it provides measurement to inform the clearance required beneath the underside of tables.

+ Popliteal height is the measurement from the floor to the popliteal angle at the underside of the knee where the tendon insertion of the biceps femoris muscle is located. This dimension defines the maximum acceptable height of the seat.

+ Hip width is the maximum horizontal distance across the hips in the seated position, and this information relates to the minimum width of a seat.

+ Hand width is measured across the palm of the hand and includes a measurement of the distal ends of the carpal bones to provide information on clearance for hand access to handles or rails.

+ Depth of the area between the popliteal area at the underside of the knee to the rear of the buttocks provides information to inform the design of the depth of a seat (Figures 8-4 and 8-5).

Measurements to note in Figure 8-4:
+ A = Shoulder width
+ B = Seat to the top of the shoulders
+ C = Seat to the top of the head
+ D = Width of the buttocks
+ E = Width of the seat
+ F = Bottom of buttocks to the elbow
+ G = Seat to the lumbar area
+ H = Rear of the buttocks to the popliteal area of the leg
+ I = Floor to the popliteal area

Measurements to note in Figure 8-5:
+ A = Chest to toe
+ B = Edge of armrest to end of toe or footplate (whichever protrudes the most)
+ C = End of armrest to end of toe
+ D = Floor to toe with foot on footplate
+ E = Floor to seat of wheelchair (or top of cushion on wheelchair)
+ F = Floor to knee with foot on footplate
+ G = Floor to eye level

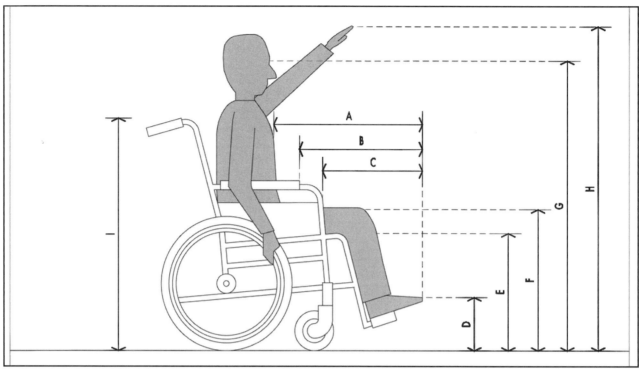

Figure 8-5. Occupied wheelchair. (Adapted from Goldsmith, S. (2000). *Universal design: A manual of practical guidance for architects*. London, UK: Elsevier.)

+ H = Diagonal forward reach
+ I = Height of wheelchair

Eye Height

The therapist also measures eye height, which is measured from the floor to the inner canthus (corner) of the eye. This dimension defines the maximum acceptable height for visual obstructions and defines sight lines (Pheasant & Haslegrave, 2006; see Figures 8-2 through 8-6).

Reach Ranges

The measurement of an individual's functional reach ranges, when positioned in various postures, is important in determining the width and height of environmental features, such as storage cupboards, benches, and clothes lines. The therapist considers the location of the features in the environment and asks clients to move and reach either forward or sideways with the arm they are most likely to use. This activity could also be undertaken in a natural environment in which the various features are positioned, or the therapist might need to simulate the location of the various features during the measurement exercise. Refer to Figures 8-2 through 8-12.

Measurements to note in Figure 8-7:

+ A to G = Side reach

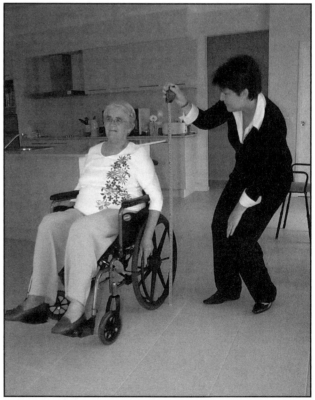

Figure 8-6. Measuring eye height above floor level.

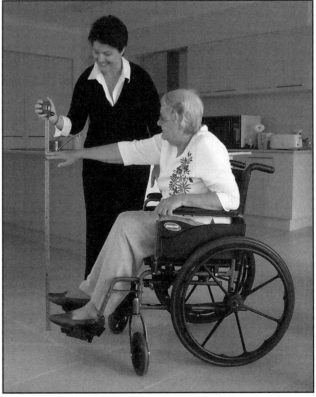

Figure 8-7. Occupied wheelchair. Side reach. (Adapted from Goldsmith, S. (2000). *Universal design: A manual of practical guidance for architects*. London, UK: Elsevier.)

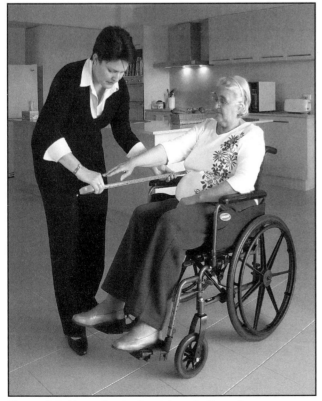

Figure 8-8. Measuring horizontal reach dimension.

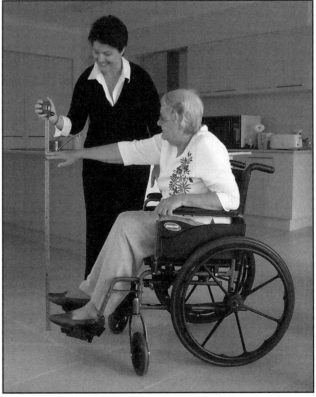

Figure 8-9. Measuring forward horizontal functional reach dimension.

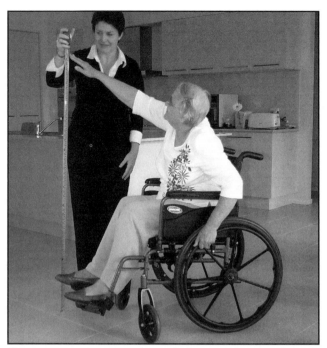

Figure 8-10. Measuring forward diagonal functional reach dimension.

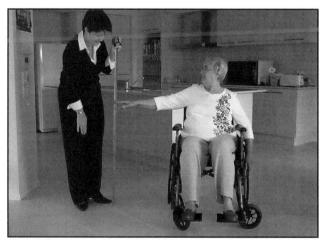

Figure 8-11. Measuring side horizontal functional reach above floor level.

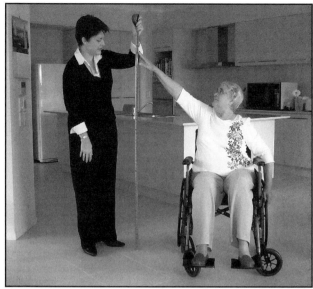

Figure 8-12. Measuring side diagonal functional reach above floor level.

Determining Size of Spaces for Transfer and Mobility Equipment

Reflecting the distinction between static or dynamic studies in anthropometrics, two strategies for determining the size of spaces for occupied or unoccupied mobility equipment such as wheelchairs, scooters, or wheeled walking aids, can be differentiated, depending upon whether the person is stationary or moving. The distinction is made here because sizes of spaces for stationary equipment can be determined from measurements of the occupied or unoccupied equipment itself, whereas, in practical terms, determining the sizes of spaces for moving equipment cannot. Spaces to consider when measuring equipment in motion include the following:

+ Volumetric (three-dimensional) space
+ Planar (two-dimensional) space traversed on the travel surface—the ground or floor surface.

Most rooms and spaces in the home will require consideration of the motion of equipment; however, consideration of stationary equipment is necessary for storage and parking spaces and at the start and end positions of their motion.

Measurement for Stationary Mobility Equipment

For the minimum size of spaces to store or park equipment, measurement will be required of at least the overall width, length, and height of the equipment. For more compact storage, such as under bench tops for wheelchairs, the dimensions of foot, back, and arm support assemblies and drive wheels will also be required. For even more compact storage of equipment that can be folded, measurements will be required of them in their folded state.

Occupied and unoccupied wheelchairs are typically illustrated in plan view as being symmetrical about their longitudinal and lateral axes. However, many unoccupied and especially occupied pieces of equipment are asymmetrical (Hunter, 2009). Asymmetry is attributable to the equipment, the occupant, accessories such as respirators, and loose items such as handbags and walking aids. The need

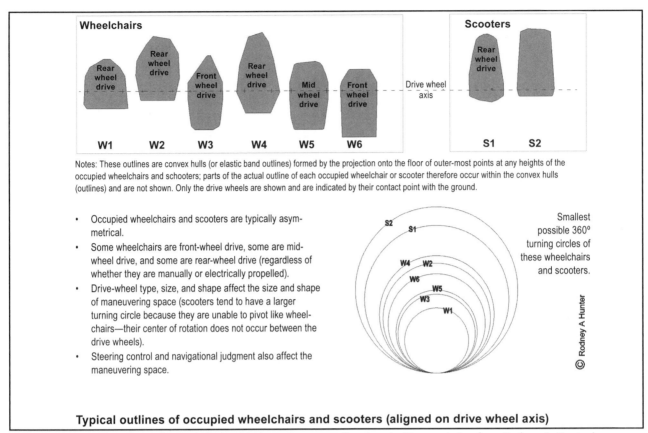

Typical outlines of occupied wheelchairs and scooters (aligned on drive wheel axis)

Figure 8-13. Typical outlines of occupied wheelchairs and scooters. (Reprinted with permission from Rodney A. Hunter.)

for consideration of loose items in space planning should be confirmed with clients. Figure 8-13 illustrates the typical asymmetry of wheelchair and scooters.

Measuring unoccupied or occupied wheelchairs and scooters requires measurement of the distance between outermost points on them. These are typically on hand rims, the rear of drive wheels, ends of handgrips, tops of back supports, and ends of arm and foot supports. Outermost points on users include, for wheelchairs, the ends of shoes and elbows, fingers, or wrists on hand rims or controls of electric wheelchairs, and the top of users' heads. Outermost points may also be on features or accessories added to the equipment by clients. Outermost points on users do not necessarily occur at the skeletal protuberances commonly used as reference points in biomechanics.

Prior knowledge of key features that typically constitute the two- and three-dimensional outlines of occupied and unoccupied equipment assists in orienting to the measuring task. Of greatest importance, however, is skill in recognizing the features that constitute the envelope of occupied or unoccupied equipment and the relevant outermost points on it.

The number of points is determined by the end use of the measuring. If the end use is to determine the size of a cube for storing equipment, only the pairs of points corresponding with overall width, length, and height of the equipment are required. For space under bench tops and the like for wheelchairs, dimensions of arm support assemblies, legs, and feet positions will also be required.

Methods for recording outermost points include photogrammetry and laser scanning; however, these can be time consuming and costly. Simple, inexpensive and sufficiently accurate methods for most home modifications are manual ones. The most common and quickest manual method is measuring between outermost points of the equipment with a tape measure.

If only the overall length and width need to be measured, movable panels can be used. Polystyrene is a suitable material for panels; the panels need to have a base that is large and heavy enough for stability of the panel. For this method, the panels are placed parallel to each other and at each side of the equipment and then moved toward it until they just touch it. The procedure is repeated at the ends of the equipment. There are three advantages of this method: (a) the panels can be easily placed at

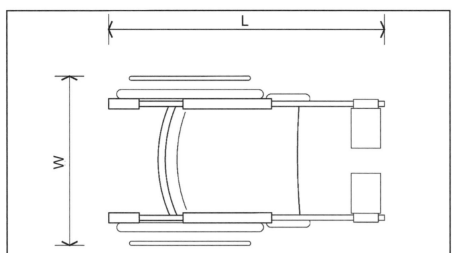

Figure 8-14. Unoccupied wheelchair.

whatever angle with respect to each other and that most snugly contains the equipment for purpose of storage space that is not rectangular in plan; (b) the panels can be used to test for the parking or storing motion of the equipment; and (c) no prior knowledge of measuring points is required.

For mobility equipment with castor wheels, a dimension that may need to be measured is the pivoting radius of the castor wheels. Castor wheels can swing outside of the envelope of equipment, especially if, after the equipment has stopped, it is suddenly moved in the opposite direction. If there is insufficient space for this, the equipment can become jammed in the storage space.

The measured width and length of the stationary equipment will need to be increased to allow for typical imperfect control of the equipment as it is driven or pushed into or out of the parking or storage space. Additional measurement will also be necessary where space is required to transfer in and out of the equipment or if space is required for another person to assist the equipment user (Figures 8-14 through 8-22).

Measurements to note in Figure 8-14:

+ L = Length of wheelchair
+ W = Width of wheelchair

Measurements to note in Figure 8-15:

+ L = Length of wheelchair
+ H = Height of wheelchair

Measurements to note in Figure 8-16:

+ W = Width of wheelchair
+ H = Height of wheelchair

Measurements to note in Figure 8-17:

+ L = Length from back of rear wheel to the front of the footplate or person's toe (edge that protrudes)

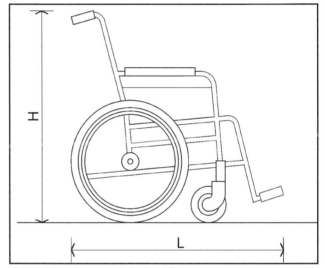

Figure 8-15. Unoccupied wheelchair.

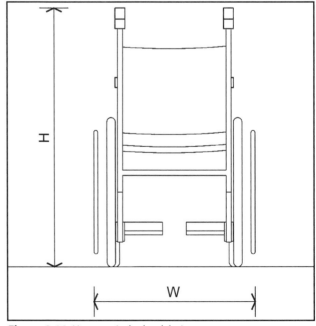

Figure 8-16. Unoccupied wheelchair.

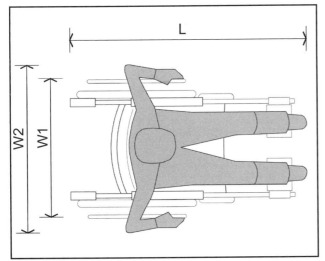

Figure 8-17. Occupied wheelchair. (Adapted from Goldsmith, S. (2000). *Universal design: A manual of practical guidance for architects*. London, UK: Elsevier.)

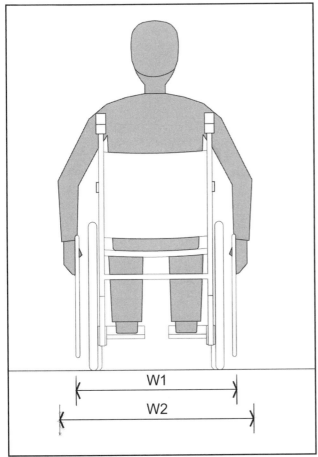

Figure 8-18. Occupied wheelchair. (Adapted from Goldsmith, S. (2000). *Universal design: A manual of practical guidance for architects*. London, UK: Elsevier.)

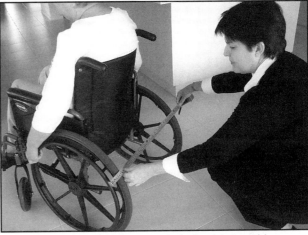

Figure 8-19. Measuring the occupied wheelchair width.

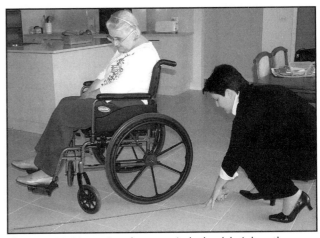

Figure 8-20. Measuring the occupied wheelchair length.

+ W1 = Width of the wheelchair without the person's hands on the wheel rims; width from wheel rim to wheel rim

+ W2 = Width of the wheelchair; person's hands on the wheel rims; width measurement to include widest point (knuckles or elbows protruding)

Measurements to note in Figure 8-18:

+ W1 = Width of the wheelchair without the person's hands on the wheel rims; width from wheel rim to wheel rim

+ W2 = Width of the wheelchair; person's hands on the wheel rims; width measurement to include widest point (knuckles or elbows protruding)

It must be noted that some people with disabilities have different body shapes, reach, and movement patterns that do not correlate with these diagrams. In such cases, an individualized measurement approach would be required.

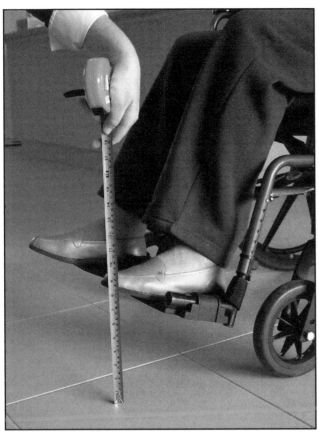

Figure 8-21. Measuring the height of the toe above floor level.

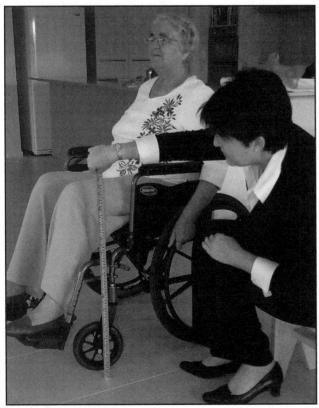

Figure 8-22. Measuring knee height above floor level.

Measurement for Mobility Equipment in Use

Mobility equipment moves between stationary states corresponding with parked or stored positions; the path between these positions are straight, curved, or partly both. Parked positions that typically need to be considered in relation to equipment motion include those in showers and at toilet pans, hand basins, and kitchen sinks.

Measuring for Straight Paths or Curved Paths of Large Diameter

For the cross-sectional dimensions of straight paths or curved paths of large diameter, such as height and width of paths, the minimum required dimensions and the techniques for obtaining them may be the same as those for stationary occupied equipment.

Curved paths of large diameter can be treated similarly to straight paths because the relevant outermost points on the occupied equipment will tend to be the same in each case.

Therapists should be aware that, even if path widths can be determined from the dimensions of stationary equipment, widths will need to be increased for typical imperfect control of equipment and hence avoidance of damage and injury. The additional width will need to be estimated or measured by trial-and-error using techniques discussed below. Additionally, for long footpaths and corridors (and for lifts), space might also be required for a 180-degree turn, for which the required space will need to be established as discussed below.

Measuring for Maneuvering and Curved Paths of Small Diameter

The term *maneuvering* here denotes motion comprised of turns having very small diameter, including reversing turns that involve alternating forward and backward motion.

Determining the size of spaces from measurements of stationary equipment is much more difficult for maneuvering and for curved paths of small diameter than it is for straight travel or curved paths of large diameter. This is because the relevant outermost points tend to be different between the two cases and different for different maneuvers. This is illustrated in Appendix A. The detail in the appendix illustrates that, for four types of 90-degree clockwise turns, there are three different pairs of outermost points that determine the width of the space.

Because of the complexity of estimating or calculating space for equipment in motion by using measurements of the occupied equipment when they are stationary, it may be much better to measure the spaces occupied by the moving equipment.

Two methods for determining the size of space for maneuvering are (a) recording the space traversed on the floor by the moving equipment and then measuring that space and (b) using barriers as measuring datums between which to measure dimensions of the space. In this latter method, the barriers act as a large measuring tool having adjustable reference planes (datums).

The first method does not require barriers; however, barriers add greater realism and possibly greater accuracy to path recording. For the second method, the barriers are incrementally positioned closer to or farther away from the occupied equipment until the client reports or it is observed that the maneuver occurs in the least space with reasonable ease and without touching the barriers.

The space traversed by moving equipment can be recorded using a physical scale model fitted with pens (Bails & Public Buildings Department of South Australia, 1983); actual occupied equipment fitted with pens (Ringaert, Rapson, Qiu, Cooper, & Shwedyk, 2001); sonar or video recording devices; pressure-sensitive mats that record electronically or physically (Hunter, 2003); or computer simulation (Han, Law, Latombe, & Kunz, 2002; Hunter, 2005). For home modifications, these techniques may be too costly and time consuming. Furthermore, physical scale modeling and computer simulation require additional information for estimates about spatial allowances for steering control and navigational judgments by equipment users and about the space occupied by people assisting the user (this additional information would need to be obtained by one of the other methods using actual equipment).

Barriers as a Measuring Tool

The use of incrementally adjustable barriers as a measuring tool is a simple method suitable for home modifications. The barriers may be simplified ones (Hunter, 2002), replicated or actual barriers (Steinfeld, Schroeder, & Bishop, 1979), or simple panels as previously noted. An advantage of this method is that knowledge of the dimensions of the occupied or unoccupied equipment or of equipment users' steering control or navigational judgments is not required, although the latter may need to be specified as part of the testing. The method can also readily incorporate the contribution to space requirements of people assisting the equipment user. Measuring may be easier in premises other than the home but may incur logistical difficulties.

Measuring may be more feasible in homes if chalked or taped lines on the floor are used instead of moveable panels. If the maneuvering overlaps lines,

they can be replaced or augmented by lines alongside them. Care is required to identify whether any part of the occupied wheelchair overlaps the lines.

Understanding an Individual's Space Needs

A measuring project for a home is facilitated by first learning how clients move about in their homes, in particular how areas are approached, activities in them carried out, and the areas departed. For example, when examining the space requirements of a wheelchair user during toileting, observations need to be made of the client's capacity to wheel to the room, negotiate the doorway, wheel beside the toilet, transfer on and off the toilet, access and use the hand basin, and then depart from the area. Movement must be possible without having to move furniture or inflicting damage to walls and doorways and other fittings and fixtures.

Consideration may also need to be given to the circumstance where more than one wheelchair is used in the home and whether a wheelchair may be changed in size or type after a period. The equipment that requires the greatest space will therefore probably have to take priority over the others in determining space requirements.

The Geometry of Curvilinear Travel

Understanding the basic geometry (shapes) of curvilinear travel can be useful for measurement projects. The geometry of curvilinear travel is infinitely variable, but some generalizations are possible.

In terms of geometry of travel, common types of wheelchairs and scooters are rear-, mid-, and front-wheel drive wheelchairs and three- and four-wheel scooters. The geometry of scooter travel is similar to tricycles. The type, size, and shape of wheelchairs determines the least possible space required for them; that is, the space required by them as if they were perfectly driven. There can be a pronounced variation between the spaces traversed by different wheelchairs in terms of sizes and shapes and the location of the spaces in relation to the physical feature with which the turn is associated.

Curvilinear travel and maneuvers are typically comprised of (a) circular turns and (b) noncircular turns such as hyperbolic-shaped turns (the diameter of the turn path becomes successively bigger, or smaller, throughout the turn). Each of these turn types may be performed as a single motion in the one direction (clockwise or counterclockwise) or as several motions in different directions as occurs in reversing turns. Most maneuvers involve reversing turns of varying complexity. A predominantly single motion turn can also incorporate a very small reversing turn (see Figure 8-23 showing an imperfect turn around a bollard).

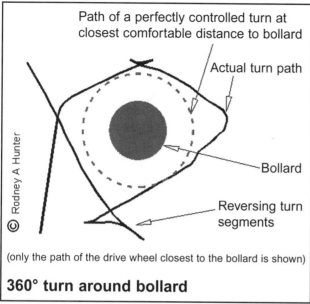

Path of a perfectly controlled turn at closest comfortable distance to bollard

Actual turn path

© Rodney A Hunter

Bollard

Reversing turn segments

(only the path of the drive wheel closest to the bollard is shown)

360° turn around bollard

Figure 8-23. Imperfect turn around bollard. (Reprinted with permission from Rodney A. Hunter.)

Motion at a feature can be regarded as a single maneuver, with start and end stationary positions (even though the equipment may be stationary for a barely measurable period). Approach and departure travel paths need to be considered additionally to this maneuver because of their contribution to the overall size of space required at the feature and, importantly, because of their influence on the type and therefore size and shape of the space traversed by the maneuvering.

Of relevance to the conventional incorporation of right-angled room layouts in buildings is categorization of compact turns of wheelchairs and scooters in terms of a small number of fundamental types. These are 360-, 180-, and 90-degree turns about the mid-point between the drive wheels of wheelchairs; 90-degree turns about either of the drive wheels of wheelchairs; 360-, 180-, and 90-degree turns about the center of the smallest turning circle of scooters (or tricycles); and noncircular turns. Reversing turns can be categorized as 180-degree turns, of which two types can also be differentiated, although reversing turns are really just successive 90-degree turns. Examples of these fundamental types of turns are indicated and further explained in Appendix B. In reality, the variety of turns employed by wheelchair and scooter users, knowingly or otherwise, is infinite. Nevertheless, knowledge of the fundamental types of turns allows an approximation or initial estimation of maneuvering space requirements.

Turns of 360 degrees are applicable to general living areas or other spaces in which there is no predominant direction of travel. Spaces for 180-degree turns are smaller than spaces for 360-degree turns and may be acceptable to clients. Turns of 90 degrees apply to doorways and corners of corridors or footpaths.

The fundamental turns should not be regarded as absolute bases for determining sizes and shapes of spaces for equipment use. Rather, they should be used as initial approximations in designing, or for the initial setup of panels or floor lines for maneuvering trials. Whether the size of spaces should be determined with reference to any one of the fundamental turns will be a matter of trial-and-error and collaboration with the client.

Procedures for Measuring Maneuvering Spaces

360-Degree turn Test

The occupied equipment is positioned in a corner formed by fixed panels or the walls of a room; two relocatable panels or other barriers or floor lines are placed parallel and opposite these walls to enclose the occupied equipment. Starting from a position facing one of the fixed elements, the person operating the equipment then performs a 360-degree turn. If space is insufficient or excessive, the moveable elements are gradually and successively positioned until the turn can be performed without the equipment or the person's body touching the walls or overlapping the barriers (International Organization for Standardization, 2005) as per Figure 8-24.

180-Degree turn Test

A fixed panel or wall of a room is used as one side of a corridor, and a moveable panel or other barrier or line marking is placed parallel with it as the other side. Starting from a position between the panels and facing along the corridor, the person operating the equipment performs a 180-degree turn. If space is insufficient or excessive, the moveable element is gradually and successively positioned until the turn can be successfully performed.

Two trial procedures should be conducted: one where the 180-degree turn is performed as a single turn in a clockwise or counterclockwise direction, or both, and the other as a reversing turn as illustrated in Appendix B. Two reversing turn trials should also be undertaken: one where the initial motion is forward and one where the initial motion is backward as shown in Diagrams 9 and 10 in Appendix B.

90-Degree Turn Test

Two types of 90-degree turns should be tested: (a) around the corner of a corridor (or through a doorway into a corridor) or (b) from a corridor through a

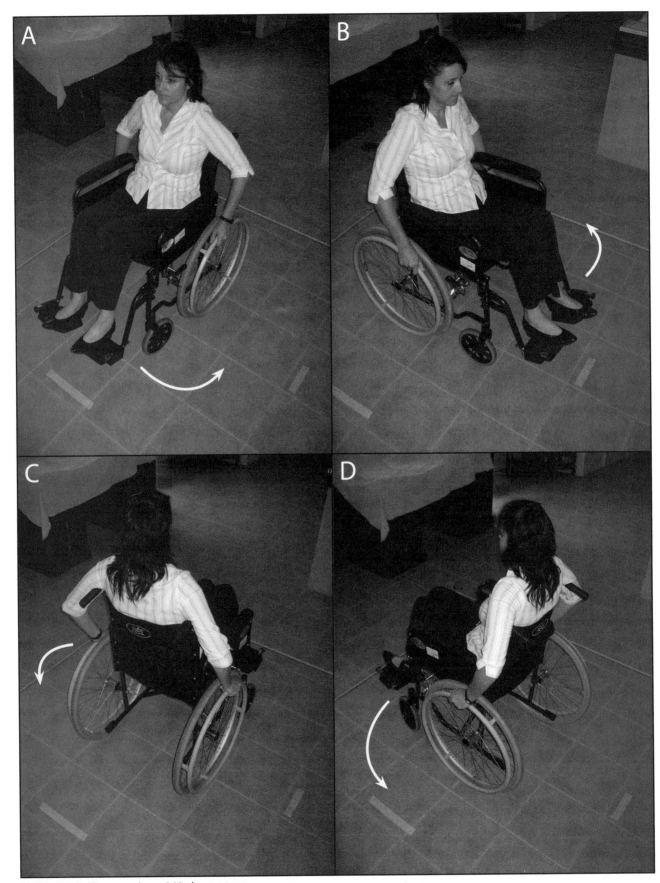

Figure 8-24. Commencing a 360-degree turn.

doorway. Instead of or as well as the corridor corner test, turns around the outside and inside of wall corners (that is, not in a corridor) will yield additional information. The procedures are similar to those for 360- and 180-degree turns. For the outside and inside corner tests, the wheelchair users should be asked to stay as close to the corner as possible. There are a large number of other configurations and maneuvers that might also need to be tested.

Specifying Circular or Noncircular Turns

Though it is easy to distinguish between circular and noncircular turns on a drawing for 180 degree reversing turns and 90-degree turns, actually testing separately for these turns will probably be impracticable. What is important is that clients employ whatever strategy is most effective for them in performing turns in as little space as comfortably possible.

Weight

The weight of the person and his or her equipment can be measured using specifically designed weight scales. Alternatively, the client might be able to report his or her own weight at the time of the home visit, and the weight of the equipment may be documented in the technical specifications available from medical equipment suppliers. This information is important in designing ramps and other structures that need to take the load of the person and his or her equipment, and these weights can be particularly important if the client has bariatric equipment requirements.

Recording Measurement Information

The measurement information can be recorded in a form similar to Table 8-1, which has been compiled from figures and information from Goldsmith (1976, 2000), Pheasant and Haslegrave (2006), Bridge (1996), and Steinfeld, Maisel, and Feathers (2005).

Measuring Features in the Built Environment

The aspects measured in the environment depend on the nature of the environmental barrier or issue that is presented at the time of the home visit. Therapists measure the observable aspects of the home environment to gather information to assist in the redesign of the area. Environmental features typically measured include the length and width of rooms and the height and location of fixtures and fittings. Distances and gradients can also be measured when the person's ability to mobilize around the property needs to be addressed. In addition, therapists may wish to establish noise and lighting levels throughout the home and the force required to open and close doors and drawers.

At times, it might be necessary for a technical specialist to visit the home to undertake more formal and specific measurement activities, particularly in cases where major modifications are to be undertaken or the therapist does not have the skill, training, and technical expertise in specific measurement techniques. For example, a builder can be engaged to measure the levels of external areas around the home in order to design a ramp, or an acoustic engineer might be required to measure the sound levels of a household.

The following section provides information on the various tools and resources used to measure features in the built environment.

Dimensions

Dimensions include measures of length, width, and height and are taken using key reference points within the built environment. These reference points are conventions documented in publications such as access standards for consistency and to establish the start and finish of a measure. For example, the reference point for measuring dimensions of walls is the finished face of the wall; that is, the plaster sheeting or tiling, which can be placed on the face of the plaster sheet. The reference points for doorways are in the inside face of the door jamb on the latch side of the doorway and the face of the door leaf in the 90 degree open position. The top of the hand rail or grab bar is the reference point for measuring their height above the nosing of the stair or floor. The center of the operable part of the power or light switch is the reference point for measuring the height above the bench or floor. The centerline of the toilet is the reference point for measuring the distance of the toilet from the side wall. Figures 8-25 through 8-28 provide examples of reference points in the built environment that are used during the measurement process.

A number of resources are available to guide therapists in measuring specific features in the built environment and identifying specific reference points. Illustrations of the location of reference points and corresponding dimension lines can guide measurement practice, and they can be found in resources such as the Comprehensive Assessment and Solution Process for Aging Residents (CASPAR; Extended Home Living Service, n.d.), which provides detailed illustrations of the essential measurements for a range of architectural features important to home modifications, such as stairs at entrances and within the home (Figures 8-29 through 8-32).

There are a range of tools that are used to measure dimension as illustrated in Figure 8-33.

Table 8-1. Measuring a Person and His or Her Mobility Equipment

FEATURE	MEASUREMENT	HOUSING FEATURES (examples)	BUILT ENVIRONMENT DIMENSION REQUIRED
General Measurements of the Person—Seated or Standing			
Height		Clearance below overhead obstructions	
Width		Width of doors, hallways	
Depth		Depth of shower seat	
Height above floor level standing—Head height		Height of window awnings	
Height above floor level seated—Head height		Height of window sills, mirror above the vanity	
Height above floor level standing—Shoulder height		Height of fittings, fixtures	
Height above floor level seated—Shoulder height		Height of fittings, fixtures	
Height above floor level seated—knee height		Height to the underside of sink	
Popliteal height—Seated position		Height of toilet, shower seat	
Hip width		Width of shower seat	
Hand width		Diameter of rails	
Popliteal crease to back of buttocks		Depth of shower seat	
Height above floor level standing—Eye height		Height of window sills, mirror above the vanity	
Height above floor level seated—Eye height		Height of window sills, mirror above the vanity	
Functional Reach Range Measurements of the Person—Seated or Standing			
Distance between chest and edge of fingertips—Horizontal reach		Width of counters	
Height above floor level—Forward horizontal reach		Height of power point above bench, door handles, light switches, shelving, towel rails	
Height above floor level—Side horizontal reach		Height of power point above bench, height of shelving, width of laundry hub, height of door handles, height of window latches	
Height above floor level—Forward diagonal (up) reach		Height of hanging rail, clothesline, power points, or cupboards, etc., with straight on approach	
Height above floor level—Forward diagonal (down)		Height of power points or cupboards, etc., with side on approach	
Height above floor level—Side diagonal (up) reach		Height of hanging rail, clothesline, power points, or cupboards, etc., with straight on approach	
Height above floor level—Side diagonal (down) reach		Height of power points or cupboards, etc., with side-on approach	

(continued)

Table 8-1. Measuring a Person and His or Her Mobility Equipment (continued)

FEATURE	MEASUREMENT	HOUSING FEATURES (examples)	BUILT ENVIRONMENT DIMENSION REQUIRED
Unoccupied and Occupied Equipment Measurements			
Unoccupied device			
Width of device (unfolded)		Space for storing device	
Folded device width		Space for storing device	
Length of device		Space for storing device	
Height of device		Space for storing device	
Occupied device			
Width of device (unfolded)		Circulation space required at doorways off of corridors, corridor width, ramp width, path width, area required between kitchen counters and in front of appliances	
Length of device (unfolded)		Circulation space required at doorways off of corridors and on ramps that turn 90 degrees to 180 degrees; area required between kitchen counters, in front of appliances	
Height above floor level—Floor to toe with foot on wheelchair or shower chair footplate		Height and depth of toe recesses on cupboards	
Height above floor level—Floor to knee with foot on wheelchair or shower chair footplate		Under sink clearance (bathroom and kitchen)	
Height above floor level—Wheelchair or shower chair seat height		To compare to toilet seat height (for side or front-on transfers)	
Height above floor level—Floor to wheelchair or shower chair armrest		Under-counter clearance	
Height above floor level—Floor to hand on wheelchair control on armrest		Under-counter clearance	
Height of hoist legs		Under bath clearance	
Turning circles: • 90-degree turn • 180-degree turn • 360-degree turn		Circulation space required at doorways off of corridors and on ramps that turn 90 degrees or 180 degrees; area required between kitchen counters, within a bathroom and bedroom, in front of appliances and cupboards, and at mailbox, clothesline, and garden shed areas	
Weight			
Weight of person		Weight load for lift capacity	
Weight of device		Structural weight load for ramps	
Other			

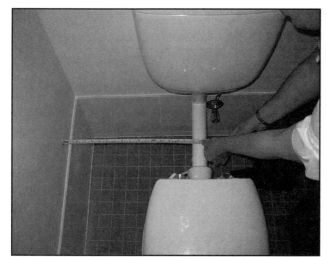

Figure 8-25. Measuring the center line of the toilet.

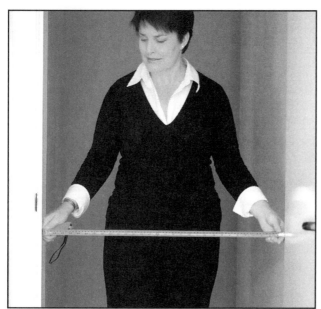

Figure 8-26. Measuring the clearance of the doorway.

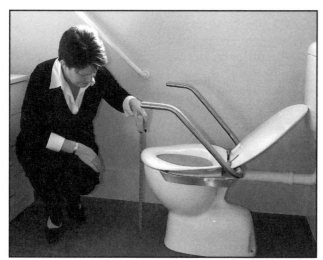

Figure 8-27. Measuring the datum point of the toilet.

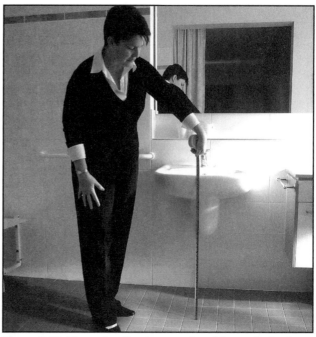

Figure 8-28. Measuring the datum point of the vanity basin.

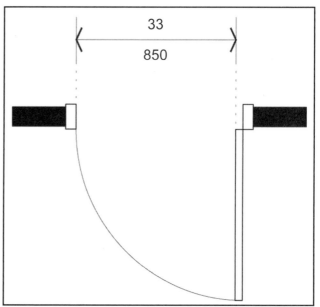

33
850

Figure 8-29. Measuring the clearance of a doorway with a swing door. The measurement on top of the line is in inches (imperial measurement) and the measurement below the line is in mm (metric measurement).

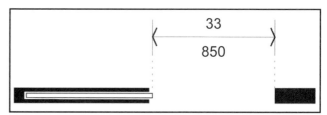

33
850

Figure 8-30. Measuring the clearance of a doorway with a sliding door. The measurement on top of the line is in inches (imperial measurement) and the measurement below the line is in mm (metric measurement).

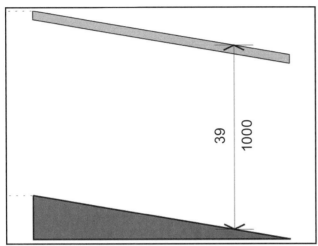

Figure 8-31. Measuring the height of a handrail above the surface of a ramp. The measurement on top of the line is in inches (imperial measurement) and the measurement below the line is in mm (metric measurement).

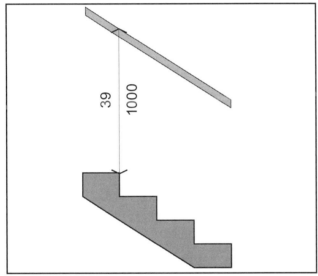

Figure 8-32. Measuring the height of a handrail above the nosing of a step. The measurement on top of the line is in inches (imperial measurement) and the measurement below the line is in mm (metric measurement).

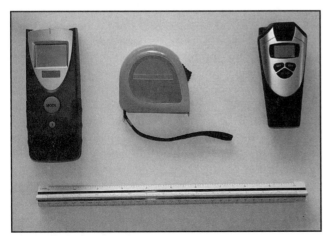

Figure 8-33. Tools to measure dimension.

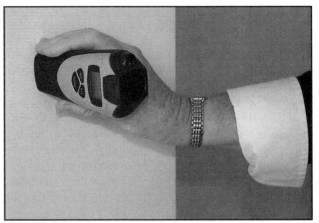

Figure 8-34. Using a distance meter to measure the length of a room.

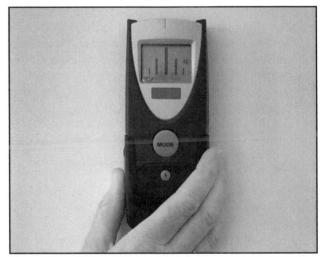

Figure 8-35. Tool used to locate studs.

The most commonly used tools to measure dimensions are the tape measure, distance meter (Figure 8-34), and stud finder (Figure 8-35).

A tape measure should:

+ Be at least 16 f/5000 mm long to measure features in the residential environment, such as the length and width of the room and the height of the ceiling

+ Be made of metal rather than plastic or woven plastic to ensure that this does not stretch, twist, buckle, or sag and result in inaccurate measurements

+ Have markings that can be clearly understood and recognized (Bridge, 1996)

+ Have a wide tape blade so that it can be aligned to a feature in the home without sagging

When measuring:

+ A tape measure is easier used on flat surfaces and in an environment that is well lit

+ The area should be measured at least two or three times to ensure the information is accurate and to establish the average measurement

+ Wall lengths should be measured at floor level and at 35.5 in/900 mm above floor level because walls are not always straight (Bridge, 1996)

A battery-powered distance meter can be used to measure horizontal or vertical distances in rooms. The distance meter is particularly useful when measuring distances greater than 197 in/5 m—for example, a vertical clearance such as floor to ceiling or between two walls in a large room. Many distance meters incorporate a laser pointer to assist in accurately positioning the beam for measurement.

When using a distance meter, ensure:

+ The tool sits squarely on a wall or floor surface

+ The beam is aimed at a solid feature, such as a wall or ceiling, and don't have plants, windows, wall furnishings, lights, or other floating matter interfere with the line of sight

+ Three sets of measurements are taken and an average established to ensure the accuracy of the data (Bridge, 1996)

Locating Structural Framing

The safe use of load-bearing aids in the home such as grab rails and hoists typically requires that they be fixed to wall or ceiling structural members, such as wall studs or ceiling joists. Wall studs are vertical structural framing members that occur at intervals of, typically, 18 in (450 mm) or 24 in (600 mm) and to which the wall lining or sheeting is fixed (Figure 8-36). Where such members do not occur or are structurally inadequate for the aid, a new structural member will need to be installed within the framing or on the face of the wall or ceiling lining but fixed to the underlying structure.

Therapists may wish to determine the feasibility of soundly fixing load-bearing aids in the preferred locations for the client and therefore to identify the location of framing members. Though this can assist in designing the recommendation, it is preferable that the tradesperson undertake an accurate assessment of the position and integrity of the structural supports behind the wall facings. For this reason, therapists might locate the position of studs but not include this information in their drawings, so that the builder retains responsibility for determining the capacity of the wall structure to support the grab bar in the recommended location.

Framing members can be found by:

+ Looking for joints in wall or ceiling lining that indicates the direction of the framing members

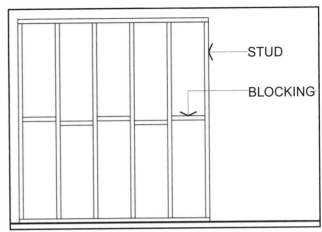

Figure 8-36. Diagram showing studs on a wall.

(they will typically run at right angles to the joints)

+ Looking for lines of nails or screws

+ Tapping along wall or ceiling lining to hear changes from hollow to solid knocking sounds (this may be ineffective for dense lining)

+ A magnetic or electronic stud finder

Greater accuracy can be achieved by using two or more of these methods. A knowledge of the era in which the home building occurred and the typical spacing and thickness of framing members will expedite finding the framing members.

Electronic stud finders may be much more useful than magnetic ones. There are several different types of electronic stud finders, including ones that can be used for timber or metal framing and that identify the presence of electrical wiring and metal piping.

Tapping and stud finders should be employed along a line at right angles to the direction of the framing member. This will also confirm responses of the stud finder to electrical wiring and metal piping. For example, to find a wall stud, the stud finder should be moved horizontally until a stud is found. The method should continue past the stud or else be repeated in the opposite direction so that the thickness and hence mid-line of the stud can be established. The procedure should be repeated at two or more heights above the floor because the wall studs will not be perfectly parallel with each other or at right angles to floor and to avoid false readings from noggings between studs and electrical wiring or metal piping. Noggings are short horizontal members located between and at approximately mid-height of studs; they impart greater rigidity to framed walls.

For ceilings, care is required to ensure that ceiling battens are not detected instead of ceiling joists. Ceiling joists are small-sectioned members that are fixed to the underside of ceiling joists to achieve, among other reasons, greater planarity of the ceiling lining (the ceiling lining is fixed to the ceiling battens, not the joists).

Therapists should bear in mind that noggings and ceiling battens are unlikely to be adequate for fixing load-bearing aids. It would be prudent for therapists to seek confirmation from suitable architects or other building designers, tradespeople, or builders about the suitability and load-bearing capacity of wall and ceiling structures for the fixing of grab bars, hoists, and other aids.

Gradient

The gradient, or slope, of surfaces influences the ability of a person to walk or wheel around the home and whether water will accumulate on the surfaces. Obtaining measurements of gradients of ramps, paths, landings, or shower floors enables comparison with design guides and standards and thereby the determination of the suitability of the inclined surfaces for ease and safety of movement.

Two methods for determining gradients can be differentiated by trigonometric calculation and by use of a gradient measuring device (Figures 8-37 through 8-39).

To determine gradients by trigonometric calculations, at least two dimensions are required: the horizontal and vertical dimension, or either of the horizontal or vertical dimensions plus the inclined length. Part of the horizontal or inclined length and the corresponding vertical dimension can be used to calculate the gradient, but this will tend to be less accurate than using the whole length of the inclined surface. Similarly, for greater accuracy, using the vertical dimension with either the horizontal or inclined length is preferable for calculations than use of the horizontal and inclined lengths.

A gradient measuring device indicates the angular difference of a surface with respect to the vertical. Using a gradient measuring device is generally quicker and may be more convenient to determine gradients than by trigonometric calculation. Measuring devices are available in various forms and are called by a variety of names, including clinometers, slope gauges, and gradient meters. Two commonly available devices are the clock-like device whereby the gradient is indicated by a pointer with respect to a perimeter scale and, increasingly commonly, the electronic digital gradient indicator. The former device is commonly smaller and may therefore need to be with a straight edge; it is also prone to inaccurate readings from parallax error.

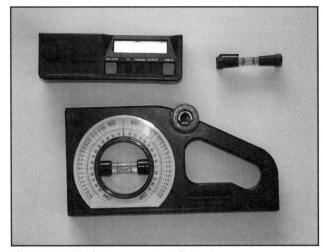

Figure 8-37. Tools to measure gradient.

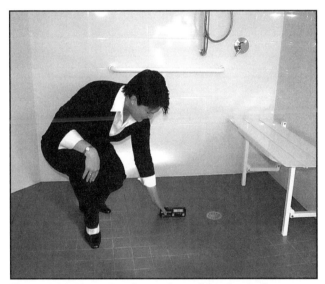

Figure 8-38. Measuring the gradient of the shower floor.

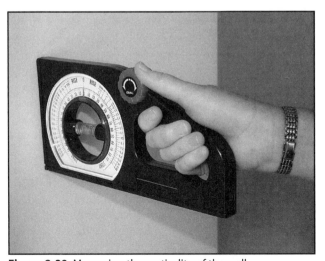

Figure 8-39. Measuring the verticality of the wall.

Table 8-2. Conversion of Angle Data to Gradient Ratios

(Using trigonometric calculations – tan = opposite/adjacent)

INCLINE IN DEGREES	GRADIENT RATIO OF 1:X	EXAMPLES OF USE OF GRADIENTS IN RELATION TO ARCHITECTURAL FEATURES (MINIMUM GRADIENT)
7.13	1:8	Ramp
5.71	1:10	
4.76	1:12	Ramp
4.09	1:14	Ramp
2.86	1:20	Path
1.91	1:30	
1.43	1:40	Landing, sideways slope of a path, ramp, car park area, or landing
1.15	1:50	1:50 to 1:60 shower recess floor
0.95	1:60	
0.82	1:70	1:70 to 1:80 bathroom floor to the edge of the shower recess
0.72	1:80	
0.64	1:90	
0.57	1:100	
0.27	1:200	

(Adapted from Bridge, C. (1996). *Environmental measurement. A handbook for the subject OCCP 5051 (15488x).* The University of Sydney, School of Occupation and Leisure Sciences, Faculty of Health Sciences, Cumberland Campus, Lidcombe, Australia.)

Units of measure of measuring devices are degrees, percentage, or both. Inter-conversion of degrees and percentages, or of either of these and ratios (for example, 1 in 20 or 1:20), is readily obtainable from Web sites or by using published tables such as that in Table 8-2.

Measurement procedure:

+ take at least three sets of measurements to ensure they are accurate and to gain an average reading

+ ensure the measuring devices are well illuminated and that they are appropriately aligned on the surfaces whose gradients are to be measured. For example, to determine the verticality of walls, the device should be aligned vertically; to determine the gradient of a ramp, the device should be aligned in the direction of travel (or the intended or most common direction of travel), and at right angles to it to establish the cross-fall; to establish the gradient of a four-sided shower floor having four facets sloping to a drainage outlet, the device should be aligned along the shortest distance between the drain and each of the sides; that is, along a line from the center of the outlet and at right angles to each side

Irregularity of surface gradient is not uncommon and needs careful consideration. Obtaining several measurements and using a straight edge enables an average or overall gradient to be determined. However, any localized gradients should also be measured because gradient irregularities can impede travel on inclined surfaces. Moreover, there might be two relevant lengths, or scale, of localized gradient that need to be considered: that over which a wheel has to travel in, say, part of its revolution, or the length corresponding with the wheel base of wheeled equipment (the distance between the ground contact points of front and rear wheels). Three gradients may therefore need to be obtained: (a) that of the steepest "small" irregularity on the inclined surface; (b) that of the steepest "medium" irregularity on the inclined surface; and (c) the overall or average gradient.

Gradient is particularly relevant in the design of ramps. Instructions on how to determine the location and configuration of external ramps can be found in Appendix C.

Light

Lighting can facilitate a person's ability to see. However, if it is not set at the correct level, it can impede function and eventually damage vision

(Spaulding, 2008b). In an indoor environment, lighting is provided by both ambient and artificial light. Ambient light can vary, depending on the season of the year and the time of day. It generally comes from outside through windows, whereas artificial light is emitted from fittings such as light bulbs (Spaulding).

Lighting must be provided, by natural or artificial light sources, so that there is sufficient illumination of the activity area but without glare causation. People vary in their requirements for levels of illumination and in their sensitivity to glare.

To determine whether lighting levels are adequate, therapists examine lighting levels in different areas of the home where people mobilize and undertake specific tasks. Measurements are generally taken on stairs and ramps, in entries and hallways, and in kitchens, living areas, bathrooms, and bedrooms. A light meter is used to measure the level of lighting, and this is recorded in lux (Figure 8-40). Recommended lux measures for various areas of the home may be found in design guides and standards. Further information on suitable lighting conditions for people with specific vision impairments should be sought from vision impairment experts or organizations such as Lighthouse International (www.lighthouse.org).

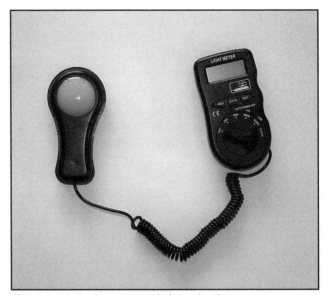

Figure 8-40. Tool to measure lighting levels.

When measuring:

+ Take three readings to ensure data are reliable and to establish an average measurement

+ Take readings at different times of the day when activities are more likely to occur in the area to ensure a true reading of variation in lighting

+ Be aware that the accuracy of these readings can vary as a result of daylight and adjacent reflective surfaces or if the batteries are low

+ Place the light meter on the work or viewing surface. For example, if the task was writing at a desk, the light meter would be placed flat on the desk. Where the task is viewing an item on the wall, the light meter would be placed vertically on the wall (Bridge, 1996)

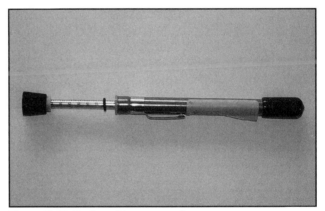

Figure 8-41. Tool used to measure force.

Force

Force is required to open, hold, or swing features such as doors, drawers, and windows. Although door-force gauges are mainly used to measure forces required to push moving features in the public access arena, they can also be used in the home environment if people are experiencing difficulty with specific features (Figures 8-41 and 8-42). Spring-load measures are used to measure the amount of force required to open features such as drawers. These gauges measure force in Newtons and/or pounds.

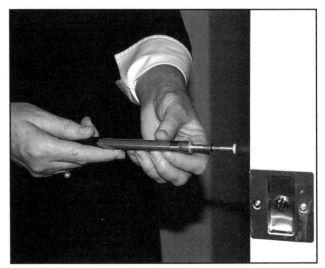

Figure 8-42. Measuring door force.

When measuring push force:

+ Place the device at the point on the door where the force is to be applied

+ Move the feature using force uniformly and slowly, in a consistent horizontal/vertical/oblique direction as required

+ Take three sets of measurements to ensure reliability and to get an average measurement (Bridge, 1996)

When measuring pull force:

+ Position the hook in the middle of the handle on the drawer where pull force is applied

+ Use a perpendicular line of action to gain a reading at the point of maximal force to stretch the load measure

+ Take measurements three times to ensure reliability and to get an average reading (Bridge, 1996)

Sound

Sound is a combination of either simple or complex waveforms (Spaulding, 2008b) and can interfere with how a person manages in the home environment. Factors affecting the individual may relate to noise level, duration of exposure, or frequency of the sound (Spaulding). Sound meters are used to measure sound levels. The formal testing of sound in the home environment is usually completed by an ergonomist or acoustic engineer rather than a therapist.

Recording Measurements of the Home Environment

Occupational therapists can develop specific forms to record the information gathered using tools to measure the built environment or add the information into existing forms such as the CASPAR (Extended Home Living Service, n.d.).

General Considerations in Measurement Practice

There may be changes in a person's measurements and capacity as he or she ages, which might affect his or her height, hand/arm and leg strength, body breadth, visual acuity, and weight. Over time, people might experience changes in their health and capacities and change the type or dimensions of the equipment or caregiver support they use. Therapists need to anticipate possible changes, accommodate variability in individual performance and household structure, and adjust measurements accordingly. In some situations, for example, with a growing child, therapists will need to plan regular reviews as the child develops and acquires new equipment.

Factors Influencing Accuracy of Measurement

There are a range of factors influencing occupational therapy measurement practice, including the following:

+ the competence of the person taking the measurements

+ tool selection use and training

+ time allocated for the visit

+ the nature of the measure or feature

+ the condition of the measurement tools

+ the timing of measurement

The Competence of the Person Taking the Measurements

Measurement error is described as having four components: error in the measuring equipment itself, error in locating the landmark or reference point, error in standardizing the posture of the person or positioning of the measuring tool, and error in the client's understanding or response to instructions on adopting the required posture or obstacles in the environment (Pheasant & Haslegrave, 2006).

To prevent measurement error, occupational therapists need to be competent and well trained in measurement practice. This includes understanding measurement practice, knowing how to take accurate measurements, and recording measurements in a meaningful format. Therapists should ensure that the measurement process generates consistent, quality information by using reliable tools and being comprehensive when gathering data.

Tool Selection, Use, and Training

Therapists can use various sophisticated devices and techniques to measure body dimensions, including calipers, tape scales, weight scales, protractors, and computer-aided anthropometric tools. Occupational therapists generally do not have access to such equipment and will need to observe the client and use a tape measure to measure basic body dimensions, reach, and clearances. For analysis, therapists could also take digital footage of the client reaching and moving. Alternatively, therapists might want to undertake training in specific measurement techniques to enhance their competencies in the area.

The environmental measurement tools selected by therapists generally provide operating instructions.

Although this information might be included when tools are first purchased, it is important that the therapist checks with people providing any technical design or building advice on how they measure features in the environment. For example, a tape measure is used to check the height and size of the light switch plate, but the therapist needs to confirm the reference point for light switches with an electrician, designer, or building professional.

Time Allocated for the Visit

Therapists must allocate sufficient time for taking measurements during the visit. This includes time for measuring the client as well as the environment. The therapist will need to allocate 1 to 2 hours to observe and measure the client, the equipment, and the environment depending on the extent of modifications required. If time is limited at the initial visit, a subsequent appointment might be required to complete the measurement process. If there are insufficient resources, such as time and money, to undertake repeated measures, therapists are to make sure the method chosen is valid, has been tested rigorously, and compares with other measures (Steinfeld & Danford, 1997). This requires an understanding of which tool or technique to use in relation to the factors to be measured in the person-environment fit. It can be time consuming to measure all dimensions of the existing room, the person, caregiver, and all equipment used in the house; however, taking thorough measurements at the initial visit can reduce the need for a repeat visit and avoid the difficulties faced when working with incomplete information.

The Nature of the Measure or Feature

The type of measurements taken by therapists can include, for example, static measurements of the client standing and using various postures to reach or bend or dynamic measurements of the client completing a movement to determine the space or clearance required for the activity. Some features, such as the diameter of grab bars or handrails or the width of lips on baths, are difficult to measure accurately having a round surface.

The Condition of the Measurement Tools

For accuracy and ease of use, measurement tools need to be kept in good working order, be regularly calibrated, and, for battery-powered devices, batteries regularly checked or replaced.

Timing of the Measurement

A person's performance can vary between different times of day, week, or season, depending upon factors such as fatigue, temperature, and the level and type of illuminance. Variance in posture can also occur (Pheasant & Haslegrave, 2006). Measurements of performance and posture may therefore also vary, and this should be considered in deciding upon the time and/or frequency of home visits for measuring purposes.

Variations in measurement may need to be recorded, with specific reference to those factors influencing the data (Dunn, 2005; Law & Baum, 2005; Law, Baum, & Dunn, 2005). Knowledge of this variation can lead to an enhanced understanding of the individual's specific situation and ensure that the modification is designed to work for the client at all times (Dunn).

CONCLUSION

This chapter has provided the reader with information on the role of measurement in improving the person-environment fit. The contribution of anthropometrics, biomechanics, and ergonomics to measurement practice has been described in addition to how each is used by occupational therapists to inform home modification practice. The value of taking an individualized approach to measuring clients and their environment has been emphasized, and the range of tools and resources that are available to assist this process has been described. Also discussed is the importance of considering the range of factors that can affect the measurement process.

Although occupational therapists need to work collaboratively with building industry stakeholders to understand the building industry's approach to measurement of the environment, it is recognized that they do not have the expertise to undertake such a technical and detailed approach. Occupational therapy training in the use of various tools and measurement techniques is highly recommended to ensure that clinical reasoning about changes to the home environment is based on sound evidence rather than guesswork.

REFERENCES

Australian Safety and Compensation Council. (2009). *Sizing up Australia: How contemporary is the anthropometric data Australian designers use.* Commonwealth of Australia. Retrieved from http://www.safeworkaustralia.gov.au/NR/rdonlyres/95EED167-56D7-41EA-9E17-51A0121F8EC9/0/Sizing_up_Australia_report.pdf

Bails, J. H., & Public Buildings Department of South Australia. (1983). *A80 wheelchair and variance: Detailed report no 22, project report on the field testing of AS1428.1-1977, Part 2, Vol 5.* Australian Uniform Building Regulations Co-coordinating Council.

Baker, N. A. (2008). Anthropometry. In K. Jacobs (Ed.), *Ergonomics for therapists* (pp. 73-93). St. Louis, MO: Mosby Incorporated.

Berg Rice, V. J. (2008). Ergonomics and therapy: An introduction. In K. Jacobs & C. M. Bettencourt (Eds.), *Ergonomics for therapists* (pp. 1-16). Newton, MA: Butterworth-Heinemann.

Bridge, C. (1996). *Environmental measurement. A handbook for the subject OCCP 5051* (15488x). Lidcombe, Australia: The University of Sydney, School of Occupation and Leisure Sciences, Faculty of Health Sciences, Cumberland Campus.

Bridge, C. (2005). *Computational case-based redesign for people with ability impairment: Rethinking, reuse and redesign learning for home modification practice.* Unpublished thesis. University of Sydney, Sydney, Australia.

Chan, D., Laporte, D. M., & Sveistrup, H. (1999). Rising from sitting in elderly people, part 2: Strategies to facilitate rising. *British Journal of Occupational Therapy, 62*(2), 64-68.

Ching, F. D. K. (1995). *A visual dictionary of architecture.* New York, NY: Van Nostrand Reinhold.

Connell, B. R., & Sanford, J. A. (1999). Research implications of universal design. In E. Steinfeld & G. S. Danford (Eds.), *Enabling environments: Measuring the impact of the environment on disability and rehabilitation* (pp. 35-57). New York, NY: Kluwer Academic/Plenum Publishers.

Conway, M. (2008). *Occupational therapy and inclusive design: Principles for practice.* Oxford, UK: John Wiley & Sons.

Cooper, R. A. (1998). *Wheelchair selection and configuration.* New York, NY: Demos Medical Publishing.

Diffrient, N., Tilley, A. R., & Bardagjy, J. (1974). *Humanscale 1-3.* Cambridge, MA: MIT Press.

Dunn, W. (2005). Measurement issues and practices. In M. Law, C. Baum, & W. Dunn (Eds.), *Measuring occupational performance: Supporting best practice in occupational therapy* (pp. 21-32). Thorofare, NJ: SLACK Incorporated.

Extended Home Living Service. (n.d.). *CASPAR: Comprehensive assessment and solution process for aging residents.* Retrieved from http://www.ehls.com/CASPAROverview.pdf

Goldsmith, S. (1976). *Designing for the disabled.* London, UK: RIBA Publications.

Goldsmith, S. (2000). *Universal design.* Oxford, UK: Architectural Press.

Han, C. S., Law, K. H., Latombe, J. C., & Kunz, J. C. (2002). A performance-based approach to wheelchair accessible route analysis. *Advanced Engineering Informatics, 16*(1), 53-71.

Hunter, R. A. (2002). *Testing wheelchair driving skills: The slalom.* Retrieved from http://www.hunarch.com.au/Articles/The%20slalom.pdf

Hunter, R. A. (2003). *Vehicle tracking with corrugated paper.* Retrieved from http://www.hunarch.com.au/Articles/Veh%20tracking%20wi%20Corrug%20Paper.pdf

Hunter, R. A. (2005). *Automated reconfiguration of path boundaries for wheelchair access.* Paper presented at Include 2005 Conference, Royal College of Art, April 5-8, 2005; London, UK.

Hunter, R. A. (2009). *Asymmetry of occupied wheelchairs and scooters.* Retrieved from http://www.hunarch.com.au/Articles/Shapes%20of%20occupied%20wheelchairs%20and%20scooters.pdf

International Organization for Standardization. (2005). Draft ISO/DIS 7176-5: *Wheelchairs—Part 5: Determination of dimensions, mass and maneuvering space.*

Kreighbaum, E., & Barthels, K. M. (1996). *Biomechanics: A qualitative approach to studying human movement.* Needham Heights, MA: Allyn & Bacon.

Kroemer, K. H. E. (1987). Biomechanics of the human body. In G. Salvendy (Ed.), *Handbook of human factors* (pp. 169-181). New York, NY: John Wiley & Sons.

Laporte, D. M., Chan, D., & Sveistrup, H. (1999). Rising from sitting in elderly people, part 1: Implications of biomechanics and physiology. *British Journal of Occupational Therapy, 62*(1), 36-42.

Law, M., & Baum, C. (2005). Measurement in occupational therapy. In M. Law, C. Baum, & W. Dunn (Eds.), *Measuring occupational performance: Supporting best practice in occupational therapy* (pp. 3-20). Thorofare, NJ: SLACK Incorporated.

Law, M., Baum, C., & Dunn, W. (2005). *Measuring occupational performance: Supporting best practice in occupational therapy.* Thorofare, NJ: SLACK Incorporated.

Panero, J., & Zelnik, M. (1979). *Human dimension and interior space: A sourcebook of design reference standards.* London, UK: Architectural Press Ltd.

Paquet, V., & Feathers, D. (2004). An anthropometric study of manual and powered wheelchair users. *International Journal of Industrial Ergonomics, 33*, 191-204.

Pedretti, L. W. (1996). Occupational performance: A model for practice in physical dysfunction. In L. W. Pedretti (Ed.), *Occupational therapy: Practice skills for physical dysfunction* (pp. 3-12). St. Louis, MO: Mosby.

Pheasant, S. (1987). *Ergonomics—Standards and guidelines for designers.* Suffolk, UK: Richard Clay Ltd.

Pheasant, S. (1996). *Bodyspace: Anthropometry, ergonomics and the design of work.* London, UK: T. J. Press.

Pheasant, S., & Haslegrave, C. M. (2006). *Bodyspace: Anthropometry, ergonomics and the design of work* (3rd ed.). London, UK: Taylor & Francis Group.

Ringaert, L., Rapson, D., Qiu, J., Cooper, J., & Shwedyk, E. (2001). *Determination of new dimensions for universal design codes and standards with consideration of powered wheelchair and scooter users.* Manitoba, CA: Universal Design Institute.

Spaulding, S. J. (2008a). Basic biomechanics. In K. Jacobs (Ed.), *Ergonomics for therapists* (pp. 94-102). St. Louis, MO: Mosby.

Spaulding, S. J. (2008b). Physical environment. In K. Jacobs (Ed.), *Ergonomics for therapists* (pp. 137-150). St. Louis, MO: Mosby.

Standards Australia. (1994). *Glossary of building terms.* Sydney, Australia: Author.

Stein, F., Soderback, I., Cutler, S. K., & Larson, B. (2006). *Occupational therapy and ergonomics: Applying ergonomic principles to everyday occupation in the home and at work.* Chichester, West Sussex, England: Whurr Publishers Inc.

Steinfeld, E. (2004). Modeling spatial interaction through full scale modeling. *International Journal of Industrial Ergonomics, 33*, 265-278.

Steinfeld, E., & Danford, S. (1997). Environment as a mediating factor in functional assessment. In S. S. Dittmar & G. E. Gresham (Eds.), *Functional assessment and outcome measures for the rehabilitation health professional* (pp. 37-56). Gaithersburg, MD: Aspen Publishers.

Steinfeld, E., Lenker, J., & Paquet, V. (2002). *The anthropometrics of disability.* Retrieved from http://www.ap.buffalo.edu/idea/anthro/the%20anthropometrics%20of%20disability.pdf

Steinfeld, E., Maisel, J., & Feathers, D. (2005). *Standards and anthropometry for wheeled mobility.* Buffalo, NY: Center for Inclusive Design and Environmental Access (IDEA), School of Architecture and Planning, University of Buffalo. Retrieved from http://www.ap.buffalo.edu/idea/Anthro/FinalAccessReport.pdf

Steinfeld, E., Schroeder, S., & Bishop, M. (1979). *Accessible buildings for people with walking and reaching limitations.* Washington, DC: US Department of Housing and Urban Development.

Steinfeld, E., Schroeder, S., Duncan, J., Faste, R., Chollet, D., Bishop, M., ... Cardell, P. (1979). *Access to the built environment: A review of literature* (pp. 98-128). Washington, DC: US Department of Housing and Urban Development, Office of Policy Development and Research.

9

Drawing the Built Environment

Elizabeth Ainsworth, MOccThy, Grad Cert Health Sci and Desleigh de Jonge, MPhil (OccThy), Grad Cert Soc Sci

Once measurements have been taken of the existing home environment, this information needs to be put into a format that can be understood by the person approving the recommendations, developing the architectural drawings, or undertaking the modification work. Occupational therapists need to know how to read and use drawings and have an understanding of their basic components in order to communicate effectively with others in the home modification field. Therapists need to know the different stages of plan development and the alternative types of plan views and be familiar with the technical drawing conventions used in the design profession in order to communicate with construction personnel. An understanding of how and when to draw to scale and being familiar with the various types of drawing tools and technologies can enhance the professionalism and credibility of therapists as they work with others in the design and building profession.

CHAPTER OBJECTIVES

By the end of this chapter, the reader will be able to:

+ Recognize the value of knowing how to read drawings and draw using various tools and technologies

+ Describe the purpose of drawings and the drawing requirements for occupational therapy home modification reports

+ Describe the range of tools and resources available for developing home modification drawings

+ Recognize the importance of clear documentation to inform the work of the design or construction professional

RECORDING ENVIRONMENTAL MEASUREMENT INFORMATION

The Purpose of Drawings

Drawings are a means of communicating ideas to all parties involved in the planning, design, and construction of the building represented. These ideas are set out in a pictorial format that incorporates spaces filled with shapes and objects (Housing Industry Association & Illaring Pty Ltd., 2006). Being the language of the building design and construction industry, drawings are used to visualize possibilities, study alternatives, and present design ideas about the form and spaces of a building (Ching & Adams, 1991). To be useful for this purpose, they need to be clear, consistent, easy to comprehend, and free of ambiguity.

Ainsworth, E., & de Jonge, D.
An Occupational Therapists's Guide to Home Modification Practice (pp. 171-188)
© 2011 SLACK Incorporated

Occupational therapy drawings are not architectural drawings, because therapists do not have professional training in this field. Rather, therapists develop concept drawings to clearly detail what is required for the home modification and to complement the individual's background information and circumstances in their report. Concept drawings describe the basic elements and approximate dimensions in the current and proposed environment using basic technical drawing conventions. Depending on the type and complexity of the home modification work, concept drawings can be drawn by hand or developed using basic computer software. Concept drawings differ from architectural drawings, which are more precise and detailed and adhere to strict technical drawing conventions.

Concept drawings are used to communicate with a broad range of people from a variety of backgrounds and interests in the home modification process. These include clients, other health professionals, people involved in the design and construction industry, and staff in organizations providing funding for the modifications. Primarily, these drawings are used by occupational therapists to describe clients' requirements; however, they are often used as the basis of the tendering and quoting process for home modifications or for the development of more detailed architectural drawings. Concept drawings can provide a foundation for the following:

+ Communicating the intent of the building work

+ Discussing design and construction issues

+ Illustrating proposed changes or variations

When minor changes are required to be made to the design, they can be noted directly on the drawing; however, if major changes are needed, a new set of drawings is usually developed. This allows the design to be evolved and the final option to be documented clearly. Concept drawings also serve as a useful audit tool during and after the home modification works have been completed to ensure that the work has been done as planned.

Resources to Assist Drawing Practice

Organizations such as the International Organization for Standardization (ISO), American National Standards Institute (ANSI), Standards Australia (SA), the British Standards Institution (BSI), and the Canadian Standards Association (CSA) establish common practice across the industry and contribute to the development of rules or manuals for the preparation and presentation of drawing documents. These standards describe the technical drawing conventions used in drawings to denote the overall layout of the design and the various objects in the built environment.

Textbooks by Bielefeld and Skiba (2007); Ching (1995, 1996); Ching and Adams (1991); Clutton, Grisbrooke, and Pengelly (2006); and Thorpe (1994) can also be used to guide occupational therapy drawing practice. These books include recommendations for drawing practice relating to dimensioning, lines, symbols, abbreviations, scales, layout of drawing sheets, orientation of drawings, architectural conventions for cross-referencing drawings, coordinates, grids, and material representation. They also provide architects, building designers, contractors, and occupational therapists with information about methods of presenting drawings before, during, and after the modification of a building.

Reading and Understanding Drawings

Development of Architectural Drawings

Reading and understanding the different types of architectural drawings enables occupational therapists to communicate more efficiently and effectively with design and construction professionals. Once therapists learn the language and practice of the design and construction industry, they can critically appraise plans to assess their suitability in relation to the design needs of their clients (Ashlee, Clutton, Pengelly, & Cowderoy, 2006).

There are three types of architectural drawings in home modification practice that therapists are likely to encounter and to be able to read and understand: sketch design drawings, developed designs, and working drawings.

Sketch Design Drawings

These are simple or quickly executed drawings representing the essential features of an object or scene. Lacking detail, they are often used as a preliminary study (Ching, 1995). In outline form, these drawings depict the designer's general intention. They give an overall picture of the scheme but do not show constructional details and are usually prepared early in the development of a design with the aim to give those involved some general information on how things ultimately go together in the bigger picture. These plans indicate space but do not provide significant detail or dimensions. An occupational therapist, architect, or builder might do a range of sketch drawings of a room or area of the house to show the client how the various features might be laid out (Figure 9-1). This type of drawing can stimulate discussion about different design layouts to create the best possible option for the area being built or modified.

Developed Design Drawings

These are more complex than sketch design drawings. They provide detailed information about the overall layout of the built environment and the relationships of the spaces within and around the building. They can include, for example, illustrations of furniture within the home, a wheelchair turning circle, and other features using specific technical design conventions. The plans include specific illustrations and technical design conventions but are not as developed as those used at the working drawing stage. They are more pictorial than technical in nature and are less likely to feature the drawing conventions of the working drawings that are produced for construction or modification work. Developed design drawings are usually done by an architect or licensed building contractor.

Sketch designs and developed design drawings are often done freehand or, if computer generated, are presented to appear freehand. The reader can feel more comfortable offering feedback if drawings are "only" freehand than if they have the "firmed up" look of technically drafted drawings.

Working Drawings

These drawings show, in graphical or pictorial form, the design, location, dimensions, and relationships of elements of a building (Ching, 1995). They describe the constituent parts of a building, articulate their relationships, and reveal how they go together (Ching & Adams, 1991). Using different technical drawing conventions than those of developed drawings, working drawings are usually developed by the architect or licensed building designer and are used to guide contractors as they undertake the building work (Figure 9-2). For example, developed drawings might show an illustration of a bathroom in pictorial form using simple lines, whereas working drawings would be more technical and use specific lines to represent the features in this area in more detail on the plan.

There are usually various sets of drawings at this stage, each describing in detail different aspects of the design, such as site plans, floor plans, elevations, sections, and drainage plans. Such complex drawings are usually drawn using drafting equipment or computer software rather than freehand.

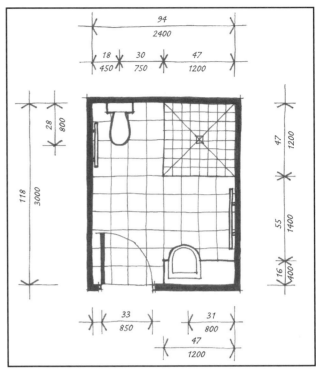

Figure 9-1. Sketch drawing of a bathroom floor plan, not to scale. The measurement on top of the line is in inches (imperial measurement) and the measurement below the line is in mm (metric measurement).

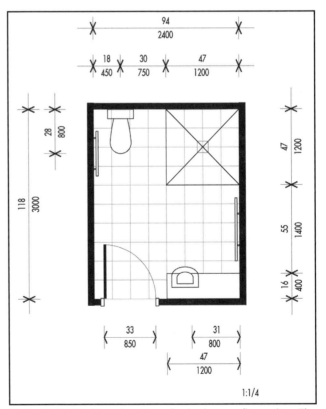

Figure 9-2. Working drawing of a bathroom floor plan. The measurement on top of the line is in inches (imperial measurement) and the measurement below the line is in mm (metric measurement).

Plan Documentation Process for Home Modification Work

Drawings can be documented and classified according to the type of information presented. A design process for home modifications might include the development of sketch and/or working drawings for the tender, quoting, and construction processes (Wang, 1996).

Because home modification work can be extensive, costly, and time consuming to draw to scale, it is preferable that therapists rely on an architect or building designer for these complex drawings. The completion of drawings by an architect or building designer may be a mandatory requirement under legislation, depending on the nature and extent of work to be completed. This practice needs to be checked with local authorities to ensure that therapists who choose to do their own drawings are not operating outside their area of professional expertise or beyond the extent of their qualifications.

TYPES OF VIEWS USED IN DRAWINGS

Various types of views can be incorporated into the drawings to understand and depict the total 3D configuration of the built environment. The most common drawing types designers use to communicate their design ideas are plans, elevations, and sections (Wang, 1996). Occupational therapists also use plan, elevation, and section views in their home modification drawing, depending on the size and complexity of the home modification work to be undertaken and the amount of detail to be provided for design or construction professionals. For example:

+ An elevation might be drawn for the installation of a grab bar beside the toilet
+ An elevation and floor plan view might be drawn for a bathroom undergoing extensive home modifications
+ A section might be drawn of a set of stairs or a vanity to illustrate the location of the shelving in the cupboard underneath

Site Plan

The site plan is a view looking down on a site from above, illustrating location and orientation of the building on a parcel of land, providing information about the site's topography, landscaping, utilities,

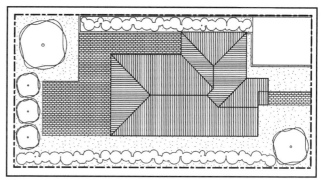

Figure 9-3. Site plan.

and site work (Ching & Adams, 1991). The site plan also details site boundaries and the location of the street, paths, and existing and adjacent buildings. There are various styles of lines used in drawings—for example, thick lines to denote the external walls of the home and covered outdoor areas; thinner lines to represent the planted areas, pavements, and driveways; and dotted lines to indicate the line of the roof of the building.

From the site plan, a reader can glean the indoor/outdoor relationship between the landscape and the building and the orientation of the building in relation to the direction of the sunrise and sunset and the prevailing breezes (Figure 9-3).

Floor Plan

Of all of the working drawings, the floor plan is one of the most important because it includes the greatest amount of information. It is a sectional drawing obtained by passing an imaginary cutting plane through the walls above the floor, usually at a height that allows windows to be located. The floor plan is a view looking down from above, and it illustrates the dimensions of a building's spaces, as well as the thickness and construction of the vertical walls and columns that define these spaces (Figure 9-4). Among other features, it will show the building layout, room sizes, door and window placement, and bathroom and kitchen design (Ching & Adams, 1991; Weidhaas, 1999). The floor plan illustrates distance, circulation space, width, depth, length of areas, and features (see Figure 9-4).

Elevation

An elevation is a horizontal or side view of a building's interior or exterior, usually taken from a point of view perpendicular to the principal vertical surfaces. It illustrates the size, shape, and materials of the interior or exterior surfaces as well as the size, proportion, and nature of the door and

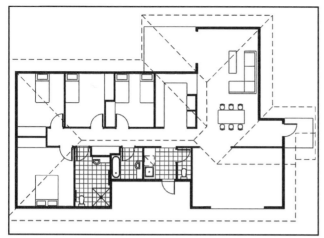

Figure 9-4. Example of the floor plan of a domestic home.

window openings in the design (Ching & Adams, 1991). Elevations show distance, length, width, and height dimensions of areas and features and are named by the direction they face—for example, a north elevation faces north. Internal elevations may be cross-referenced and named through a diagram on the floor plan—for example, four arrows labeled A to D in the center of the floor plan can each point to four internal walls represented in the corresponding elevation view (Figures 9-5 through 9-10).

Section

A building section is a cross-sectional or horizontal view after a vertical plane is cut through a building and the front portion is removed. It reveals the vertical and, in one direction, the horizontal dimensions of a building's spaces and can illustrate the thickness of floors, roofs, and walls. Sections can also include exterior and interior elevations seen beyond the plane of the cut (Figure 9-11; Ching & Adams, 1991).

Overall, sections add depth and meaning to the drawings, as well as interest. These types of drawings can take on a variety of appearances due to the evolutionary nature of the design process (Wang, 1996).

SPECIFICATIONS

Once finalized, plans form the basis from which the agreed building work is undertaken. They can be used with, or as an alternative to, a written specification (Ashlee et al., 2006). Because drawings in themselves might not convey all of the information, written specifications can be developed to provide

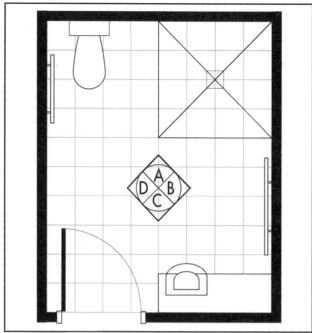

Figure 9-5. Bathroom floor plan.

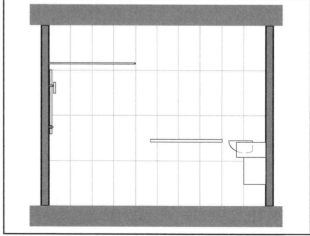

Figure 9-6. Bathroom, elevation A.

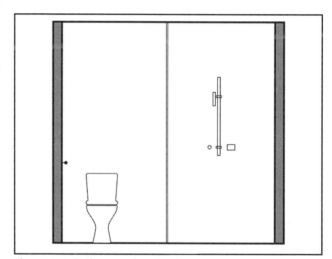

Figure 9-7. Bathroom, elevation B

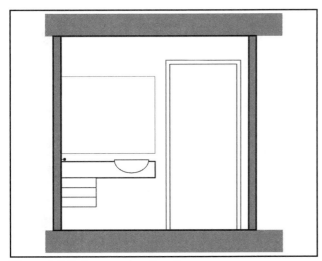

Figure 9-8. Bathroom, elevation C.

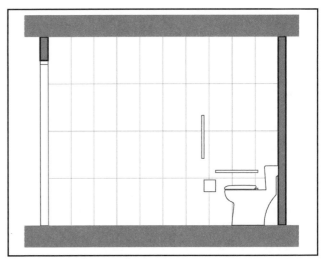

Figure 9-9. Bathroom, elevation D.

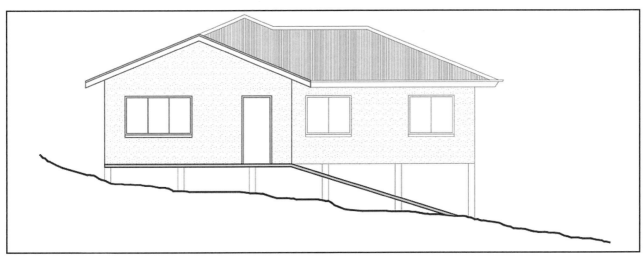

Figure 9-10. External house elevation.

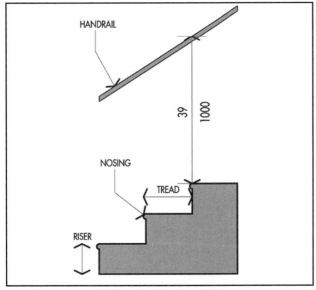

Figure 9-11. Stairs. Section view. The measurement on top of the line is in inches (imperial measurement) and the measurement below the line is in mm (metric measurement).

a detailed description of the technical nature of the materials, standards, and quality of execution of the work. The specifications are a business document, a contract document, and a working document, and they serve a diversity of readers (Standen, 1995). They provide the following:

+ Evidence to the person paying for the construction that the building will include his or her requirements

+ Information on items to be priced that are not indicated on the drawings

+ A record of what has been built

+ A reference during inspections to check that the correct products, designs, and features have been incorporated into the design (Standen, 1995)

The drawings should be used to show whatever is best displayed by the drawings, and the specification should be used to communicate information that is best described by words (Standen, 1995). By way of example, a drawing might indicate the need for tiles in a bathroom and the pattern in which they are to be laid. A specification will identify the tile manufacturer, the color, the slip resistance, the method of installation, and the type and color of the grout. The specification can be prepared by a builder, engineer, architect, or licensed building designer to advise a contractor about the materials and workmanship that cannot be displayed on the plans.

Building access standards can be referred to in a specification to direct the reader to review the most appropriate section when completing the construction. It is essential that occupational therapists and the reader of the specification understand the application and intent of the access standards to ensure that they are referred to appropriately during the design and modification process. If the therapist is requesting complex or extensive home modifications, a design or construction professional might be required to develop a detailed building specification to provide the required level of technical detail for quoting and construction purposes. If required, therapists should refer the design and construction professional to specific figures or clauses in the access standards that describe the specific performance criteria for the work.

UNDERSTANDING SCALE

Scale drawings allow therapists to examine the layout, dimensions, and spaces in the drawing to determine whether the person (the caregiver and/or the equipment he or she uses) can move between buildings and external areas or into and within the home and utilize the space, fittings, and fixtures effectively. It is a means of transferring information from actual size to a more convenient size with which to work and represent on a suitably proportioned piece of paper (Ashlee et al., 2006).

Scales are used to reproduce a large object on a sheet of paper in its correct proportions. Scale uses a ratio to show the size of a real object in relation to the size of the drawn object. A full-size drawing is one with a scale ratio of 1:1 (International Organization for Standardization, 1979). The scale chosen for the drawn object depends on the size of the real object, the amount of detail required, the complexity of the object, the purpose of the presentation (International Organization for Standardization), and the size of the piece of paper being used (Ashlee et al., 2006).

Drawings will indicate both scale and unit of measurement in either imperial or metric language. For example, ¼-inch equals 1 f or 12 in (1/4"=1'-0" indicates that the real object is 48 times larger [1:48] than the drawn object, or in metric 1:50 indicates that the real object is 50 times larger than the drawn object).

Architectural scales used in the US are generally grouped in pairs using the same dual-numbered index line, including the following:

+ 3" = 1'0" (ratio equivalent 1:4) 1½" = 1'0" (1:8)
+ 1" = 1'0" (1:12) ½" = 1'0" (1:24)
+ ¾" = 1'0" (1:16) 3/8" = 1'0" (1:32)
+ 1/4" = 1'0" (1:48) 1/8" = 1'0" (1:96)
+ 3/16" = 1'0" (1:64) 3/32" = 1'0" (1:128)

In the UK, Canada, and Australia, the architectural scales are as follows:

+ 1:1/1:10
+ 1:2/1:20
+ 1:5/1:50
+ 1:100/1:200

Scale changes might occur between section and elevation drawings. Table 9-1 shows common scales used in architectural plans.

Small or detailed objects, such as a door sill or door furniture, are often drawn to a larger scale ratio—for example, 1½" = 1'0" (1:10) or larger. The detail on the larger scale drawing takes precedence or overrides the detail on the smaller scale drawing of the same area or object. For example, the detail in the floor plan area of the bathroom (½" = 1' or 1:20) overrides the detail provided for the same bathroom as drawn in the floor plan of the house or apartment (3/16" = 1' or 1:100). The scale ½" = 1' or 1:20 is a "larger" scale than 3/16" = 1' or 1:100 because the drawing itself is larger than the same object (Figures 9-12 and 9-13).

TECHNICAL DRAWING CONVENTIONS

To read a plan, occupational therapists need to understand how objects are illustrated and labeled. This involves understanding the technical drawing conventions and symbols that are used by the design or construction professional to describe the building design (Weidhaas, 1999). Technical drawing standards contain specific information about the conventions and symbols, and they are used by the building and construction industry. Ensuring

Table 9-1.

TYPES OF DRAWINGS	IMPERIAL	METRIC
Site or dwelling floor plan	3/16″ = 1′	1:100
	¼″ = 1′	1:50
Floor plan of a room (for example, a bathroom, kitchen, or bedroom)	½″ = 1′	1:20

Figure 9-12. Example of scales (metric).

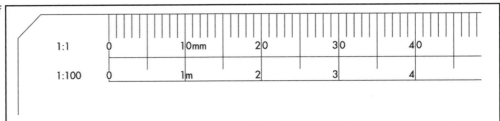

Figure 9-13. Examples of floor plan views drawn at different scales.

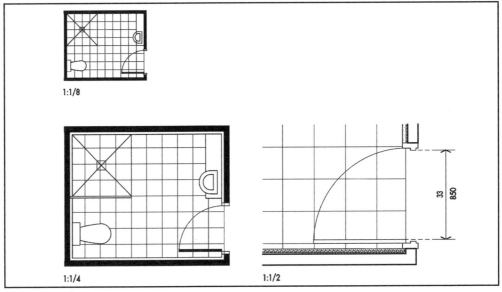

that design and construction professionals use the same terminology and symbols assists in establishing common design and construction practice. The standards are not a mandatory requirement for architectural drawings but they are a useful guide. Publications such as ISO standards, access standards—for example, ICC/ANSI A117.1 (ANSI, 2003)—or architectural books (Bielefeld & Skiba, 2007; Ching, 1995, 1996; Ching & Adams, 1991) set out examples of technical drawing conventions and symbols that occupational therapists can use as a guide when they develop concept drawings. In many instances, design and building professionals might further stylize the basic elements described in the technical drawing standards to increase the readability and attractiveness of the image.

Technical drawing standards may contain basic conventions—for example, dimension lines (Table 9-2) and symbols for architectural features (Figure 9-14). These conventions and symbols vary because there is no set requirement for them to be drawn a specific way.

Lines

The basic graphic symbol for all drawings is the line, which defines spatial edges, renders volume, creates textures, and connects to form words and numbers (Wang, 1996). Creating lines is a major element of a drawing, and good line work is critical to the development of an accurate and neat drawing (Bielefeld & Skiba, 2007; Housing Industry Association & Illaring Pty Ltd., 2006). Line work in

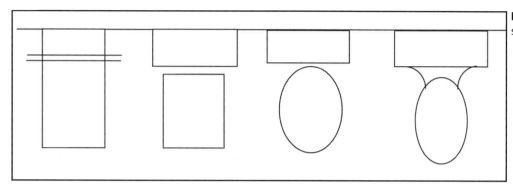

Figure 9-14. Examples of symbols for toilets.

Table 9-2. Examples of Conventions

CONVENTION	DESCRIPTION
Min	Minimum
Max	Maximum
>	Greater than
≥	Greater than or equal to
<	Less than
≤	Less than or equal to
- - - - - - - - - - - -	Boundary of clear floor space or maneuvering clearance
— · — · — · — · — ℄	Center line
⇨	Direction of travel or approach
(hatched rectangle)	Location zone of element, control, or feature

(Graphic convention for figures from American National Standards Institute. (2003). *ICC/ANSI A117.1-2003: Accessible and Usable Buildings and Facilities.* New York, NY: Author.)

plan, elevation, and section views should be sharp, dense, of uniform width, and consistent for the purpose of legibility (Wang, 1996). The specific types and thickness of each line and their application are often set out in technical drawing standards or textbooks.

There are common line and dimensioning standards for home design (Figure 9-15).

There are seven major types of lines used in drawings that have specific meanings:

1. *Visible object line*: A solid line representing the contour of an object or the visible edges

2. *Hidden object line*: Hidden or unseen objects below or in front of the reader

3. *Dimension*: A line terminated by arrows, short slashes, or dots indicating the extent or magnitude of a part or whole along which dimensions are scaled and indicated

4. *Center line*: A broken line with relatively long segments separated by single dashes and dots to represent the axis of a symmetrical element or composition

5. *Break line*: Broken line segments joined by short zigzag strokes to show a portion of the drawing that has been cut off

6. *Overhead line*: Hidden or unseen objects behind or above the observer (Ching, 1995)

Dimensioning

Dimensions are used on drawings in conjunction with dimension lines to denote the length, height, or width of the object being represented. Although the imperial system of measurement is commonly used in the United States, a combination of metric and imperial measurements is generally noted in various U.S. design standards. When imperial dimensions are used, they are expressed as feet and inches while metric dimensions are expressed in mm, never cm. In some instances, dimensions may be written in meters (e.g., 1.50 m) particularly at the sketch and developed design stages. The actual dimension number is conventionally written along the lines and placed above it (Figures 9-16 and 9-17; Bielefeld & Skiba, 2007).

CREATING CONCEPT DRAWINGS

Design or construction professionals undergo specific technical drawing training to develop the skills to create drawings that are technically sound and provide significant construction detail. These drawings have a technical detail and accuracy that cannot be achieved by therapists who have not had formal technical drawing training.

Figure 9-15. Types of lines used in plans or drawings.

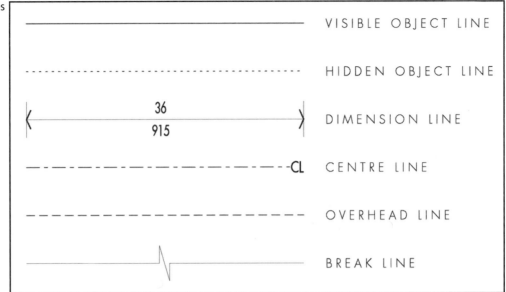

VISIBLE OBJECT LINE

HIDDEN OBJECT LINE

36
915
DIMENSION LINE

CL   CENTRE LINE

OVERHEAD LINE

BREAK LINE

Figure 9-16. Dimension line that shows imperial and metric measurements.

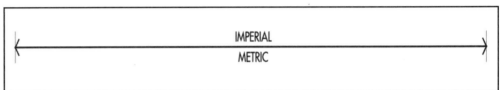

IMPERIAL
METRIC

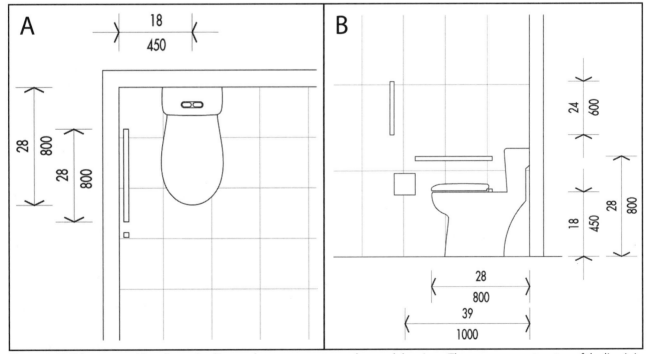

Figure 9-17. Where to position dimension lines and measurements on plans and drawings. The measurement on top of the line is in inches (imperial measurement) and the measurement below the line is in mm (metric measurement). (A) Toilet floor plan; (B) toilet elevation; (C) vanity floor plan; (D) vanity elevation; (E) bath floor plan; (F) bath elevation; (G) stairs elevation (continued).

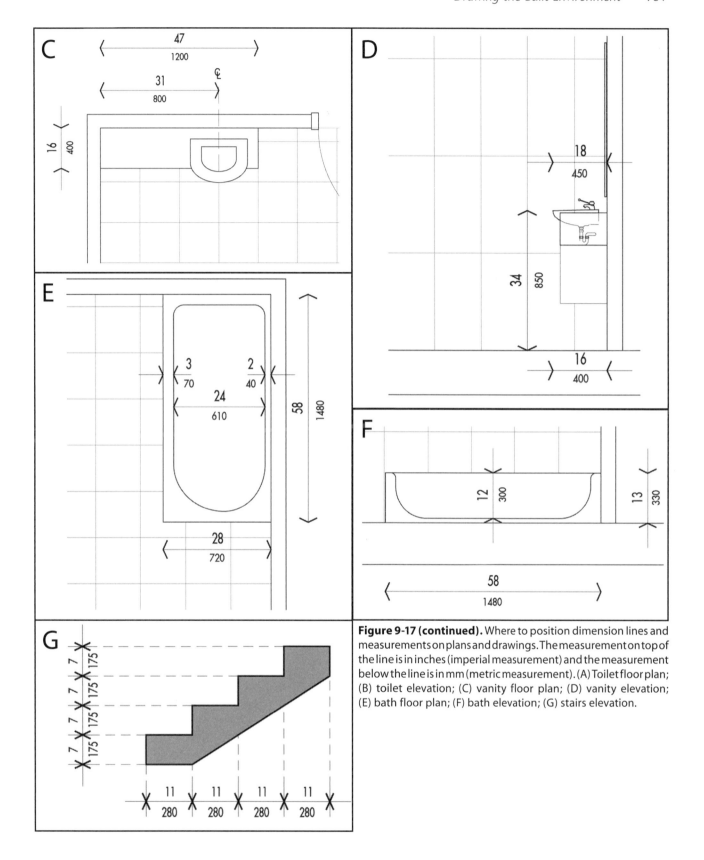

Figure 9-17 (continued). Where to position dimension lines and measurements on plans and drawings. The measurement on top of the line is in inches (imperial measurement) and the measurement below the line is in mm (metric measurement). (A) Toilet floor plan; (B) toilet elevation; (C) vanity floor plan; (D) vanity elevation; (E) bath floor plan; (F) bath elevation; (G) stairs elevation.

Therapists can create preliminary or concept sketch drawings to develop design ideas for home modifications in advance of an architect or building designer's more detailed designs. If therapists want to incorporate more developed drawings into their reports, they should refer the work to a design professional. If they would like to become skilled in any of these forms of drawing, they need to undertake formal training in architectural drawing.

Concept Drawing Information for Builders

The concept drawings provide more detail to the written wording that is contained in the occupational therapy report. If home modification work is simple and straightforward to undertake, such as the installation of grab rails, handrails, stairs, or small ramps, a concept drawing may be sufficient to guide the builder. If the home modification work is complex, such as the renovation of the bathroom or kitchen or the installation of a lift, lengthy ramp, or additional room, the concept drawing may be used as the basis for a more detailed technical drawing that is completed by the design or construction professional. It is sometimes helpful to include photos and drawings of the existing areas to be modified as well as the drawing of the proposed changes to provide the design or construction with a more comprehensive picture of the area, particularly if they are developing a more detailed technical drawing for the proposed home modifications.

When to Draw to Scale

Drawings of minor modifications, such as grab bar installations and handrails on stairs, do not generally need to be drawn to scale. If they are not drawn to scale, this should be noted on the drawing. However, the figures should always be proportionate to ensure that the reader has a good understanding of the relationship of items and areas to one another.

When developing drawings for a major modification, scale drawings enable therapists to determine which fittings, fixtures, equipment, or furniture can reasonably fit into a room and whether the space is adequate for items to be placed and for the circulation of individuals with and without their equipment. Scale drawings can also be used to indicate the precise location and assess the ease of access to existing fixtures, such as doors and windows. However, drawing to scale is time consuming because it requires that relevant dimensions of the person and the environment are accurately measured and then translated into a scale drawing.

Drawing by Hand

Although drawing can be completed with the assistance of computer technology, therapists can make concept drawings by hand quickly and easily if they are skilled in drawing. They can translate measurements of clients, their equipment and caregiver, and the home environment into a simple sketch, particularly if computer technology is unavailable. However, drawings developed by hand using pencils, rulers, scale rulers, pens, and paper are often labor intensive and take significant time. These drawings can also vary in quality, depending on the drawing skills of the person completing the drawings and the type of drawing equipment used. They cannot be edited, saved, or adjusted as easily as computer-assisted drafting (CAD) or computer-assisted drawings—for example, Microsoft Word drawings.

Tools for Drawing by Hand

Hand drawing can be completed with the aid of drafting equipment, such as a drafting board, squares, rulers, scale rulers, and other tools, for the systematic representation and dimensional specification of architectural features in the home (Bielefeld & Skiba, 2007; Ching, 1995). Quality equipment and materials make the act of drawing a more enjoyable experience, and the achievement of quality work becomes much easier in the long term (Ching, 1996). The equipment and materials need to be good quality, clean, and appropriate to the task. The following items can be used by therapists when hand drawing.

Paper

There are various types of paper that can be used when doing drawings—plain paper, graph paper, and drafting film. Although plain paper is the medium most regularly used by therapists, they might need to talk to representatives from local drawing and drafting companies about the most appropriate paper for their drawing requirements. Sketch-grade paper is suitable for quick sketches and overlays on drawings. For a quality finish to a drawing, drafting film is used. It is translucent and has a matte textured surface on one side and a plain smooth textured surface on the other. Made of a plastic that is more dimensionally stable, it resists humidity that can affect the sheet size. Although it is more expensive and resists tearing, it is also "harder" on equipment (for example, pens wear out more quickly). Grid paper is also useful if drawings are being done to scale. It provides therapists with a good visual guide, but it has the disadvantage of the extra lines, making the drawings look "busy."

Pencils

The most common pencils used for drawing are 2H and H (hard), F or HB (medium), and B (soft). Often 2B, or even softer, pencils are used for sketches (the *B* stands for *black*). The choice of pencil depends on the user's preference and drawing skills. Sharp pencils or propelling (clutch) pencils using a narrow lead are ideal for drafting. These enable the user to continue drawing without having to stop and sharpen the tool. A soft eraser is also essential to clean markings off of the drawing sheets.

Pens

Final drawings should always be in ink. Although pencil may be used initially to draw the lines, once complete, they should be drawn over in ink or in felt pen. Felt-tipped technical drafting pens are available in various thicknesses and are generally used to draw specific line widths. Ballpoint pens are not appropriate for drawing work because the lines produced by these types of pen are not clean and clear on paper.

Templates and Other Drawing Tools

Templates and a compass can save time when drawing. Templates are generally made of plastic and have geometric shapes and shapes of plumbing fixtures and furnishings. They also have lettering, numerals, and other symbols, all of which can provide a guide for drawing objects accurately and to scale. Circles are drawn with a pair of compasses.

Scale Ruler and Set Square or T-Square

Scale rulers are used to draw in a precise ratio to the original (Housing Industry Association & Illaring Pty Ltd., 2006). These rulers vary in style, quality, and scale. There are common scales used for specific plans. As indicated previously, common scales used by therapists when drawing include 3/16" = 1' (1:100); ¼" = 1' (1:50) for site or dwelling floor plans; and ½" = 1' (1:20) for floor plans of rooms or for internal elevations. Scale rulers also vary in style (Figures 9-18 and 9-19).

Scale rulers need to be kept clean by washing with a mild soap and water. They should only be used to measure drawings and not to draw lines because scale rulers become worn and the divisions of the scale can affect the quality of the line drawn. Routinely, a set square or T-square is used to rule

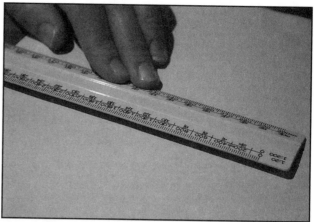

Figure 9-18. A flat scale ruler does not hold to the paper tightly unless the user tilts the ruler to the paper.

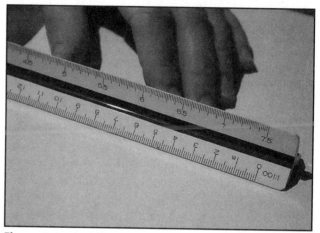

Figure 9-19. A different type of ruler that grips the paper tightly.

lines. Scale rulers should not be used as a cutting edge or be used with color markers because these will destroy the edge and markings.

Drafting Board

This is a flat working surface to which paper can be secured with clips or tape. Drafting boards vary in size but should be at least 25% larger than the largest piece of paper that will be regularly used on the board (Housing Industry Association & Illaring Pty Ltd., 2006). The paper is attached to the board so that it sits squarely to a T-square or straight-edge or, if preprinted, the border is used to square up the paper (Housing Industry Association & Illaring Pty Ltd.). Plastic drafting boards with parallel rules are reasonably priced and will generally suit therapists' drawing needs.

Square

The T-square is held firm on one edge of the drafting board—for example, to the left—and can move up and down on the page to draw horizontal lines. The T-square can also be used as a surface against which to place set squares to create vertical and angled lines. Most drafting boards have sliding rulers in place of the T-square (Housing Industry Association & Illaring Pty Ltd., 2006). The clear plastic T-square enables the user to see through to the paper.

Set Squares

Set squares are manufactured from clear plastic, and the most commonly used in home modification drawing are those that are 45/45/90 degrees and 60/30/90 degrees to assist with drawing angled and horizontal or vertical lines.

The Drawing Process

The process for completing a drawing includes the following:

+ Selecting the view(s) to be drawn
+ Choosing the paper type and size
+ Drawing the view(s)
+ Checking that all information included in the drawing is accurate
+ Providing the title block on the right side or bottom of the page
+ Dating and signing the drawing

The drawing might need to include a range of different views of the area to be modified—for example, the floor plan (to show distance, circulation space, width, depth, length) and elevation view (to show distance, heights, width, length). Therapists should ensure that each different view, or plan, of the same area contains consistent information. In particular, the measurements need to be compared to ensure that there are no discrepancies between the drawings. For example, the location of the grab bar beside the toilet—the distance from the back wall—in the floor plan view needs to be identical to its location in the elevation view.

Before starting their final scale drawings, therapists might sketch them out roughly on a piece of paper first. This allows them to get a clear picture in their mind of what they want to draw. For drawings that are not drawn not to scale, they can draw directly onto white paper, using black pen to build on the final pencil drawings. All lines should be drawn using a ruler, and figures should be recognizable using conventional symbols, be clearly labeled, and be in proportion.

If drawing to scale, therapists need to select an appropriately sized scale for the area being drawn,

as per the earlier discussion on scale. For example, a floor plan of a bathroom may be drawn ½"=1' or 1:20.

There are three different ways of completing the scale drawing using the pens or pencils and various types of paper (Figure 9-20):

1. Therapists can draw directly onto white paper or drafting film using a pencil or pen. The drafting film illustration can be photocopied onto white paper when finished.

2. Therapists can lay drafting film over grid paper, which has been set out according to a scale, to guide their drawings, using pencil and pen and a scale ruler as described previously. The grid paper provides therapists with an inbuilt reference scale during the drafting process. It helps correct alignment and guides them as they use their ruler (International Organization for Standardization, 1979). Space needs to be left around the drawing for listing lines and measurements, which requires that the drafting film be offset from the grid paper.

3. Therapists can draw directly onto grid paper.

When drawing a room, therapists first outline the overall shape of the area—for example, the walls, windows, and doors. All permanent fixtures or fittings are then drawn in their respective locations using appropriate conventions and symbols, starting with the larger items and working down to the smaller. For example, a drawing of a bathroom would include bath/shower, vanity, toilet, taps, spouts/shower roses, soap/toilet roll holder, light switches, electrical fittings, and power outlets. Dimension lines are then drawn on the outside of the drawing in line with the items they are representing. This ensures that the inside of the drawing remains uncluttered and clear. The smaller dimensions are usually recorded closest to the outside of the drawing with dimensions increasing incrementally away from the drawing. This creates a hierarchy of dimensions. The area drawn can be divided horizontally and vertically to guide the set of the dimension lines (Figure 9-21). Further, the dimension lines should be written in such a way that the page is turned only once—for example, clockwise—to read the figures on the dimension lines along the sides of the drawing (see Figure 9-21).

Drawings are initially developed using pencil. Once the drawing has been finalized, pencil lines are built on using a felt-tip pen, and the pencil lines are removed with a soft rubber eraser.

When developing a drawing, therapists should be mindful to include all of the required information in the drawing or accompanying recommendations.

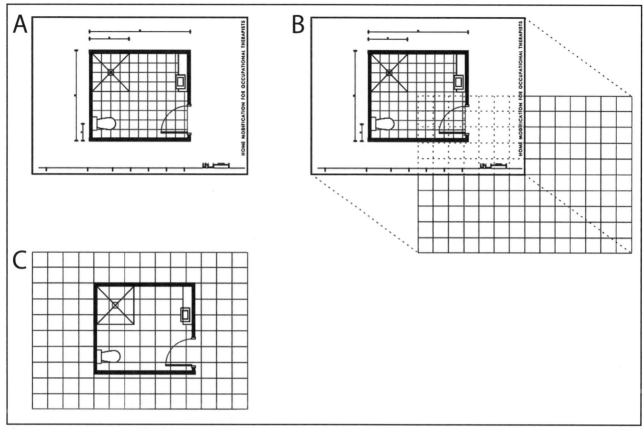

Figure 9-20. Paper options for drawing concept drawings. (A) Using drafting paper for drawings. (B) Combining drafting paper on top of grid paper for drawings. (C) Using grid paper for drawings.

For example, in an elevation of a grab bar on a wall, essential elements include the following:

+ Configuration of bar

+ Diameter of bar

+ Length of bar

+ Height of bar above floor level (AFL)

+ Wall the bar is to be located on

+ Distance of end of the bar from the back wall

+ Structure/surface of mounting wall

+ Whether studs have been located

+ Other elements described in the standards that are relevant to the client's specific requirements

A title block may be included at the side or bottom of the page to enable all relevant details about the drawing to be recorded, including the client's name and address, project name/type, the name of the area, the type of view, whether the drawing has been drawn to scale and the size of the scale, the page number or set total, the date of drawing, the review date and/or number, and the name of the designer/draftsman/occupational therapist (Housing Industry Association & Illaring Pty Ltd., 2006). Other information can include the name of the area drawn, the type of view—for example, the floor plan view or elevation, the scale, and whether measurements are in feet and in/mm if the abbreviation for these measurements is not included with the dimensions. A title block at the bottom of the page or on the right side of the page allows large sheets to be folded into sections and clipped to the left, and the drawing remains easy to read. For future reference, the therapist should sign and date plans to provide evidence of the authorship and the date they were finalized.

Lettering on Hand Drawings

Therapists are required to incorporate neat lettering into their drawings to ensure that items are clearly labeled and the document is professionally presented. Some of the most important characteristics of a lettering style are readability and consistency in both style and spacing (Ching, 1996). Skillful lettering enhances the appearance and clarity of the drawing, whereas poor lettering can be difficult to read and can detract from the drawing.

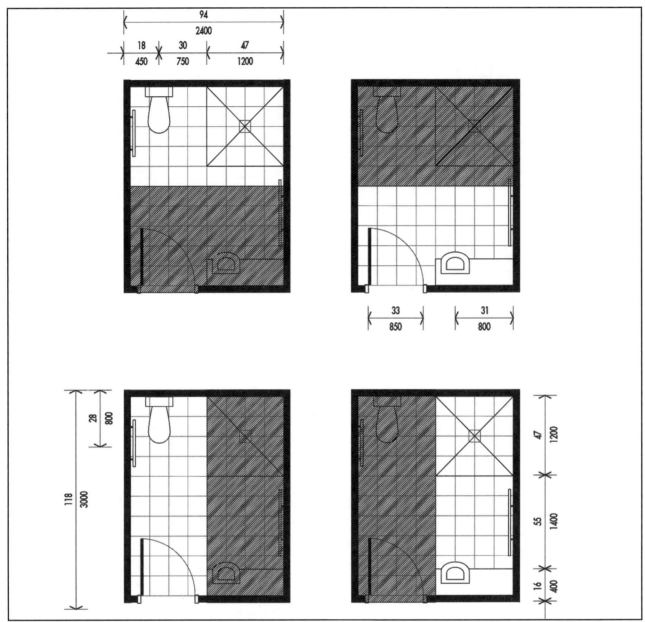

Figure 9-21. Floor plan of a bathroom area showing the horizontal and vertical division of the illustration to guide the set-out of measurements and dimension lines. The measurement on top of the line is in inches (imperial measurement) and the measurement below the line is in mm (metric measurement).

Lettering needs to be consistent, dark, crisp, and sharp for the best presentation. It can be in pencil, spaced equally to the height of letters, and finished in pen. Lettering must be neat, brief, straight, and completed horizontally on drawings. It is not to be placed over part of a space or a drawn object. Numerals are to be placed outside the view shown to ensure the drawing remains uncluttered.

Therapists can find more information on the placement of lettering and lines from local architects or building designers, through completing an architectural drawing course, or by referring to texts such as books by Ching (1995, 1996).

DRAWING USING COMPUTER TECHNOLOGY

In order to anticipate expected changes, home modification documents need to be flexible and inexpensive to revise (Wang, 1996). To accommodate minor changes and to avoid redrawing the entire sheet of documentation, Wang notes that computer technology has become popular in preparing drawings.

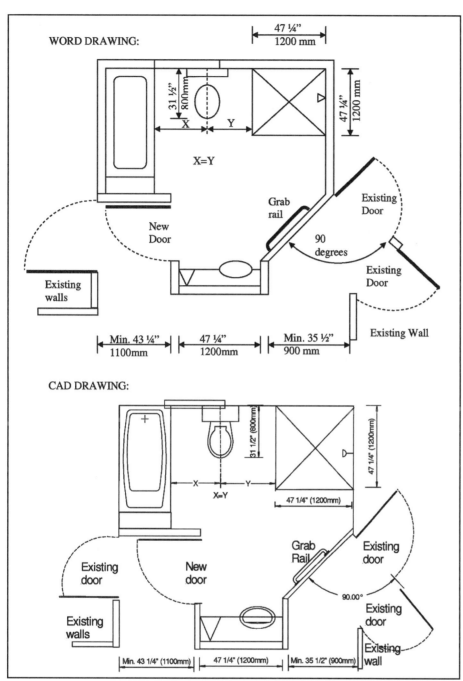

Figure 9-22. Occupational therapist's concept drawing of the floor plan of a bathroom, using Microsoft Word and Autosketch. Reprinted with permission from Nicholas Smith.

Computer Tools for Drawing

Once mastered, drawings using computer technology are faster to draw, store, and retrieve. They can be created using drawing features in existing Microsoft business software, such as Word and PowerPoint, general drawing programs such as Paint and VisioPro, or dedicated CAD software of varying levels of sophistication—for example, AutoCad, Autosketch, SmartDraw, and Google Sketch-Up (Figure 9-22). Items drawn using computer technology can be edited, saved, copied, resized, colored, and manipulated in a range of ways. Templates for areas around the home can be created that can be easily modified through the use of drawing tools to add more detail to the illustration. For example, therapists might create templates of bathroom or toilet areas for quick and easy retrieval to add in illustrations of grab rails. Further, photos, cutouts, photocopies, and other documents can be uploaded and manipulated using software tools. Software packages provide a variety of tools, including pens, airbrushes, drafting tools, and texture maps (Montague, 2005).

Drawings developed using CAD programs appear professional and stylish and make it easier to achieve accuracy of scale (see Figure 9-22). These programs have additional desirable features, including the ability to draw to scale and to import symbols that adapt to the scale. Further, some CAD programs allow scaled drawings to be converted to 3D images with walk-through views. However, to be able to make full use of such computer software, therapists require training. The more sophisticated the program, the more features and drawing options provided and the greater the level of skill and expertise required to operate them. Experienced draftsmen and women and architects are the main users of this technology, although there are industry training and packages available that range from simple to complex. Further, the packages usually contain training tutorials. It is often assumed that CAD-based drawings have been developed by people with building and design knowledge and expertise. Bearing this in mind, therapists who use CAD to develop concept drawings should state that they are to provide an overview of the area only and do not provide the specific technical detail required for building works. They should be careful to clarify that they do not have professional knowledge and expertise in design and construction.

CONCLUSION

This chapter has discussed how a client's home modification requirements can be represented in concept drawings that complement photos and other information that has been put in writing in the occupational therapy report. Though occupational therapy concept drawings are not architectural drawings, they can become the basis for the development of more detailed technical drawings by design or construction professionals. This chapter has described the resources to guide occupational therapy drawing practice, the basic requirements for drawings, and tools and technology that can provide further information to guide knowledge and skill development in the area.

This chapter has not sought to provide comprehensive information to ensure occupational therapists are competent in drawing. Rather, it has reinforced the need for therapists to consider training in the area to ensure that home visit documentation that is produced is clear and concise and communicates information that is easily understood by people working in the design and construction industry. This chapter has discussed how occupational therapists should take advantage of industry training courses in the field to become familiar with construction industry requirements and to ensure good communication with those completing the home modification work.

REFERENCES

American National Standards Institute. (2003). *ICC/ANSI A117.1-2003: Accessible and Usable Buildings and Facilities.* New York, NY: Author.

Ashlee, P., Clutton, S., Pengelly, S., & Cowderoy, J. (2006). Conveying information through drawing. In S. Clutton, J. Grisbrooke, & S. Pengelly (Eds.), *Occupational therapy in housing: Building on firm foundations* (pp. 83-108). London, UK: Whurr Publishers.

Bielefeld, B., & Skiba, I. (2007). *Basics: Technical drawing.* Boston, MA: Birkhauser.

Ching, F. D. K. (1995). *A visual dictionary of architecture.* New York, NY: Van Nostrand Reinhold.

Ching, F. D. K. (1996). *Architectural graphics.* New York, NY: Van Nostrand Reinhold.

Ching, F. D. K., & Adams, C. (1991). *Building construction illustrated.* New York, NY: Van Nostrand Reinhold.

Clutton, S., Grisbrooke, J., & Pengelly, S. (2006). *Occupational therapy in housing: Building on firm foundations.* London, UK: Whurr Publishers.

Housing Industry Association & Illaring Pty Ltd. (2006). *Introduction to drafting: participant guide.* Brisbane, Australia: Author

International Organization for Standardization. (1979). *International Standard ISO 5455.* West Conshohocken, PA: ASTM International.

Montague, J. (2005). *Basic perspective drawing: A visual approach.* Hoboken, NJ: John Wiley & Sons.

Standen, D. (1995). *Construction industry specifications.* Victoria, Australia: The Royal Australian Institute of Architects.

Thorpe, S. (1994). *Reading and using plans.* London, UK: Center for Accessible Environments.

Wang, T. C. (1996). *Plan and section drawing.* Hoboken, NJ: John Wiley & Sons.

Weidhaas, E. R. (1999). *Reading architectural plans for residential and commercial construction.* Upper Saddle River, NJ: Prentice Hall.

Developing and Tailoring Interventions

Desleigh de Jonge, MPhil (OccThy), Grad Cert Soc Sci

Occupational therapists address a variety of occupational performance issues in the home using a range of interventions. Based on an analysis of the person-environment-occupation transaction and the home environment, therapists identify alternative strategies, assistive devices, social supports, and modifications to the environment to promote occupational performance. In developing an intervention strategy, the therapist collaborates with the client to find the solution that best fits with the person and the way he or she engages in occupations in the home environment. This chapter will outline the various approaches therapists use to enhance occupational performance in the home and provide a structure for analyzing the suitability of various interventions. The role of clinical reasoning in determining the best intervention will also be discussed. In addition, the chapter will introduce practitioners to architectural elements of the built environment that might be considered when tailoring interventions to suit the person-environment fit and will present a framework for developing and tailoring environmental interventions.

CHAPTER OBJECTIVES

By the end of this chapter, the reader will be able to:

+ Describe the typical occupational performance issues faced by people in the home

+ Describe the range of interventions that occupational therapy practitioners use to enhance occupational performance in the home

+ Describe a systematic approach to identifying potential interventions

+ Discuss the potential interaction between interventions and the person, the nature of the occupation, and the environment

+ Discuss the use of clinical reasoning in determining the best intervention option

+ Describe the use of architectural elements in developing environmental interventions

IDENTIFYING OCCUPATIONAL PERFORMANCE ISSUES IN THE HOME

Occupational therapists commonly address occupational performance issues that result from a poor fit between the person's capacities and what he or she needs or wants to do and the demands of the environment where the performance takes place. Occupational performance difficulties can arise as a consequence of the following:

+ Changes in a person's functional capacities as a result of aging, injury, impairment, or a health condition

Ainsworth, E., & de Jonge, D.
An Occupational Therapists's Guide to Home Modification Practice (pp. 189-212)

+ Variations in occupational demands or the way activities are undertaken

+ Barriers or challenges presented by the environment

When evaluating occupational performance of various valued and required activities in and around the home, practitioners analyze the person-environment-occupation transaction to identify a specific cause of any difficulties experienced and determine how occupational performance can be further enabled. From this analysis, therapists are able to develop a number of alternative intervention options to address the identified concern and to further enhance performance.

Traditionally, therapists have focused on the impact of various impairments and functional deficits on daily activities and sought to maintain or enhance health, safety, and independence by recommending assistive devices or alternative methods of undertaking activities. Until recently, little attention has been given to the environment and the demands it places on people. Conventional housing design creates a number of challenges for older people and people with disabilities as they go about their daily activities. Houses with stairs, narrow doorways and corridors, inaccessible toilets and bathrooms, and limited space "create" disability (Heywood, 2004; Oldman & Beresford, 2000) and can compromise a person's health, safety (Stone, 1998; Trickey, Maltais, Gosslein, & Robitaille, 1993), independence (Frain & Carr, 1996), and well-being (Heywood). Studies undertaken by Connell and Sanford (1997); Mann, Hurren, Tomita, Bengali, and Steinfeld (1994); and Gitlin, Mann, Tomita, and Marcus (2001) have identified a number of problems experienced by older people in the home environment that would be equally relevant for people with various impairments and health conditions (Box 10-1).

The design of the residence can:

+ Place people at risk of incidents or accidents resulting in injury

+ Make it difficult for people to carry out daily activities in and around the home

+ Place unnecessary demands on people in terms of managing and maintaining the environment

People need to feel well supported by their home environment. When the home provides too many challenges, it can place people at risk of injury arising from incidents or accidents. A challenging home environment can also undermine confidence and make people apprehensive and even fearful as they go about routine activities in the home and community. People also need to be able to manage their home environment—open windows, operate

---

Box 10-1. Problems Reported by Older People in the Home

- *External access*—Difficulty walking on uneven pavements, dealing with slopes, steps, clutter, and ground surfaces

- *Entry*—Difficulty with stairs, locks, keys, and doorknobs

- *Internal mobility*—Stairs, clutter, obstacles, level changes, slippery surfaces

- *Interior (general)*—Poor lighting, difficulty managing control and outlets, hearing doorbell, and using telephone

- *Living room*—Getting up from chairs

- *Bathroom*—Getting into and out of tub, toilet too low, difficulty with taps

- *Kitchen*—Cabinets too high, too low, difficulty using appliances, trash disposal

- *Bedroom*—Getting in and out of bed

(Adapted from Connell & Sanford, 1997; Gitlin et al., 2001; Mann et al., 1994.)

---

controls, answer the telephone and doorbell (Connell & Sanford, 1997), and maintain the home in order to feel comfortable and safe. Older people and people with disabilities often experience difficulties cleaning and maintaining their homes (Peace & Holland, 2001). Homes that are unkempt and poorly maintained can create further hazards and can also increase the vulnerability of the occupants to home invasions when passers-by realize that residents would not be able to defend themselves (Jones, de Jonge, & Phillips, 2008).

INTERVENTIONS USED TO ADDRESS OCCUPATIONAL PERFORMANCE ISSUES

In the home environment, therapists aim to assist people to find ways to perform routine activities of daily living and household tasks that, however inconsequential they might seem, can be integral to leading a full and satisfying life (Crepeau & Schell, 2009). Interventions can address a presenting problem by establishing or restoring the person's capacities; altering the way the task is undertaken; or adapting or modifying the existing environment

(Dunn, Brown, & McGuigan, 1994). Alternatively, the person-environment-occupation fit can be altered (Dunn et al.) by moving the person to a more supportive environment or providing additional support in the way of informal or formal assistance. In some cases, therapists support other people in caring for or assisting people with severe or degenerative conditions (Rogers & Holm, 2009). This type of intervention is referred to as a palliative intervention (Rogers & Holm). Occupational performance difficulties can also be prevented by anticipating potential problems before they occur (Dunn et al.). Furthermore, occupational performance can be enriched by creating enabling environments that promote activity engagement and well-being (Dunn et al.). When providing interventions in the home, therapists need to not only address identified problems, but also be mindful of preventing future problems and creating environments that enrich occupational performance.

Interventions can be focused on the person, task, or environment (Rogers & Holm, 2009). Person-oriented interventions attempt to remediate the person's capacity or manage his or her performance difficulties when undertaking activities by:

+ Maintaining or restoring functions such as muscle strength, endurance, attention, and visual scanning

+ Managing issues such fatigue, attention, and short-term memory difficulties

+ Establishing habits and routines for activities that need to be undertaken regularly

These interventions usually require education, training, and, in some cases, regular involvement with a practitioner. Consequently, they are mostly recommended for clients who can modify their usual approach to tasks, follow a prescribed program independently, or regularly access a rehabilitation program. In contrast, environment-focused interventions, such as home modifications, recognize the person's existing capacities and seek to optimize occupational performance by creating a more supportive environment.

CONCEPTUAL FRAMEWORK FOR DEVELOPING INTERVENTIONS

Everyday activities are commonly undertaken using a combination of strategies, tools, and social and physical supports in the environment (Dunn et al., 1994; Enders & Leech, 1996). Each individual uses a unique blend of these resources to carry out activities in a preferred way. Changes in the person's capacities, the demands of the activity, or the resources available usually prompt people to modify their approach to the task (the strategy), the tools they use, or the way they use the social and physical elements in the environment. For example, there is enormous variation in the way people undertake a simple activity such as cooking scrambled eggs:

+ First, the activity is guided by the preferred outcome—that is, whether the individual prefers eggs light and fluffy, creamy, firm, with a natural flavor, lightly salted, or spicy.

+ How the task is undertaken is governed by the person's cooking skills, experience, knowledge, and how he or she was shown to scramble eggs.

+ The nature of tools available, such as whisk, pans, and cook-top, dictates how the tasks will be performed.

+ Finally, the people available to help and the space and layout of the kitchen will shape the way those tasks are undertaken. If the person is cooking for a number of guests with varying preferences, has an injured hand, breaks the whisk, is offered assistance, or is cooking in a different kitchen, he or she will need to alter the strategy, reconsider the tools, or structure the social and physical environment differently.

Litvak and Enders (2001) described a generic support system for human accomplishment as including strategies, tools, and cooperation and described the function of people with disabilities as being variously supported by adaptive strategies (AS), assistive devices (AD; tools), and personal assistance (PAS) or social support (Figure 10-1).

This is a useful framework for thinking about ways in which occupational performance can be supported when people encounter difficulties. As highlighted in the ecological models, such as Person-Environment-Occupation-Performance (PEOP; Christiansen & Baum, 1997) and the Person-Environment-Occupation (PEO; Law et al., 1996), occupational performance is a function of the dynamic and reciprocal interaction between the person, occupation, and environment. Therapists seek to optimize occupational performance by improving the fit between the person and his or her occupations and roles and pertinent environments. Working with the unique capacities, skills preferences, and experiences of each individual, therapists examine how strategies, tools, and the social and physical environment are currently working to support occupational performance and how they might be modified to optimize that performance.

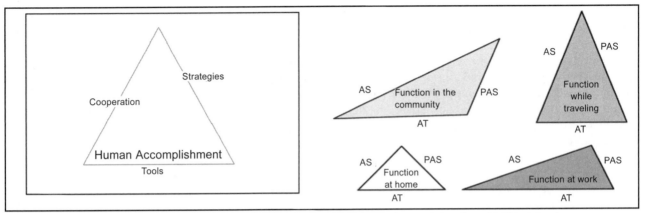

Figure 10-1. Generic support system for human accomplishment. Reprinted with permission from SAGE Publications.

To illustrate the relationship between the person-environment-occupation transaction and these supports, Litvak and Ender's model of support systems (2001) has been modified and superimposed on the Venn diagram of the person-environment-occupation interaction (Figure 10-2).

The curved/reuleaux triangle created by the intersection of the person, occupation, and environment represents occupational performance. Each side of this triangle represents the resources that support occupational performance—namely, strategies (the way the person approaches the occupation), tools (the devices in the environment used to support the occupation), and the physical and social environmental supports (the resources the person avails him- or herself of in the environment). This simple graphic representation provides therapists with a mechanism for examining and acknowledging the current supports available and exploring alternative ways of supporting and enhancing occupational performance. It also recognizes the role of occupational analysis in evaluating the person-environment-occupation transaction and the contribution of strategies, tools, and social and physical environmental supports to occupational performance.

Strategies or Adaptive Approaches to Enhance Occupational Performance

Occupational therapists have a long tradition of making activities more manageable by altering the way they are undertaken. Activities can be done in a different way using energy conservation or work simplification techniques to reduce the physical demands on the person. People can sit to undertake parts of a task or take regular rest breaks to conserve energy. Rescheduling activities to another time when the person is more energetic and mobile—for example, in the morning—can also enhance

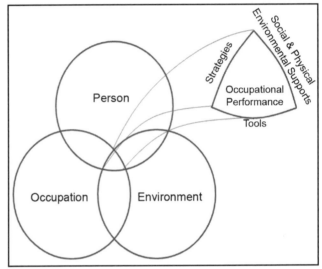

Figure 10-2. Framework for developing interventions.

performance. Activities can also be scheduled at specific time intervals to remove the complexity or urgency of performance—for example, establishing regular times for toileting to reduce accidents and the need to rush to the toilet. Sometimes, activities can be simplified and broken into a number of tasks to reduce the cognitive load. They can also be reordered or relocated to make them easier to perform. For example, during bathing, it might be easier to sit in the bedroom when undressing and dressing rather than attempting this task while standing in what might be the cluttered and slippery environment of the bathroom.

People often develop their own alternative strategies to address difficulties in occupational performance. For example, when getting up from a low toilet, many people grab hold of fixtures and fittings in the room, such as the toilet roll holder, towel rail, or door handle to assist. Though it is important to acknowledge people's resourcefulness in solving everyday problems, some of these strategies are not safe, practical, or sustainable and can place the person at risk of injury. Therapists might suggest a range of alternative strategies to keep the person safe during such a transfer, such as placing hands on knees to assist with lift-off or "keeping nose over toes" to maintain the center of gravity over the base of support (Chan, Laporte, & Sveistrup, 1999; Deane, Ellis-Hill, Dekker, Davies, & Clarke, 2003). However, it is often difficult to change entrenched patterns of behavior. Many occupations in the home are undertaken using individual and unique approaches that have been honed over many years and have become almost instinctive. Because people are often unable or unwilling to change the way they undertake tasks, therapists need to work closely with them to find alternative methods that are comfortable and acceptable. Alternatively, therapists can explore the use of other supports, such as tools or environmental interventions, which can promote a change in approach and decrease reliance on unsafe methods.

Tools or Assistive Devices to Enhance Occupational Performance

Alternative tools or assistive devices are another intervention strategy used by therapists to address occupational performance issues in the home. This intervention strategy is often easiest for therapists to use because there are myriad devices available to address a variety of performance and troublesome task components. Information on specialized devices is readily available through catalogues and equipment databases. For a number of health conditions, assistive devices are viewed as a routine element in the treatment protocol. Assistive devices are frequently funded through a range of schemes because they are generally more affordable and more readily available than environmental interventions. However, assistive devices can often change the way tasks are undertaken and, in some cases, can increase the complexity of the task. For example, transfer benches and shower chairs require people to sit to shower. This changes the nature of the task, removing the relaxation experienced when standing under a shower head and having warm water spraying down the back. Sitting to shower also creates difficulties in washing the peritoneal area. Transfer benches are frequently removed because they get in the way of others who use the bathroom. The task of then replacing the bench and fitting it safely can often prove challenging for the user.

Assistive devices are not always easy to use. For example, it might be easier for some people to walk through the house leaning on the walls for support rather than to navigate a wheeled walker through narrow hallways and doorways. Useful devices are not always at hand when needed. Reachers are very useful for retrieving items out of reach; however, they need to be nearby when required. This means keeping a reacher in each room of the house or carrying it around in case it is needed. With abandonment of assistive devices a major concern (Batavia & Hammer, 1990; Hocking, 1999; Mann & Tomita, 1998; Phillips, 1993; Scherer, 2005), it is evident that many people are receiving devices they do not need or are unable or unwilling to use long term.

Social Supports to Enhance Occupational Performance

People with significant physical, psychological, or cognitive difficulties often receive formal and informal personal assistance to assist them to successfully complete activities. Support can be provided in the form of organizational, verbal, or physical support or assistance. Assistance might be required prior to, during, or after the activity is completed. For example, a family member could prepare the area for the activity, supervise performance, prompt the person through the tasks, or physically assist the person at various stages or throughout the entire activity. Where he or she is no longer able to undertake the activity, another family member might assume complete responsibility for completing the task—for example, doing the laundry or mowing the lawn.

Therapists need to understand the informal supports available to the person and determine whether caregivers are willing, or have the capacity, to provide the required assistance. If appropriate support is available, therapists need to ensure that assistance is provided in a way that maintains the person's autonomy and safety and, wherever possible, that the meaning of the occupation to the person is retained. For example, people might bathe before bed to relax. When a caregiver is assisting with this task, the focus often shifts to cleaning the person as efficiently as possible. The activity becomes centered on the availability and needs of the caregiver rather than the needs of the person being bathed. This is understandable but, when someone is always dependent on others for assistance, the loss of control over daily routine and the relaxing pre-bed routine (or the routine of that whole day) can be distressing and might even have implications for long-term health and well-being.

Therapists are also concerned with the health and well-being of caregivers, especially when they are providing support over an extended period of time. The occupation of caring can also become a focus of intervention, with alternative strategies, assistive devices, and environmental modifications used to minimize the demands on the caregiver and reduce the risk of injury.

Formal caregiver assistance can also be used to support the completion of a range of activities; however, the amount and type of assistance available can vary from one location to another. Therapists need to be aware of the resources available within the local community and use these effectively. Formal assistance removes the demands on the family and frees the client from being dependent on family members for his or her daily needs. When clients receive assistance with routine tasks, such as bathing, it allows them to invest their limited time and energies in more highly valued occupations, such as parenting or work.

However, these formal caregiver services can be costly and often determine when and how activities are completed. Care staff can also intrude on personal spaces and disrupt personal routines. Formal support can disrupt social relationships and routines in the household and extended family. For example, a client once declined the offer of a formal service to do the weekly washing of her bed linen and larger items. The client was able to manage washing her smaller items but had her daughter wash the bed linen when she visited each week. She was concerned that if she removed the daughter's reason for visiting, she may not visit as regularly or might cease to visit at all. This task provided an opportunity for the client to prepare a snack for her daughter while she stripped the bed and put the linen in the washing machine. She could then watch television with her while they waited for the washing to dry. Further, it allowed the daughter to do something concrete and meaningful for her mother. The mother-daughter relationship required the structure of these activities because the client appeared to be a very practical and matter-of-fact woman who did not engage easily in idle chatter.

Environmental Supports to Enhance Occupational Performance

Occupational performance can also be enhanced by modifying the environment. Spaces can be reallocated, expanded, rearranged, remodeled, or redesigned to allow the client to perform activities more effectively. In addition, fixtures and fittings can be removed, relocated, replaced, or added to enhance performance. Sometimes, a room on the first floor—a study, for example—can be reassigned as a bedroom so that the client does not have to climb the stairs to go to bed. A separate and adjacent toilet and bathroom are often combined by removing the dividing wall to allow greater circulation space for both activities. The orientation or position of furniture or fixtures and fittings can also be changed to facilitate access and performance in the room. For example, vanity units may be relocated, baths may be removed, and the swing of the door into the toilet may be reversed to increase circulation space.

Home modifications can include repairs, maintenance, nonstructural and structural adaptations, and smart technologies. Repairs and maintenance are essential to ensuring the ongoing integrity of the environment and the safety and well-being of the occupants. Common repairs and maintenance tasks include the following:

+ Mending stairs, handrails, paths, and flooring

+ Removing clutter and trip hazards

+ Installing and/or replacing lighting, locks, security screens, smoke alarms and carbon monoxide detectors, and taps

Nonstructural modifications include the following:

+ Installing grab bars, rails, shower hoses, door wedges, stair climbers, and privacy screens

+ Altering door swings and window openings

+ Replacing toilets and cisterns, taps, and door handles with accessible alternatives

+ Installing slip-resistant treads in baths and showers and on stairs

+ Installing slip-resistant flooring

+ Inserting solid risers between open steps

+ Repainting walls, frames, and steps to increase color contrast

+ Repositioning fixtures and fittings

+ Introducing specialized shelving, drawers, and hanging rails into storage cupboards and closets

+ Adding and/or relocating controls, light fittings, and power and telephone outlets

Structural modifications include the following:

+ Widening doorways and passages

+ Increasing the size of rooms by moving or removing walls and combining spaces

+ Redesigning bathrooms and kitchens

+ Installing ramps, pathways, roll-in shower recesses, and elevators

+ Replacing toilets with accessible pans and cisterns

+ Fitting shower seats into shower recesses

+ Removing shelving and cupboards under sinks and hotplates

+ Installing additional height-adjustable pantries and shelving

+ Lowering countertops, cupboards, and windows

+ Raising flowerbeds

+ Adding or reassigning rooms

Increasingly, smart technologies are being used to help people maintain their health and well-being and remain living safely and independently in their own homes. These technologies may or may not require structural work or changes to the home's plumbing and electrical systems. Security and home automation systems provide older people and people with disabilities with improved safety and security and an efficient means of managing their home environment. Alarms and call devices ensure that people are able to call for assistance, whereas environmental and remote control systems and devices allow people to manage their environment and the fixture and fittings within it. A growing number of home entertainment options afford people many different ways of enjoying their time at home. Mobile phones, video conferencing, and emergency call systems allow people to maintain contact with friends and relatives and access assistance when required. A range of high- and low-tech assistive devices enable people and their caregivers to undertake their daily activities with greater ease. Emerging technologies can also be used to assist people to manage their routines by prompting them through various tasks such as cooking and taking medications. Those who need to monitor the whereabouts or safety of a loved one can use technologies to oversee or monitor movement remotely. Various remote devices and sensors also assist people and their health care teams to monitor vital signs, identify changes in performance and/or behavior, or record or predict an adverse event.

Modifications to the environment can make it easier and safer for people to engage in valued occupations and to participate actively in family and community life. They can remove the burden of using an unfamiliar strategy and specialized devices or relying on others to be available for support. However, on the negative side, they can be disruptive and change the way the home is used by other household members and visitors. They can also change the look and feel of spaces in the home, the associated memories, and the personal identity derived from the design and décor. Modifications can also be costly. People mostly rely on social services or their own personal resources to fund modifications, so therapists need to be familiar with the building and funding resources available within the community to access environmental interventions effectively (Rigby, Stark, Letts, & Ringaert, 2009).

DEVELOPING INTERVENTION STRATEGIES

Identifying a range of suitable interventions to address occupational performance difficulties is a complex task. Each person has unique expectations, preferences, and experiences and has a distinctive way of undertaking activities. In addition, the home environment has cultural, personal, temporal, physical, and social elements that need to be considered when proposing and developing any type of intervention. Therapists traditionally use occupational analysis, reasoning, and problem solving in developing their understanding of occupational performance difficulties and the range of possible interventions. Additionally, they tailor interventions to suit each situation, drawing on their knowledge of strategies, assistive devices, products, and design as well as their professional experience.

USE OF OCCUPATIONAL ANALYSIS

Therapists use occupational analysis to develop a clear and detailed understanding of the occupation and the specific way it is performed; to identify where task breakdowns occur; and to analyze factors that contribute to the breakdown. They then generate a list of alternative strategies, assistive devices, social support, and modification options that have the potential to address the identified occupational performance difficulty. Building on the example of going to the toilet discussed earlier in this chapter and in Chapter 7, Table 10-1 details the range of alternative interventions for breakdowns at each stage of the activity. Note that this is a theoretical analysis and, as such, does not claim to be comprehensive or account for the variation that may occur in the way the activity is undertaken by an individual or the unique characteristics of a home environment.

When analyzing activities, therapists are encouraged to consider the whole activity—that is, access to and egress from the activity area and all of the stages or elements of the activity from start to finish. Practitioners sometimes restrict analysis to select parts of the activity, focusing on the transfer on and off the toilet. Problems can arise when

Table 10-1. Interventions to Address Breakdowns in Going to the Toilet

TASK	STRATEGY	ASSISTIVE DEVICE	ENVIRONMENTAL MODIFICATION
Register need to go to the toilet	Set at regular intervals	Use an alarm to remind or register moisture	Have a clock visible with marker
Locate and find way to toilet	Feel way along the wall	Install sensor lights	Use lighting or colored line to illuminate way
Open the door	Leave door open	Install sensor opener	Install lever handle or reverse opening
Enter the room	Leave mobility device outside of toilet	Place threshold ramp at doorway	Widen doorway Remove level change
Turn on the light	Leave light on permanently	Install sensor light	Large switch
Close the door	Leave door open		Install self-closing hinge
Travel, turn, and position at front of pedestal	Use cues or markers on the floor	Use walking frame	Increase circulation space
Undress		Wear pants with elastic waist	Hold onto grab bar
Sit down onto toilet	Use supportive lowering technique	Use raised toilet frame	Raise pedestal Install grab bar
Reach for toilet paper/ release sheet	Use pre-torn sheets	Use extend-a-hand	Install automatic sheet dispenser
Transfer weight for wiping	Stand to wipe		Lean onto grab bar
Attend to personal hygiene		Use toilet duck or other wiping aid	Bidet
Move from sitting to standing	Push up on knees	Use toilet frame	Push up on grab bar
Don and adjust clothing	Pull up to thighs while seated	Use easy reacher	Hold onto grab bar
Turn and flush toilet	Leave unflushed	Modify button/lever	Auto flush
Clean toilet bowl		Brush with extended handle	
Open door	Leave door open	Install sensor opener	Install lever handle or reverse opening
Negotiate doorway	Leave mobility device outside of toilet	Place threshold ramp at doorway	Widen doorway Remove level change
Find way to sink to wash hands	Feel way along the wall	Install sensor lights	Use lighting or colored line to illuminate way
Turn on taps	Use moist wipes/antiseptic hand wash	Use tap turner	Level handles
Wash hands			
Dry hands			Use electric hand dryer
NB collapse or need assistance	Leave door open	Use emergency call system	Lift off hinges

designing a support, such as a grab bar, to assist with only one stage of the activity. The therapist is likely to overlook the impact of this support when the person is attending to personal hygiene while seated on the toilet. The grab bar might not provide the person with the support he or she requires when shifting his or her weight while seated and, more importantly, could be an obstruction to the person when performing this action.

The type of intervention used is, in part, dependent on the nature of the identified problem. Experienced clinicians can often generate a number of alternative solutions for any one difficulty. This provides the client with the opportunity to select the interventions that best fit his or her style and preferences and demands of the environment. Therapists with limited knowledge of alternative options can have difficulty problem solving unique situations and responding to the specific requirements of the individual and household. Because occupational therapists have traditionally used alternative strategies or assistive devices to address occupational performance issues, they are less familiar with ways the environment can be modified to support performance.

USE OF REASONING

The nature of the intervention chosen is dependent on a range of factors. First, the person is likely to have past experience, preferences, and capacities that influence how receptive he or she is to an intervention. Second, although some tasks are more conducive to a change in strategy, others are better supported by an assistive device, social support, or modification. Third, other people in the home environment are likely to influence decisions when interventions impact on how they use the home environment. Finally, the home environment might also constrain what can be achieved as a result of the design and physical structure of the house.

Therapists rely on professional reasoning to determine the potential effectiveness and impact of proposed interventions by using a combination of scientific, narrative, pragmatic, and ethical reasoning to design acceptable, effective, and workable home modifications. Refer to Chapter 7 for a definition of each of these reasoning styles and the contribution each makes to the evaluation process. A description of the role reasoning styles play in developing interventions follows.

Therapists use scientific reasoning to identify a range of suitable interventions and tailor them to each client's specific requirements. Knowledge of

interventions and their effectiveness—derived from databases, professional literature, and professional experience—guides therapists in selecting suitable options. Therapists also review research to ascertain the level of support for proposed interventions and the applicability of this information to each client's situation (Chapter 11 has further information on the use of evidence in designing interventions). In addition, therapists are able to design individualized solutions using their expertise in anthropometrics, biomechanics, ergonomics, health conditions and impairments, occupational performance, and various aspects of the environment.

Working within a person-environment-occupation theoretical framework, therapists examine the potential impact of each option on the associated interaction. For each alternative strategy, assistive device, social support, or environmental intervention, the therapist asks the following questions.

Person

+ Can the client manage the alternative strategy, device, or approach to the occupation?

+ Is he or she willing or able to do the activity in a different way?

+ Is he or she satisfied with the recommended changes?

Occupation

+ How will the recommended option affect the nature of the occupation?

+ Is the recommended option well suited to the unique way the person undertakes the occupation?

+ In what way does the recommended option alter the occupation procedure, meaning, or routine?

Environment

+ How well will the environment support the recommended option?

+ Are resources available in the environment to support the recommended option?

+ How does the recommended option impact on other people in the environment?

+ How does the recommended option impact on the personal, physical, social, cultural, and temporal aspects of the environment?

Therapists use narrative reasoning to explore each client's preferences and perceptions of the effectiveness of the recommended options in addressing the identified problem and the potential impact of each solution on the identified goal, the meaning of the occupation, and the various dimensions of the home environment. It is essential that therapists discuss the proposed interventions with all household members to fully explore the impact of these on the household.

Therapists use pragmatic reasoning to examine the relative costs and availability of resources to implement each option. The physical structure of the house and immediate environment can often define the suitability of interventions, particularly modifications. The focus and policies of the service can also impact on what, and how, resources are made available. However, because clients retain the right to decline the options on offer, they can also access their own resources or an alternative service to address their needs in their preferred way. It is also important to remember that installation or construction might disrupt the household temporarily and that the potential impact of these disturbances on the household needs to be considered when deciding the best option.

Therapists also use ethical reasoning to evaluate the potential value of options and to identify the best solution for each situation. While therapists have a duty of care to deliver the best possible intervention, they frequently use ethical reasoning to wrestle with inadequate resources to implement an effective solution. When clients and therapists differ in their understanding of the effectiveness and impact of various solutions, therapists seek to fully understand the person's perceptions of each option and provide him or her with a deeper understanding of their professional perspective. An exchange of information and understanding generally results in the development of a workable solution that meets the person's goals and preferences and addresses the therapist's concerns. Ultimately, clients have the right to do what they think is best in their own homes, but therapists also have a responsibility to inform them of the potential risks in choosing a less-than-ideal option.

Determining the Best Option

There are usually any number of potentially useful alternative solutions to occupational performance problems in the home; however, there are several issues that can impact on decision making, including economic, architectural, and social barriers (Rigby et al., 2009). Cost is often a consideration when designing environmental interventions. It is important to work responsibly within a budget, but therapists should also be mindful of the potential long-term costs of interventions. For example, some assistive devices, such as a transfer bench for the bath or over-toilet frame, cost less to install than a shower recess or an accessible toilet with grab bars. However, these interventions can prove to be more costly in the long term if the client requires additional supervision or assistance to complete the task or sustains an injury because he or she is incapable of using the assistive device safely. It is well recognized in the occupational health and safety arena and in the area of workplace accommodations that there is a hierarchy of interventions in terms of their anticipated effectiveness. It is proposed that environmental interventions are more effective in managing risk and reducing incidents and accidents than alternative methods because it is difficult for people to change entrenched behaviors in familiar environments.

The design and structure of the home also poses a number of challenges when designing environmental interventions (Rigby et al., 2009). Therapists need to understand the constraints presented by the built environment in order to determine what is feasible. Because this is not an occupational therapist's area of expertise, it is advisable to access a design or construction professional to advise on the suitability of the building for modification. Further information will be provided later in this chapter to assist therapists in understanding the complexities they are likely to encounter when working with the built environment.

While home visits provide therapists with an enriched understanding of clients and their home environment, therapists, in reality, experience only a snapshot of people's lives. It is therefore critical to examine solutions thoroughly with clients to ensure that they will fit well with them, their families, their routines, their lifestyles, and their home environments. Collaboration is required if interventions are to be effectively designed to suit the goals and preferences of clients and their families.

The nature of interventions considered is also likely to be influenced by factors related to therapists' experiences and models of practice and the service and information resources available. Each therapist tends to have particular expertise and experience that impacts on the options identified. Therapists who have worked with particular products or designs are likely to favor these over unfamiliar options. The models of practice therapists employ also predispose them to using some interventions in preference to others. For example, therapists using a rehabilitation framework are likely to focus on remediating function before compensating for lost function by using assistive devices or removing barriers in the environment to accommodate specific impairments and activity limitations. On the other hand, therapists using a person-environment-occupation model would focus primarily on enabling occupational performance by ensuring that the environment was designed to promote engagement in personally meaningful activities in the home and community.

Therapists might work within a particular service with its own specific focus, policy, procedures, or protocols that dictate the resources therapists have readily available to them. Some services and agencies fund assistive devices more readily than environment interventions, which defines the intervention options available. The availability of technical advice can also vary between services, which impacts on therapists' capacity to consider modifications that require structural changes or building expertise. Though research and industry standards provide information on the safety and effectiveness of some interventions, there can be limited information on other options. This can result in options such as exercise, education, and assistive devices being favored in the absence of evidence on environmental interventions. Further, the detail provided in the access standards on the design requirements of young adult wheelchair users often predominates because there is little known about the design requirements of people with severe and multiple impairments who use other devices and rely on caregiver support to complete activities in areas of the home.

TAILORING INTERVENTIONS

Environmental interventions in the home need to be practicable and acceptable to the residents and accommodate everyone who lives in or visits the home regularly. They should not only address the identified problem but should also promote occupational performance and ensure that the essential qualities and meaning of activities and the home environment are retained. Therapists should also ensure that the interventions will not cause any unexpected stress or discomfort and will not create new issues for the person in the home environment.

Therapists generally tailor the intervention to the specific requirements of the person, the occupation, and the environment, giving consideration to the following:

+ The characteristics of the person

+ The way the activity is undertaken and specifically where performance breakdowns or difficulties occur and/or where the activity could be further supported

+ Whether the environment can accommodate an intervention or places any constraints on its availability, usefulness, or location

CHARACTERISTICS OF THE PERSON

When tailoring an intervention for a specific situation, therapists consider the person's goals, preferences, his or her specific impairments and occupational performance difficulties, ability to cope with the intended change, and general capacities that include the anthropometrics of the person(s) likely to use the intervention. People have preferred ways of approaching activities and also personal experiences and tastes that can impact on their decisions. Some people find it difficult to approach a task in a different way so it is important that occupational therapy works with their preferred approach. Other household members using the space will also be affected by the changes and will need to be consulted during the planning process.

Therapists determine whether the individual has specific impairments in his or her sensory, motor, cognitive, or psychosocial function that may present additional difficulties and ensure these are accommodated in the design of the solution. For example, when designing a grab bar to assist during toileting, the therapist would consider the following:

+ Static balance in the seated and standing positions and dynamic balance when moving determines the amount and type of support required

+ Strength and coordination of the upper limbs to determine whether the grab bar can be used for pushing or pulling

+ Sensation to establish whether additional grip is required

+ Vision and visual perception to determine the degree of color contrast required

+ Cognition to establish whether the person requires any training, prompting, supervision, or assistance in using the grab bar

+ The person's confidence and self-efficacy during the activity

Anthropometrics, which uses standardized methods of measurement, can also assist therapists in determining the best configuration and position for a grab bar. Chapter 8 provides a detailed description of this methodology. Therapists often use anthropometrics to tailor the intervention to suit each client. They assess their:

+ Weight—to determine whether the load capacity of the grab bar needs to be increased

+ Height when seated and standing—to determine the required height of the bar above the floor

+ Arm length, reach range, and length of forearm—to establish the best location for the rail and the preferred length

+ Hand size—to guide the size of the diameter of the grab bar

+ Grip strength—to guide the size of the diameter of the grab bar and the finish on the surface of the bar

+ Right or left dominance—to determine the side of the toilet on which the bar should be placed

CHARACTERISTICS OF THE ACTIVITY AND OCCUPATION

Therapists customize solutions to support clients through troublesome aspects of activities while ensuring that other aspects of the activity are not disrupted. For example, when designing a grab bar to assist an individual to transfer on and off the toilet, the therapist observes the client's posture, movement, and center of gravity in relation to his or her base of support and notes specific aspects of the transfer that are problematic. With an understanding of the biomechanical factors that impact on the sit-to-stand transfer, the therapist determines whether the client is experiencing difficulty with flexion momentum, lift-off, extension, and stabilization (Laporte, Chan, & Sveistrup, 1999; Figure 10-3) and designs the grab bar accordingly. If a client is having difficulty bending forward, the therapist might provide a vertical grab bar that he or she can pull on to move forward. If lift-off is problematic, the therapist might provide a horizontal grab bar to push up on. To assist the client in the extension or stabilization stage of the transfer, the therapist might provide a diagonal or vertical bar that the client can hold on to while transitioning and standing. However, if the client experiences difficulty at each stage of the transfer, the grab bar configuration would need to incorporate each of these elements.

The therapist would also determine other aspects of the activity where the client could benefit from grab bar support and ensure that the solution is adequate for these aspects of the activity. For example, male clients might require support when standing to urinate, or clients might require support when shifting their weight while seated to attend to their hygiene. In addition, the therapist would need to ensure that the proposed design does not interfere with other actions or tasks the person performs during this activity—for example, that the person will not knock his or her elbow on the grab bar when donning his or her clothes. The therapist would also remain mindful of the value of the activity to the person and, in particular, the unique elements and methods he or she should aim to retain when tailoring the intervention to the occupation—for example, a rail might be required in front of the toilet cistern to enable the client to rest against the toilet lid to lean back and relax during toileting.

CHARACTERISTICS OF THE ENVIRONMENT

In addition to the personal, temporal, social, and cultural aspects of the environment discussed previously, the physical environment also requires careful consideration when designing interventions. Often, the environment can constrain the design of a solution because there is insufficient space or structural support for the proposed modification. For example, therapists are commonly interested in maximizing circulation space in the bathroom. This is often achieved by removing other fixtures, such as the bath, or annexing spaces adjacent to the bathroom, such as the toilet, and incorporating this space into the bathroom. If the wall between the bathroom and toilet has to support the roof or upper floor, costly structural work can preclude this option. The positioning of grab bars can also be limited by the location of studs, because grab bars need to be anchored directly into studs that sit behind the wall sheeting or onto solid blocking mounted onto the studs (Adaptive Environment Center, 2002).

Therapists should consult with building and design professionals if they are uncertain whether the environment can support the proposed intervention because there are often ways to modify spaces and provide additional structural support. Figure 10-4 shows that there are a number of alternatives to securing grab bars directly into studs:

+ Using special fasteners

+ Fixing a backing board onto the studs

+ Installing blocking between studs

+ Replacing the wall sheeting with ¾-inch (19-mm) plywood

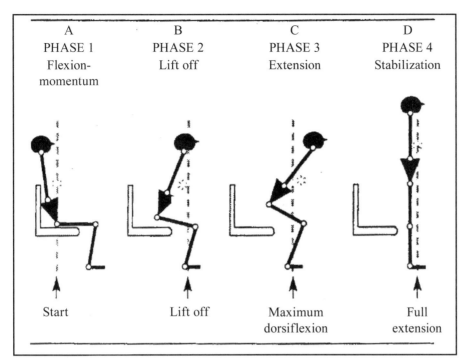

Figure 10-3. Phases of rising. (Reprinted from *British Journal of Occupational Therapy, 62*(1), 36-42 with permission from the College of Occupational Therapists Ltd.)

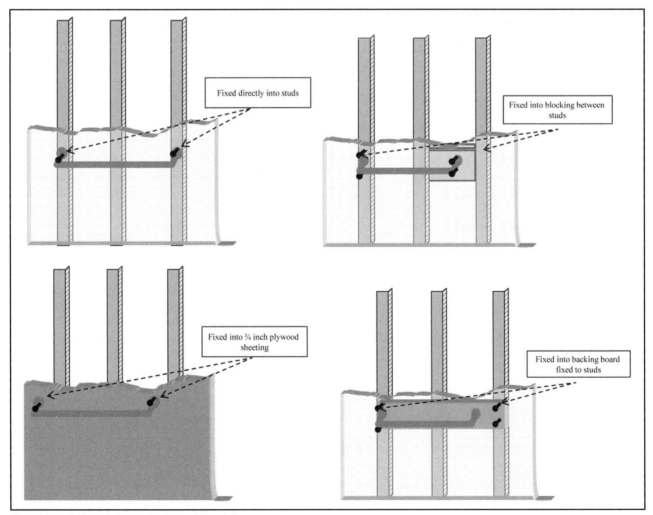

Figure 10-4. Alternative ways to secure grab bars.

Therapists are encouraged to develop an understanding of the built environment so that they understand the constraints on designing environmental interventions and can effectively discuss alternatives with building and design professionals.

The home is not just a physical structure. Consideration also needs to be given to the personal, temporal, social, and cultural dimensions of the home when determining the best option. Each of these dimensions impacts how they are viewed by the clients, their families, and other householders and whether they are accepted, used, or rejected. The personal dimension reflects the sense of identity gained from places, objects, routines, roles, and activities (Despres, 1991; Dovey, 1985; Rubinstein, 1989; Sixsmith, 1986). People can have strong reactions to foreign objects or changes to the home environment that do not reflect the image they have of themselves. The temporal dimension of the home involves routines, activities, places, and things that may be important to the person because they evoke memories of the past, provide links with the present, or reflect hopes for the future (Fisher, 1998). People can be reluctant to make changes to the home they built and raised their children in. They are often resistant to preparing for the likelihood of disability because many are fearful of anticipating this as an outcome. The social dimension incorporates the other people in the home, relationships, and collaboration that occurs during activities (Fisher). When making changes to the home, it is important to consider the other people who also use the area as well as any caregiver involved in the completion of the activity. The cultural dimension takes into account customs, beliefs, activity patterns, behavior standards, and societal expectations (American Occupational Therapy Association [AOTA], 2008). Householders are often wary about introducing items and changes into the home that vary too greatly from what other houses in their community or culture look like or contain.

DEVELOPING ENVIRONMENTAL INTERVENTIONS

As noted earlier in this and other chapters, the capacity and potential of the environment to support occupational performance is well recognized. Changes to the environment can reduce demands on the person; enhance health; increase safety, independence, and effectiveness of performance; improve the quality of the experience; and promote further occupational engagement. Environmental changes can also reduce the need to learn new ways of performing activities and can limit reliance on assistive devices and other people.

Although therapists are experts in promoting occupational performance, they tend to be less familiar with environmental interventions and the architectural aspects of the built environment. Consequently, they can feel uncomfortable making and designing environmental recommendations, seeing themselves as ill-equipped to assess the viability of an environmental modification. Therapists can address this in a number of ways. They can:

+ Liaise with specialists who can advise them on environmental options

+ Use resources targeted specifically at common occupational performance problems in the home and typical environmental interventions

+ Use tools that direct them to specific environmental problems and how these can be addressed

+ Familiarize themselves with general resources on designing safe and accessible environments

+ Develop expertise in the technical aspects of the built environment

+ Use a framework for considering elements in the built environment

Liaising With Specialists

Therapists can refer clients to specialist services for an environmental intervention or seek advice from other experts, such as more experienced therapists or design and building professionals. When referring clients to a specialist service, it is important to provide them with appropriate information and liaise with them about alternative strategies and assistive devices that have been recommended.

It is often necessary for occupational therapists to access the expertise of an experienced colleague or building or design professional when designing an environmental intervention. Ideally, it is useful for the therapist and builder/designer to attend the property together because there are often constraints when attempting to modify an existing structure. The best solution is often achieved when the therapist and builder/architect collaborate with the client to identify the environmental intervention that will achieve the best person-environment-occupation fit. Remote strategies, such as video teleconferencing, have also been used to enable building and design specialists to direct measurement and observe activity in the environment (Sanford & Butterfield, 2005). This technology allows the therapist, client, and specialists to discuss concerns in real time and draw on the experience and expertise of all parties in negotiating an acceptable solution.

If it is not possible to visit the property with the building and design professional or negotiate a remote consultation, tools such as the Comprehensive Assessment and Solutions Process for Aging Residents (CASPAR; Sanford, Pynoos, Tejral, & Browne, 2002) can guide therapists to measure aspects of the environment that designers and builders need to redesign or modify the area (Figure 10-5).

Targeted Resources

Targeted resources are generally aimed at assisting consumers in identifying problems in the home and informing them of potential solutions. For example, the Adaptive Environments Center (2002) has developed the *Consumer's Guide to Home Adaptation*, which can be used by a consumer, community care worker, or building and design professional to evaluate needs, identify solutions, plan, and undertake environmental modifications (Figure 10-6).

Similarly, the Canada Mortgage and Housing Corporation (CMHC) has developed a number of useful publications to assist with making homes accessible and safe, including *Accessible Housing by Design Series* (2010) and *Maintaining Seniors' Independence Through Home Adaptation: A Self Assessment Guide* (2007).

Box 10-2 provides an excerpt from the CMHC 2007 publication detailing recommendations for people who experience difficulty stepping into or out of the bathtub.

These publications introduce therapists to the broad range of environmental interventions available to address specific occupational performance difficulties in the home for older people and for people who mobilize using wheelchairs.

Tools for Identifying and Addressing Specific Environmental Problems

Tools such as the Housing Enabler (HE; Iwarsson & Slaugh, 2010) assist therapists in identifying and measuring problematic design elements in the built environment, while BUILDEASE (www.lifease.com/lifease-buildease.html) assists in selecting appropriate home modification products and design solutions for older people or people with disabilities. The HE provides therapists with details of environmental design elements that interfere with the performance of people with a range of identified functional and mobility impairments. It also provides the minimum design requirements, according to Swedish accessibility standards. As noted in Chapter 7, the HE alerts therapists to elements in the physical environment that present challenges to people with varying functional and mobility impairments, such as difficulty interpreting information; severe loss of sight; complete loss of sight; severe loss of hearing; prevalence of poor balance; incoordination; limitations of stamina; difficulty in moving head; difficulty in reaching with arms; difficulty in handling and fingering; loss of upper extremity skills; difficulty bending, kneeling, etc.; reliance on walking aids; reliance on wheelchair; and extremes of size and weight (see Figure 7-3).

Once potential barriers have been identified, therapists can focus on removing or modifying the environment to be more accessible (Figure 10-7).

BUILDEASE is a multifaceted software tool that assists in identifying environmental features that are likely to be difficult for clients given their current functional abilities. It guides the user in measuring the client and the environment and designing home modification solutions by providing a database of more than 1,500 suggestions and building product solutions. A report can then be downloaded and edited, allowing graphics, pictures, photographs, floor plans, and so forth to be added as required.

General Environmental Intervention Resources

General resources on accessible design, such as the Americans with Disabilities Act (ADA)/American Building Act (ABA) access standards and the Accessible Housing Design File (Barrier Free Environments, 1991), assist therapists in understanding the design requirements for people with disabilities and, in particular, people with mobility impairments. Therapists often refer to the standards to identify the recommended specifications for particular design elements—for example, the circulation spaces around various fixtures and fittings, heights of power points and light switches, and grab rail specifications, such as diameter, wall clearance, load capacity, and clearance from the centerline of the toilet. However, these standards were designed for public buildings and were aimed to suit the majority of users. Based on the anthropometrics of young adults who mobilize independently using a wheelchair, the specifications in these standards are not always appropriate for occupational therapy clients, many of whom do not fit the profile on which these standards were founded. Further discussion on how the standards are used in home modification practice is provided in Chapter 12.

There are also a number of resources dedicated to designing for specific groups:

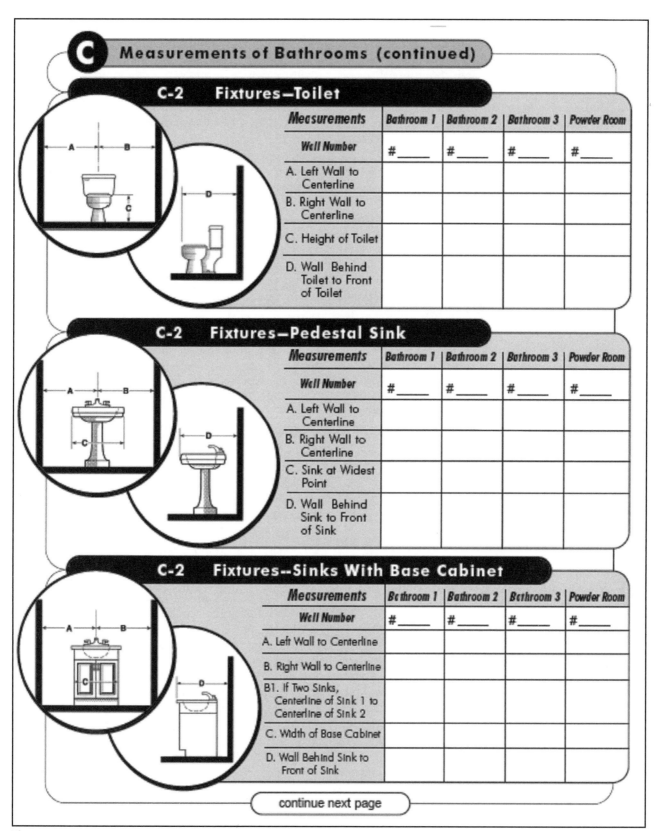

C-2 Fixtures—Toilet				
Measurements	Bathroom 1	Bathroom 2	Bathroom 3	Powder Room
Wall Number	#_____	#_____	#_____	#_____
A. Left Wall to Centerline				
B. Right Wall to Centerline				
C. Height of Toilet				
D. Wall Behind Toilet to Front of Toilet				

C-2 Fixtures—Pedestal Sink				
Measurements	Bathroom 1	Bathroom 2	Bathroom 3	Powder Room
Wall Number	#_____	#_____	#_____	#_____
A. Left Wall to Centerline				
B. Right Wall to Centerline				
C. Sink at Widest Point				
D. Wall Behind Sink to Front of Sink				

C-2 Fixtures--Sinks With Base Cabinet				
Measurements	Bathroom 1	Bathroom 2	Bathroom 3	Powder Room
Wall Number	#_____	#_____	#_____	#_____
A. Left Wall to Centerline				
B. Right Wall to Centerline				
B1. If Two Sinks, Centerline of Sink 1 to Centerline of Sink 2				
C. Width of Base Cabinet				
D. Wall Behind Sink to Front of Sink				

continue next page

Figure 10-5. CASPAR Part 5, Description of the Home—C Measurement of Bathrooms. (Permission to reproduce CASPAR item provided by Extended Home Living Services, Wheeling, IL.)

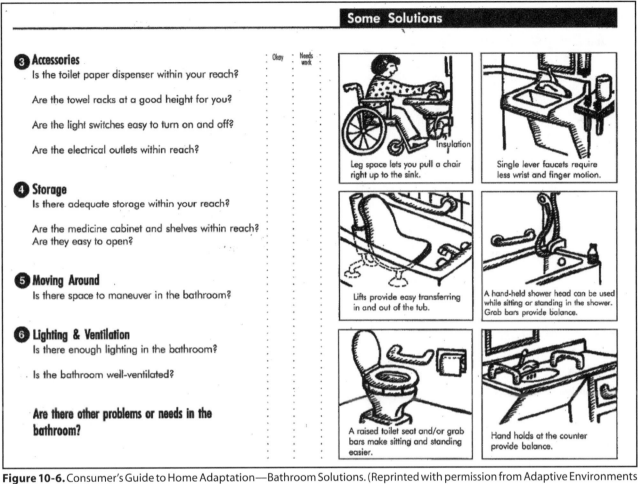

Some Solutions

❸ Accessories
Is the toilet paper dispenser within your reach?

Are the towel racks at a good height for you?

Are the light switches easy to turn on and off?

Are the electrical outlets within reach?

❹ Storage
Is there adequate storage within your reach?

Are the medicine cabinet and shelves within reach?
Are they easy to open?

❺ Moving Around
Is there space to maneuver in the bathroom?

❻ Lighting & Ventilation
Is there enough lighting in the bathroom?

Is the bathroom well-ventilated?

Are there other problems or needs in the bathroom?

Okay   Needs work

Leg space lets you pull a chair right up to the sink.

Single lever faucets require less wrist and finger motion.

Lifts provide easy transferring in and out of the tub.

A hand-held shower head can be used while sitting or standing in the shower. Grab bars provide balance.

A raised toilet seat and/or grab bars make sitting and standing easier.

Hand holds at the counter provide balance.

Figure 10-6. Consumer's Guide to Home Adaptation—Bathroom Solutions. (Reprinted with permission from Adaptive Environments Center. (2002). *Consumer's guide to home adaptation.* Boston, MA: Author.)

+ *Residential Design for Aging in Place* (Lawlor & Thomas, 2008), which discusses design considerations for older people

+ *Making Life More Livable: Simple Adaptations for Living at Home* (Duffy, 2002), which details how to make homes more livable for individuals with visual impairments

+ *Alzheimer's and Related Dementias Homes That Help: Advice From Caregivers for Creating a Supportive Home* (Olsen, Ehrenkrantz, & Hutchings, 1993)

Increasingly, there is an emphasis on designing homes using a universal approach. Universal design (UD) ensures that features in the home are usable, comfortable, and convenient for everyone in the home, regardless of ability or life stage. There are a growing number of resources that describe universal design features for residential buildings. One such resource is *Practical Guide to Universal Home Design* (Wilder Research Center, 2002). This 19-page booklet illustrates essential UD features for various

areas of the home, including entrance, kitchen, bathroom, laundry, bedrooms, living and dining rooms, storage, garage, doorways and hallways, floors, windows, and stairs.

These resources provide therapists with a vision of what is possible and also an understanding of specific design requirements. However, they do not assist the therapist in determining the specific design requirements for an individual or whether the existing environment is able to accommodate the proposed design elements.

Developing Expertise in the Technical Aspects of the Built Environment

Some therapists find it useful to invest time reading or studying the technical aspects of the built environment to assist them in understanding building structures and systems that impact on modification design. Additional knowledge assists therapists to communicate more effectively with building and design professionals and enables them to identify

---

Box 10-2. Maintaining Seniors' Independence Through Home Adaptation: A Self-Assessment Guide Item— Canada Mortgage and Housing Corporation

Canada Mortgage and Housing Corporation has developed *Maintaining Seniors' Independence Through Home Adaptation: A Self-Assessment Guide*, which is designed to assist older people in addressing specific problems in the home environment. This guide details a range of activities that older people typically experience difficulties with in the home and describes adaptations to address these difficulties. Activities addressed include getting in and out of the home, using the stairs, moving around the home, using the kitchen, using the bathroom, getting out of a bed or chair, using closets and storage areas, doing laundry, using the telephone or answering the door, and controlling light and ventilation. This tool does not attempt to diagnose the specific cause of the difficulty but provides a range of environmental interventions aimed at reducing difficulty in performing the tasks such as removing, moving, modifying, replacing, or adding various fixtures and fittings.

Example of *Maintaining Seniors' Independence Through Home Adaptation: A Self-Assessment Guide* item:

5. Using the Bathroom

    5.3. Do you have any difficulty stepping into or out of the bathtub?

No >> If no, go to next question

Yes >> If yes, check the adaptations below that would help you

☐ Install a vertical and a horizontal or angled grab bar by the tub

☐ Install non-slip flooring throughout the bathroom

☐ Install a non-slip surface in the bathtub

☐ Install a commercial or custom-made transfer bench so that the tub can be entered from a seated position

☐ Replace bathtub with a shower stall, if difficulty is severe

☐ Install a separate shower stall, if difficulty is severe

☐ Other (describe)

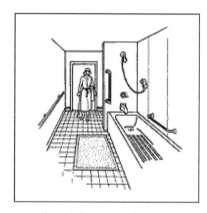

A vertical grab bar provides support when entering the tub, while a horizontal (or angled) bar helps you to complete the entrance and lower yourself onto a shower seat or to the bottom of the tub.

---

whether a solution is viable before referring on to a builder/architect for a work design or quote. For example, if the therapist knows that the existing wall in the toilet is unable to support the installation of grab bars in the required location, he or she can discuss alternative options with the client or prepare him or her for the structural work required to install the grab rails. It is, however, unwise for therapists who do not have formal building qualifications to provide advice that is outside of their area of expertise. Occupational therapists understand the person-environment-occupation transaction but do not necessarily have expertise in building systems

and structures or building legislation. It is always advisable for therapists to seek further advice when environmental interventions require building or design expertise.

Framework for Dealing With Elements in the Built Environment

A deeper understanding of the built environment will assist therapists to appreciate the impact of the environment on the person-environment-occupation transaction. Therapists have a sound understanding of body structures and functions that allows them to

C. Indoor environment General (p. 128)	A	B1	B2	C	D	E	F	G	H	I	J	K	L	M	N	NOTES
																Note that the indoor assessment is linked to "necessary housing functions" (in particular stairs, door widths).
1. Stairs/thresholds/differences in level between rooms/floor spaces (more than 25 mm).		3	3		3	3		1					3	4		
2. Complicated/illogical circulation routes (p. 129).	3	3	3				4						1	1		
3. Narrow passages/corridors in relation to fixtures/design of building (less than 1.3 m, p. 131).													3	4	1	*Note the difference between C3 and C9.*
4. Narrow doors (clearance less than 0.80 m, pp. 146–47).													4	4	1	
5. Slippery walking surface (hygiene rooms are rated separately) (pp. 96–97).		3	3		3	3	1						3		1	
6. High-pile/loose-weave/soft floor covering (pp. 96–97).							1						1	3		
7. Loose small mats.				3	2	1							2	3		
8. Loose cables etc. on the floor.				3	2	1							2	3		
9. Insufficient manoeuvring areas in relation to movable furnishings (pp. 26–27)		2	3		3	3							3	4	1	*Note the difference between C3 and C9.*

Figure 10-7. Housing Enabler Environmental Assessment. (Reprinted with permission from Iwarsson, S., & Slaug, B. (2010). *The Housing Enabler: A method for rating/screening and analysing accessibility problems in housing* (2nd ed.). Lund & Staffanstorp, Sweden: Veten & Skapen HB and Slaug Enabling Development.)

understand the impact of impairments on function. They also possess a deep understanding of occupational performance that allows them to analyze the value and elements of various activities. A richer understanding of the environment and the elements within an occupational performance space and how they are structured will help therapists understand the limitations of the existing environment and what and how it can be altered to support occupational performance. This understanding will also enable therapists to collaborate with builders and designers in developing modifications that fit with the person, the occupations he or she undertakes in the space, as well as the realities of the built environment.

Elements in the built environment that need to be considered when designing modifications include the following:

+ Building structures
+ Service systems
+ Spaces and places
+ Products, devices, and technologies
+ User interfaces

Building Structures

Therapists need to appreciate the importance of structures in the built environment when developing environmental interventions. The structure of a house is found in the framework, which is comprised of three basic parts: the floors, walls, and roof.

In modification work, therapists are mostly interested in moving or removing walls or adding, modifying, or repositioning fixtures and fittings on walls, so it is important to understand how they are constructed and the functions that walls perform.

In most houses, walls are constructed using 2-in by 4-in (50-mm by 75-mm) timber. They consist of a frame with studs or vertical lengths every 16 in (450 mm) along the length of the wall. This frame is then covered with some type of sheeting, such as plywood, particleboard, fiberboard, plasterboard, or some other drywall material (Figure 10-8).

Increasingly, stud walls are being constructed from steel rather than timber, which has implications for how easily they can be modified and how fixtures and fittings can be attached. Walls can also be constructed of concrete blocking or masonry (brickwork), which is more difficult to remove or

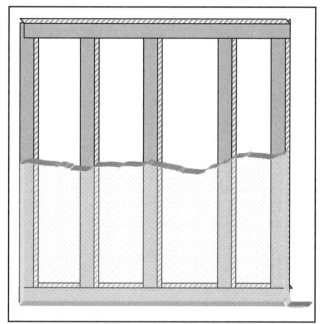

Figure 10-8. Structure of a stud wall.

modify and requires special tools and fasteners to install fittings and fixtures. When items such as grab bars are installed on a wall, they need to be secured into the studs or other structural supports in the wall. The nature and location of these structures can determine whether a grab bar can be safely attached and where it or other accessories can be located. Alternative structural supports can be put in place if the wall structure is inadequate or if the studs are not located in the required positions; however, the advice of a suitably qualified building contractor or designer should be sought if there are concerns about the capacity of the wall to support these fittings.

Walls often house electrical and plumbing lines and heating and cooling ducts. Although they are mostly used to divide up interior spaces, some walls are load bearing and serve the additional function of supporting an upper floor, ceiling, and/or roof. Therapists need to be aware that a supporting or load-bearing wall cannot be removed without being replaced by a suitable support structure. This type of alteration requires the expertise of a building or design professional and can be costly.

When considering any structural modification, it is advisable to employ a building or design professional to inspect the building to ensure that it is in good repair and able to accommodate the recommended changes. It is also essential to know what is behind the surfaces of walls, floors, and ceilings before work begins.

Service Systems

The service systems within a home include plumbing; wiring or the electrical system; and heating, ventilation, and air-conditioning (HVAC) system. Plumbing in residential structures involves the water supply system as well as a drain system. The home's electrical system is made up of wiring, outlets, and switches and has many circuits, each of which starts from a main service panel. The HVAC, the home's heating and cooling system, includes the heating or cooling unit as well as a series of ducts leading to and from various rooms in the house. Each of these systems has lines (pipes, wiring, and ducts) that run through the wall, floor, and ceiling cavities, which need to be considered when proposing changes.

In some buildings, it is extremely costly or impossible to relocate systems, such as electrical wiring, power outlets, water pipes, and sewage and waste outlets. For example, relocating a toilet or a waste in the bathroom would require the drainage pipes and outlets in the floor to be repositioned. Where this is possible, it can be costly, and, in some constructions, such as a slab-on-ground construction, it is not reasonable to undertake such changes. Consequently, when looking to remodel a bathroom, for example, it is advisable to note the location of existing fixtures and fittings and plan to keep them in those locations or to account for the cost in relocating them when discussing the relative merit of designs and installations.

Though therapists are not required to possess this building knowledge, it is important that they are aware of some of the limits to what is possible and seek the advice of a suitably qualified builder, designer, or contractor when investigating modifications that require changes to the building structures or systems.

When working within the existing structure of a home, there are a number of design elements that can impact on occupational performance. These elements, or attributes, of the physical environment have been identified as spaces and places; products, devices, and technologies; and user interfaces (Table 10-2) (Sanford & Bruce, 2010).

Spaces and Places

When considering the impact of the environment on occupational performance, it is useful to examine the spatial elements of the environment and whether these elements need to be altered to promote performance. Sanford and Bruce (2010) identify key spatial considerations to include the following:

+ *Entry*: Can the person approach the entry and negotiate the clearance through the doorway safely and efficiently?

Table 10-2. Common Attributes of Physical Environment Features Proposed by Sanford and Bruce

SPACES AND PLACES	PRODUCTS, DEVICES, AND TECHNOLOGIES	USER INTERFACES
• Entry • Circulation/level changes • Orientation cues • Configuration/layout • Location of products, devices, and technologies • Location of environmental controls • Ground/floor and wall materials/finishes • Ambient conditions	• Product type • Dimensions • Weight • Location of user interfaces • Materials/finishes	• Type of interface • Minimum approach distance and angle • Dimensions • Activation force required • Operational attributes • Materials/finishes • Feedback mechanisms

(Reprinted with permission from Sanford, J., & Bruce, C. (2010). Measuring the impact of the physical environment. In E. Mpofu & T. Oakland (Eds.), *Rehabilitation and health assessment* (pp. 207-228). New York, NY: Springer.)

+ *Circulation/level changes*: Is there adequate room for the person to move, approach, reach, and use various fixtures and fittings in the room? Are there any changes in levels to negotiate between areas?

+ *Orientation cues*: Is signage clear and appropriately located? Are key landmarks well lit, visible, and located in a logical position?

+ *Configuration/layout*: Is the layout logical in terms of the way the person uses the space? Does the size of the spaces, configuration, or layout allow the person and/or caregivers to maneuver equipment? Do these allow flexibility in use of space?

+ *Location of products, devices, and technologies*: Are the switches, outlets, and fixtures visible, accessible, and located in a logical place?

+ *Location of environmental controls*: Are the controls visible, accessible, and located in a logical place? Can they be operated or adjusted easily?

+ *Ground/floor and wall materials/finishes*: Are the floor materials appropriate for the activities being undertaken and the people using the space? Do the materials used create a suitable look and feel? Do the materials used assist in differentiating spaces for different purposes? Do the wall materials provide flexibility in supporting future fixtures and fittings?

+ *Ambient conditions*: Is the lighting adequate for the tasks being undertaken and is it located in the appropriate area? Is the room a comfortable temperature for the activity being undertaken?

Products, Devices, and Technologies

Products such as fixtures, appliances, and building elements—for example, flooring, doors, and windows—have characteristics that impact on ease of use. Considerations identified by Sanford and Bruce (2010) include the following:

+ Product type: What products does the user need to interact with?

+ Dimensions: Do the fixtures fit into the space or location available (leaving adequate room for approach and operation)?

+ Weight: Can the fixtures and fittings be moved if required?

+ Location and size of user interfaces: Can the controls on the fixture be reached and operated easily? Are they visible and well lit? Can they be easily read?

+ Materials/finishes: Do the materials and finishes provide appropriate contrast, friction, or resistance? Can the fixtures and fittings be operated using limited force/dexterity? Do the fixtures and fittings provide adequate auditory and/or visual information to the user? Are they comfortable to use (temperature and texture of the surface against the skin, etc.)? Will materials and finishes stand up to the anticipated wear (to suit heavy equipment use or impact by equipment)?

User Interfaces

User interfaces include controls and hardware such as handles, knobs, taps, locks, and handrails and grab bars; electronic and mechanical controls and dispensers also affect use. Key considerations identified by Sanford and Bruce (2010) include the following:

+ Type of interface: What controls and hardware does the user need to interact with?

+ Minimum approach distance and angle: Can the controls/hardware be accessed easily?

+ Dimensions: Do the controls fit into the space and location available (leaving adequate room for approach and operation)?

+ Activation force required: Can the controls/hardware be operated using limited force/dexterity?

+ Operational attributes: What is the direction and distance that controls/hardware need to be moved? Can they be easily read and operated?

+ Materials/finishes: Do the controls/hardware provide adequate contrast/friction? Are they comfortable to use (temperature and texture of the surface against the skin, etc.)? Will they tolerate the way they are likely to be used?

+ Feedback mechanisms: Do the controls/hardware provide adequate auditory and/or visual information to the user?

The number of design elements that require consideration can be overwhelming for new therapists. Consequently, checklists and frameworks for considering these elements systematically are quite useful. However, when attempting major modifications, the expertise of a designer or builder is essential. Therapists should not take responsibility for determining the suitability or integrity of the existing building for modification. They should, however, have sufficient understanding of the built environment to be alert to its limitations to enable them to collaborate effectively with builders and designers and to ensure that their recommendations are reasonable, the needs of the client are adequately addressed in the redesign, and the modifications do not present any unanticipated difficulties or complexities for the people living in the home.

CONCLUSION

This chapter has described the range of performance issues that older people and people with disabilities experience in the home and the range of intervention strategies occupational therapists use to address these issues. It has introduced a framework for analyzing the resources used during activities and identifying ways in which alternative strategies, assistive devices, social supports, and environmental modifications can address occupational

performance concerns and further facilitate the person-environment-occupation transaction. The role of occupational analysis and clinical reasoning in designing client-centered interventions has also been examined. In particular, this chapter described considerations in determining the best intervention and tailoring it to the specific needs of the person, activity, occupation, and environment. Finally, this chapter has detailed the range of environmental interventions used to address occupational performance issues in the home and provided therapists with mechanisms for developing their understanding of the built environment.

REFERENCES

Adaptive Environment Center. (2002). *Consumer's guide to home adaptation.* Boston, MA: Author.

American Occupational Therapy Association. (2008). Occupational therapy practice framework: Domain and process (2nd ed.). *American Journal of Occupational Therapy, 62,* 625-683.

Americans with Disabilities Act and Architectural Barriers Act Accessibility Guidelines. (2004). Retrieved from http://www.access-board.gov/ada-aba/final.cfm

Barrier Free Environments. (1991). *The accessible housing design file: Barrier free environments.* New York, NY: Van Nostrand Reinhold.

Batavia, A. I., & Hammer, G. S. (1990). Toward the development of consumer-based criteria for the evaluation of assistive devices. *Journal of Rehabilitation Research and Development, 27*(4), 425-436.

Canada Mortgage and Housing Corporation. (2007). *Maintaining seniors' independence through home adaptation: A self assessment guide.* Ottawa, ON: Author. Retrieved from http://www.cmhc-schl.gc.ca/en/co/maho/adse/masein/masein_005.cfm#CP_JUMP_44995

Canada Mortgage and Housing Corporation. (2010). *Accessible housing design series.* Ottawa, ON: Author. Retrieved from http://www.cmhc-schl.gc.ca/en/co/renoho/refash/refash_033.cfm

Chan, D., Laporte, D. M., & Sveistrup, H. (1999). Rising from sitting in elderly people, part 2: Strategies to facilitate rising. *British Journal of Occupational Therapy, 62*(2), 64-68.

Christiansen, C., & Baum, C. (Eds.). (1997). *Occupational therapy: Enabling function and well-being* (2nd ed.). Thorofare, NJ: SLACK Incorporated.

Connell, B. R., & Sanford, J. A. (1997). Individualizing home modification recommendations to facilitate performance of routine activities. In S. Lanspery & J. Hyde (Eds.), *Staying put: Adapting the places instead of the people* (pp. 113-131). Amityville, NY: Baywood.

Crepeau, E., & Schell, B. (2009). Analyzing occupations and activity: A way of thinking about occupational performance. In E. B. Crepeau, E. S. Cohn, & B. A. Boyt Schell (Eds.), *Willard & Spackman's occupational therapy* (11th ed., pp. 359-374). Philadelphia, PA: Wolters Kluwer Lippincott Williams & Wilkins.

Deane, K. H. O., Ellis-Hill, C., Dekker, K., Davies, P., & Clarke, C. E. (2003). A Delphi survey of best practice occupational therapy for Parkinson's disease in the United Kingdom. *British Journal of Occupational Therapy, 66*(6), 247-254.

Despres, C. (1991). The meaning of home: Literature review and directions for future research and theoretical development. *Journal of Architectural and Planning Research, 8*(2), 96-115.

Dovey, K. (1985). Home and homelessness. In I. Altman & C. M. Werner (Eds.), *Home environments* (Vol. 8, pp. 33-61). New York, NY: Plenum Press.

Duffy, M. A. (2002). *Making life more livable: Simple adaptations for living at home.* New York, NY: AFB Press.

Dunn, W., Brown, C., & McGuigan, A. (1994). The ecology of human performance: A framework for considering the impact of context. *American Journal of Occupational Therapy, 48*, 595-607.

Enders, A., & Leech, P. (1996). Low-technology aids for daily living and do-it-yourself devices. In J. C. Galvin & M. J. Scherer (Eds.), *Evaluating, selecting and using appropriate assistive technology* (pp. 30-39). Gaithersburg, MD: Aspen Publishers, Inc.

Fisher, A. G. (1998). Uniting practice and theory in an occupational framework. *American Journal of Occupational Therapy, 52*(7), 509-520.

Frain, J. P., & Carr, P. H. (1996). Is the typical modern house designed for future adaptation for disabled older people? *Age and Ageing, 25*(5), 398.

Gitlin, L. N., Mann, W., Tomita, M., & Marcus, S. M. (2001). Factors associated with home environmental problems among community-living older people. *Disability and Rehabilitation, 23*(17), 777-787.

Heywood, F. (2004). The health outcomes of housing adaptations. *Disability and Society, 19*(2), 129-143.

Hocking, C. (1999). Function or feelings: Factors in abandonment of assistive devices. *Technology and Disability, 11*, 3-11.

Iwarsson, S., & Slaug, B. (2010). *The Housing Enabler: A method for rating/screening and analysing accessibility problems in housing* (2nd ed.). Lund & Staffanstorp, Sweden: Veten & Skapen HB and Slaug Enabling Development.

Jones, A., de Jonge, D., & Phillips, R. (2008). *The role of home maintenance and modification services in achieving health, community care and housing outcomes in later life* (Research Report). Melbourne, Australia: Australian Housing and Urban Research Institute.

Laporte, D. M., Chan, D., & Sveistrup, H. (1999). Rising from sitting in elderly people, part 1: Implications of biomechanics and physiology. *British Journal of Occupational Therapy, 62*(1), 36-42.

Law, M., Cooper, B., Strong, S., Stewart, D., Rigby, P., & Letts, L. (1996). The person-environment-occupation model: A transactive approach to occupational performance. *Canadian Journal of Occupational Therapy, 63*, 9-23.

Lawlor, D., & Thomas, M. A. (2008). *Residential design for aging in place.* Hoboken, NJ: Wiley & Sons.

Litvak, S., & Enders, A. (2001). Support systems: The interface between individuals and environments. In G. L. Albrecht, K. D. Seelman, & M. Bury (Eds.), *Handbook of disability studies* (pp. 711-733). Thousand Oaks, CA: Sage Publications.

Mann, W., Hurren, D., Tomita, M., Bengali, M., & Steinfeld, E. (1994). Environmental problems in homes of elders with disabilities. *Occupational Therapy Journal of Research, 14*(3), 191-211.

Mann, W. C., & Tomita, M. (1998). Perspectives on assistive devices among elderly persons with disabilities. *Technology and Disability, 9*, 119-148.

Oldman, C., & Beresford, B. (2000). Home sick home: Using housing experiences of disabled children to suggest a new theoretical framework. *Housing Studies, 15*(3), 429-442.

Olsen, R., Ehrenkrantz, E., & Hutchings, B. (1993). *Alzheimer's and related dementias homes that help: Advice from caregivers for creating a supportive home.* Newark, NJ: New Jersey Institute of Technology.

Peace, S. M., & Holland, C. (2001). *Inclusive housing in an ageing society: Innovative approaches.* Bristol, UK: Policy Press.

Phillips, B. (1993). Technology abandonment from the consumer point of view. *NARIC Quarterly, 3*(2-3), 4-91.

Rigby, P., Stark, S., Letts, L., & Ringaert, L. (2009). Physical environments. In E. B. Crepeau, E. S. Cohn, & B. A. Boyt Schell (Eds.), *Willard & Spackman's occupational therapy* (11th ed., pp. 820-849). Philadelphia, PA: Wolters Kluwer Lippincott Williams & Wilkins.

Rogers, J. C., & Holm, M. B. (2009). The occupational therapy process. In E. B. Crepeau, E. S. Cohn, & B. A. Boyt Schell (Eds.), *Willard & Spackman's occupational therapy* (11th ed., pp. 478-518). Philadelphia, PA: Wolters Kluwer Lippincott Williams & Wilkins.

Rubinstein, R. L. (1989). The home environments of older people: A description of the psychosocial processes linking person to place. *Journal of Gerontology: Social Sciences, 44*(2), 545-553.

Sanford, J. & Bruce, C. (2010). Measuring the impact of the physical environment. In E. Mpofu & T. Oakland (Eds.), *Rehabilitation and health assessment* (pp. 207-228). New York, NY: Springer.

Sanford, J. A., & Butterfield, T. (2005). Using remote assessment to provide home modification services to underserved elders. *Gerontologist, 45*(3), 389-398.

Sanford, J. A., Pynoos, J., Tejral, A., & Browne, A. (2002). Development of a comprehensive assessment for delivery of home modifications. *Physical and Occupational Therapy in Geriatrics, 20*(2), 43-55.

Scherer, M. J. (2005). *Living in a state of stuck: How technology impacts on the lives of people with disabilities* (2nd ed.). Cambridge, MA: Brookline Books.

Sixsmith, J. (1986). The meaning of home: An exploratory study of environmental experience. *Journal of Environmental Psychology, 6*, 281-298.

Stone, J. H. (1998). Housing for older persons: An international overview. *Technology and Disability, 8*(1-2), 91-97.

Trickey, F., Maltais, D., Gosslein, C., & Robitaille, Y. (1993). Adapting older persons' homes to promote independence. *Physical and Occupational Therapy in Geriatrics, 12*(1), 1-14.

Wilder Research Center (2002). *Practical guide to universal home design.* Saint Paul, MN: East Metro Seniors Agenda for Independent Living. Retrieved from http://www.lifease.com/PracticalGuideToUniversalHomeDesign.pdf

11

Sourcing and Evaluating Products and Designs

Desleigh de Jonge, MPhil (OccThy), Grad Cert Soc Sci

Therapists use a wide range of mainstream and specialized products and design solutions to address a variety of occupational performance concerns and difficulties. Consequently, they need access to a number of different information systems to locate information on what is available. They also need to be able to evaluate the relative benefits of each option to determine the best solution for each client and his or her household. The first section of this chapter overviews the information systems therapists can use to gain an understanding of environmental interventions and then examines the nature of information provided by each of these systems. Therapists can use these resources to locate suitable options for individual clients, to enable them to remain informed about developments in the area, and to build a body of knowledge about the range of interventions available.

The second section of this chapter outlines a systematic process for reviewing and comparing products and designs and details a number of considerations when evaluating the relative merits of various options. It identifies the information therapists require to undertake a thorough comparison of options and discusses the unique perspective clients bring to the decision-making process. It also highlights the benefits of drawing on the experiences of other therapists, designers, builders, and clients to understand the advantages and disadvantages of various products and designs. The role of evidence and design and product standards in reviewing the suitability of options is also discussed in this

chapter, as are the principles of good design, which aim to ensure that products and designs used for older people and people with disabilities are aesthetic, flexible, and functional in the long term.

CHAPTER OBJECTIVES

By the end of this chapter, the reader will be able to:

+ Identify and discuss the benefits and limitations of various information systems used to gather information on products and designs

+ Describe a systematic process for reviewing products and designs

+ Identify key issues in evaluating the potential value and effectiveness of product and design solutions

SOURCING AND EVALUATING PRODUCT AND DESIGN OPTIONS

When developing environmental interventions, therapists draw from a broad range of products and design solutions, including specialized and mainstream options. Consequently, they need access to information on specialized assistive devices for people with various functional impairments as well as the many generic building products on the market.

Ainsworth, E., & de Jonge, D.
An Occupational Therapists's Guide to Home Modification Practice (pp. 213-228)

They also need to understand various design approaches and be able to evaluate their suitability for each situation. Because there is an ever-increasing number and range of options and information on these is scattered across industries, information systems, and suppliers, it is often difficult for therapists to feel confident that they have a good understanding of all of the options available.

Information on Products and Designs

To develop effective interventions, therapists need to actively develop their understanding of the broad range of specialized and mainstream options available. They need to know where to find information on products and designs and how to search for solutions suited to the unique requirements of each client. It is therefore important that therapists are aware of the information systems available and can use these effectively to locate suitable options for individual clients.

When searching for potential options, a number of questions come to mind:

+ What products and design options exist?

+ Where are they available?

+ Who were they designed for?

+ How well will they suit the person's identified needs? How long have they been tested and available in the marketplace?

+ Why choose one product over another?

Therapists need a good understanding of the range of options available and their specifications—that is, size, shape, weight, and finish. They need to know where they are available and how much they cost. It is also important to know who the product was designed for because this gives therapists an indication of its potential strengths and limitations and the situations it best suits. Therapists also need to know how the product can be adjusted or customized as well as its installation, maintenance, and service requirements. Ultimately, therapists need to be able to explain why they would choose one product over another so they can justify that they have recommended the best. In the case of a legal challenge, therapists need to be able to defend their choices. In order to answer these questions, therapists need to access a range of resources to gather information. These include the following:

+ Company catalogues

+ Trade exhibits or display centers

+ Databases

+ Online resources: dedicated home modification Web sites, as well as building, government, and community Web sites concerned with home renovation, modification, repair, and maintenance—for example, checklists, buyers' guides, renovation guides, and product reviews

+ Professional publications and resources: books, journals, and newsletters

+ Conferences and workshops

+ People with experience: clients, professional colleagues, builders, and designers

A list of resources is available in Appendix D.

Company Catalogues

Many specialist and mainstream building suppliers provide catalogues of their products, either in hard copy or online. These resources answer the "what" and "where" questions well because they can provide good graphics and specifications of the products in their range. They can also provide an up-to-date price list and the contact details of suppliers in various locations. Generally, companies supply a defined range of goods, which means that therapists need to access a number of companies' catalogues to understand the full range of options available. Catalogues generally provide clear photos or drawings of each product, which can be used when describing alternatives to clients. Sales representatives might also be able to provide a sample of the product to view or test in various situations. It is important to remember that sales representatives are paid to promote their products, so they will be able to describe all of the features and identify all of the advantages of their products. A discussion with representatives from a number of companies is usually required to develop a full understanding of the strengths and limitations of all options on the market. Company representatives may also be able to provide information on whom the product was specifically designed for or situations where it is best suited. Therapists would then need to ascertain whether the product would meet the specific requirements of each client. Catalogues are useful for therapists who have a clear understanding of the requirements of the client and well-developed professional reasoning skills that allow them to filter and analyze the information provided. Therapists with a good understanding of the range of options should also ensure that they access catalogues from all relevant suppliers and not limit themselves to a restricted range of options. It is also advantageous to have some experience with the application of the products or access to people who have used them so that sales information can be balanced with an understanding of how well products work in various situations.

Trade Exhibits or Display Centers

Trade exhibits or display centers are an excellent way for therapists to develop an overview of the range of products available and to keep up to date with recent developments. These resources provide therapists with similar benefits and challenges; however, having a number of companies and products co-located makes it easier to gather information on a range of options and to view and compare alternatives. It should be noted that, although these exhibits and display centers have a number of products on display, they might not be comprehensive or representative of all of the products available on the market. They are likely, however, to showcase local suppliers and contractors, which is advantageous to people who are unfamiliar with resources in the area or who live in more remote areas where such resources are often scattered.

Databases

There are a number of specialist and mainstream databases that allow therapists to search for specific products. Most of these are now available online. The advantage of using a database is that many of them feature consistent fields to describe the various products they have on file. This allows therapists to quickly access information on a range of options and compare specifications and costs. It is sometimes possible to search for products with specific features, thus allowing therapists to define their search and locate suitable products quickly. The amount of information and graphics provided varies, and the currency of the information depends on how regularly the database is updated. Some of the information provided may be location specific, so it is important to use databases that have information on products from the appropriate region. Therapists with sound clinical skills and a clear idea of what they want from products are well placed to maximize the use of these resources. The volume of information available can be overwhelming for therapists who are new to the area. Once again, it is advantageous to have some experience with the application of the products or access to people who have used them so that information can be augmented with an understanding of how well the products work in various situations.

Online Resources

There are many dedicated home modification and building Web sites, as well as government and community Web sites, that display a variety of resources related to home renovation, modification, repair, and maintenance. With the country's aging population, there has been an explosion of resources designed to assist older people in identifying and addressing their home modification and maintenance needs. Many checklists, buyers' and renovation guides, and product reviews can be uncovered with a simple or advanced Google search. Several of these resources have been written specifically to assist older people to identify and address their safety and function in the home as they age. In addition, a number of resources outline how to make homes accessible for people using wheelchairs or manageable when caring for someone with dementia. These resources can be particularly useful for clients and therapists because they provide an overview of issues and an introduction to potential solutions, especially low-cost options. They may or may not provide details of specific solutions or products and, if they do, the information may be location-specific. These resources can be useful for clients and novice therapists; however, it is important that therapists check the authority of these sites by confirming, against other resources, the expertise of the authors and the validity of the information provided. It is also advisable to be aware of the domain of the Web site and to interpret the information accordingly. For example:

+ .com is a commercial site
+ .org is a community organization
+ .edu is an educational institution
+ .gov is a government site

Each of these sites has a particular function and perspective that need to be considered when assessing the authority and validity of the information provided. Therapists need to dedicate time to becoming familiar with, and regularly reviewing, resources on the Internet. Experienced therapists are well placed to piece together these scattered resources and direct new therapists and clients to the best resources available.

Professional Publications and Resources

There are an increasing number of books, journals, newsletters, and Web sites that provide information related to home modifications. Books written by occupational therapists and others on home modifications provide therapists with an understanding of a range of solutions; however, the qualifications and experience of the authors, the frames of reference from which they operate, and the focus of the book can define the range of options presented. For example, occupational therapists will generally seek to define the specific needs of the client before detailing the potential options. They also see environmental interventions as part of a suite of interventions and will, therefore, discuss these in conjunction with alternative strategies, assistive devices, and supports. On the other hand, books written by building and design specialists will provide details of alternative designs without necessarily identifying who they best suit or alternatives to costly renovations. However, these texts allow therapists to develop their understanding of the range of options and considerations when designing environmental solutions. Books do not generally refer to specific products but might provide a list of suppliers relevant to the location of the publication. It is important, however, to be aware that the information may be dated, given that books generally are not frequently revised. A range of books has been written on aspects of home design for people with specific requirements, including older people, people with dementia or vision impairment, or wheelchair users. Some books focus exclusively on low-cost modifications to existing premises and others describe design elements that need to be incorporated into the design of a new home or in extensive renovations of an existing home.

Journals and newsletters might also discuss and evaluate various intervention approaches or provide reviews of products. A number of Web sites are dedicated to home design, construction, and modification. These sites are a repository for publications, reviews, and information on training and education opportunities, and they often provide links to other relevant sites.

By monitoring these information resources, therapists can develop a broader understanding of the effectiveness or usefulness of various interventions and products and can search for more specific details when relevant situations arise. Therapists who need an overview of the area and an understanding of the range of possible solutions available will find such resources invaluable; however, they would also need to ensure they are well informed about current products and design approaches in their local area.

Conferences and Workshops

Conferences and workshops are useful in assisting therapists to understand the range of interventions, approaches, and products available and in helping them develop an awareness of existing services and expertise. The location of the conference or workshop and the background and experience of the presenters might be considerations in applying the information directly to clinical practice. Therapists might need to evaluate whether the approach, products, or designs are well suited to the needs of their client group and location. These resources provide therapists with benefits and challenges similar to those provided by professional publications and resources; however, novice therapists might find workshops a more efficient way of getting the basic knowledge and skills they require because the expert presenters often collate current information from a range of resources and tailor it to the background and level of experience of the workshop participants. More experienced therapists are well equipped to use information presented at conferences and will benefit from having access to a range of home modification experts and exhibitors at international, national, and regional conferences.

Specialist Education and Training

Home modification practice requires therapists to develop specialist skills and knowledge. In addition to identifying occupational performance difficulties in the home and addressing these using alternative strategies, assistive devices, and caregiver support, therapists are required to understand how and when the environment can be modified. Many therapists seek additional training or courses to extend their knowledge of the built environment. These courses introduce therapists to building practices, various design approaches, products, and finishes and show how to navigate funding systems and modification services and to manage building processes. This understanding complements the clinical knowledge therapists have and the reasoning they use to address occupational performance difficulties and concerns in the home. Additionally, it enables them to work more effectively with designers and builders in developing effective home design solutions.

People With Experience

Clients, professional colleagues, builders and designers, and suppliers with experience designing, supplying, or using home modifications can be invaluable in assisting therapists to identify alternatives or select and tailor environmental interventions to individuals' needs. Discussing situations with professional colleagues or building and design professionals can help clarify issues and solve problems associated with difficult scenarios. People with special skills and knowledge or experience using products and designs over extended periods can provide insights into what does and doesn't work well in different situations. They often have extensive knowledge of the products and designs that can be supported locally and the quality of after-sales service and maintenance services for various products. These resources are of value to novice and experienced therapists alike, allowing them to draw on the experience of others to complement their own skills and knowledge to develop the best possible solution for their clients.

Reviewing Product and Design Alternatives

Once the range of alternative products and designs has been identified and located, each option has to be evaluated to determine the best one for each situation. When evaluating the suitability of designs or products, therapists need to ask the following:

+ Who has the product/design been developed for?

+ How well will the product/design meet the client's specific requirements?

+ How long has the product/design been tested and available in the marketplace?

+ Why choose one product/design over others?

There are a number of considerations when examining the origin of products and designs. First, design and product requirements can vary between countries and some regions. Therapists need to ensure that designs and products they recommend meet the requirements of their national and local standards or building codes. For example, design standards or building codes for a region with a low-density population, high winds, or low rainfall might not reflect the standards of a region with a high-density population and heavy snowfall. Second, commercially available products are generally designed for the mainstream market and might not acknowledge the diversity of function in the broader population. Therapists therefore need to be mindful of the needs of their particular client group and individual clients when assessing the suitability of various mainstream products and designs. For example, many fittings require fine motor control that can be problematic for older people and people with disabilities. In addition, labels or indicators are often difficult to see or read, and even specialized products or designs can be developed with one particular disability group in mind. For example, products and designs developed to address the needs of wheelchair users with full upper limb function might not readily address the needs of people with other disabilities.

When choosing the best product for a particular client or situation, therapists think about the client's specific requirements and consider the strengths and limitations of each option in relation to these requirements. Each product or design should be evaluated in terms of how well they:

+ Will be used by the client, given his or her physical, cognitive, sensory, and emotional capacities

+ Will enable the client to complete the occupation in his or her preferred manner

+ Will fit with the physical, personal, social, cultural, and temporal aspects of the environment.

In addition, each option needs to be compared in terms of the following:

+ Product features and specifications

+ Clients' priorities and preferences

+ Experience of the product or design

+ Existing evidence of the benefits of the product or design

+ Conformity with design or product standards or building code requirements

+ Good design practice or inclusive design

How long have the products and designs been available in the marketplace? This will provide information about whether the product, for example, has been tried and tested extensively, whether there is likely to be service support for setup and maintenance/servicing, whether parts are available, and whether there are people who can comment on its suitability for their circumstance. Such knowledge will guide practice decisions about a product's application and use.

Product Features and Specifications

When reviewing products and designs, it is useful for therapists to gather information on the features, specifications, and cost of each option so that they can be systematically compared. Therapists often develop templates that allow them to gather all of the information they need when considering the suitability of options. This template can include:

+ Name of product and a description

+ Models

+ Appearance—a graphic

+ Specifications

+ Price range

+ Construction (what the product is made of)

+ Installation requirements

+ Care and maintenance requirements

+ Advantages and limitations

+ Compliance with relevant standards or building codes

+ Suppliers and services able to fit and maintain the product

+ Notes regarding supply (e.g., availability and after-sales support)

When considering the cost of interventions, as well as the original purchase price, it is also important to consider the installation, maintenance, and replacement costs (Andrich, 2002). Further, the social cost of various options also needs to be examined (Andrich). For example, the cost of formal or informal support as an alternative to the product or design can be prohibitive. Although the cost of formal support can be readily calculated, the cost of informal support can be overlooked. Therapists need to be mindful that it might be more cost-effective to install a product or design rather than recommend the provision of formal or informal support as an alternative. These issues are important when comparing options and ensure that the comparisons consider the long-term impact of solutions as well as immediate expenses.

Consumers' Priorities and Preferences

Clients are often not afforded sufficient choice and control over the home modification process, which can result in them feeling disempowered (Hawkins & Stewart, 2002; Heywood, 2004; Sapey, 1995) and dissatisfied that their priorities and preferences are not reflected in the outcome. Professionals often have knowledge of and experience with a range of products and designs and have assessed their functional suitability. However, clients are best placed to evaluate how suitable the products or designs would be for their situation and, in particular, how well they will fit with the look and feel of the home, the people who live there, and the many activities that are undertaken in it. Clients can often have quite different views of their homes and needs than service providers, and this can impact on how they value advice and their willingness to proceed with recommendations (Auriemma, Faust, Sibrian, & Jimenez, 1999).

When clients are evaluating products and designs, they are most often concerned with the following:

+ Appearance

+ Cost

+ Availability

+ Functionality or usability

+ Impact on other household members or visitors

+ Adaptability and suitability

+ Installation or construction requirements

+ Care requirements

+ After-sales support

+ Anticipated lifespan

Modifications can sometimes have a clinical appearance, which might not fit well in the home environment (Duncan, 1998). Complying with design standards or building codes designed for public buildings and spaces can also result in modifications having an institutional appearance, which is not generally in keeping with residential environments (Lund & Nygard, 2004). It is therefore important that products and designs are well suited to a domestic situation, are in keeping with the style and décor of the client's home, and reflect personal preferences.

Though clients are often mindful of the costs associated with home modifications, they are also likely to want quality products, designs, and finishes in their home. Many therapists can let the expectations and restricted financial resources of the subsidizing organization determine their choice of products and designs (Rousseau, Potvin, Dutil, & Falta, 2001). However, the cheapest option is not always the best value. Modifications that do not fully satisfy the current and anticipated needs of the household can result in wasted expenditure (Department for Communities and Local Government, 2006).

Householders often have pragmatic concerns when reviewing alternative options. Once they decide to proceed with the modification, they want to ensure minimal delay and disruption. Consequently, they might show a preference for products that are readily available and choose designs that have been used locally, especially if they can view the finished product prior to confirming choice. Another important consideration is usability, or the extent to which an individual's performance and activity patterns can be fulfilled in a particular environment (Bernt & Skar, 2006). Potential usability is best judged by the individual who will be using the product or space and is likely to be influenced by his or her experiences and expectations (Steinfeld & Danford, 1999). Because performance and activity patterns can vary from day to day or throughout the day, it is important to consider the capacity of the product to support or to be adjusted to account for these variations. In addition, when a number of people are using the product or space, its ability to accommodate all users needs to be examined. This includes the potential impact of the product or design on other household members as well as regular visitors.

The installation or construction requirements might also be a matter for consideration when reviewing alternatives. Some clients find it difficult to tolerate major disruptions to their routines or households and might prefer an option that is less intrusive in the short term. It is therefore important that they are made aware of potential disturbances associated with product and design choices. In addition, the care requirements may prove problematic for some clients. For example, although textured flooring provides good grip and reduces the risk of slipping, it is more difficult to clean, especially for people with reduced mobility and upper limb strength. Over time, the buildup of soap and grime can make these floors more hazardous.

The availability of after-sales support for products or the construction is also of interest to clients, who are often responsible for the repair and replacement of the modification to their home. Clients wanting value for money will also be concerned with the lifespan of the product. Selecting a product with a longer lifespan, even if it costs more initially, might be preferable and less expensive in the long term.

Experience of the Product or Design

Therapists, designers, and builders with extensive experience in home modifications can draw on this wealth of knowledge when selecting products and designs. They usually know how well a product or design works in various situations and the range of people who have used the intervention successfully. These professionals might also have an understanding of difficulties encountered in acquiring, installing, adapting, or getting approval for a solution in a variety of situations or locations. Experienced therapists, designers, and builders can also have a good understanding of the lifespan of products and designs that have been used over a period of time. This information also assists in anticipating how well certain materials and finishes can stand up to wear and tear in a range of situations.

Follow-up with clients provides therapists with information on the usability of interventions, care requirements, and the responsiveness of after-sales support. Seeking feedback from clients and monitoring their experience over variable periods is an effective way of accumulating experience of various products and designs. Therapists can gain a richer understanding of the application of products and designs in a range of situations. It is especially valuable in identifying any unexpected issues in relation to the following:

+ Acceptance
+ Cost
+ Functionality or usability
+ Adaptability and suitability
+ Installation or construction
+ Care
+ After-sales support
+ Lifespan

As noted previously, these issues are also important considerations for clients.

Therapists often encounter challenging situations that require products or designs with specific features and functions. Those with limited experience can benefit greatly from discussing options with their more experienced colleagues. Listservs, where people come together online to discuss issues, can be an effective medium for therapists seeking information and opinions from a wide range of experienced people. Useful information can also be gained from examining products and designs in public environments that receive extensive use. Products and designs commonly used in the building industry can also give an indication of their reliability and cost-effectiveness.

Existing Evidence of the Benefits of the Product or Design

Therapists draw on a range of evidence when designing interventions and evaluating the suitability of various products and designs. Evidence-based practice requires that the best available information or evidence is integrated with clinical experiences and expertise and with due consideration of the clients' priorities and preferences (Sackett, 2000; Turpin & Higgs, 2009). It is therefore important that therapists review the nature of evidence they are accessing—its dependability and generalizability—and consider this information carefully in light of their own experience and expertise and the priorities and preferences of their clients.

There are various types of evidence, including the following:

+ Anecdotal material (e.g., home modification listservs)
+ Expert opinion or theoretical or unsystematic literature reviews or standards
+ Case (i.e., case series and case comparative)
+ Observational (i.e., cohort studies, pre- and post-test studies, and cross-sectional and longitudinal studies)
+ Quasi experimental (i.e., no randomization)
+ Randomized controlled trial (RCT)
+ Systematic review (Bridge & Phibbs, 2003)

Each of these types of evidence provides a different type of information, which varies in terms of its applicability to specific situations, level of dependability, and ability to demonstrate the benefits of a particular intervention (Turpin & Higgs, 2009). Anecdotal information and expert opinion can be based on accumulated experience and often provides the detailed and practical information required when considering specific situations and local products and designs. Therapists should be aware, however, that these sources are prone to bias; the information is likely to be shaped by personal preferences and unique experiences. Similarly, case-based, observational, and quasi-experimental studies can provide detailed information about interventions, the contexts in which they have been applied, and the changes that resulted from these. It is important to note, however, that the observed changes might also be attributable to other variables that have not been controlled for. RCTs and systematic reviews provide dependable information about the outcomes of interventions because they are structured to control for confounding variables and to minimize potential bias. However, to date, these studies have tended to examine the impact of home modifications generally and in combination with a range of other interventions, and they have not examined specific home modification interventions and their relative impact in a variety of situations. Table 11-1 reviews the advantages and disadvantages of various types of evidence as described by Bridge and Phibbs (2003).

Although applied research comparing the effectiveness of various environmental interventions for particular populations is limited, research on home modifications is increasing. Literature about many traditional occupational therapy interventions is located in the category of health; however, home modification and related literature can also be found in other fields of study, such as social sciences and architecture. The following databases can be useful for locating literature on home modifications and environmental design:

+ Health-related databases, such as Pubmed (www.pubmed.gov), OTseeker (www.otseeker.com), OTDbase (www.otdbase.org), or Cinahl (nursing and allied health)

+ Social-sciences databases, such as social services abstracts, sociological abstracts, Ageline (aging-related information in psychological, health-related, social, economics, public policy, and the health sciences)

+ Architectural databases, such as the Avery index to architectural periodicals, API (Architectural Publications Index)

These databases access literature on theoretical frameworks, literature reviews, and research published in refereed journals and can be searched using keywords or broad search terms. In areas of practice with vast quantities of research, it can be useful to confine searches using specific terms related to the particular problem, client group, intervention, and outcome (PICO). For example, if searching for research on grab bars to assist older people into and out of the bath, the search would be defined as follows:

+ *Problem*: Getting in and out of the bath

+ *Client group*: Older people

+ *Intervention*: Grab bar

+ *Outcome*: Increased safety and independence

Other terms would also need to be included in the search to ensure that all relevant literature was identified. For example, the bath might be referred to in some studies as a tub; older people are also referred to as elders; grab bars are called grab rails in some countries; and some studies might also identify outcomes as reduced falls or hospitalizations. It is useful to seek the assistance of a librarian when developing a list of search terms because they are aware of alternative terms and particular terms used in different databases, such as the MeSH (Medical Subject Headings). Some databases also provide advanced search strategies that allow the user to define the age range of the subjects and nature of the studies (e.g., RCTs).

Using specific PICO search terms assists in narrowing the search to the most relevant studies; however, targeted research is limited in many areas of occupational therapy practice. In home modification practice, it is advisable to use broad terms to ensure that all relevant literature is located.

Systematic reviews of research can be located in the Cochrane Collaboration (www.cochrane.org/reviews). Cochrane reviews examine the evidence for and against the appropriateness and effectiveness of a range of interventions in specific circumstances based on the best available information (www.cochrane.org/reviews/clibintro.htm). For example, recent reviews have examined the impact of home modifications on the reduction of injuries (Lyons et al., 2006) and interventions for preventing falls in older people (Gillespie et al., 2009).

The Home Modification Information Clearing House (www.homemods.info) is also a valuable resource, providing evidence-based reviews on a range of home modification-related interventions, such as coatings for tiled floors (Whitfield, Bridge, & Mathews, 2005), designing home environments for people who experience problems with cognition and who display aggressive or self-injurious behavior (Hodges, Bridge, Donelly, & Chaudhary, 2007), and selecting diameters for grab rails (Oram, Cameron, & Bridge, 2006).

There is also a wealth of information of relevance to home modification practice in legislative and regulatory documents and on the Internet—in particular, on Web sites dedicated to home design and modification, as well as in the grey literature such as nonrefereed publications posted on the Web, industry newsletters, and manufacturers' specifications (Bridge & Phibbs, 2003).

Table 11-1. Advantages and Disadvantages of Various Types of Evidence

TYPE OF EVIDENCE	ADVANTAGES	DISADVANTAGES
Anecdotal material	• May be based on hearsay • May not clearly indicate assumptions or method • May be faulty or inaccurate	• May assist in reconceptualization of problem area • May add to knowledge in terms of scoping variables or measurement methods
Expert opinion/theoretical/unsystematic literature review/standards	• May be based on hearsay • May not clearly indicate assumptions or method • May be faulty or inaccurate	• May assist in reconceptualization of problem area • May add to knowledge in terms of scoping variables or measurement methods
Case (i.e., case series and case comparative)	• No statistical validity • Hard to control for confounders as no controls • Subject to recall bias as retrospective. • Difficult to demonstrate causality	• May generate hypotheses • Less expensive than other research designs • Can have large sample sizes
Observational (i.e., cohort studies, pre- and posttest studies, cross-sectional and longitudinal studies)	• Can take a long time • Can be an expensive, large-scale undertaking • Useful when randomized studies are inappropriate • External factors can change over time with panel or longitudinal data	• Most reliable observational data are cohort studies because there is no recall bias and can ensure baseline similarities between groups • More reliable answers and less statistical problems than case control
Quasi-experimental (i.e., no randomization)	• Because variables not fully controlled may exhibit selection, performance, and measurement bias	• Remains experimenter controlled • Most reliable when variables of interest and controls for these made explicit
Randomized control trial (RCT)	• Assumes variables can be controlled and groups appropriately matched • Assumes randomized blind allocation of intervention is given ethical clearance by relevant human ethics review board • Very expensive in terms of time and money • May be compliance and participant attrition problems • Blinding and random allocation can be problematic	• Provides evidence with causality • Considered "gold standard" in health research • Random allocation balances known, unknown, and unmeasurable confounding variables • Greater confidence that conclusions are attributable solely to intervention manipulation • Reduces selection bias • Blinding reduces measurement and performance bias • Provides evidence of causality
Systematic review	• Cutoffs for inclusion may be too high or too low • Question under consideration may not be specified properly (i.e., it may be too broad or too specific) • Results capture a snapshot of published research at a particular time interval so results must be interpreted in relation to currency of information and change in the body of knowledge being reviewed	• Attempts to answer a particular research question in an evidence-based manner • Provides policymakers with a summary of available evidence • Effectively maps the inputs and outcomes under review

(Reprinted with permission from Bridge, C., & Phibbs, P. (2003). Protocol guidelines for systematic reviews of home modification information to inform best practice. Sydney, Australia: Home Modification Information Clearinghouse, University of Sydney. Retrieved from http://test.homemods.info/files/SysRevProtocolJune%202k3.pdf. Table 4: Study design definitions.)

It is important that therapists carefully evaluate information for its relevance, dependability, and generalizability and consider it in light of their own experience and expertise and the priorities and preferences of their clients before applying it in practice.

Conformity With Standards, Guidelines, and Codes

Legislative and regulatory documents are particularly important when selecting and designing environmental interventions and evaluating the suitability of various options. Many products and designs are governed by design and installation requirements detailed in various standards, guidelines, and codes. Therapists need to be aware of these documents and ensure that proposed products or designs meet the appropriate requirements of their region or country.

The three national standards that guide the accessible design of buildings in the United States include the following:

1. Americans with Disabilities Act and Architectural Barriers Act (ADA-ABA) Accessibility Guidelines for Buildings and Facilities—Commercial facilities and public accommodation

2. The Fair Housing Accessibility Guidelines— Multifamily housing

3. American National Standards Institute ANSI A117.1—Units and Apartments

Because the specifications in these standards relate specifically to the design of public buildings and multifamily dwellings and units, they do not apply directly to the design of single-family houses, except where particular elements are included in local building codes. Model building codes that serve as a basis for local codes might include accessibility requirements for specific building projects within their jurisdiction.

Elements of these standards can sometimes be used in the design of new homes or the modification of existing homes to promote access and mobility within the dwelling. Designers can depart from particular technical and scoping requirements in these guidelines when they can demonstrate that alternative designs and technologies can provide equivalent or greater access to, and usability of, the facility. In addition, variations to the specifications detailed in building standards are often required in residential settings when residents have particular requirements or when design is limited by existing topography of the land, building structures, service systems, and space restrictions.

There are several design elements specified in these standards, which include the following:

+ Dimensions (e.g., the height, width, depth of clearances and spaces, and size and location of various fixtures and fittings

+ Features of fixtures and fittings (e.g., level handles on doors and drawers or taps

+ Structural and technical requirements (e.g., sheer forces, maximum slope, maximum length of ramps, minimum height of edgings, minimum space between rail and wall

+ Materials and finishes (e.g., the nature of surfaces and edges)

Dimensions and the features of fixtures and fittings detailed in these accessibility standards allow adults with disabilities to function in buildings. In particular, the standards are designed to ensure adult wheelchair users can independently move into and through the structure and use various controls. These specifications provide a useful reference when designing modifications for individuals similar in stature, size, and functional ability to those for whom the standards were designed. However, many young clients with multiple and severe impairments and older clients with comorbidities and secondary conditions do not fit this profile and require dimensions and features to be tailored to their specific requirements (Sanford, 2001; Steinfeld & Shea, 1993).

Therapists are often well placed to assist in customizing designs to the specific requirements of an individual because they can determine the circulation space each person requires to move throughout the home and maneuver in various areas. They are also able to measure each individual and his or her equipment to determine the best location for various fixtures and fittings. Therapists' understanding of function and occupational performance allows them to define and identify design features that promote better performance. In addition, their observations of daily routines assist them in understanding how spaces and controls are used and when and where people are provided with assistance. Because the standards do not consider the requirements of people who rely on assistance (Sanford, 2001), dimensions detailed in these documents often need to be modified to accommodate the spatial requirements of caregivers during tasks and the equipment they might use in their routine with the client.

The structural and technical specifications in the standards ensure the safety of people using the building. Engineering evaluations have determined the structural strength requirements of fixtures and fittings, such as grab bars, tub and shower seats, fasteners, and mounting devices, under regular use by people within the average weight range.

It is inadvisable to select products or design modifications that do not meet these requirements without the advice of an engineer or suitably qualified consultant. Therapists should check that products have been certified as meeting these specifications and that contractors are aware of the requirements when installing these fixtures and fittings. Promotional materials produced by suppliers that make a general statement that their products meet accessibility standards are not sufficient proof. Therapists should seek supporting documentation and ensure that the product meets all of the specifications. For example, some products might meet the requirements in terms of dimensions but may not meet, or only partially meet, the structural strength requirements. In the ADA-ABA, specifications relating to the structural strength of shower seats state that "allowable stresses shall not be exceeded for materials used when a vertical or horizontal force of 250 lb (1112 N) is applied at any point on the seat, fastener, mounting device, or supporting structure" (ANSI, 2003, p. 61) For example, therapists would want to ensure that shower seats under consideration are able to substantiate their claims for meeting both the vertical and horizontal force requirements. Further, therapists working with people who are outside of the average weight range would need to select products that have been designed to withstand the additional forces to which they are likely to be subjected.

It is particularly important that any imported products meet the requirements of the country where they are to be installed. For example, many grab bars made in the United States designed to meet the ADA-ABA would withstand a lateral load of 250 lb (1112 N). However, these would not meet the requirements set out in Australia where the accessibility standards require grab bars to withstand 1100 N in all directions.

The gradient or slope and maximum height and length of ramps detailed in the design standards have been determined as being functionally appropriate for most adults with disabilities (Sanford, Story, & Jones, 1997). It is therefore advisable to design ramps to these requirements unless it is determined that the client or the attendant is unable to manage a ramp with these specifications. In these situations, therapists can recommend that the ramp be designed to specifications greater than the minimum required by the standards if this is practicable in the environment. In some situations, the ramp might need to be made steeper or the length shortened as a result of environmental constraints. In these situations, the therapist would need to demonstrate that the client has the capacity to traverse a steeper or shorter ramp and provide justification for deviating from the standard. Support for varying from the standard might include a description of the existing environmental limitations, a statement of intended usage and potential users, a report on the user's performance when trialing a ramp of the proposed gradient, or research evidence on the effect of ramp slope on performance, such as that undertaken by Sanford et al. Though it is reasonable to tailor an environmental intervention to the specific needs of the current resident, therapists should also be mindful of the person's long-term capacities, visitors to the property, and future residents when designing permanent modifications.

Design elements, such as the presence and height of edging to ramps, the space between grab bars or handrails and the adjacent wall, also improve people's safety and promote effective use of the built environment. It is important that these elements or suitable alternatives are reflected in product choices and are incorporated into the design of modifications. Materials and finishes might also have safety and/or functional implications; for example, insulating exposed pipes or removing sharp and abrasive surfaces under sinks ensures that wheelchair users' knees and thighs are not injured when they wheel under sinks. Grab bars that rotate in their fittings can also be hazardous to users. The recommended level of slip resistance for walkways and ramps is also an important consideration when designing modifications for the home environment to ensure the safety of householders walking or wheeling on the surface.

By understanding the specifications in the accessibility standards and their intent, therapists can ensure that elements relating to safety are incorporated into the design of modifications.

However, where a client's age, stature, size, and functional abilities and equipment type and dimensions lie outside of those covered by the standards, the dimensions and functional elements of the product and design should be reviewed in light of the functional requirements of each individual. Therapists also need to be mindful that there are a number of standards governing the design of domestic dwellings that need to be adhered to when redesigning areas of the home, and they will need to liaise closely with designers and building professionals to ensure that designs and products conform to these. In some instances, these standards might impede the design of accessible features, resulting in therapists having to work closely with building and design professionals to negotiate a mutually acceptable outcome. Further information on these is provided in Chapter 12.

Good Design Practice and Inclusive Design

Traditionally, therapists have focused on achieving independence using alternative strategies and devices designed within a medical context. Many of these are made of metal and plastic with cold, hard surfaces and have a clinical appearance. Similarly, early home modifications tended to have an institutional appearance (Sanford & Butterfield, 2005). Such devices and modifications often do not fit well with the ambience of a home environment where soft surfaces and warm colors often predominate. Further, when the appearance of devices and modifications provoke strong negative reactions from the user and visitors to the home, it can influence acceptance and use (Hocking, 1999; Wessels, Dijcks, Soede, Gelderblom, & De Witte, 2003; Wielandt & Strong, 2000).

With the emergence of universal design (UD), there has been an increased emphasis on designing products and environments for the broader community rather than being designed specifically for people with special requirements. UD recognizes the diversity of capabilities of users (Wylde, 1995) and aims to make products and environments inclusive, spanning age, gender, and ability (Center for Universal Design, 1997). Universally designed products and environments have been described by Wylde as being:

+ *Usable and useful*: Can be used successfully to perform the intended function simply and expediently

+ *Neutral*: Do not demand right- or left-handed performance

+ *Inclusive*: Built to include a diverse population of users—that is, of differing sizes and abilities

+ *Visible*: Provide clear, visible clues as to how they are to be used

+ *Elegant*: Are aesthetically pleasing

+ *Redundant*: Provide additional cues to the user—for example, acoustic, tactile, and visual information

+ *Simple*: Avoid superfluous controls, ornamentation, and embellishments

+ *Accessible, adaptable, and adjustable*: Accessible to individuals of varying abilities and designed to be adjusted or adapted for those whose abilities fall beyond the ranges of practical design considerations

+ *Logical*: Built purposefully with each component and feature, and placement and function consistent with expectations

In light of these principles, Wylde (1995) developed the *Enabling Products Sourcebook 2*, which provides criteria for a "head-to-toe" evaluation of products, including the following:

+ The head—Cognition, vision, audition, and olfaction

+ The upper body—Manual dexterity

+ Strength and stamina of the lower body

+ Overall safety features

+ Product features related to cleaning and maintenance

While not every criterion will be relevant to every product, the criteria assist in evaluating the range of users who will be able to use product effectively (Wylde, 1995). For example, when reviewing the visual demands of a product, Wylde examines whether:

+ Functions with a visual output are accompanied by audible and/or tactile output

+ The surface of the product has a non-glare finish in areas where vision is required

+ All graphics, signage, and coding are legible under adverse viewing conditions

+ The print and symbols provide color contrasting with the background

+ Use of colors as indicators is purposeful and visible

+ Indicator lights relate directly to the function they control

+ An integral light source is provided where vision is required for safe operation

+ Raised lettering is used where possible

+ Where audible and tactile cues are not feasible, the product accommodates Braille overlays on functions requiring vision

By designing modifications universally, therapists can ensure that the products and design are usable by everyone who lives in or visits the home. Further, attention to the design ensures that modifications continue to be useful as the needs of clients and other householders change over time. Universally designed products and environments have also been found to be considered more functional, accessible, safe, and attractive by users and less visible than specialized options (Park, 2006).

The seven principles of universal design proposed by the Center of Universal Design (1997) were developed to promote products and environments designed to be usable by all people, to the greatest extent possible, without the need for adaptation or specialized design.

Universal Design Performance Measures for Products

VERSION 1.0

		Not Applicable	Strongly Disagree	Disagree	Neutral	Agree	Strongly Agree	Comments
PRINCIPLE ONE	**EQUITABLE USE**							
1A.	All potential users could use this product in essentially the same way, regardless of differences in their abilities.							
1B.	Potential users could use this product without feeling segregated or stigmatized because of differences in personal capabilities.							
1C.	Potential users of this product have access to all features of privacy, security, and safety regardless of personal capabilities.							
1D.	This product appeals to all potential users.							
PRINCIPLE TWO	**FLEXIBILITY IN USE**							
2A.	Every potential user can find at least one way to use this product effectively.							
2B.	This product can be used with either the right or left hand alone.							
2C.	This product facilitates (or does not require) user accuracy and precision.							
2D.	This product can be used at whatever pace (quickly or slowly) the user prefers.							

Figure 11-1. Universal Design Performance Measures for products. (Reprinted with permission from Center for Universal Design. (2000). *Evaluating the universal design performance of products*. Raleigh, NC, The Center for Universal Design, North Carolina State University. Retrieved from www.design.ncsu.edu/cud/pubs_p/docs/UDPP.pdf.)

The principles encourage designers to develop products and environments that allow the following:

+ *Equitable use*: Useful and marketable to people with diverse abilities

+ *Flexibility in use*: Accommodates a wide range of individual preferences and abilities

+ *Simple and intuitive use*: Easy to understand, regardless of the user's experience, knowledge, language skills, or current concentration level

+ *Perceptible information*: Communicates necessary information effectively to the user, regardless of ambient conditions or the user's sensory abilities

+ *Tolerance for error*: Minimizes hazards and the adverse consequences of accidental or unintended actions

+ *Low physical effort*: Can be used efficiently and comfortably and with a minimum of fatigue

+ *Size and space for approach and use*: Appropriate size and space for approach, reach, manipulation, and use regardless of user's body size, posture, or mobility (Center for Universal Design, 1997)

Therapists can use these principles to evaluate products and designs under consideration for home modifications. The Center for Universal Design (2000) has developed the Universal Design Performance Measure (Figure 11-1), which designers and therapists can use to evaluate the design characteristics of options and compare the universality of various products and designs. The measure is not intended to replace user evaluation or experience with a product or design but offers assistance to therapists and designers in evaluating the border usability of interventions.

Although these principles appear to be simple, in reality, people vary enormously in terms of height, weight, endurance, strength, balance, mobility, and visual and hearing acuity (Conway, 2008). When considering the suitability of design, therapists need to draw on their understanding of this diversity and aim to maximize the usability of the product and environment for as many people as possible while ensuring that they continue to support clients' occupational performance. The knowledge of diversity that occupational therapists possess can be invaluable in reviewing the potential of product and design solutions. Furthermore, this expertise allows therapists to make a significant contribution to the development of products and designs.

CONCLUSION

There is a range of resources available to assist therapists in locating and sourcing products and designs. Each of these contributes different information and allows therapists to develop a portfolio of products and designs suited to the needs of an individual in a range of situations. Initially, therapists need to establish a broad understanding of the diverse range of options available. They can then build on this solid foundation to undertake a targeted search of resources to identify products and designs suited to the specific needs of each client. It is often difficult for therapists who are new to the field or undertake modifications only as a small part of their work to establish and maintain the expertise required to do modifications well. In these situations, therapists need to consult with colleagues with greater expertise to ensure the best outcomes for their clients.

To determine the best solution for each case, therapists review and evaluate options by comparing the features and specification of each, with due consideration to client priorities and preferences. Therapists also draw on available evidence and use professional reasoning to collect and interpret different types of information to determine the best option for each situation, assessing the quality and relevance of information and applying it judiciously. Therapists also need to be conscious of the standards when selecting and evaluating products and designs while remaining mindful of the specific needs of each client and his or her situation. Finally, therapists need to ensure that products and designs incorporated into modifications are aesthetic and recognize the diverse and changing abilities of all residents of the household while reflecting the expectations of society in terms of what a home should look and feel like.

REFERENCES

American National Standards Institute. (2003). *ICC/ANSI A117.1-2003: Accessible and Usable Buildings and Facilities*. New York, NY: Author.

Americans with Disabilities Act and Architectural Barriers Act Accessibility Guidelines. (2004). Retrieved from http://www.access-board.gov/ada-aba/final.cfm

Andrich, R. (2002). The SCAI instrument: Measuring costs of individual assistive technology programmes. *Technology and Disability, 14*, 95-99.

Auriemma, D., Faust, S., Sibrian, K., & Jimenez, J. (1999). Home modifications for the elderly: Implications for the occupational therapist. *Physical and Occupational Therapy in Geriatrics, 16*(2-4), 135-144.

Bernt, N., & Skar, L. (2006). A pilot study of the activity patterns of five elderly persons after a housing adaptation. *Occupational Therapy International, 13*(1), 21-34.

Bridge, C., & Phibbs, P. (2003). *Protocol guidelines for systematic reviews of home modification information to inform best practice*. Sydney, Australia: Home Modification Information Clearinghouse, University of Sydney. Retrieved from http://test.homemods.info/files/SysRevProtocolJune%202k3.pdf

Center for Universal Design. (1997). *The principles of universal design Version 2.0*. Raleigh, NC: Author. Retrieved from http://www.design.ncsu.edu/cud/about_ud/udprinciplesht-mlformat.html#top

Center for Universal Design. (2000). *Evaluating the universal design performance of products*. Raleigh, NC: Author. Retrieved from http://www.design.ncsu.edu/cud/pubs_p/docs/UDPP.pdf

Conway, M. (2008). *Occupational therapy and inclusive design: Principles for practice*. Oxford, UK: Blackwell Publishing Incorporated.

Department for Communities and Local Government. (2006). *Delivering housing adaptations for disabled people: A good practice guide*. London, UK: Author.

Duncan, R. (1998). Blueprint for action: The National Home Modifications Action Coalition. *Technology and Disability, 8*(1-2), 85-89.

Gillespie, L. D., Robertson, M. C., Gillespie, W. J., Lamb, S. E., Gates, S., Cumming, R. G., & Rowe, B. H. (2009). Interventions for preventing falls in older people living in the community. *Cochrane Database of Systematic Reviews,* Issue 2, Art. No.: CD007146. DOI: 10.1002/14651858.CD007146.pub2

Hawkins, R., & Stewart, S. (2002). Changing rooms: The impact of adaptations on the meaning of home for a disabled person and the role of occupational therapists in the process. *British Journal of Occupational Therapy, 65*(2), 81-87.

Heywood, F. (2004). The health outcomes of housing adaptations. *Disability and Society, 19*(2), 129-143.

Hocking, C. (1999). Function or feelings: Factors in abandonment of assistive devices. *Technology and Disability, 11*, 3-11.

Hodges, L., Bridge, C., Donelly, M., & Chaudhary, K. (2007). *Evidence based research bulletin: Designing home environments for people who experience problems with cognition who display aggressive or self-injurious behaviours*. Sydney, Australia: Home Modification Information Clearinghouse, University of Sydney.

Lund, M. L., & Nygard, L. (2004). Occupational life in the home environment: The experiences of people with disabilities. *Canadian Journal of Occupational Therapy, 71*(4), 243-251.

Lyons, R. A., John, A., Brophy, S., Jones, S. J., Johansen, A., Kemp, A., ... Weightman, A. (2006). Modification of the home environment for the reduction of injuries. *Cochrane Database of Systematic Reviews, 18*(4), CD003600. doi: 10.1002/14651858.CD003600.pub2

Oram, L., Cameron, J., & Bridge, C. (2006). *Evidence based research: Selecting diameters for grabrails.* Sydney, Australia: Home Modification Information Clearinghouse, University of Sydney, Australia. Retrieved from http://www.homemods.info/resource/bibliography/selecting_diameters_for_grabrails_evidence_based_research

Park, D. (2006). Universal design in aging in place senior housing: A pilot study of residents' perspectives. In W. C. Mann & A. A. Helal (Eds.), *Promoting independence for older persons with disabilities* (pp. 193-203). Fairfax, VA: IOS Press.

Rousseau, J., Potvin, L., Dutil, E., & Falta, P. (2001). A critical review of assessment tools related to home adaptation issues. *Occupational Therapy in Health Care, 14*(3-4), 93-104.

Sackett, D. L. (2000). *Evidence based medicine: How to practice and teach EBM.* Edinburgh, UK: Churchill-Livingstone.

Sanford, J. (2001). *Best practices in the design of toileting and bathing facilities for assisted transfer* (Research report). Washington, DC: United States Access Board. Retrieved from http://www.access-board.gov/research/toilet-bath/report.htm

Sanford, J. A., & Butterfield, T. (2005). Using remote assessment to provide home modification services to underserved elders. *The Gerontologist, 45*(3), 389-398.

Sanford, J. A., Story, M. F., & Jones, M. L. (1997). An analysis of the effects of ramp slope on people with mobility impairments. *Assistive Technology, 9*(1), 22-33.

Sapey, B. (1995). Disabling homes: A study of the housing needs of disabled people in Cornwall. *Disability and Society, 10*(1), 71-85.

Steinfeld, E., & Danford, G. S. (1999). Theory as a basis for research on enabling environments. In E. Steinfeld & G. S. Danford (Eds.), *Enabling environments: Measuring the impact of environment on disability and rehabilitation* (pp. 11-33). New York, NY: Kluwer Academic/Plenum Publishers.

Steinfeld, E., & Shea, S. (1993). Enabling home environments: Identifying barriers to independence. *Technology and Disability, 2*(4), 69-79.

Turpin, M., & Higgs, J. (2009). Clinical reasoning and evidence-based practice. In T. Hoffman, S. Bennett, & C. Del Mar (Eds.), *Evidence-based practice across the health professions* (pp. 300-317). Melbourne, Australia: Elsevier.

Wessels, R., Dijcks, B., Soede, M., Gelderblom, G. J., & De Witte, L. (2003). Non-use of provided assistive technology devices: A literature overview. *Technology and Disability, 15*, 231-238.

Whitfield, K., Bridge C., & Mathews, S. (2005). *Coatings: Evidence based research: Selecting coatings for tiled floors.* Sydney, Australia: Home Modification and Maintenance Information Clearinghouse, University of Sydney. Retrieved from http://www.homemods.info/resource/evidence/coatings_evidence_based_research_selecting_coatings_for_tiled_floors

Wielandt, T., & Strong, J. (2000). Compliance with prescribed adaptive equipment: A literature review. *British Journal of Occupational Therapy, 63*(2), 65-75.

Wylde, M. (1995). *Enabling products sourcebook 2.* Hackettstown, NJ: National Kitchen and Bath Association and Promatura. Retrieved from http://www.homemods.org/resources/pages/enabling.shtml

12

Access Standards and Their Role in Guiding Interventions

Elizabeth Ainsworth, MOccThy, Grad Cert Health Sci;
Desleigh de Jonge, MPhil (OccThy), Grad Cert Soc Sci;
and Bronwyn Tanner, BOccThy, Grad Cert OccThy,
Grad Cert Soc Planning, MPhil

There is much confusion and debate about the relevance and application of access standards to home modification practice. Although access standards were created in response to public access requirements in the community, occupational therapists in home modification practice often use them as a reference, particularly with regard to major modifications. The primary focus of occupational therapy home modification practice is a thorough understanding of the needs of the individual and the unique fit between the individual and his or her home environment. However, sound practice also requires an understanding of the relevance and the appropriateness of the application of access standards when recommending modifications to the home environment. This chapter seeks to inform occupational therapists about access standards—how they are developed, their benefits and limitations, and their use in the design of public buildings—as well as their applications to home modification practice. Therapists will find this information useful with working with other stakeholders involved in the home modifications process as there can be confusion about the application of access standards to modification of domestic homes.

CHAPTER OBJECTIVES

By the end of this chapter, the reader will be able to:

+ Describe access standards, their development, and how and when they are relevant reference guides to home modification practice

+ Describe the benefits and limitations associated with the application of access standards in home modification practice

INTRODUCTION

The following discussion includes general information on standards, their development, their general benefits for society, and the specific benefits for people with disabilities.

Standards are described as documents that define best practice. Information provided by standards include dimensions, ratings, terminology, symbols, test methods, and performance and safety requirements for personnel, products, systems, and services in a wide range of industries (American National Service Institute [ANSI], 2009).

Ainsworth, E., & de Jonge, D.
An Occupational Therapists's Guide to Home Modification Practice (pp. 229-238)
© 2011 SLACK Incorporated

Specifications and procedures are detailed in standards with the objective of ensuring that a material, product, method, or service is fit for its purpose and consistently performs in the way that it was intended (ANSI). These documents are generally established by consensus and are approved by a recognized body, such as ANSI, the BSI British Standards (BSI), or Standards Australia (SAA). They provide a common language to describe quality and safety criteria (SAA, 2007) and define terms to ensure that there is no misunderstanding among those using the standard (ANSI).

Standards can be voluntary or mandatory. While voluntary standards, by themselves, impose no obligations regarding use, mandatory standards are generally published as part of a code, rule, or regulation by a regulatory government body and impose an obligation on specific parties to conform to them (Breitenberg, 1987). Specifications detailed in the standards are described as being either prescriptive or performance based. Prescriptive standards detail or prescribe specifically what is required—for example, the location of the center line of the toilet from the side wall (International Code Council [ICC] & ANSI, 2003). Performance-based standards identify a function or an operation that needs to be met—for example, the grab bar to be installed has to be able to take 1112 N of force (ICC & ANSI, 2003).

There are a range of standards that govern the safety, amenity, and integrity of public and residential built environments as well as the consistency and quality of products.

Standards relating to the built environment are specific technical guidelines that encompass the entire process of construction and assembly of buildings; structural, plumbing, electrical, and mechanical systems; and fire protection and energy conservation and consumption within and around commercial and residential buildings (Lawlor & Thomas, 2008). Standards related to public buildings detail the design requirements to address wind resistance; structural load; fire safety and egress; and electrical, plumbing, and mechanical systems. Depending on the jurisdiction and type of construction, standards may also address safety, accessibility, and indoor quality (Lawlor & Thomas).

Residential buildings are governed by similar standards relating to the structure and safety of the building, but these are tailored to the specific building type, geographic location, and use of various areas within the building. For example, there are a range of standards that govern the design and construction of domestic dwellings, including standards having to do with electrical and wiring installation, slip resistance in wet areas, and waterproofing requirements. Various standards also guide the design of fixtures and fittings and materials used within the home. Many of these standards are mandatory, especially when they are incorporated into building legislation. Consequently, there are a number of standards that can influence the outcome of the home modification process. For example, compliance with plumbing and electrical standards is a requirement when undertaking modification work in a bathroom area. Further, products and equipment such as mobile over-toilet shower chairs, scooters, wheelchairs, and stair and platform lifts are generally required to meet specific standards. Therapists therefore need to be aware of the range of standards that exist and their influence on design, construction products, and equipment.

DEVELOPMENT OF STANDARDS

Nearly all countries have standards, which are developed by specific standards organizations consisting of expert committees set up and supported by government (Bridge & Kendig, 2005). These organizations seek to serve the interests of a range of industry sectors, as well as government, individuals in the community, employees, and society in general. They aim to ensure the various standards are useful, relevant, and authoritative in their country (BSI, 2007).

There are various benefits of having standards to guide practice. They can:

+ Provide protection for businesses and consumers to ensure that goods and services are safe, reliable, and will do the intended job

+ Provide a yardstick for the measurement of public health, safety, and environmental policies

+ Provide a platform on which to build new and innovative ideas relating to the latest technologies and industry practices

+ Boost production and productivity to save businesses time and money and to foster new technologies

+ Enhance the competitive nature of businesses nationally and internationally

+ Provide linkages with international markets and enhance international competition through the manufacturing of products to suit other countries

+ Complement regulation and enhance consistency across the marketplace (SAA, 2007)

Various countries have bodies that develop standards, which include the following:

+ United States—ANSI

+ Australia—SAA

+ Canada—Standards Council of Canada (SCC)

+ Finland—Finnish Standards Association (SFS)

+ France—Association Française de Normalization (AFNOR)

+ Germany—Deutsches Institut fur Normung (DIN)

+ Italy—Ente Nazionale Italiano di Unificazione (UNI)

+ Japan—Japanese Industrial Standards Committee (JISC)

+ Malaysia—Standards and Industrial Research of Malaysia (SIRIM)

+ Netherlands—Nederlands Normalisatie-instituut (NEN)

+ Norway—Norwegian Standards Association

+ Philippines—Bureau of Product Standards

+ United Kingdom—BSI

These organizations can be a useful resource for therapists. Further information on these organizations can be found in Appendix E.

Expert committees that operate on national, continental, or international levels develop standards in response to a defined market need (BSI, 2007). Some standards committees use a consortium model, where consultation involves steering groups, review panels, and standing committees to fast-track the development of standards, while others use a model of consensus whereby national committees form to develop documents (BSI). Most standards committees rely on expertise from a wide range of sources, including researchers, experts from design disciplines, code officials, and other interested parties, such as consumer groups. Standards are researched, developed, and revised by committees made up of people from government, business and industry, community, and academia (SAA, 2007). For example, committee members involved in the development of standards related to access and mobility within public buildings include representatives from the design and construction industry, the disability sector, and health professionals. To provide their professional perspective, occupational therapists sit on committees related to the design of buildings, products, and fixtures and fittings for people with disabilities. Standards are under continuous review, being updated regularly to take account of changing technology, industry practices, and community

expectations (Bridge & Kendig, 2005). Amendments may be issued between editions (SAA, 2001), and they may also be withdrawn from circulation as required (BSI).

There are specific processes associated with the development and ongoing revision of standards. Formal British (BS), European (EN), and international standards (ISO/IEC) are developed according to strict rules to ensure they are transparent and fair. This involves a technical committee proceeding through the following stages:

+ Proposal for new work

+ Project acceptance

+ Drafting

+ Public comment period

+ Approval

+ Publication (BSI, 2007)

Such stages are similar in other countries, such as the United States and Australia. The central body responsible for the identification of a single consistent set of voluntary standards in the United States is ANSI, a not-for-profit organization. ANSI accredits organizations that develop standards, publishes procedures for standards development, and approves standards according to its procedures (Steinfeld & Levine, 1998). ANSI specifically indicates that it has a positive role in enhancing the global competitiveness of U.S. business and U.S. quality of life by promoting and facilitating voluntary consensus standards and conformity assessment systems and safeguarding their integrity (ANSI, 2009).

In the United States, standards can develop in three ways: through an accredited committee, an accredited organization, or a community group (Steinfeld & Levine, 1998). Discussions at the committee level are documented, which assists in tracing the rationale and decision-making process in relation to particular items proposed for inclusion in the standards. The various organizations that develop standards have the main role of preparing these documents and reviewing them on a regular basis to keep up to date with industry requirements. It is estimated that there are more than 200 accredited ANSI bodies that develop consensus standards in different sectors (ANSI, 2005).

LANGUAGE OF STANDARDS

A list of terminology is usually provided in the introduction to a standard. This acts as a reference for various people using the documentation to guide design practice. A review of this list will ensure clear understanding of the industry wording and language and design requirements because there are differences between standards in various countries in terms of terminology and measurement conventions (imperial/metric; Steinfeld, Maisel, & Feathers, 2005). For example, the U.S. standard ICC/ANSI A117.1 (2003) describes a ramp as "a walking surface that has a running slope steeper than 1:20." In the comparative Australian standard AS 1428.1 (SAA, 2001), a ramp is described as "an inclined access way with a gradient steeper than 1 in 20 but not steeper than 1:14."

In access standards, there are words used to describe various design features that might not be explained in the terminology guide. For example, it would be assumed that people reading the access standards would be familiar with standard building terms like *switch back* or *dog leg* stairs. To ensure there is clear understanding of the meaning of the terms used in the access standards, it is useful to refer to a glossary of building terms (ICC & ANSI, 2003).

Some words have a very specific meaning when used in the standards. For example, the U.S. standards use terms such as *shall* when referring to an essential or mandatory requirement. With respect to water temperature, for example, bathtubs shall deliver water that is 120°F (49°C) maximum (ICC& ANSI, 2003, Section 607.8). Other standards use additional terminology such as *should*, which refers to a desirable requirement, and *may*, which indicates an option to guide the reader. It is important for occupational therapists to check the definitions of the various terms used in the standards to ensure that they understand how they are being used to direct designers and others using these documents.

ACCESS STANDARDS FOR PUBLIC BUILDINGS

The creation and use of access standards grew out of the recognition that the design and construction of much of the built environment is inaccessible to a significant sector of the population and that people with disabilities are "entitled to have their special needs taken into consideration at all stages of economic and social planning" (United Nations [UN], 1975). Access standards for public buildings or federally funded buildings have therefore been created to improve access for people with disabilities in the general community and to provide the greatest access for the greatest number of people.

In countries where access standards exist, such as the United States, public buildings such as libraries, hospitals, office spaces, meeting halls, schools, and retail areas are designed to provide external and internal wheelchair access. Design features include accessible paths of travel within and outside of a building, ramp designs, car parking, bathroom design, circulation space for access to and through doorways and within rooms, grab bar and handrail installation, electrical switch location, the location of blocking or reinforcement behind walls for supporting grab bars, and other features. These standards might also provide information on spatial requirements and reach ranges relating to the person in a wheelchair or ambulant people with mobility impairment who sit and stand during activities (Steinfeld et al., 2005). In the United States, access standards have emerged that govern accessible design, such as ICC & ANSI A117.1 (2003).

ACCESS STANDARDS FOR RESIDENTIAL PREMISES

Until recently, developing and implementing access standards in most countries had little to do with residential building design and construction. The increasing proportion of older people and people with disabilities within populations across the world has heightened awareness of the need for housing construction that is accessible. In general, however, the creation of design standards for newly constructed domestic premises has not been well supported by governments. This is in part due to the perception that monitoring compliance with these standards would be problematic. As well, the perspective that private homeowners have a right to choose how they wish to spend their own money and design their own homes has contributed to a lack of legislative action regarding the construction of accessible residential housing (Imrie, 2006a).

However, a number of countries have developed standards or design guidelines for accessible and adaptable residential premises that people can refer to. These include the Fair Housing Accessibility Guidelines (United States), the Adaptable Housing Standard (Australia), and Lifetime Homes Standards (United Kingdom). The United States is one of the few countries to have a requirement for residential design in the Fair Housing Amendment Act (1988); however, this does not require full accessibility and is only mandatory in select building types. The United Kingdom is aiming to incorporate the Lifetime Home Standards in the design of new residential buildings in the near future. The U.K. "Lifetime Homes, Lifetime Neighbourhoods Strategy" includes the

Lifetime Homes Standard in its Code for Sustainable Homes and sets out a plan for all new public and private housing to be built to the Standard by 2013 (Victorian Council of Social Services, 2008).

BENEFITS OF ACCESS STANDARDS

Access standards describe the performance criteria for access and mobility and establish design expectations for the building industry (Harrison, 2004). They contain agreed-upon solutions that have already been time tested and proven (Breitenberg, 2009). Standards provide detailed diagrams and minimum performance criteria that can be used by designers and builders, thus saving money, time, and effort in design and construction and reducing costly errors and poor design and construction outcomes (Harrison; Imrie, 2006a). By providing clear and precise specifications, access standards reduce uncertainty in expectation about accessible design and make it easier and less costly for developers to create accessible environments (Harrison).

A product or design's conformance with accepted standards allows the manufacturer or designer to efficiently convey complex information on the product or design (Breitenberg, 1987). It also affords consumers with certainty about the product and its performance, quality, safety, and suitability.

Standards provide a number of benefits, namely:

+ A description of the minimum requirements for equipment, appliances, products, finishes, and designs

+ Criteria relating to the level of quality, safety, reliability, and functionality of equipment, appliances, products, finishes, and designs to ensure the health and safety of people using them

+ Detail on the technical aspects of equipment, appliances, products, finishes, and designs

+ A degree of legal certainty regarding quality for all parties, especially if they are referred to in legislation

Access standards are publicly available and are a practical tool to facilitate access and mobility in the built environment. Access standards, particularly those referred to in legislation, are regularly reviewed in response to research, the introduction of new equipment onto the market, and the change in design approaches over time.

Standards also stimulate the innovation of products, services, and systems, just as innovation stimulates standardization (Breitenberg, 2009). They foster innovation by establishing a baseline for design and performance that will satisfy user requirements. The performance criteria and minimum standards outlined in the standards allow suppliers or manufacturers some creativity and flexibility to vary features, function, or price, which means they can establish their own niche in the marketplace (Breitenberg). Standards are the baseline for improvements and can help elevate the expectation of users, who then demand improvements to current practice (Breitenberg).

LIMITATIONS OF ACCESS STANDARDS

The specifications in access standards from a range of countries have largely been based on limited research that, in some instances, dates back to the 1960s. For example, the anthropometric research on wheeled mobility users that underlies the technical requirements of the ICC & ANSI A 117.1 (2003) *Accessible and Usable Buildings and Facilities and the Americans With Disabilities Act Accessibility Guidelines* were generated from research completed between 1974 and 1978 on a sample of 60 individuals who used wheelchairs (Steinfeld et al., 2005). Research informing many of the prescribed standards (of physical dimension and performance) has been criticized as being poorly designed and using small sample sizes that are not representative of the population of older people and people with disabilities in terms of age range, type of disability, stature, and other factors that impact on design (Harrison, 2004; Imrie & Hall, 2001; Imrie & Kumar, 1998; Steinfeld et al.). Various access standards around the world have been developed on anthropometric data of populations of people where their bodies have been reduced to a universal type or standard, characterized by fixed body parts (Imrie & Hall).

The standards have been developed using a generalized view of the needs of the population of people with disabilities rather than a view that acknowledges the true diversity of the population (Imrie, 2006a; Imrie & Kumar, 1998). Concerns have also been raised about the profile of the people used as a basis to create the dimensions and performance criteria of the access standards. It has been argued that access standards have been based on the capabilities of young people who mobilize independently in standard manual or electric wheelchairs and thus do not reflect the requirements of children, many young people with multiple and severe impairments, or older people with co-morbidities and secondary conditions (Czaja, 1984; Faletti, 1984; Sanford, 2001; Sanford, Echt, & Malassigné, 1999; Steinfeld & Shea, 1993). In addition, standards do not consider the requirements of people who rely on caregiver assistance (Sanford).

Though some information in standards might have been considered accurate at a particular moment in time, there has been little attention to advances in wheeled mobility technology that influences the accuracy of the current standards (Steinfeld et al., 2005). New wheelchair technology for manual and electric wheelchairs is resulting in different performance characteristics and new environmental design requirements (Steinfeld, Lenker, & Paquet, 2002). Further, different styles of mobility devices are affecting the design requirements for environments—for example, motorized scooters and floor-based and ceiling track hoists—which have not been included in the design of the access standards.

Research methods also have not been clearly documented, leading to questions about the reliability and validity of studies (Steinfeld et al., 2005). Furthermore, studies across various countries have not always used the same terms, definitions, standards, or variables in the respective countries (Steinfeld et al., 2005). This limits the likelihood of combining findings from around the world into a single database for generalization (Steinfeld et al., 2002). An international approach to access design would be advantageous in assisting people as they travel and interact in different communities around the world (Steinfeld et al., 2005). This would require the development of an international consensus on standards and research methods and the use of terminology, definitions, and measurements to prevent divergent approaches during the review of standards, as well as consideration of cultural differences in economic development and expectations of independence between various countries (Steinfeld et al., 2005).

Finally, access standards can constrain design (Imrie, 2006b). Minimum access standards tend to be about "building down to something" rather than maximum standards, which are about "building to the highest quality" (Imrie & Kumar, 1998, p. 359). Imrie and Hall (2001) indicate that design professionals rarely exceed the legislative minimum in providing access and regard the provision of access as a significant cost. Adherence to access standards can therefore result in a design solution that is only minimally acceptable but viewed, incorrectly, as best practice and perhaps the only solution possible (Imrie, 2006a). Access standards that are conservative in their design tend to be rigid and incomplete (Steinfeld et al., 2002). Designers tend to over-rely on these documents to define access requirements, rather than creatively designing to optimize access and utility and incorporate flexibility and options within designs.

ACCESS STANDARDS AND HOME MODIFICATION PRACTICE

Though the design information contained in access standards can be useful to the design of home modifications, there are a number of issues related to the use of such standards in a residential setting. There has been continued debate in the literature over the use of access standards as the basis of home modification design (Danford & Steinfeld, 1999; Pynoos & Regnier, 1997; Pynoos, Sanford, & Rosenfelt, 2002; Steinfeld & Shea, 1993; Tanner, Tilse, & de Jonge, 2008). The debate centers on the relevance of standards developed for public access and intended to provide the greatest access for a range of people (that is, a faceless population) to the unique and individual home environment. Accessibility standards are typically designed to determine minimal legal guidelines and have very little to do with the needs, aspirations, desires, and uniqueness of a particular individual (Danford & Steinfeld). A danger in approaching home modifications from a public access agenda is that the meaning of home as a private, personalized space can be undermined and the individual's needs can become compromised. Using access standards in residential settings has also resulted in a physical or technical approach to building design (Imrie, 2006a). Within access standards, there is little emphasis on or information about domestic design and, where it does exist, there is little consideration about using flexible features, such as demountable walls, smart technologies, and design of multifunctional rooms with integrated elements, such as bathing or sleeping areas (Imrie, 2006b).

Because the building sector operates in an environment governed by regulations, codes, and standards, contractors are required to comply with a range of national, state, or local codes and standards in many aspects of their work. When any remodeling work is being undertaken, additional maintenance or repair work may be required to address noncompliance, such as old electrical wiring and replumbing old pipe work. This additional work can add substantially to the cost (Jones, de Jonge, & Phillips, 2008; Steinfeld, Levine, & Shea, 1998). In addition, building contractors often mistakenly apply public access standards to the remodeling of domestic premises, which can impact on the nature and overall cost of a solution (Steinfeld et al.) and the considerable expense of reverting the work when the house is sold (Balandin & Chapman, 2001). Further, inappropriate adherence to the standards, which were not created with the older person in mind, can result in inadequate solutions (Klein, Rosage, & Shaw, 1999).

The rigid and variable interpretation of standards can also result in a lack of both creativity and flexibility when negotiating a design solution that meets the needs of both the code and the householder (Pynoos, Liebig, Alley, & Nishita, 2004). When access standards are used in residential settings, features are inflexible and noticeable, and their appearance can be clinical, oversized, and inelegant (Lund & Nygard, 2004). Dimensional standards are said to be based on dated lifestyle assumptions and not on a sophisticated understanding of interactions between people and their home environments (Imrie, 2006b).

HOW THERAPISTS CAN USE ACCESS STANDARDS

In most countries, it is not a mandatory requirement for existing domestic premises to incorporate public access provisions for people with disabilities into domestic designs or modifications. However, in countries such as the United States, some local building regulations can require compliance to aspects of the access standard in the construction of new dwellings or major modification work on an existing dwelling.

In occupational therapy practice, the application of access standards to home modifications is best understood in terms of where in the home modification process they are referred. Access standards should not be the starting point of the home modification process nor should they drive the design of the modification. However, they can be a useful reference when exploring physical changes to the environment and striving for accessibility. Specifications detailed in public access standards, such as circulation spaces, door clearances, changes in level between floor surfaces, width of corridors and paths, vertical height clearance of features, and other criteria, could be of use when developing options for individuals with characteristics similar to those in the population on whom the standards have been based. For example, the specifications in the standards for a roll-in shower can assist in designing a bathroom for a young adult who mobilizes independently in a wheelchair. The standards are also a useful guide for ensuring the safety and long-term viability of home modifications. For example, if a person has a degenerative health condition and is likely to become a wheelchair user in the future, the standards can assist in anticipating the minimum design requirements when redesigning areas of the home.

Occupational therapists might use public access standards to do the following:

+ Audit the built environment to identify features that are inaccessible

+ Identify key landmarks for measuring and drawing the environment

+ Assess the suitability of the access specifications, including the performance criteria for individuals using simulated spaces, layout, and measurements to provide information to clients on accessible features and their specifications

+ Act as a reference to inform the redesign of structures, spaces, fixtures, and fittings to stimulate ideas and develop alternative solutions

+ Alert designers and contractors to the specific design and construction criteria required for design and modification work

+ Guide the development of specifications, drawings, and wording for home modification reports

The access standards provide detail on specific design features for accessibility, such as circulation spaces, door widths or clearances, and bench heights. The measurements in the standards can be used to identify changes required in the environment to accommodate a wheelchair user. The drawings in the standards illustrate the landmarks that identify the points between which the measurement should be taken. For example, door clearance is measured between the door stop (the door stop is the part the door hits against when it closes) and the face of the door on the hinge side. Therapists then compare these measures against the dimensions of the clients and their equipment and their ability to maneuver in a simulated environment. For example, as detailed in Chapter 8, recommended circulation spaces can be marked out on the floor using masking tape to test the client's ability to maneuver in the proposed area. Therapists refer to the specifications and drawings in the standard to explain to clients the characteristics of the proposed changes—for example, ramp slope and hand rail design. Alternative options, such as bathroom layouts, detailed in the standards, can be used to guide discussions and decision making about the best option, given the proposed use of the area and the existing space and structures in the built environment.

Therapists can direct contractors and designers to the specific design, construction, and installation criteria related to their recommendations. It is important that therapists ensure designers and contractors are aware of the defined scope and parameters of the standards; that is, that these have been developed to address the access and mobility requirements of adult wheelchair users in public buildings.

They should also confirm that designers and contractors understand that occupational therapy recommendations are based on a thorough assessment of the individual and the activities he or she undertakes within his or her particular home environment. Therapists can draw on the wording and diagrams used in the standards to document their recommendations. The use of industry language in the standards minimizes misunderstandings and ensures that the desired outcome is achieved.

The relevance of the specifications in the access standards to each situation depends greatly on the following:

+ Whether the person and his or her equipment fits the profile on which the standards have been based

+ The activities to be undertaken in the area

+ Characteristics of the existing built environment and the household

Before therapists consider using aspects of the access standards in developing home modification recommendations, it is important to determine whether the client fits the profile on which the standards are based, including his or her age, body dimensions, the nature of the disability, level of independence and mobility, and equipment type and size. The standards do not address the design requirements of older people, people outside the average range for weight and height, people with severe and multiple disabilities, or people who require caregiver assistance. In addition, equipment such as mobile over-toilet and over-shower chairs, common to many people requiring home modifications, is not a consideration in access standards because such devices normally would not be used in a public toilet. Homes may also accommodate floor-based or ceiling track hoists to enable people to move within or between rooms, whereas hoists are unlikely to be used in public facilities.

The standards provide detailed specifications for areas where functional tasks, such as toileting, are performed but provide limited guidance on the overall layout of the internal and external areas of the home or other domestic areas, such as the kitchen, bedroom, laundry, and car park, where many home-based activities are undertaken. Further, specific areas have been designed with only limited activities in mind. For example, in public buildings, the vanity has been designed for independent hand washing; however, in the home environment, people use the vanity for a range of activities, including shaving or brushing teeth.

Being primarily for new public buildings, the standards are not designed to apply to the design or modification of residential environments. Existing domestic premises have physical constraints; that is, they do not have the footprint or floor area to accommodate the public access standards design and layout requirements. For example, many bathrooms in existing older dwellings will have insufficient space to incorporate a fully accessible bathroom. Further, a range of people use areas of the home in a variety of ways, which is not a consideration of public access standards.

When tailoring modifications to the specific requirements of individuals, the activities they perform, and their home environment, therapists first determine the functional requirements of the individuals and then ensure that the designs and products recommended are safe and reliable. Occupational therapists use their expertise to tailor interventions to suit the individual—body dimensions, abilities, limitations, goals, preferences, and equipment used—to enable the person to undertake the task safely and independently, using his or her preferred method given the opportunities offered by the environment. Consequently, therapists might determine that the specifications in the standards do not adequately address the design requirement of the individual. For example, when recommending a grab bar to assist an older person in getting on and off a low toilet, the therapist would determine the best height, configuration, and location of grab bars for this particular situation. The relevance of public access standards to this modification is extremely limited because the height and position of grab bars in public toilet facilities is designed primarily to assist wheelchair users to transfer on and off a higher accessible toilet. Another example of the limited relevance of the public access standards is in recommending a ramp for someone using a powered wheelchair. The length and turning space requirements of the equipment might necessitate a greater landing dimension compared with the recommendations in the standard.

Once the functional elements have been determined, therapists then consider the safety and reliability of interventions. The standards contain specifications related to the safety and reliability of a number of design features that are based on technical expertise and population anthropometric studies. These can assist therapists in selecting safe and reliable products and designs and ensuring that these can be installed appropriately. For example, a number of specifications contained in the access standards relate to the safety characteristics of grab bars, such as the amount of vertical and horizontal force a grab bar, fastener mounting device, or supporting structure should support and the horizontal space between the wall and grab bar to allow for safe hand placement and movement. Therapists should comply with these specifications unless the client's requirements are outside of the scope of the standards. For example, people who have bariatric requirements will require grab bars that are installed to withstand greater forces. Therapists do not have the technical expertise to determine the vertical and horizontal force requirements in this situation and should seek appropriate advice. Further, therapists are advised to comply with the stipulated ramp gradient in the standards unless they can produce supporting evidence to justify a steeper ramp installation. This may be achieved through providing research evidence to support the recommendation for the particular client, producing specification details on gradient capabilities of the powered mobility device, or testing the client's ability to mobilize on a steeper gradient under various conditions. Technical advice or evidence should be documented in the client's report to support recommendations that vary from technical specifications in the standards.

CONCLUSION

This chapter has provided an introduction to the concept of standards generally and an overview of how standards are developed by expert committees in various countries and supported by governments. A review of access standards and their development and applicability to the home modification process has also been discussed. Access standards for public buildings can be a useful resource for occupational therapists when determining the design of a home modification in certain instances, particularly if the individual home dweller is of similar profile to the population on which the standards were originally based. Caution needs to be taken in the indiscriminate use of access standards to inform home modification design. Therapists need to ensure that the starting point of all home modification interventions is a good understanding of the needs, desires, and goals of the individual home dweller and that it is this, and not the access standards, that drives the home modification design process. While there are benefits associated with the use of standards as a reference or guide, therapists need to be mindful of their limitations. This will ensure that occupational therapy practice in this field is not constrained by a poor understanding of the intent and application of standards to home modification scenarios, which can result in poor designs and poor outcomes for people with specific needs.

REFERENCES

American National Standards Institute. (2003). *ICC/ANSI A117.1-2003: Accessible and Usable Buildings and Facilities*. New York, NY: Author.

American National Standards Institute. (2005). *The American National Standards Process*. Retrieved from http://publicaa.ansi.org/sites/apdl/Documents/Standards%20Activities/American%20National%20Standards/Procedures,%20Guides,%20and%20Forms/ANSexplanation.doc

American National Standards Institute. (2009). *Consumer affairs overview: How standardization helps consumers*. Retrieved from http://www.ansi.org/consumer_affairs/overview.aspx?menuid=5

Balandin, S., & Chapman, R. (2001). Aging with a developmental disability at home: An Australian perspective. In W. F. E. Preiser & E. Ostroff (Eds.), *Universal design handbook* (pp. 38.1-38.15). New York, NY: McGraw Hill Handbooks.

Breitenberg, M. A. (1987). *The ABC's of standards-related activities in the United States*. Retrieved from http://ts.nist.gov/Standards/Conformity/stdpmr.cfm

Breitenberg, M. A. (2009). *The ABCs of standards activities*. Gaithersburg, MD: National Institute of Standards and Technology. Retrieved from http://www.nist.gov/customcf/get_pdf.cfm?pub_id=903219

Bridge, K., & Kendig, H. (2005). Housing and older people: Environments, professionals and positive ageing. In V. Minichiello & I. Coulson (Eds.), *Contemporary issues in gerontology: Promoting positive aging* (pp. 144-166). New York, NY: Allen & Unwin.

BSI British Standards. (2007). *Introducing standards*. Retrieved from http://www.bsigroup.com/upload/Standards%20&%20Publications/Committee%20members/BSI_introducing_standards.pdf

Czaja, S. (1984). *Hand anthropometrics*. Technical paper prepared for the U.S. Architectural and Transportation Barriers Compliance Board, Washington, DC.

Danford, G. S., & Steinfeld, E. (1999). Measuring the influences of physical environments on the behaviors of people with impairments. In E. Steinfeld & G. S. Danford (Eds.), *Enabling environments: Measuring the impact of environment on disability and rehabilitation* (pp. 111-137). New York, NY: Plenum Publishers.

Fair Housing Amendments Act of 1988, 42 U.S.C. §§ 3601 et seq. (1988).

Faletti, M. V. (1984). Human factors research and functional environments for the aged. In I. Altman, M. P. Lawton, & J. F. Wohlwill (Eds.), *Elderly people and the environment* (pp. 191-237). New York, NY: Plenum Press.

Harrison, M. (2004). Defining quality and environment: Disability standards and social factors. *Housing Studies, 19*(5), 691-708.

Imrie, R. (2006a). *Accessible housing: Quality, disability and design*. London, UK: Routledge Taylor and Francis Group.

Imrie, R. (2006b). Independent lives and the relevance of Lifetime Homes. *Disability and Society, 21*(4), 359-374.

Imrie, R., & Hall, P. (2001). *Inclusive design: Designing and developing accessible environments*. London, UK: Spon Press.

Imrie, R., & Kumar, M. (1998). Focusing on disability and access in the built environment. *Disability and Society, 13*(3), 357-374.

International Code Council & American National Standards Institute. (2003). *ICC/ANSI A 117.1–2003. American National Standard—Accessible and Usable Buildings and Facilities*. New York, NY: Author.

Jones, A., de Jonge, D., & Phillips, R. (2008). *The impact of home maintenance and modification services on health, community care and housing outcomes in later life.* Melbourne, Australia: Australian Housing and Urban Research Institute.

Klien, S.K., Rosage, L., & Shaw, G. (1999). The role of occupational therapists in home modification programs at an area agency on aging. In E. D. Taira & J. L. Carlson (Eds.), *Aging in place: Designing, adapting, and enhancing the home environment* (pp.19-38). Binghampton, NY: The Haworth Press.

Lawlor, D., & Thomas, M. A. (2008). *Residential design for aging in place.* Hoboken, NJ: John Wiley & Sons.

Lund, M. L., & Nygard, L. (2004). Occupational life in the home environment: The experiences of people with disabilities. *Canadian Journal of Occupational Therapy, 71*(41), 243-251.

Pynoos, J., Liebig, P., Alley, D., & Nishita, C. M. (2004). Homes of choice: Towards more effective linkages between housing and services. *Journal of Housing for the Elderly, 18*(3/4), 5-49.

Pynoos, J., & Regnier, V. (1997). Design directives in home adaptation. In S. Lanspery & J. Hyde (Eds.), *Staying put: Adapting the places instead of the people* (pp. 41-54). Amityville, NY: Baywood Publishing Company Inc.

Pynoos, J., Sanford, J. A., & Rosenfelt, T. (2002). A team approach to home modifications. *OT Practice, 8,* 15-19.

Sanford, J. A. (2001). *Best practices in the design of toileting and bathing facilities for assisted transfers.* Final report US Access Board. Retrieved from http://www.access-board.gov/research/Toilet-Bath/report.htm

Sanford, J. A., Echt, K., & Malassigné, P. (1999). An E for ADAAG: The case for accessibility guidelines for the elderly based on three studies of toilet transfer. *Journal of Physical and Occupational Therapy in Geriatrics, 16*(3,4), 39-58.

Standards Australia. (2001). *Design for access and mobility. Part 1: General requirement for access—New building work (AS 1428.1).* Sydney, Australia: Author.

Standards Australia. (2007). *What is a standard?* Retrieved from http://www.standards.org.au

Steinfeld, D., Lenker, J., & Paquet, V. (2002). *The anthropometrics of disability.* Report prepared for the US Access Board. Retrieved from http://www.ap.buffalo.edu/idea/Anthro/The%20Anthropometrics%20of%20Disability.html

Steinfeld, E., & Levine, D. (1998). *Technical report: CABO/ANSI A117.1 Standard.* Buffalo, NY: IDEA, University of Buffalo. Retrieved from http://www.ap.buffalo.edu/idea/Publications/technical%20reports.htm#CABO

Steinfeld, E., Levine, D., & Shea, S. (1998). Home modifications and the Fair Housing Law. *Technology and Disability, 8,* 15-35.

Steinfeld, E., Maisel, J., & Feathers, D. (2005). *Standards and anthropometry for wheeled mobility.* Buffalo, NY: Centre for Inclusive Design and Environmental Access, School of Architecture and Planning, University of Buffalo. Retrieved from http://www.ap.buffalo.edu/idea/Anthro/FinalAccessReport.pdf

Steinfeld, E., & Shea, S. (1993). Enabling home environments: Identifying barriers to independence. *Technology and Disability, 2*(4), 69-79.

Tanner, B., Tilse, C., & de Jonge, D. (2008). Restoring and sustaining home: The impact of home modifications on the meaning of home for older people. *Journal of Housing for the Elderly, 22*(3), 195-215.

United Nations. (1975). *Declaration on the rights of disabled persons.* Retrieved from http://www1.umn.edu/humanrts/instree/t3drdp.htm

Victorian Council of Social Services. (2008). *Universal housing, universal benefits.* Melbourne, Australia: Author.

13

Ethical, Legal, and Reporting Variables— Pathways to Best Practice

Elizabeth Ainsworth, MOccThy, Grad Cert Health Sci and Barbara Kornblau, JD, OT/L, FAOTA, ABDA, DAAPM, CDMS, CCM

This chapter provides an overview of the potential ethical and legal issues that can arise in home modification practice, which occupational therapists should carefully consider when carrying out home visits and providing home modification recommendations to clients and services. Practitioners require an understanding of legal, ethical, and reporting issues to ensure effective working relationships with recipients of their services and to achieve best practice. This includes knowledge of frameworks and tools to analyze ethical issues and to evaluate decision making, and an awareness of their subsequent obligations and responsibilities as service providers (Doherty, 2009).

The chapter discusses the potential liability issues of occupational therapists who provide home modification services. It reviews basic principles and provides details on actions that clinicians can take to prevent litigation to lead them down the pathway to best practice. Further, there is advice on best practice with respect to good documentation, particularly in instances where the client, family member, guardian and/or conservator, or funding body might not accept the home modification recommendations.

Also examined in this chapter is the role of the occupational therapist as an expert witness in court, where judges make decisions about damage awards to clients for future home modification and care services. The chapter provides information

on how the occupational therapy report becomes evidence and a source of information for the court on the person's future needs and contributes to the decision-making process the court uses to make its final judgement on the case.

CHAPTER OBJECTIVES

By the end of this chapter, the reader will be able to:

+ Recognize and discuss some of the basic ethical and legal concepts, issues, and approaches relevant to home modification practice

+ Identify sources of information relating to ethics and legal issues to guide professional practice

+ Describe and apply a basic problem-solving framework for ethical issues in occupational therapy home modification practice

+ Acknowledge the importance of good report writing by incorporating specific techniques to ensure protection from litigation, to aid court decisions, and to facilitate excellent clinical competence

+ Explain the role of the occupational therapist as an expert witness and the process in preparing and presenting in court

Ainsworth, E., & de Jonge, D.
An Occupational Therapists's Guide to Home Modification Practice (pp. 239-260)
© 2011 SLACK Incorporated

ETHICAL AND LEGAL OBLIGATIONS

Contemporary professional life presents challenges that require occupational therapists to consider their actions and decisions in terms of their ethical and legal obligations (Opacich, 2003). Occupational therapy assistants must also consider ethical and legal obligations in practice. However, because assistants carry out their work under the supervision of occupational therapists, and because the practice of home modifications is an advanced area, this chapter addresses the responsibilities of occupational therapists.

Occupational therapists must work within the context of ethics and law. Therefore, they must understand basic legal principles that constrict or empower them and ethical reasoning and decision making that affect practice (Dimond, 2004; Doherty, 2009). Ethical and legal obligations are rules of conduct grounded in moral theory, and ignorance of these rules does not abrogate therapists of these responsibilities (Scott, 1997).

Ethical Issues

Ethical rules govern the conduct of professionals. They delineate the proprietary of official conduct, especially in relation to business dealings with people (Scott, 1997). Those areas of conduct regulated by codes of ethics include the nature of the professional-person relationship and the scope of business relationships.

Occupational therapists, as a group, have professional organizations such as the American Occupational Therapy Association (AOTA) that guide and maintain the ethics and values of the profession through standard setting and resources that explain the standards (Van Denend & Finlayson, 2007). The AOTA document, the *Occupational Therapy Code of Ethics and Ethics Standards* (2010) sets the ethical standards of the profession. It serves as a guide for practitioners to determine appropriate moral and professional behavior toward clients and others that abides by laws and regulations. It also acts as a contract with the society that occupational therapists serve (Mosey, 1981). To ensure compliance with this ethical standard, AOTA established *Enforcement Procedures for the Occupational Therapy Code of Ethics* (2007), with oversight and enforcement provided by AOTA's Commission on Standards and Ethics (SEC):

A professional code of ethics sets out the rules or principles intended to express the values of the profession as a whole (Kornblau & Starling, 2000). The professional code of ethics provides the minimum standard for the occupational therapy profession (Kornblau & Starling). A person's membership in a professional association means the occupational therapist accepts the responsibility to abide by the association's code of ethics (Kornblau & Starling). Licensing or registration boards may embrace, adopt, or incorporate the code of ethics into their licensure or registration rules or regulations, requiring occupational therapists who are not members of the association to abide by the code of ethics pursuant to those rules or regulations (Kornblau & Starling).

Similar to other codes of ethics for the profession around the world, the AOTA *Code of Ethics* is a public statement of principles used to promote high standards of professional conduct. Occupational therapists are required to promote inclusion, diversity, independence, and safety for all people at all stages of their lives, health, and illness, and to empower those who benefit from occupational therapy services (AOTA, 2010).

The AOTA Code is an aspirational guide to professional conduct when ethical issues emerge in day-to-day practice with recipients of services as well as with other members of society (AOTA, 2010). The code is based on ethical reasoning surrounding practice and professional issues and empathic reflection regarding practice situations (AOTA). The AOTA Code:

+ Identifies and describes the principles supported by the occupational therapy profession

+ Educates the public and members about the various principles to which occupational therapists are accountable

+ Orients new occupational therapy practitioners to expected standards of conduct

+ Assists in the recognition and resolution of ethical dilemmas (AOTA, 2010)

The various principles described in the AOTA Code relate to beneficence, nonmaleficence, autonomy, confidentiality, social justice, procedural justice, veracity, and fidelity.

Ethical Principles and Approaches

Various ethical approaches and theories support clinical decision making and provide assistance when solving ethical dilemmas, such as adopting a principle-based approach (Shannon, 1993). The principle-based approach relates to the following fundamental ethical principles:

+ Respect for autonomy

+ Nonmaleficence

+ Beneficence

+ Justice (Beauchamp & Childress, 2001)

Autonomy

Autonomy means different things in different contexts in relationship to privacy, individual choice, freedom of will, decisions about one's own behavior, and being one's own person (Beauchamp & Childress, 2001; Shannon, 1993). Autonomy refers to one's moral right to make choices and decisions about one's own life plan and course of action (Jonsen, Siegler, & Winslade, 2006; Kornblau & Starling, 2000; Shannon). It involves freedom from controlling interference of others and limitations, such as inadequate cognitive functioning, which limits personal choice.

To exercise one's autonomy, an individual must have the ability to analyze alternatives, make responsible choices, and undertake intentional actions (Beauchamp & Childress, 2001). In contrast, others can limit the autonomy of people incapable of deliberating or acting on the basis of their desires and plans (Beauchamp & Childress). In home modification practice, occupational therapists should provide clients with a choice to participate in the assessment process to respect their autonomy and should give clients choices of interventions where feasible. Therapists might have to constrain a person's freely chosen actions when that person's preferences and actions infringe on the rights and welfare of others (Jonsen et al., 2006).

Nonmaleficence

The principle of nonmaleficence asserts the obligation not to inflict harm on others (Beauchamp & Childress, 2001; Shannon, 1993). In medical ethics, it is associated with the Hippocratic Oath, which states, "I will use treatment to help the sick according to my ability and judgment but will never use it to injure or wrong them" (Beauchamp & Childress, p. 113). This means occupational therapists may not intentionally cause harm to individuals they serve (AOTA, 2010; Bailey & Schwartzberg, 2003; Costa, 2007; Doherty, 2009; Opacich, 2003). This includes ensuring they do not cause injuries extending beyond physical or psychological harm, such as harm to one's property, liberty, or reputation (Kornblau & Starling, 2000). For example, in order to prevent falls during the home visit, the principle of nonmaleficence requires that therapists lock wheelchair wheels before clients attempt to transfer.

Beneficence

Some philosophers combine nonmaleficence with beneficence into a single principle (Beauchamp & Childress, 2001). Beneficence assures that a professional will treat individuals autonomously and refrain from harming them, but also will contribute to their welfare (Beauchamp & Childress; Jonsen et al., 2006; Shannon, 1993). It relates not only to refraining from doing harm but to taking positive steps to ensure the well-being of others (Beauchamp & Childress; Shannon). This ensures that people receive quality occupational therapy services in accordance with best practice (AOTA, 2010; Bailey & Schwartzberg, 2003; Costa, 2007; Doherty, 2009; Opacich, 2003). For example, an occupational therapist who does a home visit must evaluate the potential benefits of any proposed intervention in relation to its risks, make recommendations to the client, and solicit the client's preferences about whether to proceed with the intervention (Jonsen et al.). Beneficence would also require therapists to recommend interventions, such as assistive devices, should they see a client with a disability experiencing difficulty rising from the toilet.

Justice

Justice relates to fairness, entitlement, and what one deserves. It is viewed as fair, equitable, and appropriate treatment in light of what is due or owed to the individual (Beauchamp & Childress, 2001; Shannon, 1993). Injustice relates to wrongful acts or omissions that deny individuals the benefits to which they have a right and/or distribute burdens unfairly (Beauchamp & Childress).

Ethicists identify various forms of justice:

+ Distributive justice relates to fair, equitable, and appropriate distribution of benefits of society determined by justified norms that structure terms of social cooperation.

+ Criminal justice relates to the just infliction of punishment.

+ Rectificatory justice relates to just compensation for transactional problems, such as malpractice (Beauchamp & Childress, 2001).

During tough economic times involving budget constraints and debates over the appropriate allocation of funds to programs for older people and people with disabilities, distributive justice can be a significant issue in home modification practice.

Occupational therapy professional societies universally embrace the principles contained in the AOTA Code. For example, the World Federation of Occupational Therapists' (WFOT) *Code of Ethics* (2005), which sets standards for general categories of appropriate professional conduct, states that occupational therapists should exhibit personal attributes, such as personal integrity, reliability, open-mindedness, and loyalty, in all aspects of their professional role. On appropriate conduct, the WFOT *Code of Ethics* states that occupational therapists shall work responsibly with individuals and show respect and regard for their individual situations. It also stipulates that therapists not discriminate against individuals and that they take into consideration a person's values, preferences, and abilities when providing services. This includes ensuring the confidentiality of information. According to the code, therapists can provide information to others only with that person's consent.

The WFOT *Code of Ethics* also states that occupational therapists participate in lifelong learning and seek knowledge based on best available evidence. Further, it proscribes that when therapists participate in research activities, they respect the ethical implications of this work. The code advocates that therapists aim to improve, develop, and promote the profession in an ethical manner (WFOT, 2005).

Codes of ethics rarely provide professionals with an absolute guide to behavior or decision making in any given circumstance. However, according to Kornblau and Starling (2000), they do provide a starting point to seek guidance on professional practice and decisions. The occupational therapy profession itself imposes three major responsibilities with respect to ethics. Occupational therapists must:

+ Keep faith with the tenets and principles of the discipline by ensuring services continue to embrace client-centered, occupation-based practice

+ Preserve the integrity of the professional community through clearly established guidance on the competencies and professional development required for practitioners

+ Ensure the integrity of individual practitioners by encouraging ethical contemplation, reflection, and clinical reasoning based on perception, understanding, accountability, and sensitivity (Doherty, 2009; Opacich, 2003)

Problem-Solving Frameworks for Ethical Issues

An ethical problem occurs when one believes a situation might question cherished moral values and duties and might involve difficult choices to determine a course of action (Doherty, 2009). An ethical dilemma occurs when the occupational therapist's response or actions can cause negative consequences or nullify the benefits of good consequences (Kornblau & Starling, 2000). A true dilemma occurs when therapists face a strong persuasive argument both for and against a course of action, posing a moral conflict (Doherty; Kornblau & Starling).

Ethical dilemmas can be viewed from personal, organizational, and societal perspectives, all of which should be given consideration (Kornblau & Starling, 2000). A personal dilemma might relate to concern for the good of the individual. For example, a therapist might experience conflict when the client declines his or her recommendations. An organizational dilemma might relate to issues affecting institutions, such as businesses, professional associations, health care services or agencies, or the family. For example, the home modification service might experience conflict when deciding whether to provide limited services to a large number of clients or a more comprehensive service to a limited number of clients. Societal dilemmas consider the well-being of the community or society as a whole (Kornblau & Starling). An example is when a government experiences conflict over priorities for allocation of resources in health and social care services. The ethical dilemmas that occupational therapists might encounter in the home modification field include the following:

+ Confidentiality and disclosure of the person's private information

+ Resource allocation and priorities in home modification practice

+ Client's decision-making capacity

+ Personal and professional boundaries

+ Use of power

+ Cultural, religious, or family considerations

Confidentiality and Disclosure of Private Information

After a home modification visit, do occupational therapists respect the client's right to privacy or do they report that he or she is living in a state of neglect? Does it make a difference whether paid caregivers or family members provide the care in the home? Does the law require such a disclosure?

Resource Allocation and Priorities

Should home modification programs finance all types of modifications or only those alterations that improve the person's health and safety in the home? During tough economic times, should publicly or grant-funded programs still fund adaptations to enhance the individual's independence, community participation, and quality of life? How can occupational therapists provide services if they are working in settings with limited resources, while at the same time ethics and regulatory bodies require they provide quality care (Kinsella, Ji-Sun Park, Appiagyei, Chang, & Chow, 2008)?

Client's Decision-Making Capacity

Should occupational therapists rely solely on the self-report of people whom they believe are in the early stages of dementia or should they contact others to assist with decision making?

Personal and Professional Boundaries

How can occupational therapists deliver home modification services in a diagnostically driven health care system that conflicts with occupational therapists' values rooted in client-centered practice, social justice, enabling occupation, and, in some places, social models of care (Kinsella et al., 2008)?

Use of Power

Should occupational therapists place their clients and their families in situations that compel them to agree with professional recommendations, even in those instances where clients and their families do not feel comfortable with the proposed changes, or should they acquiesce to the views of clients and their families?

Cultural, Religious, or Family Considerations

Should occupational therapists alter their modification recommendations to suit another family member who also has a disability, or should they provide modifications only to benefit the client? Should occupational therapists consider the needs of caregivers in developing modification recommendations in addition to the needs of the client?

Ethical Terminology

Ethical terminology of relevance to occupational therapists includes the following:

+ Informed consent
+ Veracity
+ Confidentiality
+ Fidelity
+ Duty
+ Rights
+ Paternalism

Informed Consent

Informed consent obligates occupational therapists to provide clients with truthful, comprehensive information on all assessment and intervention strategies to ensure they can make willing, informed decisions (Kornblau & Starling, 2000; Shannon, 1993).

Informed consent is defined as a client's willing acceptance of an intervention after adequate disclosure of the nature of the intervention and its risks and benefits and the alternatives and their risks and benefits (Jonsen et al., 2006; Shannon, 1993). One can determine the adequacy of disclosure by exploring what a reasonably prudent therapist would tell a client under similar circumstances (health professional-centered approach) or which information reasonable clients need to know to make rational decisions (client-centered approach; Jonsen et al.).

Codes of ethics and licensure laws and federal and state laws and regulations require occupational therapists to seek informed consent (Kornblau & Starling, 2000).

The requirements of informed consent as described by Biano and Hirsh (1995, cited in Kornblau & Starling, 2000, p. 28) include the following:

+ Occupational therapists must ensure the client understands the procedure or treatment and its risks, potential benefits, and any available alternatives.

+ Clients must freely give consent, willingly and without duress.

+ Clients must possess the capacity to give consent.

If clients have impaired decision-making capacity, the therapist must seek consent from a parent, guardian, or conservator. Further, clients who do not wish to participate in the occupational therapy process might refuse to give informed consent (Kornblau & Starling, 2000).

Veracity

Veracity in occupational therapy practice involves the comprehensive, accurate, and objective transmission of information to individuals and the manner in which the occupational therapist fosters their understanding (Beauchamp & Childress, 2001). It stems from respect for others; the obligations of fidelity, truth, and promise keeping; and trust (Beauchamp & Childress).

Occupational therapists must speak and act truthfully in all communication with clients. If the therapist fails to speak truthfully, it may interfere with the client's ability to make an informed decision (Kornblau & Starling, 2000). When occupational therapists seek informed consent for assessment, treatment, or intervention, they must provide clients with comprehensive, accurate, and objective information as part of this process. For example, veracity can include providing clients and their caregivers accurate and complete information about the use of assistive devices in the home. Veracity also includes accurately representing one's occupational therapy qualifications to students seeking a home modification fieldwork experience (Costa, 2007).

Confidentiality

Privacy entails respecting a person's right to limit access to his or her personal sphere. In contrast, confidentiality focuses on informational privacy. It prevents disclosure of information previously disclosed within a confidential relationship (Beauchamp & Childress, 2001; Jonsen et al., 2006; Opacich, 2003; Stallard, 2005). Occupational therapists need to ensure that they familiarize themselves with practice requirements relevant to privacy and confidentiality. For example, in the United States (US), the Health Insurance Portability and Accountability Act of 1996 (HIPAA) creates a comprehensive system that defines the value, scope, and limits of confidentiality (Jonsen et al.). Regulatory bodies, codes of ethics, and standards of practice usually require that occupational therapists—including those who practice home modifications—keep records of their interventions. They must maintain these records according to HIPAA's confidentiality requirements. The Summary of the HIPAA Privacy Rule (US Department of Health and Human Services [HHS], 2003) provides particularly useful information regarding HIPAA's application to occupational therapy practice.

A breach in confidentiality occurs when professionals fail to protect information about people who have shared that information in confidence or they share it without permission (Beauchamp & Childress, 2001; Stallard, 2005). Breaches in confidentiality can result in various actions, such as:

+ Employer disciplinary proceedings

+ Termination of contract of employment

+ Referral to the professional body for ethics violations

+ Legal proceedings for compensation

+ Criminal proceedings if the breach is prohibited by law (Stallard, 2005)

Occupational therapists might justify breaches in confidentiality if there is specific concern for the safety of others, such as instances of child or elder abuse, or where a person is mortally threatened, or where there is concern for public welfare (Jonsen et al., 2006; Kornblau & Starling, 2000). Occupational therapists may disclose information where clients agree to the disclosure and provide a HIPAA release or consent. Disclosure may be in the best interest of people with disabilities to ensure their health, safety, and independence in the home. In such instances, statutes or court orders might require the disclosure (Dimond, 2004; Stallard, 2005). For example, in the US, state laws often require that occupational therapists and other health professionals report suspected elder abuse. Therapists who practice home modifications might find circumstances in the home that lead them to suspect possible elder abuse. Reporting this suspected elder abuse falls under an exception to HIPAA's confidentiality requirements.

Where someone has impaired decision-making capacity, therapists might need to obtain consent for release of information from a guardian, conservator, or health care surrogate. Clients or substitute decision makers must sign written documentation as evidence of their agreement to release the information (Stallard, 2005). In the US, the client or substitute decision maker must sign a HIPAA release. Further, the HIPAA release form must stipulate contents of the information and to whom it is being released. If therapists are in doubt about the process of sharing information with other parties, they should check with their employers or relevant others and review the HIPAA requirements.

Fidelity

Fidelity refers to faithfulness of one human being to another, in implicit or explicit promises and commitments (AOTA, 2010; Bailey & Schwartzberg, 2003; Beauchamp & Childress, 2001; Costa, 2007; Doherty, 2009; Opacich, 2003). This principle justifies the obligation to act in good faith to keep vows and promises, fulfill agreements, maintain relationships, and discharge fiduciary responsibilities (Beauchamp & Childress). In occupational therapy, fidelity means upholding responsibilities to clients. This might include, for example, a program or department following through with its commitment to perform scheduled home modification evaluations or to keep shared information confidential (Kornblau & Starling, 2000).

Duty

A duty is a responsibility therapists have to their patients or clients. It refers to obligations required of professionals by society, codes of ethics, laws, and regulations, or self-imposed actions. For example, occupational therapists have a duty to their patients and clients to maintain their level of competence in their area of practice through lifelong learning, so they can deliver quality care (Costa, 2007).

Rights

Rights refer to a justified claim or entitlement warranted by moral principles and rules (Beauchamp & Childress, 2001). Rights relate to the moral entitlement to protect life, liberty, expression, and property. When respected, rights can provide a basis to protect against oppression, unequal treatment, intolerance, and invasion of privacy, among others (Beauchamp & Childress; Shannon, 1993). For example, during their interactions in home modification practice, occupational therapists must ensure clients' rights to autonomy, privacy, and confidentiality.

Paternalism

Historically, decision making in the medical field has been "paternalistic." Physicians made diagnoses, prescribed treatments, and gave "orders," providing the patient with limited information (Jonsen et al., 2006). In occupational therapy practice, paternalism occurs when occupational therapists fail to respect clients' autonomy and act with no regard of the person's individual rights (Kornblau & Starling, 2000).

Paternalism may emerge when there is conflict between beneficence and autonomy. It can involve interference with, or refusal to conform to, individual clients' preferences regarding their own good (Beauchamp & Childress, 2001; Shannon, 1993). Paternalistic acts can involve force, coercion, deception, lying, manipulation, or nondisclosure of information; overriding one's known preferences; or restricting a person's autonomous choice (Beauchamp & Childress). For example, paternalism would occur in home modification practice if therapists coerced clients into accepting home modification recommendations, insisting that they knew best.

In the middle of the 20th century, this pattern of paternalism shifted, in theory, to patient autonomy in which the person was seen as the authoritative decision maker (Jonsen et al., 2006). The current view sees shared decision making between the health professional and the client as the preferred relationship (Jonsen et al.).

Problem-Solving Tools for Ethical Issues

Although the study of ethical theory provides the basis for formulating solutions, it might not readily solve the problem identified. Instead of easy answers, it can raise a variety of questions and issues. Occupational therapists require knowledge of a range of resources and tools that help translate their judgments into specific action steps to solve ethical dilemmas (Kornblau & Starling, 2000). Resources and tools help analyze the situation in a structured and systematic way, including, for example, referring to the profession's codes of ethics, such as the AOTA's code (AOTA, 2010), which incorporates ethical principles. It might also include referring to textbooks in the field that provide guidance and information to assist in the analysis of ethical issues (Van Denend & Finlayson, 2007).

Analysis of ethical dilemmas is a multistep process guided by various sets of values and principles (Kornblau & Starling, 2000). Though there are various methods or processing tools available to analyze ethical dilemmas, the CELIBATE Method (Clinical Ethics and Legal Issues Bait All Therapists Equally) for Analyzing Ethical Dilemmas provides occupational therapists in home modification practice with a workable tool for addressing problems they might come across. This method, developed by Kornblau and Starling, provides therapists with a clear framework that considers both legal and ethical issues (Table 13-1). The title of the method is an acronym where each letter provides a cue for the user of the framework:

+ C is for clinical situation.
+ E is for ethical issues.
+ L is for legal issues.
+ I is for information.
+ B is for brainstorming actions.
+ A is for analyzing actions.
+ T is for taking action.
+ E is for evaluating the results.

Occupational therapists need not use the CELIBATE method alone. In fact, working with other members of the team, therapists can ensure a range of insights into ethical problem solving. Kornblau and Starling (2000) provide further information on the application of this approach (pp. 54-60).

Tymchuck (1982) developed another model for resolving dilemmas, whereby it provides steps on how to describe the ethical issues and assess this information. The process for making ethical decisions is a seven-step procedure.

1. Describe the parameters of the situation.
2. Describe the potential issues involved.
3. Describe the guidelines already available that might affect each issue—for example, values, laws, codes, practice, and research.
4. Enumerate the alternative decisions for each issue.
5. Enumerate the short-term, ongoing, and long-term consequences for each alternative.
6. Present evidence (or the lack thereof) for those consequences as well as the probability of their occurrence.
7. Rank order, and vote on the decisions (Tymchuck, 1982, p. 170).

Table 13-1. CELIBATE Method for Analyzing Ethical Dilemmas

1. What is the problem?
2. What are the facts of the situation?
3. Who are the interested parties? • Facility, patient, other therapists, observers, payers, etc.
4. What is the nature of the interest? Why is this a problem? • Professional • Personal • Business • Economic • Intellectual • Societal
5. Ethical? • Does it violate a professional code of ethics? • Which section(s)?
6. Legal? Is there a legal issue? • Practice act/licensure law & regulations? • Other laws: Check the CELIBATE Checklist

7. Do I need more information?
• What information do I need?
  ◦ Is there a treatment, policy, procedure, law, regulation, or document that I do not know about?
  ◦ Can I obtain a copy of the treatment, policy, procedure, law, regulation, or document in writing?
  ◦ Do I need to research the issue further?
  ◦ Do I need to consult with a mentor, an expert in this area, and/or a lawyer?

8. Brainstorm possible action steps.

9. Analyze action steps.
• Eliminate obvious wrong or impossible choices.
  ◦ How will each alternative affect my patients, other interest parties, and me?
  ◦ Do your choices abide by the Code of Ethics?
  ◦ Do your choices abide by the practice act & regulations?
  ◦ Are my choices consistent with my moral, religious, and social beliefs?

10. Choose your course of action
• The Rotary Four-Way Test
  ◦ Is it the truth?
  ◦ Is it fair to all concerned?
  ◦ Will it build goodwill and better friendships?
  ◦ Will it be beneficial to all concerned?
• Is it win-win?
• How do you feel about your course of action?

(Reprinted with permission from Kornblau, B. L., & Starling, S. P. (2000). *Ethics in rehabilitation: A clinical perspective*. Thorofare, NJ: SLACK Incorporated.)

Ethical Breaches and Consequences

Unethical practice is practice that fails to conform to established professional standards (Kornblau & Starling, 2000). This can include unreasonable, unjustified, ineffective, immoral, questionable, and knowingly harmful or wrong practice (Kornblau & Starling). Clients, colleagues, employers, family members, and others can raise breaches of the code of ethics with the various registration or certification bodies that monitor professional conduct.

Employers can also have codes of conduct that impose professional and/or contractual duties on occupational therapists as workplace requirements. Employers might respond to ethics complaints with disciplinary proceedings, which could result in demotion or dismissal. Therapists who are self-employed or working on a contractual basis might find their contract terminated.

Numerous rules and regulations govern the basic ethical and legal requirements of professional conduct. These include the following:

+ The profession's *Occupational Therapy Code of Ethics and Ethics Standards* (AOTA, 2010)

+ State licensure laws

+ Malpractice standards

+ State and federal criminal or civil statutes

+ Case law (Bailey & Schwartzberg, 2003)

Ethical and legal matters differ in the types of penalties professionals can face as a result of their behaviors (Table 13-2).

Therapists who violate the professional code of ethics may also violate a criminal law and find themselves subject to legal action (Costa, 2007; Scott, 1997). While ethics and law are not synonymous, occupational therapists need to be aware of the effect of law on decisions they make in practice because not all legal actions are ethical and not all ethical actions are legal (Opacich, 2003). At times, therapists might consider a law wrong or contrary to their ethical principles (Dimond, 2004). Under these circumstances, they need to determine what personal action to take, in full awareness that they subject themselves to penalties (Dimond). For example, a therapist receives a request for a home modification intervention and, during the initial visit, discovers that the client has a guardian/conservator who must approve the visit. The therapist calls the guardian to explain the need and seek consent. However, the guardian refuses to allow the visit to proceed and tells the therapist "to stay out of family business." According to the law, without the consent of the guardian, the therapist cannot visit the client and provide the service. However, the therapist may feel an ethical and moral obligation to not abandon the client and to provide the services. At the same time, the law and ethical obligations require the therapist not to see the client without informed consent. The therapist needs to decide what action to take, which may include petitioning the court for permission to see the client.

When ethical conflicts occur in practice, legal rules might sometimes set limits to ethical options or can even create ethical conflicts (Jonsen et al., 2006). For example, therapists might feel conflicted between their ethical duty to protect confidential information and their legal duty to report required information in order to protect a person or community's health and safety (Jonsen et al.). For example, an occupational therapist visiting a client to undertake a home modification assessment may find that he or she is living in a state of abuse and neglect despite residing with family. The occupational therapist may feel conflicted between his or her ethical duty to respect the confidentiality of the client's circumstances as per the family's wishes and his or her legal duty to report the client's suspected state of abuse and neglect.

Occupational therapists in home modification practice can face situations that raise both ethical and legal concerns. It is important that therapists problem solve ethical issues using ethical concepts and reasoning because the law, though relevant to various cases, rarely settles ethical problems (Jonsen et al., 2006).

LEGAL ISSUES

The law has been described as "a collection of rules and regulations by which society is governed" (Bailey & Schwartzberg, 2003, p. 4). They are generally manmade and involve the blending of court decisions, state and federal statutes, regulations, and procedures to ensure people's rights are protected (Bailey & Schwartzberg). Laws commonly reflect society's needs, attitudes, and mores and serve to regulate social conduct in a formal and binding manner.

The two legal issues that are commonly raised in relation to the negligence of occupational therapists include professional standard of care and professional negligence.

Professional Standard of Care

A health professional must practice according to a specific standard of care, which is the standard that

Table 13-2. Possible Ethical and Legal Penalties in the United States

FEATURE	ETHICS	LAW
Compromised of:	Standards of practice	Federal statutes
	Codes of ethics	State statutes
	Social values	State regulations
	Religious values	Federal regulations
	Cultural values	Case law
	Moral value	(Licensure laws)
Penalties	Fines	Fines
	Loss of provisional privilege, license, or certification	Monetary damages (punitive, compensatory, or restitution)
	Relinquishment of membership in professional organization	Imprisonment
	Reprimand—public or private	Injunctions
	Censure—usually public	Revocation or suspension of license
	Publication of the ethical violation and penalty imposed	Publication of revocation or suspension of license
	Report to licensure or certification board	License placed in probationary status
	Termination	Termination

(Adapted with permission from Kornblau, B. L., & Starling, S. P. (2000). *Ethics in rehabilitation: A clinical perspective.* Thorofare, NJ: SLACK Incorporated.)

a reasonably prudent person in the same profession would demonstrate under similar circumstances (Ekelman Ranke & Moriarty, 1995). Under the law, occupational therapists who possess average skill and competence in the exercise of their profession establish the standard of care (Jarvis, 1983).

Standard of care comes from the person who testifies to what the standard is (the expert witness), the profession's standards of practice and codes of ethics, professional literature, standard textbooks, licensure laws and regulations, and how 51% of occupational therapists would act under similar circumstances (Simon, 2005). Failure to perform to these standards constitutes negligence or malpractice (Ekelman Ranke & Moriarty, 1995). For example, during a home modification evaluation, an occupational therapist must review a client's occupational performance in a range of areas in the home if he or she believes the client may have requirements extending beyond those indicated in the initial referral.

The law, codes of ethics, and standards of practice require that occupational therapists competently provide assessments and interventions (Neeman, 1979). The concept of competence in professional practice is important because it relates to employee expectations in the workplace and involves more than the accomplishment of a number of discrete or separate tasks (OT Australia, 1994).

Competence is described as "a complex interaction and integration of knowledge, judgment, higher order reasoning, personal qualities, skills, values and beliefs" (OT Australia, 1994, p. 5). Competent professionals recall and apply facts and skills, evaluate evidence, create explanations from available facts, develop hypotheses, and synthesize information from their own knowledge base (OT Australia). Competence also involves the capacity to generalize or transfer skills and knowledge from one situation to another (OT Australia).

The occupational therapy profession accepts responsibility for the competence of its members. It sets standards for their preparation and practice, provides a means of achieving competence, identifies those qualified as competent, and implements measures to oversee occupational therapy practice (Neeman, 1979). The *Occupational Therapy Code of Ethics and Ethics Standards* (AOTA, 2010) clearly imposes requirements for individual occupational therapists to engage in competent practice and recommends continuing competence plans (Moyers & Hinojosa, 2003).

All occupational therapists must ensure their own competence in the area in which they practice by keeping abreast of current developments in the field through the professional literature. At a minimum, they must know what other reasonable and competent occupational therapists in the same specialty know or should know (Jarvis, 1983; Neeman, 1979). Employers have a duty to hire people with appropriate qualifications, and supervisors have a duty to delegate tasks within the individual's sphere of competence (Neeman).

The consequences of incompetent performance could include occupational therapists' self-dissatisfaction with respect to their own performance, as well as clients' and employers' dissatisfaction with their work practices (Moyers & Hinojosa, 2003). Incompetent practice can result in a decline in business, a reduction in revenue for the business, limited opportunities for promotion, job loss, and difficulty obtaining new employment (Moyers & Hinojosa). Incompetent occupational therapists could face actions for malpractice or loss of their state licenses, certifications, and/or professional association memberships (Moyers & Hinojosa).

Because home modification is a specialized area, various occupational therapy professional organizations around the world, such as AOTA, have developed home modification practice competencies. While students can acquire some training through education and fieldwork, they are likely to need further training to establish competency in home modification practice, particularly after they receive a license (Yarett Slater, 2004). Occupational therapists must document their competence in home modification practice and update it regularly to ensure consistency of skill and knowledge (Yarett Slater). This is particularly important if specific countries do not have their own set of documented competencies for this area (Yarett Slater). If a patient or client is harmed, occupational therapists who perform home modification work beyond their professional knowledge, skill, and expertise might open themselves to allegations of professional incompetence or malpractice (Bull, 1998).

Legal frameworks in state practice acts, such as those in effect in the US, establish the scope of practice of occupational therapy (Yarett Slater, 2004). State licensure laws in the US—also called *practice acts*—legally define the profession's scope of practice to protect consumers of occupational therapy services (Yarett Slater). Other countries might have other frameworks that establish the domain of practice of occupational therapy. Additionally, occupational therapy professional bodies might also have specific practice guidelines for home modification

practice that can assist individuals who work in this area. Therapists can acquire information about home modification practice from professional literature, standard textbooks, licensure laws and regulations, and other occupational therapists with expertise in the field.

Professional Negligence

To appreciate the risks involved in home modification practice and to implement strategies to reduce these risks, occupational therapists will find it useful to understand the laws of negligence and professional malpractice (Ekelman Ranke & Moriarty, 1995).

In the US, two sets of laws govern behavior toward one another: criminal and civil (Ekelman Ranke & Moriarty, 1995). Under civil law, everyone in society has a duty to exercise due care or reasonable care for his or her own safety and the safety of others (Ekelman Ranke & Moriarty). Failure to ensure this safety of self or others is considered negligent, which can result in a civil lawsuit (Ekelman Ranke & Moriarty).

Negligence is a common civil action where the defendant (the occupational therapist) owed a duty of care to someone (the client); the defendant breached that duty; and the breach of the duty caused reasonably foreseeable harm to person or property (Dimond, 2004; Jarvis, 1983). The harm to the person or property results from an action that a "reasonable person" would not take or the failure to take an action that a reasonable person would take under similar circumstances (Jarvis). If an action or failure to take action occurs without damage or harm, there is no negligence. At the same time, if damage or harm occurs but the action taken meets the "reasonable person" test, then it does not constitute negligence (Jarvis).

Negligence is not synonymous with *malpractice* (Jarvis, 1983). Malpractice, a broader concept, applies to all wrongful acts against a person, such as treating without valid consent, as well as negligence (Costa, 2007; Jarvis; Stallard, 2005). Malpractice occurs when professionals participate in professional misconduct, lack reasonable skills, and fail to deliver appropriate professional services with the degree of skill and learning expected of members of the profession, which results in injury, loss, or damage to service recipients or those entitled to services (Costa; Jarvis; Stallard). Malpractice includes malicious practice or illegal and immoral conduct (Costa; Jarvis; Stallard).

The fundamental guiding principle in professional practice is the "reasonable occupational therapist standard," and the courts decide what is reasonable under the law (Jarvis, 1983). Courts have the fundamental obligation to apply the same standards to similar cases. They might look to the standard of care of a similarly situated professional, or the court may look to the profession's own standards to determine potential liability (Hertfelder & Crispen, 1990).

The "reasonable person standard" applies to all members of the general public. However, a higher standard applies to health professionals, such as occupational therapists (Jarvis, 1983). There are various reasons why the law holds professionals to a higher standard than nonprofessionals. First, the law sees the skills of professionals coming from validated, theoretical bodies of knowledge, which laypeople do not bring to the equation (Jarvis). Second, professional practice is based on research and the ongoing development of new theories compared with laypeople, who base what they do on general knowledge (Jarvis). Finally, the law views professionals as those who can provide the best solution to meet the clients' need based on their own knowledge as professionals and the needs of the client. The client is not usually in a position to question the judgment of the professional, compared with the judgment of a layperson, who may provide customer service or other nonskilled tasks (Jarvis).

The Four Elements of Malpractice

The courts consider four elements when determining whether a professional's action or lack of action constitutes malpractice (Jarvis, 1983). They include duty of care, breach of duty, harm, and causation.

Duty of Care

By the nature of the relationship, occupational therapists always owe a duty of care to the clients with whom they establish relationships. This relationship starts when the therapist first establishes contact with the client (Dimond, 2004; Jarvis, 1983; Kornblau & Starling, 2000). A duty of care arises when a person can reasonably foresee that his or her actions or omissions (the failure to do something one should do) could cause reasonably foreseeable harm to another person (Dimond; Mu, Lohman, & Scheirton, 2005).

Occupational therapists may find themselves liable for damages caused by actions they took (acts of commission) as well as the actions they failed to take (acts of ommissions; Kornblau & Starling, 2000). To achieve success in a negligence action, the person claiming the harm (the plaintiff) must show that the person he or she claims harmed him or her (the defendant) actually owed the plaintiff a duty of care (Dobbs, 2000). Occupational therapists' duties

compel them to exercise the reasonable care and skills expected of a reasonably prudent occupational therapist. In fact, the courts will inquire as to whether a reasonably prudent occupational therapist would act in a similar manner under similar circumstances (Kornblau & Starling).

Breach of Duty

After presenting evidence that the defendant had a duty of care, the plaintiff must show the defendant had to practice according to a minimum standard of practice (Dobbs, 2000). Occupational therapists breach the duty of care if they fail to meet the standard of practice required by law (Jarvis, 1983). This can be established through first determining the most appropriate standard of practice, including care and proficiency (Dimond, 2004; Wright, 1985). This involves examining the following:

+ The reasonableness of the practice
+ The degree of risk of an incident or accident occurring
+ The consequences of not providing a service (Dimond, 2004)

The expert witness' role in court is to help prove breach of duty or providing care that falls below the standards of a reasonably prudent occupational therapist (Kornblau & Starling, 2000). Expert witnesses are usually practitioners in the same field who testify to provide their opinion on the standard of care to which occupational therapists must practice in particular situations (Kornblau & Starling). Standards of practice, codes of ethics, licensure laws, professional literature, and standard texts provide evidence to the court as to the standard of care.

The type of relationship an occupational therapist has with an employer, hospital, or agency affects the determination of liability for therapists' acts of negligence (Ekelman Ranke & Moriarty, 1995). The two most common relationships involving occupational therapists include the employer/employee relationship and the relationship between occupational therapy independent contractors and the contracting entities, such as hospitals, agencies, and individual clients (Ekelman Ranke & Moriarty). In the US, under the doctrine of "respondent superior" ("let the master answer"), occupational therapists can find themselves liable for the action of subordinates unless they are independent contractors (Ekelman Ranke & Moriarty; Kornblau & Starling, 2000). Under this doctrine, the law can impute liability to occupational therapists or employers who direct and supervise employees if they delegate therapy services to staff who are not qualified or who fail to perform these services properly (Kornblau & Starling).

If occupational therapists work in a private capacity under an independent contractor agreement and their actions result in damage to the person receiving the services, the contracting agency or entity would generally not be held liable for the independent contractor's negligence (Ekelman Ranke & Moriarty, 1995). Under these circumstances, occupational therapists are liable for their own actions. Independent contractors should consider professional liability insurance to protect themselves from malpractice actions (Ekelman Ranke & Moriarty). In the US, however, attorneys are more likely to sue occupational therapists with malpractice insurance than those without.

Harm

In a negligence case, breach of duty must result in some sort of harm (Dobbs, 2000). The person to whom the duty of care was owed must prove the harm. Harm is established when the person experiences some loss or injury (Jarvis, 1983). Examples of recognizable harm include personal injury, death, lost wages, and property damage (Dimond, 2004). This harm or loss is referred to as damages and forms the basis for the claim (Dimond).

Occupational therapists might act in a manner that falls below the standard of care without causing any harm. Should no harm occur, one cannot make a case for malpractice (Kornblau & Starling, 2000). Additionally, therapists might act reasonably and provide effective services, but the person's condition does not improve. This also fails to rise to the level of malpractice (Kornblau & Starling).

Causation

The plaintiff must show that the occupational therapist's negligent conduct was responsible for the reasonably foreseeable harm to the client (Dimond, 2004). The standard is the "but for" test: But for the occupational therapist's negligence, the client's injury would not have occurred (Kornblau & Starling, 2000).

OTHER LEGAL-RELATED PRACTICE ISSUES

Assault and Battery

During home visits, occupational therapists might provide physical assistance to clients as they complete various activities to demonstrate how they manage in the home. This involves the client cooperating and giving informed consent before undertaking any activities in the home (Kornblau & Starling, 2000). Occupational therapists need to know that if they place someone in a position where he or she is apprehensive of being touched in an offensive manner without consent, this is considered assault. Intentionally touching someone without consent defines battery to the person (Dimond, 2004; Kornblau & Starling).

Occupational therapists must take reasonable care in their interactions with clients (Dimond, 2004). A chaperone could prove useful should therapists later find themselves accused of harming a client (Dimond). It is also essential that the occupational therapist clearly document any incidents that might have occurred at the time of the interaction with the client to ensure that he or she has a clear record of the event for future reference.

Breach of Fiduciary Duty

Another type of action is breach of fiduciary duty, which can apply to professionals in specific situations. Under the law, occupational therapists owe a fiduciary duty to their clients (Jonsen et al., 2006). As defined in the law, a fiduciary owes undivided loyalty to clients and must work for their benefit (Jonsen et al.). Fiduciaries have specialized expertise; are held to high standards of honesty, confidentiality, and loyalty; and must avoid all conflicts of interest that could prejudice their client's interests (Jonsen et al.).

Where professionals use their relationships to procure a benefit for themselves without disclosing the private interest to clients, the law requires that they account for those benefits to the client. For example, the law does not look kindly on therapists who recommend products and fittings for a home that come from a company in which they have a personal financial interest and fail to disclose this to the client. Additionally, the law prohibits therapists from obtaining any financial benefit from a client's acquisition of products and finishes. This creates a conflict between occupational therapists' private interest and their duty to their client. If they are receiving "kickbacks" or commissions from the company that provides the products and fittings, they could face ethical charges, criminal charges, and disciplinary action from the licensure or certification boards.

DEFENSES TO AN ACTION

Even when the plaintiff can prove all of the specific elements of negligence, the court might accept some defenses against allegations of negligence (Dobbs, 2000). This means that defendants might justify some actions, even though they were negligent and individuals suffered losses from those actions (Dobbs). If negligent actions are defensible, individuals harmed might find that they cannot pursue claims for compensation from the people who caused their harm (Dobbs).

The plaintiff must prove facts corresponding to the various acceptable legal defenses, which can include the following:

+ *Contributory negligence*: Where the claimant is partly responsible for the harm

+ *Exemption from liability for loss or damage to property or person*: Where, for example, individuals might waive their right to sue via a contract or fail to follow proper procedures; or the government limits the right to sue, such as the doctrine of sovereign immunity; or where a statute prevents suing a government employee, such as the Federal Tort Claim Act (FTCA) 28 U.S.C. §§ 1346(b), 2671–2680 (1948)

+ *Statute of limitation*: Where the claimant fails to initiate a lawsuit within the time allowed by law

+ *Assumption of risk*: Where injured parties knowingly and willingly place themselves at risk of harm (Dimond, 2004; Dobbs, 2000)

IMPLICATIONS FOR OCCUPATIONAL THERAPY PRACTICE

Occupational therapists must use diligence, care, knowledge, skill, and caution in their interactions with clients during home visits (Wright, 1985). To guard against negligence and malpractice, occupational therapists need to follow safe and acceptable work practices and procedures.

They must ensure their knowledge is up-to-date and commensurate with peers who practice in the home modification field. Therapists must use reasoned judgment in all situations (Jarvis, 1983). This can be accomplished by following the recommendations of Costa (2007), Kornblau and Starling (2000), Moyers and Hinojosa (2003), and Wright (1985). Occupational therapists are to:

+ *Maintain professional standards*: Maintain professional membership and keep abreast of ethical and legal practice requirements; comply with the profession's standards of practice and quality assurance programs; and attend conferences and workshops, read the professional literature, and participate in lifelong learning and regular professional development.

+ *Manage day-to-day practice effectively*: Request policies and instructions in writing from employers and those with whom therapists contract; provide close supervision to students on placements; establish a relationship with a mentor or professional supervisor; take time out to think through issues and seek advice; recognize when to hand over clients to another occupational therapist with more expertise.

+ *Communicate clearly and comprehensively*: Establish sound communication with individuals in their homes and provide an explanation of occupational therapy's role and the purpose of any activities undertaken in the home for the housing-needs assessment process; complete contemporaneous, complete, and comprehensive documentation accurately and truthfully, and save these documents for future reference; ensure written documentation demonstrates sound clinical reasoning, rationale, and consultation throughout the housing-needs assessment process.

+ *Deal with ethical and legal issues appropriately*: Report ethical and legal violations to ethics and licensure boards; seek counsel, support, and assistance from other experts or a legal representative if issues arise.

Preventing Occupational Therapy Errors

Given the complexities of issues that occupational therapists deal with, there is a risk of errors occurring. In the US in 1999, the Institute of Medicine (IOM) produced a report entitled *To Err is Human: Building a Safer Health System* (Kohn, Corrigan, & Donaldson, 2000). Kohn et al. reported that errors in health care professional practice cause significant harm to the population. This report defined *safety* as freedom from accidental injury and *error* as the failure to take planned action to be completed as intended or the use of a wrong plan to achieve an aim (Jonsen et al., 2006). The report highlighted personal and financial costs of errors. It noted some errors occurred because of incompetence, mistaken judgment, and unrecognized and uncorrected system failures, which resulted in a breach of the health care professional's responsibility (Jonsen et al.).

Research shows that errors occur in occupational therapy practice (Lohman, Mu, & Scheirton, 2003; Mu, Lohman, & Scheirton, 2005, 2006; Scheirton, Mu, & Lohman, 2003). Lohman et al. highlighted common occupational therapy practice errors, their causes, prevention, and other implications.

Practice errors can be physical or psychosocial in nature (Lohman et al., 2003) and can occur as a result of something the therapist does or fails to do (Lohman et al.; Mu et al., 2005). Examples of practice errors in home modification practice include causing a client unnecessary fatigue and falls during a transfer.

Research indicates a range of causes of errors, including human factors, equipment factors, controllable and uncontrollable environmental factors, and poorly structured organizations and systems (Mu et al., 2005). In occupational therapy, major causes of errors included misjudgment of situations, poor preparation, lack of experience, inadequate training and knowledge, miscommunication, poor attention, heavy workload, and inadequate supervision, or a combination of these factors (Lohman et al., 2003). Practice errors can be prevented when occupational therapists do the following:

+ *Create a supportive work environment*: Create a nonpunitive work culture to encourage reporting of errors and learning from these experiences; create policies and procedures and require staff to follow them; re-examine existing policies and procedures to improve them; conduct orientation and training of all new staff and students and highlight potential areas for errors during training; maintain appropriate staffing levels; and facilitate collaborative teamwork.

+ *Develop structures for monitoring, reporting, and analyzing errors*: Develop monitoring and reporting structures; encourage staff to become more vigilant, pay attention to all circumstances, and do not rush decisions; encourage staff honesty and error disclosure; encourage staff to seek assistance from colleagues with more expertise.

+ *Provide training*: Provide client safety and error reduction education; establish programs for areas of concern; provide in-services for different intervention approaches; provide staff assertiveness training (Lohman et al., 2003; Mu et al., 2005, 2006).

Research shows that occupational therapists need to learn from their errors and develop preventative strategies to reduce errors and improve client safety rather than feeling pressured to attain 100% perfection (Mu et al., 2006). This learning best occurs in supportive environments that have processes established to investigate, analyze, and plan improvements to occupational therapy practice. In particular, clinical practice needs therapy to be based on sound clinical reasoning and informed by consumer need, principles of best practice, and research.

Occupational therapists can minimize or prevent practice errors by careful analysis and management of potentially injurious situations. Therapists working in the area of home modifications practice are frequently exposed to situations that place their clients at risk. For example, when evaluating a person's ability to perform activities in their own environment, a therapist needs first to determine the potential risk involved in this assessment and how it can be managed. The therapist needs to determine the probability of an incident occurring and the likely consequences. He or she would then need to reduce the likelihood of an event occurring and minimize an injury by avoiding the task altogether or putting strategies in place to reduce the risk. Further, therapists should constantly monitor the client, tasks, and environment during the home visit to avoid potentially hazardous situations. Chapter 7 contains further information on risk assessment and risk management.

Therapists must understand adverse events and risks and learn how to reduce them. This promotes effective service delivery and helps prevent incidents, accidents, adverse events, or death, which can result in harm to the client and associated litigation.

DOCUMENTATION

Documentation is an essential aspect of occupational therapy practice and is critical to ensuring best practice and minimizing harm. Occupational therapists must determine the most appropriate type of documentation within their practice area and provide it in accordance with the requirements of their practice settings, agencies, external accreditation programs, referral sources, and, in the expert witness context, the requirements of the court or attorney (AOTA, 2003).

Documentation serves many purposes. First, it provides information on the rationale behind the provision of occupational therapy services. Second, documentation conveys the occupational therapist's clinical reasoning and professional judgment while communicating information about the client from an occupational therapy perspective. Third, it provides a chronological record of the client's status, the occupational therapy services provided, and the outcome of the interventions (AOTA, 2010; Stallard, 2005). Finally, adequate documentation reduces risk and legal liability (Ekelman Ranke, 1998).

AOTA's *Guidelines for Documentation of Occupational Therapy* (2003) explain different types of documentation provided by occupational therapists, the required contents of reports, and the fundamental elements of reports. According to the guidelines, therapists must be thorough in documentation of home modification assessments and must ensure information is accurate. Inadequate or incomplete documentation can lead to misunderstandings, duplication of effort, and errors that can ultimately result in harm. It is generally difficult, if not impossible, to defend poor documentation in court where the attorney's view of a medical record is adversarial (Ekelman Ranke, 1998). The plaintiff's attorney might argue that poor documentation is proof of careless judgment or poor practice. If therapists fail to document proceedings, there is no evidence to prove that it ever happened. For example, if the therapist fails to document a recommendation for grab bars and the patient falls, there is no proof that the therapist made the recommendation (Ekelman Ranke).

Occupational therapists seeking to demonstrate best practice in documenting client information can use the following list as a guideline. Reports are to contain the following:

+ All relevant demographic information about the client including his or her contact details and phone number

+ The date of the home visit and a summary of all people present at that time

+ A summary of the client's health background or disability, functional implications, prognosis, and level of risk of accident or injury and his or her past and present health history as it relates to housing needs

+ The source of the medical or disability information, including the name of the author of reports reviewed and the date of the report, information about the client's self-report, or the therapist's observation of the client

+ Information on the impact of the person's health or disability on his or her everyday roles and activities and how the person presents functionally

+ A statement about the client's anticipated future function

+ Information on the person's mobility, including how he or she manages transfers, use of equipment, and how he or she accesses community facilities

+ Detail about the person's level of independence with respect to completing his or her self-care and homemaker tasks (and any other relevant activities around the home)

+ A summary of the type and level of support services, including current and future need for medical intervention, family or caregiver support, and location of services

+ Equipment dimensions and anthropometric measurements (static and dynamic) where appropriate (including information on future equipment needs where possible)

+ A record of the use of any standardized assessment tools and a statement of the goals set by the client

+ A description of the home and the environmental barriers identified

+ A description of the options considered when discussing the various interventions

+ A list of the client's preferred options

+ Information on the person's preferences, which might differ from the occupational therapist's recommendations

+ The occupational therapist's opinions, including a discussion of concerns where the occupational therapist's and the client's preferences differ

+ A detailed list of the final interventions selected and the reasons as to why they were chosen—for example, to enhance the client's health, safety, independence, and home and community participation

+ A statement of possible risks associated with not proceeding with recommendations

+ An indication of whether the client agrees with the recommended options

+ References to relevant peer-reviewed literature that supports the modifications or specific assistive devices recommended

+ A summary list of the home modification requirements and detailed diagrams in a separate section of the report, to be used by the builder for quoting purposes

+ Information about the author of the report, including name, job title, qualifications, hours of work and contact number; the author's signature; and the date of the report (DeMaio-Feldman, 1987; Dimond, 1997)

Detailed reports are essential where there has been a compromise because of a conflict with client wishes, environmental constraints, service policy, or financial limitations. The occupational therapist must report and document to the employer, insurance company, or service that has engaged him or her any difficulties in negotiating options with the client. It is also recommended that clients sign documentation to indicate that they have declined the suggested recommendations. An example home visit checklist for collection of information in the field, a report template, and an example client report can be found in Appendices E, F, and G.

Documentation must not contain the following:

+ Inconsistencies, mistakes, and omissions that might support the claim of malpractice or raise a question of veracity

+ Inappropriate alterations or extraneous hand-written notes

+ Veiled criticisms of another service provider

+ Alterations or criticisms that may raise concerns about the care provided or the competency of the provider

+ Contradictory or inconsistent sequence of events

+ Documentation of staff shortages that could support a claim of corporate negligence (Ekelman Ranke, 1998)

The nature and type of documentation occupational therapists keep is likely to depend on who requested the home modifications and the type of documentation they want. For example, in the US, an attorney might not want the therapist to prepare a written report as part of a trial strategy; instead, he or she might hire a therapist to complete an assessment only, without any documentation or intervention.

Errors in documentation may result in duplication of effort, poor decision making, inaccurate assessments, and loss of court cases (Dimond, 2004). Inaccurate information will not help the occupational therapist's defense. In serious cases, it can lead to civil or criminal proceedings (Stallard, 2005). All documentation, including notes and reports, must be clear, factual, contemporaneous, comprehensive, relevant, and objective in style (Dimond; Ekelman Ranke, 1998; Stallard). This includes documenting the following:

+ Facts, rather than assumptions, about the situation

+ The time and date of calls therapists made to others, to whom they spoke, and the content of the discussions

+ Evidence of client compliance or non-compliance with instructions

+ Date and time of follow-up visits (Ekelman Ranke, 1998)

Further, occupational therapists should prepare documentation to suit the reporting requirements of the audience or readers (Sames, 2009). Each audience reads documentation with a different focus, depending on their practice setting, education level, understanding of medical terminology, and/or cultural background (Sames).

Occupational therapists should ensure that their documentation:

+ Is jargon-free and written at the appropriate literacy level for the reader

+ Is devoid of spelling and grammatical errors

+ Uses standard abbreviations for the practice area

+ Is legible and written in black or blue ink or typed

+ Is dated and signed and accompanied by the legible name and position of the professional (Ekelman Ranke, 1998; Stallard, 2005)

Illegible or messy handwriting makes deciphering records difficult. It also prevents the reader from discerning information that might lead to provider liability or support him or her in accusations of liability. It may cause mistakes to be made by other providers. Plaintiff's counsel or regulatory agencies can interpret illegible documentation as a deliberate attempt to disguise incorrect decisions or oversight in client care (Ekelman Ranke, 1998). However, as electronic medical records become the norm, this might not present itself as an issue any longer.

An intentional change to another person's documentation is called *spoliation*, and occupational therapists can face discipline if they change records after the fact. For example, once an attorney or a client requests copies of reports or records, the therapist cannot change them. Once therapists submit records to the service or court, including the occupational therapy report and the architect or building contractor's drawings or specifications, they cannot change them. If changes are required, therapists should send them back to the source to request changes before submitting them for use by the service or in court.

Occupational therapists must document the discontinuation of services to ensure comprehensive records of occupational therapy services (Stallard, 2005). Finally, therapists must remember that their records are legal documents that can be entered as evidence in any type of legal proceeding involving malpractice, fraud, negligence, or incompetence. Documentation includes e-mail, rough notes on paper, and any and all references to the patient. Attorneys may present any type of documentation as evidence in a proceeding, without the occupational therapist present to provide further explanation (Sames, 2009).

Recommendations Rejected by Referral Source

Occupational therapists might receive referrals for home modification evaluations where the referral source might not agree with the final proposals. Therapists should document their recommendations based on their professional assessments, client preferences, and consequences to the client if the modifications are not provided. Referral sources make the final decision if they are paying for the modifications and consequently hold the responsibility for choosing an alternative option. Therapists should not alter their recommendations or reports in light of fiscal constraints but rather identify the best option for optimizing the person's occupational performance and discuss relative benefits and limitations of the alternatives. Decisions regarding the affordability of the option should remain the responsibility of the person providing the funding.

APPEARING IN COURT AS AN EXPERT WITNESS

Occupational therapists might need to appear in court because of problems arising from their home modification practice or to provide information as an expert witness. Legal systems generally recognize two types of witnesses—fact witnesses and expert witnesses. Fact witnesses testify as to something they saw, heard, or otherwise experienced first-hand (Carson, 1990). Expert witnesses, as well as testifying as to facts, provide opinions (Carson). The courts decide who may testify as an expert (Carson). For example, occupational therapists with expertise in home modification could testify as to design and modification requirements of the individual (Forrester & Griffiths, 2001).

The right expert witnesses can make or break a case (Friedman & Klee, 2001). However, not anyone can be an expert witness. Courts use specific criteria to determine whether the person qualifies as an expert (DeMaio-Feldman, 1987). The person must possess specialized qualifications or experience, which might include relevant qualifications, such as board certifications, knowledge, experience, and specialized training. An examination of curriculum vitae will provide the court with an overview of the prospective expert witness's training, professional interests, research, and teaching experience (DeMaio-Feldman; Friedman & Klee).

Some courts in the US follow the Supreme Court's decision in the case of Daubert v. Merrell Dow Pharmaceuticals, 509 US 579 (1993). The court limited expert witness testimony to what it considered scientific knowledge that would assist the judge in making a decision. The court announced four factors to consider in determining whether to admit scientific expert witness testimony under the Federal Rules of Evidence.

1. Has the theory or technique been tested?
2. Has the theory or technique been subjected to peer review and publication?
3. In the case of a particular scientific technique, is there a known or potential rate of error and standards controlling the technique's operation?
4. Is the underlying technique generally accepted in the scientific community (Daubert, 509 US 579, 1993)?

An occupational therapist who could not pass the four-factor test as an expert witness could only testify to first-hand knowledge and facts as a fact witness. In such instances, courts would probably exclude reports from nonexperts that contain opinions.

Experts must develop unbiased conclusions as opposed to acting as a "hired gun" to advocate for one specific position (Friedman & Klee, 2001). Experts can provide opinions based on what they know and what other witnesses have told them. This includes their professional opinion about matters related to the case, such as a description of the client's needs for assistive technology in the home and how often specific devices might need replacement.

For the expert witness role, occupational therapists should prepare comprehensive resumés or curriculum vitae summarizing all relevant experience. If requested by the attorney, occupational therapists should prepare thorough reports supported by relevant peer-reviewed literature. Sometimes, because of trial strategy, attorneys might not want experts to prepare anything in writing, including notes.

Occupational therapists have a range of skills to offer the legal system. In civil cases, they can testify about the impact an injury might have on an individual's life, how he or she might manage on a day-to-day basis, and the kinds of home modifications needed to maximize independence (DeMaio-Feldman, 1987). Courts value this holistic approach to evaluating individuals, and an objective expert opinion helps relate judgments to awards of monetary damages for future housing options. Additionally, they can also contribute to, and testify about, design/modifications for future housing needs.

The entry into the expert witness role begins when an attorney (solicitor)—who represents the plaintiff or claimant—or the defendant contacts the occupational therapist to seek assistance with a person's compensation claim. The therapist must evaluate the case to determine whether it is appropriate for his or her area and level of expertise. Potential experts must decide whether they can be fair and impartial or if they have ethical or other reasons not to take the case. Occupational therapists may decline cases if, after reviewing the files, they find ethical or other reasons to turn down a particular case. They must provide clear verbal feedback to the attorney (solicitor) who requested their services so alternative assistance can be sought (DeMaio-Feldman, 1987).

Occupational therapists prepare various types of reports for use in court proceedings. For example, in claims where individuals seek compensation for injuries or losses suffered and to prevail they need to prove negligence and damages, either party's attorneys (solicitors) can request reports that outline needs (Stallard, 2005). In home modification practice, this requires therapists to make a home visit to complete a full housing needs assessment of the home. Various laws and rules exist in different countries, states, and provinces that govern how therapists proceed with their roles as expert. This includes an overriding duty to the court rather than to the person requesting the report (Stallard, 2005). Various rules might also dictate the contents of reports and the scope and duties of the expert. Experts might be subpoenaed and questioned about their expert opinions before administrative bodies, courts, tribunals, or at depositions (Allen, Carlson, Ownsworth, & Strong, 2006).

Insurance companies and employers might request reports where individuals file insurance claims for a work-related or non–work-related accident or injury. Individuals might experience difficulty carrying out their job duties. A housing-needs assessment, as part of the process, will recommend modifications to assist people with managing their work and lifestyle. For example, a person with a disability might need bathroom modifications and a ramp to enable him or her to manage his or her self-care and entrance and exit from home to the workplace.

Preparation and Information Gathering

If requested, the occupational therapist must prepare thorough documentation to help establish the facts and/or assess the person's needs. This includes a comprehensive review of all reports and records provided by the attorney or agency that requested the housing-needs assessment for either new construction or home modification solutions.

To gather information not available in reports and records, the therapist should interview and observe individuals in their homes and complete standardized assessments where possible. Before interviews, the therapist must review available documentation to ensure that he or she is familiar with the individual's situation to date. Conversation with the referral source can provide other unwritten information about the case.

If requested, the therapist must independently prepare an unbiased report. This report should detail specific, factual information that can assist organizations, agencies, or courts to establish the scope of the person's disability, medical condition resulting in disability, and the impact on function and roles. Information is also provided on the outcome of the assessment process and references to supporting research literature. This helps to provide evidence of a clear process for clinical reasoning and justification of recommendations. Therapists may complete the report in consultation with contractors or architects experienced in home modification work. They address the housing-needs assessment report to the court or the party that requested their home modification services, which might include an attorney, case manager, rehabilitation counselor, or insurance adjustor, among others.

Therapists should not imply responsibility for the actual physical modifications in their recommendations. Rather, their report should clearly indicate the needed changes to the contractor or licensed tradesman. The final report should include a description of the home and photographs of areas around the home, with a particular emphasis on the areas to be modified. Diagrams of the existing area and proposed changes also provide the reader with the necessary details of the changes.

Throughout this process, if requested, not only must therapists complete a housing-needs assessment report, but they must also keep other notes on conversations with various parties and the outcomes of any standardized assessments, research, or other activities. This ensures clear information in the record as the work progresses. For court purposes, therapists need to work with attorneys. Attorneys might not want a report or other notes because any written documents are discoverable and can be subpoenaed by the opposing party.

Based on the review of documentation, the attorney might prepare a diary of events, conduct a review of policies and procedures, perform background checks of personnel, and/or review available incident reports (Ekelman Ranke, 1998).

Appearing in Court or at a Deposition

Various authors provide guidelines for professionals who appear in court or at sworn depositions. Some examples include the following:

+ Prepare materials for the testimony carefully to ensure an orderly sequence of materials. Do not bring material to court or depositions unless specifically requested.

+ Speak slowly, loudly, and clearly to ensure the judge and jury can follow the testimony.

+ Answer only the question asked, and avoid unnecessary comments to the judge or opposing counsel.

+ Remain courteous, firm, and even tempered.

+ State qualifications fully.

+ Explain the methods used to reach conclusions and reference the literature that supports opinions presented.

+ Present the testimony convincingly, concisely, and with relevant detail to resolve any doubts in the mind of the judge.

+ Avoid unimportant details and keep to the essentials of the testimony.

+ Indicate when a question requires additional information for a response or whether the question is based on erroneous assumptions (DeMaio-Feldman, 1987).

Some helpful points for therapists to follow to prepare for the role of expert witness include the following:

+ Consult with established experts in the field

+ Visit courts and watch a trial

+ Attend criminal and civil trials to observe other health professionals testifying

+ Visualize oneself giving a high-level performance in the courtroom

+ Visit an empty courtroom to prepare psychologically

+ Prepare—especially prepare reference materials

+ Research and review the relevant peer-reviewed literature

+ Develop good knowledge through reading medico-legal material

+ Study academic literature to seek out evidence to support practice

+ Develop sound public speaking skills (Allen et al., 2006).

CONCLUSION

A range of issues contribute to the complexities of ethical, legal, and reporting practices. Occupational therapists need to familiarize themselves with these issues as described in this chapter and the resources they can use to guide them to make sound ethical and legal decisions. Through increased awareness of legal issues and measures to prevent medical errors, therapists can reduce their risk of exposure to malpractice liability (Ekelman Ranke & Moriarty, 1995). Best practice requires that therapists understand legal processes, such as court proceedings and investigation of malpractice cases, and use clear and concise documentation that comports with legal, ethical, and/or organizational requirements (Ekelman Ranke, 1998) as described in this chapter.

REFERENCES

Allen, S., Carlson, G., Ownsworth, T., & Strong, J. (2006). A framework for systematically improving occupational therapy expert options on work capacity. *Australian Journal of Occupational Therapy, 53,* 293-301.

American Occupational Therapy Association. (2003). Guidelines for documentation of occupational therapy. *American Journal of Occupational Therapy, 57*(6), 646-649.

American Occupational Therapy Association. (2007). Enforcement procedures for the occupational therapy code of ethics. *American Journal of Occupational Therapy, 61*(6), 679-685.

American Occupational Therapy Association. (2010) Occupational Therapy Code and Ehtic Standards. Retrieved from http://www.aota.org/Consumers/Ethics/39880.aspx

Bailey, D. M., & Schwartzberg, S. L. (2003). *Ethical and legal dilemmas in occupational therapy* (2nd ed.). Philadelphia, PA: FA Davis.

Beauchamp, T. L., & Childress, J. F. (2001). *Principles of biomedical ethics* (5th ed.). New York, NY: Oxford University Press.

Bull, R. (1998). Making the most of an occupational therapist's skills in housing for people with disabilities. In R. Bull (Ed.), *Housing options for disabled people* (pp. 40-77). London, UK: Jessica Kingsley Publishers Incorporated.

Carson, D. (1990). Reports to court: A role in preventing decision error. *Journal of Social Welfare Law, 12*(3), 151-163.

Costa, D. (2007). *Clinical supervision in occupational therapy: A guide for fieldwork and practice.* Bethesda, MD: AOTA Press.

Daubert v. Merrell Dow Pharmaceuticals, 509 U.S. 579 (1993).

DeMaio-Feldman, D. (1987). The occupational therapist as an expert witness. *American Journal of Occupational Therapy, 41*(9), 590-594.

Dimond, B. C. (1997). *Legal aspects of occupational therapy* (2nd ed.). Oxford, UK: Blackwell Publishing.

Dimond, B. C. (2004). *Legal aspects of occupational therapy.* Oxford, UK: Blackwell Publishing.

Dobbs, D. B. (2000). *The law of torts.* St. Paul, MN: West Group.

Doherty, R. F. (2009). Ethical decision making in occupational therapy practice. In E. Blesedell Crepeau, E. S. Cohn, & B. A. Boyt Schell (Eds.), *Willard & Spackman's occupational therapy* (11th ed., pp. 274-285). Philadelphia, PA: Lippincott, Williams & Wilkins.

Ekelman Ranke, B. A. (1998). Documentation in the age of litigation. *OT Practice*, March, 20–24.

Ekelman Ranke, B. A., & Moriarty, M. P. (1995). An overview of professional liability in occupational therapy. *American Journal of Occupational Therapy, 51*(8), 671-680.

Fair Housing Act Amendments, 24 C.F.R. § 100.204 (1989).

Federal Tort Claims Act. 28 U.S.C. §§ 1346(b),1402(b), 2401(b), 2671-2680 (1948)

Forrester, K., & Griffiths, D. (2001). *Essentials of law for health professionals.* Sydney, Australia: Harcourt.

Friedman, H. J., & Klee, C. H. (2001). The roles of experts and litigation support consultants in medical-legal claims. *Neurorehabilitation, 16*, 123-130.

Hertfelder, S. D., & Crispen, C. (1990). *Private practice: Strategies for success.* Rockville, MD: AOTA Press.

Health Insurance Portability and Accountability Act (HIPAA) of 1996. P.L.104-191 (1996)

Jarvis, H. (1983). Professional negligence and the occupational therapist. *Canadian Journal of Occupational Therapy, 50*(2), 45-48.

Jonsen, A. R., Siegler, M., & Winslade, W. J. (2006). *Clinical ethics: A practical approach to ethical decisions in clinical medicine* (6th ed.). Stamford, CT: Appleton & Lange.

Kinsella, E. A., Ji-Sun Park, A., Appiagyei, J., Chang, E., & Chow, D. (2008). Through the eyes of students: Ethical tensions in occupational therapy practice. *Canadian Journal of Occupational Therapy, 75*(3), 176-183.

Kohn, L., Corrigan, J., Donaldson, M., (Eds.). (2000). *To err Is human: Building a safer health system.* Washington, DC: Committee on Quality of Health Care in America, Institute of Medicine. National Academies Press

Kornblau, B. L., & Starling, S. P. (2000). *Ethics in rehabilitation: A clinical perspective.* Thorofare, NJ: SLACK Incorporated.

Lohman, H., Mu, K., & Scheirton, L. (2003). Occupational therapists' perspectives on practice errors in geriatric practice settings. *Physical and Occupational Therapy in Geriatrics, 21*(4), 21-39.

Mosey, A. C. (1981). *Occupational therapy: Configuration of a profession.* New York, NY: Raven Press.

Moyers, P. A., & Hinojosa, J. (2003). Continuing competency. In G. L. McCormack, E. G. Jaffe, & M. Goodman-Lavey (Eds.), *The occupational therapy manager* (pp. 461-490). Bethesda, MD: AOTA Press.

Mu, K., Lohman, H., & Scheirton, L. (2005). To err is human! Common practice errors and preventative strategies in occupational therapy. *OT Practice,* September 19, 13-17.

Mu, K., Lohman, H., & Scheirton, L. (2006). Occupational therapy practice errors in physical rehabilitation and geriatric settings: A national survey study. *American Journal of Occupational Therapy, 60*(3), 288-297.

Neeman, R. L. (1979). Specialization: Legal and administrative implications. *American Journal of Occupational Therapy, 33*(2), 118-119.

Opacich, K. J. (2003). Ethical dimensions in occupational therapy management. In G. L. McCormack, E. G. Jaffe, & M. Goodman-Lavey (Eds.), *The occupational therapy manager* (4th ed., pp. 491-511). Bethesda, MD: AOTA Press.

Occupational Therapy Australia. (1994). *Australian competency standards for entry level occupational therapists.* Melbourne, Australia: Author.

Sames, K. S. (2009). Documentation in practice. In E. Blesedell Crepeau, E. S. Cohn, & B. A. Boyt Schell (Eds.), *Willard & Spackman's occupational therapy* (11th ed., pp. 403-410). Philadelphia, PA: Lippincott, Williams & Wilkins.

Scheirton, L., Mu, K., & Lohman, H. (2003). Occupational therapists' responses to practice errors in physical rehabilitation settings. *American Journal of Occupational Therapy, 57*(3), 307-314.

Scott, R. W. (1997). *Promoting legal awareness in physical and occupational therapy.* St Louis, MO: Mosby.

Shannon, T. A. (Ed.). (1993). *Bioethics: Basic writings on the key ethical questions that surround the major modern biological possibilities and problems* (4th ed.). Mahwah, NJ: Paulist Press.

Simon, R. E. (2005). Standard-of-care testimony: Best practices or reasonable care? *Journal of the American Academy of Psychiatry and Law, 33*, 8-11.

Stallard, E. (2005). Legal influences on practice. In T. J. Clouston, L. Westcott, A. Turner, & N. Palastgna (Eds.), *Working in health and social care* (pp. 161-181). New York: Elsevier/ Churchill Livingstone.

Tannous, C. (2000). Therapists as advocates for their clients with disabilities: A conflict of roles? *Australian Occupational Therapy Journal, 47*, 41-46.

Tymchuck, A. J. (1982). Strategies for resolving value dilemmas. *The American Behavioural Scientist, 26*, 159-175.

United States Department of Health and Human Services. (2003). *Summary of the HIPAA Privacy Rule.* Retrieved from http://www.hhs.gov/ocr/privacy/hipaa/understanding/summary/privacysummary.pdf

Van Denend, T., & Finlayson, M. (2007). Ethical decision making in clinical research: Application of CELIBATE. *American Journal of Occupational Therapy, 61*(1), 92-95.

World Federation of Occupational Therapists. (2005). *Code of ethics.* Retrieved from http://www.wfot.org/office_files/WFOTCode%20of%20Ethics%202005.pdf

Wright, M. (1985). Legal liability for occupational therapists. *Canadian Journal of Occupational Therapy, 52*(1), 16-19.

Yarett Slater, D. (2004). Legal and ethical practice: A professional responsibility. *OT Practice,* September 6, 13-16.

14

Evaluating Outcomes

Desleigh de Jonge, MPhil (OccThy), Grad Cert Soc Sci

Outcomes are the end result of the occupational therapy process and describe what an intervention achieves (American Occupational Therapy Association [AOTA], 2008). Evaluating the outcomes of home modifications is an essential aspect of service delivery. At a basic level, a review of a modification immediately following installation allows evaluation of the quality and consistency of service delivery and an opportunity to determine the client's level of satisfaction with the nature and quality of service provided. An evaluation of outcomes can also confirm that the modifications fulfilled the service, client, and household goals and have not resulted in any unexpected negative outcomes. Over time, this accumulated information can inform practice and develop evidence of the efficacy of various environmental interventions. Further, specifically designed evaluations can establish the effectiveness of modification interventions for a particular client population. Systematic and consistent use of outcome measures allows the benefits and cost of environmental interventions to be established and compared with other interventions.

There is a range of measures used to evaluate the effectiveness of interventions, each with a particular focus and purpose. Some document the specific benefits of an intervention to an individual or group of clients, whereas others are designed to capture the outcomes of a particular service or the impact of a particular intervention on a sector of society. The purpose of the evaluation generally determines the type of outcome measures used.

This chapter examines why it is important to evaluate environmental interventions and discusses some of the difficulties in undertaking an evaluation of outcomes and selecting suitable outcome measures. It describes the types and levels of evaluation used to establish the quality, effectiveness, value, and impact of home modifications and the implications for the measures used. This chapter also outlines the range of tools available and their contribution to evaluating home modifications.

CHAPTER OBJECTIVES

By the end of this chapter, the reader will be able to:

+ Discuss the importance of undertaking outcome evaluations

+ Outline the issues in evaluating outcomes

+ Describe the different purposes of outcome evaluations

+ Identify a range of outcomes measures and distinguish their focus and purpose

+ Explain the psychometric properties of measures

+ Describe outcomes measures that are useful in evaluating the outcomes of home modification interventions

Ainsworth, E., & de Jonge, D.
An Occupational Therapists's Guide to Home Modification Practice (pp. 261-286)

Importance of Evaluating Outcomes of Home Modification Interventions

It has become increasingly important to evaluate the outcomes of interventions provided in health and social services, including home modification interventions. Concerns about rising costs of health and social care services, the aging population, inequities and inefficiencies in service delivery, practice errors, and inconsistencies in the quality of services has resulted in many governments establishing accreditation systems to monitor service provision. These systems require services to develop quality assurance frameworks to review, evaluate, and improve the quality and consistency of service delivery and outcomes (Arah, Westert, Hurst, & Klazinga, 2006). Further, a shift to a market-oriented approach to health and social care service delivery that places an emphasis on value for money demands interventions that are both clinically and cost-effective (Laver Fawcett, 2007). These and other developments require therapists to make a meaningful contribution to the review and documentation of processes and outcomes within the health and social care services in which they work. This necessitates that therapists develop measurement strategies to evaluate the effectiveness and impact of the interventions they provide.

Professionals also have an ethical responsibility to evaluate the outcomes of their interventions. All health professionals are bound by a code of ethics, which compels them to make a positive contribution to people's lives (beneficence) and ensures that they do not cause harm (nonmaleficence). Historically, professionals are always assumed to have behaved in an ethical manner. They were rarely questioned about their practice. However, practitioners are increasingly being required to account for decisions and to defend their actions. Occupational therapists are particularly vulnerable to complaints in home modification practice because they are working in a complex environment, and the consequences of an incident or accident resulting from a modification can be significant. Modifications have been found to be unacceptable, ineffective, and, in some cases, harmful (Heywood, 2004a; Heywood & Turner, 2007). Evaluating outcomes enables therapists to confirm that they have improved the client's situation, thus meeting their ethical responsibilities and reducing the likelihood of legal action. Outcome evaluation also provides individual therapists and services with feedback that can be used to improve service delivery and increase effectiveness. This information is essential for informing home modification practice and refining the design of future environmental interventions.

Client-centered practice also highlights the importance of outcome evaluation. A client-centered approach requires therapists to provide clients with sufficient information about interventions to make informed decisions. Clients, increasingly, are becoming well informed and frequently request information on the effectiveness of interventions (DeRuyter, 2001). Consequently, they are less likely to rely solely on professional expertise and anecdotal evidence when making decisions involving expensive changes to their homes. Documenting outcomes assists therapists to clearly communicate the effectiveness of various interventions to clients. Client-centered practice also requires therapists to address clients' priorities and goals. Outcome evaluation affords therapists an opportunity to confirm that interventions have met clients' goals and have not resulted in any unexpected issues.

The demand for evidence-based practice has also heightened the need for outcome evaluation (Laver Fawcett, 2007). Though occupational therapists currently base their modification recommendations on strong theoretical knowledge and experience (Luebben & Royeen, 2005), the profession has yet to establish a body of research to inform and refine home modification practice. In an increasingly competitive funding environment, the profession needs to establish evidence on the efficacy of home modifications and build a body of knowledge on the relative effectiveness of various interventions in order to understand how, what, when, where, and why particular interventions are most effective.

Funding for health and social care services has become increasingly dependent on establishing the cost-effectiveness of interventions. Services are likely to receive funding only if they can demonstrate that their interventions are cost-effective. To date, the effectiveness of home modification has been determined using global measures, such as morbidity, mortality, and quality of life. While these benefits are important, there has been little attention paid to the benefits gained from investing in people's well-being, safety, activity engagement, and participation in the home and community. Information gathered by therapists on the broad benefits of home modifications will assist in identifying the value of these interventions to clients and to the society as a whole and will promote environmental interventions as an investment rather than a discretionary cost (Frisch, 2000; Hurstfield, Parashar, & Schofield, 2007).

ISSUES IN EVALUATING OUTCOMES

Evaluating the outcomes of home modifications presents a number of challenges. Combining to increase the complicated nature of this task are complexities in the way home modification services are delivered, the unique approach and experience of each therapist providing advice, the diversity of people and households undertaking home modifications, and the variety of housing forms being modified.

Home modifications are generally provided in conjunction with a number of other interventions, such as assistive technologies, education and training, and personal care. Consequently, it might be difficult to ascertain the degree to which the modifications are responsible for the outcomes achieved. Service delivery is diverse and fragmented, with modifications being provided within a number of systems with very different briefs—for example, health, home, and social care, housing, and not-for-profit organizations (Jones, de Jonge, & Phillips, 2008). There is immense variation across services in terms of the nature of information collected and solutions provided. This makes it difficult to collate and meaningfully analyze any information that might be collected. Change is best measured by using consistent and standardized measures before and after an intervention. Currently, there are few standardized tools that adequately measure changes resulting from modifications, and these are not routinely used.

To date, therapists have been reluctant to engage in outcome measurement in the area of home modifications. This is largely because service managers and funders have not deemed it necessary and have not allocated time and payment for follow-up and evaluation. Consequently, little is known about the usefulness of modifications once installed. Home modifications, as with assistive devices, are regarded as a practical intervention. It is assumed that once the problem has been appropriately identified and a solution put in place, the problem has been solved and there is no need to evaluate the impact or effectiveness of the intervention. Further, therapists experience difficulties in evaluating outcomes. They often have limited time and find it easier and more informative to use nonstandardized measures, such as observation and informal client feedback (Bowman, 2006). Therapists have also reported difficulty in identifying what and how to measure the outcomes of occupational therapy interventions (Bowman). Limited knowledge of outcomes measures and skill in the use of standardized measures also hampers the evaluation of outcomes (Bowman).

Outcome evaluation is further complicated by the heterogeneity of the clients receiving home modifications, the nature and extent of their impairments, the range of individualized goals, and the variety of interventions used. This variation makes it difficult to identify measures capable of addressing the breadth and diversity in outcomes sought. The complexity of the person-environment-occupation transaction and the home environment also makes it difficult to define the expected outcomes. Further, people's needs and expectations change over time, and these might shift during the process of exploring needs and options. Expectations also influence perceptions of outcomes. The goals people begin with might not be the same as the goals they have at the end of the process, after they have learned what is possible. When developing environmental interventions, people often have to make compromises as a result of the availability of products, the suitability of the design to the existing dwelling, as well as the costs involved. Given their original expectations, these concessions can result in clients having limited appreciation of the effectiveness of the modification.

Poor outcomes can result from any number of reasons other than the suitability of the recommendation—namely, changes in the person's health or social situation since the modification, disruptions experienced during the modification process, or unexpected expenses resulting from the work or quality of the workmanship or quality of the product installed. There are also variables, such as a past negative experience or an unsupportive household, that might also contribute to the perceived failure of an intervention (Gelderblom & De Witte, 2002). Perception of effectiveness can sometimes differ from actual performance, and separating these and other issues can be a challenge when evaluating outcomes.

PURPOSES OF OUTCOME EVALUATION

Despite the complexities inherent in assessing outcomes, it is essential to evaluate the impact and consequences of modifications. Traditionally, occupational therapists have thought about evaluation predominantly in terms of determining an individual's needs. As noted in Chapter 7, therapists use a range of formal and informal evaluation strategies to understand clients' abilities and occupational performance difficulties, and they use information gained from these evaluations to develop interventions. However, evaluating and recording the consequences of occupational therapy interventions is critical to the ongoing improvement of service delivery, ensuring good outcomes for clients, "building a body of evidence to support practice" (Sells, 2005, p. 286), and establishing the value or cost-effectiveness of home modifications. To be successfully undertaken, it is important to first understand the purpose of the evaluation (Barak & Duncan, 2006) because this determines its aim and focus.

An outcome evaluation can be focused on the following:

+ Monitoring the quality and consistency of service provision

+ Determining whether service, client, or therapist goals have been met

+ Building a body of knowledge or evidence

+ Demonstrating the efficiency and value of interventions

Monitoring Service Provision

Many services have some form of quality assurance process in place to ensure the ongoing quality and consistency of service delivery. This level of evaluation is generally concerned with establishing whether the service is responding to and meeting the expectations of the client group in terms of what the service delivers and how it is delivered.

Organizations generally want to confirm that the service has been delivered in a timely manner and that all consumers are satisfied with the level and quality of service. Service managers generally monitor the ongoing responsiveness and quality of service provision using a quality assurance framework. This framework can involve the routine collection of information about the timing of service events or periodic survey of service recipients. Undertaking postmodification evaluations can assess the quality of the completed works with a view to evaluating the workmanship of the contractor and confirming that the work was carried out according to the recommendations and the appropriate building codes.

The main indicators of a quality home modification service are:

+ A timely response

+ Clients feel they are treated respectfully and consulted throughout the process

+ Clients have a clear understanding of the process and the responsibilities of the people involved

+ Clients are satisfied with the service and outcome

+ Clients are satisfied with the quality of the modification

+ Work has been completed successfully and in accordance with recommendations and building codes

+ The modification meets performance expectations in terms of reliability, maintenance, and durability (Rossi, Lipsey, & Freeman, 2004)

Generally, therapists can monitor these outcomes through the following:

+ Reviews of documentation and databases—Tracking service events from date of referral and date of completion

+ Telephone surveys and questionnaires—Seeking clients' feedback on their satisfaction with the service and the modification

+ Auditing the modification work—Designed to evaluate the workmanship of the installation and its compliance with the recommendations and relevant building codes

Therapists can assist in tracking events and developing survey questions to capture the service and outcome quality indicators that reflect the priorities of occupational therapists and their clients. For example, therapists might be interested in knowing the time taken to complete a modification work so they can advise clients of the likely timing of service events. They might also wish to know whether the work resulted in any disruptions to daily routines in the household, so that they can assist clients to prepare for modification work. Therapists would be particularly interested in finding out whether or not the work was completed according to their recommendations and reasons for any incongruencies. This feedback will assist them to understand how well their instructions were interpreted and the factors that prevent recommendations from being implemented.

By evaluating the accessibility, adequacy, appropriateness, and sustainability of the program, occupational therapists can also assist service managers with a broader view of the effectiveness of services. For example, therapists can contribute to the ongoing development of the service by examining whether the program is

+ Reaching everyone with a home modification need

+ Efficient in the delivery of services

+ Providing all of the environmental interventions that are required

+ Supplying the most effective modifications

+ Building adequate structures, resources, and capacity to support the program and the knowledge and skills of its employees long term

By reviewing the demographic data of the population in the area, waiting lists for home modifications services, and hospital admissions and discharge data, therapists can identify people at risk who may benefit from an environmental intervention. A review of the service database will also provide information about the timeliness of response times to those requests. And, by analyzing referral rates and the range of modifications provided, therapists can understand the nature of services provided and where resources need to be invested. This information can also be compared with service events in a similar service in another region so that differences can be identified and analyzed. Information gathered on the return rate of clients and the nature of return requests provides an indication of the effectiveness of previous service events. Finally, information gathered in this type of evaluation can be used to identify where the system requires improvement. These data provide a sound foundation for justifying the development of service structures and resources and building capacity within the system by improving the knowledge and skills of staff.

Determining Whether Goals Have Been Met

While it is important to ensure that the quality of home modification services is consistent, it is equally important to establish that services are making a positive contribution to the client's and family's ability to carry out activities in the home and that the environmental interventions have not resulted in any unexpected or undesirable outcomes.

This type of evaluation ensures that interventions are targeted appropriately. Most home modification services have broad goals of promoting the health, safety, independence, quality of life, home and community participation, and well-being of their clients. In particular, services are generally interested in determining whether the modifications have addressed safety issues and improved the person's independence and quality of life. It is also important at this time to affirm that the environmental interventions have not created any additional safety risks for the client or other householders or any challenges to their independence and well-being.

Occupational therapists and their clients are generally focused on reducing occupational performance difficulties and concerns in everyday activities and increasing participation in the home and community. Clients usually have particular issues they want addressed, and a postmodification evaluation provides the therapist with an opportunity to confirm that the client's specific concerns and other occupational performance difficulties have been adequately resolved. At this point, the therapist might also want to confirm that the client is using the modification successfully and that the home environment—that is, the physical, social, cultural, personal, and temporal aspects of the home—has not been unduly disrupted by the environmental changes.

Routine evaluation of home modification outcomes allows services and therapists to monitor the effectiveness of environmental interventions for individuals and groups of clients as well as their impact on other householders. The main indicators that the interventions have been effective in meeting the goals of the client (and significant others) are that they:

+ Feel their priorities were adequately addressed

+ Are using the solution as intended without adverse effects

+ Have maintained health and increased safety, and have reduced the risk of incident, accident, or injury

+ Are not experiencing any additional risk or difficulties resulting from the modification

+ Have increased independence

+ Experience less difficulty in performing activities in the home and community

+ Are satisfied with their performance of activities in the home and community

+ Have increased engagement in activities in the home and community

+ Do not feel that the home environment or activities of the household have been adversely affected by the modification.

If the therapist has the opportunity to follow up with clients, these outcomes are generally monitored through informal evaluation strategies, such as informal interview or observation. Routine follow-up is essential in allowing therapists to confirm that their recommendations have been useful in meeting the service, therapist, and client goals. Follow-up can also include the use of structured and standardized measures to assist in determining the extent to which the intended outcomes have been achieved. For example:

+ Telephone surveys/questionnaires seeking clients' feedback on their level of satisfaction with the service and modification and how well it has improved their safety, independence, and quality of life in the home and community

+ Structured observation of the client's occupational performance and of obstacles and risks in the environment

+ Standardized outcome measures—Goal attainment, measures of occupational performance and participation, or the accessibility, safety, and quality of the home and community environment. Global measures of quality of life and well-being may be of interest to the service

Building a Body of Evidence

There is a growing requirement for therapists to use evidence-based interventions. Evidence has been described as being derived from a combination of clinical expertise and knowledge and relevant published research (Cohen & Kearney, 2005; Sackett, Rosenberg, Gray, Haynes, & Richardson, 1996). Traditionally, therapists accumulated expertise and knowledge through clinical experience; however, this is not a very effective way for a profession to build a body of knowledge. Further, when a profession does not have a well-established body of evidence, clients can be repeatedly subjected to uninformed advice from novice therapists. Because there is limited research to support practice in this area, it is essential that therapists establish a mechanism for gathering evidence on the effectiveness of home medication interventions.

Therapists generate volumes of detailed data in clinical practice, which can be used as evidence if therapists are systematic in collecting and organizing evaluation data (Cohen & Kearney, 2005). For easy retrieval of this valuable information, individual data can be stored in databases with fields for client demographics (for example, age, gender, health condition, medications), specific goals and occupational performance issues, modifications provided, outcomes achieved, and unexpected events and consequences (Cohen & Kearney). With the accumulation of client information and judicious use of outcome measures, occupational therapists can build a body of evidence to support their home modification practice.

To establish evidence, therapists need information on the following:

+ The number and demographics of people requiring home modifications, the nature of issues they encounter in the home, and the type of modifications undertaken

+ The outcomes of modifications and the extent to which they met client goals and difficulties in the home and community

+ The outcomes of specific home modifications in various situations

+ Whether there were any unintended consequences of environmental interventions

By systematically evaluating the outcomes of various environmental interventions with a range of clients, therapists can gather information on where and when various interventions are most effective. They can then make comparisons between alternative options so they can generate a body of knowledge about the relative effectiveness of various modifications in a range of situations.

Evidence-based practice also requires therapists to review the literature for research on environmental interventions and their effectiveness. To date, research on home modifications has been patchy, unsystematic, and variable in quality (Jones et al., 2008). In addition, many research questions critical to informing home modification practice remain unanswered (Gitlin, 2003). There have been some studies detailing the need and demand for modifications; environmental difficulties experienced by various client groups in the home; the effectiveness of environmental interventions in terms of health, safety, and independence; and their impact on the client's well-being and the home environment. Specific evaluations of the effectiveness of particular modifications, especially in relation to alternative options, are less prevalent. More detailed data collection by therapists regarding the outcomes of home modification interventions and more focused, systematic research on the effectiveness of specific interventions would greatly assist in informing practice in this area.

The Efficacy and Value of Environmental Interventions

Therapists employ a wide variety of interventions, such as home modifications, assistive devices, and in-home care services, to address a range of difficulties experienced by older people and people with disabilities in the home. While these multifactorial interventions have been found to produce savings to health and social care (Heywood & Turner, 2007), little is known about the specific cost benefits of home modifications. Home modifications, in combination with interventions previously mentioned, have been found to reduce the cost of care and improve the outcomes for clients (Heywood & Turner), but more information is required on the cost-effectiveness of modifications specifically and whether some environmental interventions are more cost-effective than others and in which circumstances (Pynoos, Rose, Rubenstein, Choi, & Sabata, 2006).

Cost-effectiveness analysis (CEA) and cost-benefit analysis (CBA) are formal methods for comparing the costs and consequences of an intervention to determine whether the intervention is worth doing

(Rossi et al., 2004). CEA measures benefit in terms of an outcome—for example, health outcomes, quality-adjusted life years (QALYs)—whereas CBA calculates benefit in terms of money—for example, dollar outlays averted (value of reductions in re-admissions to hospitals) and value of life years saved.

Cost-effectiveness and costs benefit analyses need to:

+ Define the intervention under investigation
+ Identify relevant costs
+ Identify relevant effects and benefits
+ Measure costs (direct and indirect)
+ Measure effects and calculate benefits for individuals and the community at large (Rossi et al., 2004)

Once again, therapists can provide input into identifying the direct and indirect costs of environmental interventions and identifying and measuring the relevant effects or benefits of home modifications. Cost considerations include the cost of the investment, maintenance, and services (Andrich & Caracciolo, 2007). For home modifications, these costs are likely to be:

+ The cost of purchasing the products
+ The cost of installation
+ Ongoing maintenance, repair, running costs, and replacement costs over a specified period
+ Additional expenses incurred during the work—for example, replacing electrical wiring to bring it up to the requirements of local building codes
+ Personal support required to use the modification effectively

The benefits of interventions are generally discussed in terms of the benefits to society. For example, the benefit of home modifications is often conceptualized in terms of savings made from reduction of care costs or life years saved. It is in the interests of occupational therapists to contribute to identifying the cost benefits to society; however, therapists are most likely to be able to identify the cost benefits to the client and/or caregivers in terms of increased health, safety, independence, and participation in home and community activities. The benefits of home modification interventions could be identified as:

+ Reduced risk of incident or accident resulting in injury
+ Reduced reliance on formal and informal supports
+ Increased health and independence

+ Decreased difficulty in performing activities in the home and community
+ Increased engagement in activities in the home and community
+ Improved satisfaction with performance of activities in the home and community
+ Improved quality of life

By routinely collecting information on the outcomes of home modifications for each client, therapists can ensure that the benefits for clients (and their caregivers) can be used in CEA and CBA analyses. These outcomes are preferable to the global measure commonly used in these analyses because they acknowledge the impact of these interventions for the clients rather than their general benefit to society. These data will assist in home modifications being reconceptualized as an investment rather than a discretionary cost or substitute for care (Frisch, 2000; Hurstfield et al., 2007).

TRADITIONAL APPROACHES TO MEASURING HOME MODIFICATION OUTCOMES

As discussed earlier in this chapter, there are a number of clear reasons why home modification outcomes need to be evaluated. The question now remains: What are the best ways for this evaluation to happen? To date, most of the evaluations of home modifications have focused on the impact and cost-benefits of environmental interventions, which have been measured in terms of reduced injuries, morbidity and mortality, or the cost of ongoing care. For example, one randomized controlled trial involving 90 frail elderly home-based people found that members of the intervention group, who were systematically provided with assistive technologies and environmental interventions, were found to decline at a slower rate (experiencing reduced morbidity) than the control group and had reduced institutional and in-home personal care costs (Mann, Ottenbacher, Fraas, Tomita, & Granger, 1999). Studies have found that home modifications reduced the hours of unpaid help for wheelchair users who live alone (Allen, Resnik, & Roy, 2006). Other studies have found that home modifications, in combination with other interventions, reduce falls (Gillespie et al., 2003; Nikolaus & Bach, 2003) and other injuries (Plautz, Beck, Selmar, & Radetsky, 1996). Another retrospective study on the costs of home modifications and assistive technologies, using seven detailed case studies, found substantial savings resulting from the interventions (Andrich, Ferrario, & Moi, 1998). Although this information provides funders and policymakers with justification for funding environmental interventions, it provides only indirect evidence of the efficacy of these interventions and does not inform day-to-day clinical practice.

Quality of life has also been used to evaluate the impact of interventions, with modifications or adaptations being found to have a positive impact on people's quality of life (Andrich et al., 1998; Heywood, 2001). As a global measure, quality-of-life measures are relatively inexpensive to administer and are therefore popular in public health and social care settings. Quality-of-life outcomes are also used in the research community (Douglas, Swanson, Gee, & Bellamy, 2005; Haigh et al., 2001) and in economic analyses to review the impact of interventions and compare the cost-effectiveness of various interventions. This information is then used to inform policy, which in turn influences the allocation of funding. Although there are numerous quality-of-life measures available, they are not routinely used in clinical settings (Douglas et al.). These measures provide a mechanism for reviewing the indirect benefits of home modifications and associated interventions; however, they do little to confirm that the client, therapist, and service goals have been addressed. Further, they do not inform therapists about the effectiveness of specific modifications for particular clients.

Traditional measures of functional independence, such as the Functional Independence Measure (FIM; Uniform Data System for Medical Rehabilitation [UDS], 1997), have become benchmarks in outcome measurement in hospital settings, because they allow comparisons across client groups and care settings. Many independence measures developed in the context of rehabilitation in the 1960s and 1970s have been useful in informing and evaluating care by providing information on people's ability to perform the basic activities of daily living (ADL) independently (Jette & Haley, 2005). However, the modest goals of inpatient rehabilitation at that time do not reflect current professional, consumer, and societal expectations of community-based services and interventions (Jette & Haley). Though the values, beliefs, and principles underlying the development of these tools are not always stated explicitly, they are generally embedded in the measure's conceptual foundation, item inclusion, standardization, and scale design (Klein, Barlow, & Hollis, 2008). The purpose of these tools is not well suited to a home modification evaluation. Independence has

not been found to be an effective measure of an individual's ability in daily life or of the impact of modifications (Johansson, Lilja, Petersson, & Borell, 2007; Petersson, Lilja, Hammel, & Kottorp, 2008). In addition, generic scales, such as the FIM, are not very responsive to the impact of environmental adaptations (Klein et al.). Though ADL assessment has historically been a key aspect of occupational therapy practice, the scores on many of these tools are negatively affected by the use of a modification or device and are not sufficiently sensitive to measure changes in performance, such as reduced effort or difficulty. Outcome measures developed within a traditional medical framework are not designed to capture the complexities of the person-environment interaction (Gitlin, 2003) and do not reflect a contemporary understanding of health and well-being.

SHIFT IN FOCUS OF OUTCOMES EVALUATIONS

With the introduction of the International Classification of Function (ICF; World Health Organization [WHO], 2001), the concept of health has been expanded from being an absence of illness to being seen in terms of physical, mental, and social well-being (AOTA, 2008). Health and social care systems are interested in function, well-being, and quality of life rather than just "fixing impairments" (Law, Baum, & Dunn, 2005). Disability is no longer viewed as simply a personal problem, directly caused by disease, trauma, or health conditions, but also as resulting from barriers in the environment (WHO). The ICF has extended the concept of function to encompass engagement in activities and involvement in life (participation), which is seen as important determinants of health (WHO). This framework recognizes the dynamic interaction between the person and contextual factors (Jette & Haley, 2005). Increasingly, it is used to inform outcomes evaluation practices, resulting in a growing number of measures focused on activity engagement, participation, and the environment.

This shift in the focus aligns well with the broad and overarching outcome of occupational therapy services, identified by the *Occupational Therapy Practice Framework* as "supporting health and participation in life through engagement in occupation" (AOTA, 2008, p. 32). Occupation or "daily activities that reflect cultural values provide structure to living, and meaning to individuals; these activities meet human needs for self care, enjoyment and participation in society" (Crepeau, 2003, p. 1031).

Occupational therapy models, such as the person-environment-occupation transactional models, also recognize the role of the environment in occupational performance; however, outcome measures that capture the person-environment-occupation transaction and are responsive to changes are yet to be developed.

SELECTING OUTCOME MEASURES

To date, home modification therapists have mostly used informal and qualitative strategies to determine needs and evaluate the effectiveness of interventions. While these methods allow therapists to deal with the complexity and uniqueness of each person-environment-occupation transaction, they do not allow them to determine the extent of the need or improvement afforded by the modification for each individual or to compare the effectiveness of modifications in different situations. Reliance on informal evaluation strategies makes it difficult to communicate the impact of modifications and accumulated knowledge of the effectiveness of various modifications to colleagues, service managers, and funding bodies. An outcomes-oriented approach to delivering home modification services allows occupational therapists to monitor the impact and effectiveness of specific recommendations and inform practice by building a body of knowledge about the effectiveness of a range of modifications.

The use of standardized outcomes measures would greatly improve practice in this area and would allow data relating to the needs and outcomes of individual clients to be systematically recorded and accumulated to document the needs of the population of which the clients are a part (Sells, 2005). This information could also be used to record the outcomes of the interventions provided by the service for the population being served, which in turn could contribute to a broader understanding of the impact of modifications. A change in the way therapists understand evaluation requires them to not only think carefully about what outcomes to evaluate but to also consider how these are best evaluated.

Sometimes measures are selected because they are easy to use and are readily available, and insufficient consideration is given to their purpose and limitations (Backman, 2005). Because the tools used and the variables measured often become the operational definition for the outcome, occupational therapists need to select outcome measures carefully. For example, the FIM has become the gold standard for measuring independence in ADL. Though

the FIM might be considered to define people's levels of independence, in reality, independence is much more complex. While people who perform well on this assessment might be able to perform the defined activities independently in the hospital environment, this does not ensure that they will be independent at home. First, environmental challenges that are not present in the hospital environment might compromise their performance. Second, being independent assumes that the person can perform tasks safely, confidently, and with ease; however, the FIM does not explicitly evaluate these parameters. Finally, independence in basic self-care tasks is often not a good indication of an individual's ability to cope at home on his or her own because there are many other critical tasks required to ensure health and safety in the home environment, such as cooking, mopping up spills, and taking out the trash.

Outcome evaluations need to be undertaken carefully, ensuring that the outcome tools are:

+ Relevant to the needs and desires of clients

+ Congruent with the practitioner's theoretical model of practice

+ Psychometrically sound (AOTA, 2008)

Client-Centered Outcomes Evaluation

Outcome evaluations have conventionally focused on the person's clinical status as defined and evaluated by the therapist (Law, 1998). However, research on the acceptance and outcomes of home modifications highlight the importance of understanding the complexity of the home environment and the person-occupation-environment transaction and routinely reviewing the effectiveness of the recommended modifications for the client and other householders (Gitlin, 2003).

Many therapists have encountered clients who decline a modification suggestion or refuse the contractor entry to the property once the recommendation has been made. There are many reasons why a client might find a therapist's recommendations unacceptable. First, the client and therapist might have different priorities or concerns. For example, a client might be more concerned about the threat of a home invasion and might therefore not be as concerned with their safety and difficulty in the bathroom. Second, the client might have a specific concern that might not have been fully captured in the therapist's recommendations. Consequently, what the therapist believes to be appropriate might not be acceptable to the client (Gitlin, Luborsky, & Schemm, 1998). Third, clients might also reject a modification if they perceive that it will impact negatively on their sense of independence and autonomy (Messecar, Archbold, Stewart, & Kirschling, 2002). Overemphasis on safety and performance problems can detract attention from other important issues, such as independence, injury prevention, caregiver health, and social integration (Duncan, 1998; Pynoos, 2004). Finally, home modifications have been found to impact negatively on people's self-image and connection with the home (Heywood, 2005), as well as on their routines and sense of heritage when the needs of the person were not fully understood or considered (Heywood). Adaptations to the home can result in people being labeled as different and, more importantly, making them vulnerable to ridicule or violence (Fisher, 1998). It is therefore important that the client's priorities, goals, and preferences are not only considered in designing the modification, but that these are also incorporated into an evaluation of the intervention.

As noted in Chapter 7, evaluation methods, including outcome evaluation, should allow clients to identify their specific concerns about valued occupations, record their unique occupational performance requirements, and document the impact of interventions on their lives (Law, Baum, & Dunn, 2005). This requires that outcome evaluation strategies also:

+ Allow occupational performance issues or problems to be identified by the client and household members and not solely by the therapist and team

+ Permit the unique nature of each person's participation in occupations to be recognized

+ Provide opportunities for both the subjective experience and the observable qualities of occupational performance to be recorded

+ Afford the client (and relevant others) to have a say in evaluating the outcomes of the interventions

+ Recognize the unique qualities of the home environment

+ Assist clients and household members to develop a mutual understanding of therapists' safety, prevention, or health-maintenance concerns (Law & Baum, 2005)

Using a client-centered approach encourages clients to identify goals and outcomes that are meaningful to them (Law, 1998). It also ensures that the factors that affect the client and the way they operate in, and relate to, the home environment are acknowledged (de Jonge, Scherer, & Rodger, 2007). The personal meaningfulness of occupations is also an important consideration when evaluating

outcomes (Klein et al., 2008). Because each individual is unique, this challenges therapists to choose outcome measures that reflect an individualized perspective (Donnelly & Carswell, 2002).

Conceptual Framework for Outcome Evaluation

As noted earlier, there are numerous outcome tools, each founded on a particular theory or understanding and with a specific purpose in mind. The challenge for occupational therapists is to choose outcome measures that are in harmony with the health and social care system in which they work but also reflect the scope and focus of occupational therapy interventions (in this case environmental interventions). Increasingly, the ICF is used to define and organize outcomes and measures around the constructs of body structures and function, activity and participation, environmental conditions, and personal characteristics (Backman, 2005). The ICF aims to provide an interprofessional and international framework for studying and understanding health outcomes, having a means of collecting and comparing data across countries for research, and for developing health and social policy (Hemmingsson & Jonsson, 2005). Its recognition of the relationship between people's daily activities and health and the role of the environment in promoting health make the ICF, and tools developed using this framework, useful to occupational therapists, allowing them to communicate their understandings to others. Although there are a number of commonalities between the ICF and occupational therapy models, it is also important not to underestimate the differences (Kjeken & Lillemo, 2006).

Occupational therapists have a unique and thorough understanding of occupation and its role in promoting health. Further, they appreciate the dynamic interaction between the person, occupation, and the environment. Consequently, they need their own language, frameworks, and tools to develop and evaluate occupational therapy interventions. A number of conceptual models (see Chapter 3) have been developed in occupational therapy to understand and explain the complex reality that therapists encounter in daily practice (Stamm, Cieza, Machold, Smolen, & Stucki, 2006). Whether therapists use these models consciously or unconsciously, they direct clinical decisions and shape choice of evaluation measures and interventions. It is therefore important, when choosing outcome measures, that therapists review the theoretical foundation of the tools and ensure that they are compatible with occupational therapy's conceptual frameworks and goals

(Miller Polgar, 2009). Measures that reflect the aims and principles of occupational therapy practice allow therapists to demonstrate their unique contributions to health and social care (Klein et al., 2008). If the expected outcome of occupational therapy, namely occupational performance, is improved, then "measuring the presence, absence or magnitude of change in occupational performance should be a primary outcome measure for occupational therapy" (Backman, 2005, p. 259).

Occupational performance is variously defined as the experience of being engaged in, or the act of doing and accomplishing, everyday life activities that hold particular value and meaning to the individual, referred to as occupations. It is described as having a subjective experiential element or meaning to the person as well as an objective observable component (McColl & Pollock, 2001). Measurement of occupational performance must therefore capture both the subjective and objective aspects of occupational performance (McColl & Pollock). Occupational therapy's understanding of occupational performance is also guided by a number of pervasive values and beliefs, such as holism, client-centeredness, and the uniqueness of each individual and his or her life situation (Klein et al., 2008). These values and beliefs are reflected in transactional models that recognize the dynamic relationship between the person, the environment, and the occupations in which he or she chooses to engage (Klein et al.). Occupational therapists also see occupational performance in the home environment as an orchestration of valued activities that allow the person to fulfill meaningful roles in the home and community (Crepeau & Schell, 2009; Larson, 2000) rather than a series of disconnected routine tasks. When selecting home modification outcome measures, therapists should evaluate the capacity of each tool to capture these important occupational therapy constructs.

Klein et al. (2008) developed a construct rating review form (Figure 14-1) for reviewing the cohesion between evaluation measures and the value and principles of occupational therapy practice.

This review form alerts therapists to the elements essential to an occupational therapy evaluation of occupational performance. It enables them to select measures that are better aligned with the profession's aims and understanding of people as occupational beings; the dynamic relationship between the person, his or her occupations, and the environment; and the extent to which occupational performance or engagement is afforded by changes in the environment. In their review of existing ADL measures, Klein et al. identified six tools that adequately reflected the values and

beliefs of occupational therapy. The review of these tools explains the dissatisfaction occupational therapists have with existing measures and alert the profession to a need for measures based on conceptual foundations that are better aligned with occupational therapy practice. The profession needs to be actively involved in developing tools that fit well with occupational theory and practice rather than relying on tools developed within other frameworks.

Psychometric Properties of Outcome Measures

All selected outcome measures should have sound psychometric properties, including validity, reliability, responsiveness (Barak & Duncan, 2006; Jerosch-Herold, 2005), and clinical utility (Corr & Siddons, 2005). These properties are important because the quality of the measure impacts on the quality of the data obtained (Gelderblom & De Witte, 2002). When a tool has established validity, you can be certain that it is measuring what it purports to measure and that there is general agreement about what is being measured (Dunn, 2005). A reliable tool ensures that the measures are consistent across time and assessors (Dunn). Tools also need to be responsive to changes in the parameter being measured. Using tools with sound psychometric properties ensures that any improvements detected by the measure are the result of real change and not random error.

The psychometric properties of outcome measures and the quality of data they obtain is not just a concern for researchers. Therapists and their clients also need to be confident in the outcomes measures used. When selecting them, therapists need to consider whether the tool is:

+ Appropriate for the purpose and population for which it is being used (valid for the purpose and application)
+ Able to produce accurate information repeatedly (reliable)
+ Sensitive to small but clinically important changes (responsive)
+ Useful and easy to use (has clinical utility) (Jerosch-Herold, 2005)

Jerosch-Herold (2005) provides a useful checklist for reviewing the validity, reliability, and sensitivity of outcomes measures (Table 14-1).

It is important to remember that the validity, reliability, and responsiveness of tools are not fixed properties; rather, they are influenced by where and how the tool is used (Jerosch-Herold, 2005).

This form is intended to be used for reviewing established ADL measures for constructs identified as important for the assessment of ADL in occupational therapy practice. Please keep in mind the following:

- Each question has some examples that were raised to help illustrate this construct. This is not meant to be exhaustive, just to help recall the construct.
- Many of these measures will not have the construct you are looking for outlined clearly in the supporting documentation (that would be too easy!).

You will need to examine the measure, the way it has the tester examine ADL, and how the tester scores it to see if that particular construct is "implied" or "inherent" by the way it is structured. For example, the measure may not overtly state that they consider the environment, but it may have a place on the score sheet to describe the test environment. For this reason, we are asking you to comment on what drew you to that conclusion about that particular question. This will be very important for our review.

Score measure based on the following scale:
(0) Construct not present
(1) Some elements of construct present
(2) Construct present

	0	1	2
1. Is the measure client-centred? 1.1 Does the measure allow the tester to identify tasks important to the client? For example: • does the test have a total score or can it be done in components valued by the client? • is the measure comprised of a scoring format that allows the client to prioritize tasks where he or she wants to invest his or her energy? • does the measure acknowledge role expectations of self and others (gender, culture, age, how acceptable it is to get assistance from other family members, how the culture values independent occupational performance)? 1.2 Does the measure identify if the client is motivated to learn new ways to be independent? 1.3 Does the measure identify when the client is willing to persist with the task to complete it?			
2. Does the client have a general knowledge of task demands? 2.1 Does the measure identify the client's knowledge of the task demands? • does he or she know the steps of the task? 2.2 Does the measure recognize the client's awareness of strengths, challenges, and ability to prioritize tasks, e.g. decide what he or she wants to invest their energy in doing)? 2.3 Does the measure allow for making informed decisions about taking risks? • is the client aware that going down to the bottom of the tub may increase the risk of a fall, but that is the way he or she wants to do it.			
3. Is the client's performance competent? 3.1 Is task competence identified/defined by the client?			

Figure 14-1. ADL Construct Rating Review Form. (Reprinted with permission from Klein, S., Barlow, I., & Hollis, V. (2008). Evaluating ADL measures from an occupational perspective. *Canadian Journal of Occupational Therapy, 75*(2), 69-81.) (continued)

3.1.1 Does the measure allow for the task success to be defined by the client?
- the client has identified getting clean while bathing as a task that requires submersion in a tub bath, not showering.

3.1.2 Does the measure allow for different ways or processes for completing the task?
- task success vs. doing it "correctly"
- task process is only important if the client has identified that as a concern—such as speed of dressing.
- allows for how the culture affects the way an ADL task is done (China bowl for eating, rather than with plate, knife, fork).

3.2 Where is the performance breaking down?

3.2.1 Does the measure recognize or acknowledge interaction between the person, environment, and task?

3.2.2 Does the measure allow for qualitative observation?

3.3 Does the client have the ability (performance components)?

3.3.1 Does the measure identify or allow observation of underlying performance components (e.g., sensation, motor control, and perception)?

3.4 Are the demands/supports of the task appropriate for the person's ability and environmental situation (i.e., task modification)?

3.4.1 Does the measure recognize/identify modifications needed for success?
- does the measure identify issues related to time restraints – dressing for work/school vs. less pressured time restrictions?
- a client is unable to dress independently due to limited ROM, but would be able to if long-handled aids were available, or a different dressing technique.

3.5 Are the demands/supports of the environment appropriate for the person's ability and task difficulty?

3.5.1 Does the measure identify the "assessment" environment and the demands of the "discharge" or "typical" environment?
- hospital vs. home
- when role requires changing environments for task

3.5.2 Does the measure acknowledge the social support environment?
- does it identify who lives with the client and how much they are able to assist?
- does it identify the client's role expectations of self and others related to how acceptable it is to get assistance from another family member?

3.5.3 Does the measure identify whether financial resources/supports are available?
- does the client have the ability to pay for equipment or environmental modification that may be needed to be independent?

Total Score ____ /60

© **CAOT PUBLICATIONS ACE**

Figure 14-1 (continued). ADL Construct Rating Review Form. (Reprinted with permission from Klein, S., Barlow, I., & Hollis, V. (2008). Evaluating ADL measures from an occupational perspective. *Canadian Journal of Occupational Therapy, 75*(2), 69-81.)

Table 14-1. Checklist for Reviewing the Validity, Reliability, and Sensitivity of Outcomes Measures

RESULTS: VALIDITY YES NO RESULTS
1. Does the measure make intrinsic sense—face validity (expert opinion/consensus)?
2. Does the measure sample the content/domain adequately?
3. Is there evidence of the test's construct validity?
(i) Does the test discriminate between healthy and diseased groups (known-groups method)?
(ii) Do the test values agree with the values of a similar test or gold standard (concurrent or convergent validity) or with a future outcome (predictive validity)?
If yes, then:
(a) What is the strength of the correlation?
(b) What are the confidence limits, if given?
(iii) What is the internal consistency (relevant where scales have multiple items that sum up to a total score)?
RESULTS: RELIABILITY YES NO RESULTS
4. What is the test-retest reliability?
(i) Have appropriate statistical measures been used to assess agreement between two or more occasions using the same observer?
(ii) What is the level of agreement (for example, kappa or ICC)?
(iii) What are the confidence limits, if given?
5. What is the inter-tester reliability?
(i) Have appropriate statistical measures been used to assess agreement between two or more observers?
(ii) What is the level of agreement (for example, kappa or ICC)?
(iii) What are the confidence limits, if given?
RESULTS: RESPONSIVENESS YES NO RESULTS
6. Does the instrument capture clinical change?
(i) What is the magnitude of the responsiveness of the instrument (for example, effect size or standard response mean)?
(ii) Is there evidence of floor or ceiling effects?

(Reprinted with permission of the College of Occupational Therapists Ltd and Christina Jerosch-Herold from Jerosch-Herold, C. (2005). An evidence-based approach to choosing outcome measures: A checklist for the critical appraisal of validity, reliability and responsiveness studies. *British Journal of Occupational Therapy, 68*(8), 347-353.)

For example, a tool designed to assess falls risk in a clinical setting will not be a valid measure of falls risk in a home environment unless validated for that context. A tool designed solely for use with the frail aged is no longer valid if used with young adults. Tools designed to measure changes in quality of life following surgery are not always responsive to subtle changes that occur over time with regular therapy. Measures of independence that penalize the use of assistive technologies will respond negatively to the introduction of aids and equipment. It is therefore important that therapists select tools that are appropriate to the purpose and the population to which they will be applied. The tools also need to be used in accordance with the instructions and scored in the correct manner to retain their validity and reliability (Corr & Siddons, 2005; Sells, 2005). A "pick and mix" approach, where only sections of standardized measures are used, is also not appropriate when using standardized tools because this "invalidates the tool and renders the results meaningless" (Corr & Siddons, p. 204).

To evaluate the psychometric quality of tools, it is useful to understand each of the properties and how these are established.

Validity

As noted previously, validity refers to "the degree to which a test measures the phenomenon that it purports to measure" (Jerosch-Herold, 2005, p. 349). There are several kinds of validity. The types of concern to therapists are face, content, construct, and ecological validity. As the lowest form of validity, face validity is assessed subjectively in terms of whether the items make sense to the assessor and the client (Jerosch-Herold). This ensures that therapists and clients understand what the test is assessing, which is usually established by a number of practicing therapists reviewing the test items.

Content validity refers to the extent to which the items in the assessment fully represent the attribute being examined (Corr & Siddons, 2005). The comprehensiveness of a measure is generally established through consultation with experts and consensus (Jerosch-Herold, 2005).

Construct validity is the extent to which an assessment supports the theory on which it is founded (Crist, 2005). This is generally established by demonstrating that the measure:

+ Correlates with an established test that measures a similar construct (convergent validity)

+ Can differentiate between someone known to experience difficulties and those without concerns (discriminant validity; Crist, 2005)

Convergent and discriminant validity are usually established using a "gold standard," or established tool, as a basis for comparison, with correlations of 0.6 and above being considered excellent (Salter, Jutai, Teasell, Foley, & Bitensky, 2005).

When a test has established content and construct validity, therapists can be assured that the test has adequate theoretical foundation and that experts have confirmed all of the relevant elements. Occupational therapists using tests developed in other conceptual frameworks may, however, feel that a test does not adequately measure the attribute as they understand it or that it does not assess it appropriately. Therefore, although a test may have established validity from one perspective, it might not be adequate within an occupational therapy context. Similarly, validity of an older tool might no longer be considered adequate because understandings of the attribute being examined might have changed. For example, ADL assessments have traditionally focused on determining whether someone requires assistance (independence) in basic self-care activities. Increasingly, however, therapists are concerned with measuring the quality of performance and outcomes of a broad range of daily activities, paying particular attention to the safety and ease of performance.

In home modification practice, less structured measures are considered more suitable because they allow therapists to evaluate the uniqueness of performance within the dynamic person-environment-occupation interaction (Klein et al., 2008). The ecological validity of a measure—that is, the extent to which the assessment reflects performance in the real world (Bottari, Dutil, Dassa, & Rainville, 2006; Sbordone & Guilmette, 1999)—is very important when evaluating a person's performance in the home environment. However, even within the home environment, the use of simulated tasks can limit the ecological validity of measures, such as ADL assessments (Bottari et al.). These tasks are selected and structured by the therapist where environmental elements differ from actual performance—for example, time of day, lighting conditions, time pressures, occupational context of the tasks, and the presence of the therapist.

There have been attempts to improve a number of ADL tools by increasing their ecological validity and the accuracy of inferences based on these assessments. A less structured approach in the natural environment has been used, giving greater consideration to environmental demands and incorporating a larger sample of more complex tasks (Bottari et al., 2006). Criterion-referenced assessments, such as the *Activities of Daily Living Profile* (Dutil, Bottari, Vanier, & Gaudreault, 2005; Dutil, Forget, Vanier, & Gaudreault, 1990), *Assessment of Motor and Process Skills* (AMPS; Fisher, 2001a, 2001b), and the *Performance Assessment of Self-Care Skills* (PASS [Home]; Rogers & Holm, 2007), allow therapists to observe and record performance difficulties experienced by clients when undertaking activities in the usual way and in their natural environment. Occupational performance, therefore, can be measured more accurately than using traditional standardized independence measures (Bottari et al.).

Reliability

While ecological validity requires that measures allow for variability in task performance so that they more accurately reflect real situations, reliability is strengthened by standardization and repeatability of test items (Klein et al., 2008). As noted earlier, reliability reduces the likelihood of measurement error and ensures that the measure is used correctly (intra-rater reliability) and that measurement remains stable over time (test-retest reliability) and across different testers (inter-rater reliability) (Jerosch-Herold, 2005). Intra-rater reliability—that is, consistency in test administration and scoring—requires each therapist to undertake training in using the tool and to calibrate its use regularly

(Crist, 2005). Test-retest reliability is particularly important when measuring changes resulting from an intervention because it ensures that the change in score reflects the true change and is not a result of the instability of the measure (Crist). Inter-rater reliability is reliant on all therapists learning to use the test appropriately, adhering to published administration and scoring procedures (Crist). The reliability of tools is generally reported in terms of correlation coefficients. The closer the correlation between testing events or testers is to 1.0, the more reliable the test is considered (Laver Fawcett, 2007). Correlation scores of 0.7 or more are considered to have high reliability (Corr & Siddons, 2005; Polgar & Thomas, 2000).

A good outcome measure must have good reliability and validity if it is to measure outcomes accurately (Laver Fawcett, 2007). A target analogy, first presented by Pynsent, Fairbank, and Carr (2004), provides a useful illustration of the impact of having neither, both, or only one of these properties present on the accuracy of the outcome. In this analogy, the bulls-eye stands for the true outcome being measured and each arrow stands for a single application of the outcome tool (Laver Fawcett). When a measure is neither valid nor reliable, the arrows are scattered across the target (Figure 14-2A), indicating that the tool is not capturing the true purpose consistently. A measure that is reliable but not valid will have the arrows clustered together closely but not near the bulls-eye (Figure 14-2B), signifying that the tool is reliably measuring something but not necessarily what needs to be measured. A measure that is valid but not reliable will have the arrows near the bulls-eye, but they will be dispersed widely (Figure 14-2C), demonstrating that the tool is appropriately focused but not consistent. Finally, a measure that is both valid and reliable will have the arrows clustered closely together within the bulls-eye area (Figure 14-2D), establishing that the tool is both appropriately focused and accurate in capturing what it needs to measure.

Responsiveness

Outcome measures need to be able to detect small changes over time (Corr & Siddons, 2005; Salter et al., 2005). Some standardized tools are not responsive to changes that result from environmental interventions. For example, measures of independence such as the FIM (UDS, 1997) typically penalize reliance on assistive devices or modifications and do not register subtle changes in performance, such as reduced completion time and improved safety (Corr & Siddons). Consequently, they are not considered responsive or sensitive

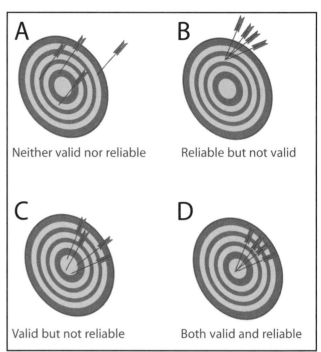

Figure 14-2. Target analogy for reliability and validity.

enough for this purpose. Responsiveness is evaluated using a variety of statistical measures, such as standardized effects size that quantify the magnitude of change (Jerosch-Herold, 2005). These calculations involve correlations where values of more than 0.8 are considered a large effect (Jerosch-Herold; Salter et al.).

Another important consideration in terms of a tool's sensitivity is its capacity to detect changes at the upper and lower ends of the scale (Jerosch-Herold, 2005). If a test is too difficult, scores will cluster at the lower end of the scale and exhibit "floor" effects (Jerosch-Herold; Salter et al., 2005). Alternatively, if a test is too easy, and scores cluster at the upper end, it is considered to show "ceiling" effects (Jerosch-Herold; Salter et al.). Consequently, tests that have floor or ceiling effects will not be sufficiently sensitive to detect changes in people at the upper and lower ends of the range. The size of the ceiling effect is examined by determining the percentage of people obtaining maximum or minimum scores (Laver Fawcett, 2007). If more than 20% of the test population score minimum or maximum scores, the test is considered to have ceiling effects (Salter et al.). It is important that the outcome measures used by therapists are able to detect changes across a broad range of people. Many existing ADL measures fail to determine the full extent of the difficulties people experience in daily activities or the tasks people need to complete safely in order to live a full life. In other words, people are considered capable of performing tasks even when they find them effortful or challenging, or they are assumed independent when there are activities they cannot do.

Clinical Utility

The overall utility of a tool is reflected in its usefulness in a clinical situation (Laver Fawcett, 2007). Therapists are interested in the availability, ease of use, acceptability, portability, cost, administrative burden, and training requirements of a measure (Laver Fawcett; Law, 2005; Miller Polgar, 2009) as well as the meaning and clinical relevance of the information it provides (Miller Polgar). Many valid and reliable tools remain unused if therapists find them too cumbersome, complicated, or time-consuming to administer (Laver Fawcett). Equally, the measure must provide information that is useful in informing clinical practice or determining the impact of the intervention. As discussed earlier, global measures, such as measures of independence, provide little information on the specific difficulties someone is experiencing in carrying out a task and cannot establish whether an intervention addresses these specific difficulties.

Existing Outcome Measures

A range of outcome measures has been developed, each with a particular focus. They come in a variety of formats: self-administered questionnaires and interviewer-administered telephone interviews, face-to-face interviews, or computerized/Web-based interviews with the client or a proxy, such as a family member (Barak & Duncan, 2006). In addition, a number of observational assessments can be undertaken by a trained assessor.

Outcome measures have been designed to measure a range of domains. Traditionally, measurement has focused on evaluating body structure and functions; however, with the introduction of the ICF, there has been an increased number of tools developed to examine activity performance and participation and aspects of the environment. In home modification practice, therapists are most interested in measuring the impact of the intervention on:

+ The person's (or caregiver's) physical and mental health and well-being

+ Occupational performance and participation

+ Aspects of the home environment and the person's experience of home

Measures of Physical and Mental Health

Modifications are designed to reduce the environmental "press" placed on people within and around the home. Environmental interventions can reduce physical and mental stress by decreasing physical or cognitive effort or the pain and difficulty an individual experiences when completing activities. For some people, especially those who spend a lot of time at home or have mental health vulnerabilities, the general ambiance of the home can also affect their mood or mental health. In addition, modifications can increase an individual's sense of safety and security, self-efficacy, general well-being, and quality of life (Jones et al., 2008).

Therapists can obtain an objective measure of the effort involved in completing tasks by various means—for example, by taking the person's pulse rate or recording the time taken to perform tasks. Some ADL assessments, used primarily to determine a person's specific performance difficulties during activities, might also be useful in identifying changes in performance once the environment has been modified. Tools, such as the AMPS (Fisher, 1995), the PASS (Rogers & Holm, 1994), and the *Activities of Daily Living Profile* (Dutil et al., 2005), allow therapists to observe how well the individual manages the physical and cognitive demands of various activities. Changes in performance might be noted if environmental barriers are removed or facilitators introduced. For example, reduced physical demands might be observed in the showering task when a step into the shower is removed and a grab rail is installed; and decreased cognitive demands might be observed during a coffee-making task when the required items are moved and stored within the person's field of vision.

There are also a number of standardized self-report measures that evaluate perceived efficacy and pain. Self-efficacy questionnaires have been found to be useful in examining people's confidence in various activities. The *Falls Efficacy Scale* (FES; Tinetti, Richman, & Powell, 1990) was modified by Sanford and colleagues (2006) to evaluate people's confidence in performing 10 household activities on a scale of 1 (not confident at all) to 10 (completely confident). Questions in the FES—such as "How confident are you in performing the following activities without falling?"—were adapted by removing the words "without falling" from the end of each question. Activities included in the measure were getting dressed and undressed, cleaning the house, preparing simple meals, bathing, shopping, going up and down stairs, reaching into cabinets or cupboards, getting in and out of a chair, walking around the neighborhood, and hurrying to answer the phone.

Pain experienced during activities can be evaluated using the dedicated pain questionnaires and various verbal, visual, and picture pain-rating scales (Patterson, Jensen, & Engel-Knowles, 2002).

Common pain measures include the *McGill Pain Questionnaire* (Melzack, 1975) and the *Faces Pain Scale* (Bieri, Reeve, Champion, Addicoat, & Ziegler, 1990). Tools have also been developed to evaluate the level of burden or stress on caregivers in terms of their physical and mental health, disruption to family life, and financial difficulties (Gupta, 2008). The *Caregiver Strain Index* (Robinson, 1983) is brief and easily administered and is one of the most commonly used scales for caregiver burden (Post, Festen, van de Port, & Visser-Meily, 2007). This tool contains 13 statements related to strain experienced by caregivers. If the caregiver agrees with seven or more statements, he or she is considered to be experiencing a high level of burden (Robinson). The *Perceived Change Index* (PCI) has also been used to examine the impact of home modification and related interventions on caregiver well-being (Gitlin, Hauck, Winter, Dennis, & Schulz, 2006). This is a 13-item scale, including, for example, change in affect, ability to manage difficult behaviors, and somatic feelings (fatigue). The caregiver rates how often in the past month things have become worse or improved, using a 5-point Likert scale (Gitlin, Winter, Dennis, & Hauck, 2006). Measures of mood states, such as the *Beck Depression Inventory II* (BDI-II; Beck, Ward, Mendelson, Mock, & Erbaugh, 1961), might also be useful in measuring changes in mood following modifications to the home. It is important, however, when using these generic measures to assess mental well-being, to be aware of the many other factors that can contribute to fluctuations in mood.

As discussed previously, global measures of quality of life and well-being have become increasingly popular in health and social settings when measuring and comparing the impact of various interventions. There are a number of quality-of-life measures available. One of the most popular is the *Short Form 36* (SF-36; Ware, Snow, Kosinski, & Gandek, 1993), a self-report survey comprising 36 questions. The scale measures eight dimensions—namely, vitality, physical functioning, bodily pain, general health perceptions, physical role functioning, emotional role functioning, social role functioning, and mental health. It provides functional health and well-being scores as well as psychometrically based physical and mental health summary measures and a preference-based health utility index (Ware & Sherbourne, 1992). However, it is important to be aware that quality-of-life measures are not without criticism. Quality of life is considered by some to be a dynamic construct, the reference value of which might not remain constant (Allison, Locker, & Feine, 1997; Carr, Gibson, & Robinson, 2001). People's expectations can have an impact on their perceptions of quality of life. Those with high expectations find changes in the environment to have less of an impact than those with low expectations. In addition, this construct has been linked to personality (DeNeve, 1999) and core affects (Davern, Cummins, & Stokes, 2007), thus making measures of quality of life vulnerable to individual interpretations of life events.

Measures of Occupational Performance and Participation

Occupational therapists need to use valid and reliable measures of occupational performance and participation if they are to establish the efficacy of their interventions (Law, Baum, & Dunn, 2005). It is believed that modifications enable people to be more independent in daily activities and to increase their participation in the home and the community. There is an ever-growing number of tools available that measure occupational performance and participation.

Some tools, such as the *Canadian Occupational Performance Measure* (COPM; Law et al., 1998), are used to gain an understanding of the client's current occupational performance goals and perceptions of performance. This individualized evaluation tool uses a semi-structured interview to identify specific problems in occupational performance areas, such as self-care, work, and leisure. It allows clients to rate the importance of each problem on a scale of 1 (not important) to 10 (very important) and their perceptions of their current level of performance and satisfaction with their performance are rated on scales of 1 (unable to perform, not satisfied) to 10 (able to perform, extremely satisfied). This tool can then be used to assess changes in their perceptions following an environmental intervention. The COPM has been used with a variety of client groups in practice and in outcomes research over the last decade (Carswell et al., 2004). More specifically, a number of studies have used it to determine the impact of rehabilitation (Donnelly et al., 2004) and home modifications (Stark, 2004). The COPM has been found to be sensitive to changes that result from home modifications and to provide information that cannot be obtained from less individualized measures (Dedding, Cardol, Eyssen, Dekker, & Beelen, 2004). A systematic review of the COPM undertaken by Parker and Sykes (2006) demonstrates the value of the COPM in promoting client-centered practice and evaluating occupational performance outcomes.

Though self-report measures provide a perception of ability, they do not provide therapists with detailed information on the quality of performance. Occupational therapists have used a range of measures to standardize their observations of occupational performance. Some tools allow therapists to rate the person's level of independence—for example, the FIM (UDS, 1997); however, as discussed previously, many of these tools are not sensitive to changes in the quality of performance that result from environmental interventions. Increasingly, therapists are seeking outcome measures that also allow them to record changes in the safety and quality of performance of everyday activities in the home. Measures such as the *Activities of Daily Living Profile* (Dutil et al., 1990, 2005), AMPS (Fisher, 2001a, 2001b), and the PASS (Home) (Rogers & Holm, 1994), which allow the therapist to observe the person undertaking relevant tasks in the usual way in his or her own environment, are best suited to evaluating home modifications. Although these tools require specialist training and have setup requirements, they do enable therapists to evaluate changes in performance.

In particular, the home version of the PASS includes 26 core tasks: functional mobility (5), personal self-care (3), instrumental activities of daily living with cognitive emphasis (14), and instrumental activities of daily living with physical emphasis (4) (Rogers & Holm, 2007). Therapists can select tasks relevant to the client's priorities or lifestyle or use a template to develop a criterion for a specific task of importance to the client. The tool allows therapists to identify the precise point of task breakdown and to record the independence, safety, adequacy of the process, and outcome of each task using a 4-point scale, where 0 = unable to complete/requires maximum assistance or unacceptable level of safety or quality and 4 = independent, safe, and acceptable performance. The PASS has been established as being a valid and reliable tool for evaluating the occupational performance of women with depression (Holm & Rogers, 1999) and has been used to describe activity outcomes for people with a range of medical conditions (Skidmore, Rogers, Chandler, & Holm, 2006).

The *Client-Clinician Assessment Protocol* (C-CAP) was also designed to assess an individual's performance in activities in terms of independence, difficulty, and safety. It uses both self-report and observation of 22 activities, including mobility and personal and instrumental activities of daily living (Thomas Jefferson University, n.d.). It has four parts: Part I is a client self-report of perceived ability to perform daily life tasks and Parts II through IV consist of performance-based assessments of the client's ability to perform daily life tasks and the impact the home environment has on occupational performance (Petersson, Fisher, Hemmingsson, & Lilja, 2007).

Measures of participation would also be useful in examining the full impact of home modifications. People have described modifications as a "godsend" (Jones et al., 2008) and as releasing them from being a prisoner in their own home (Heywood, 2004b). This suggests that modifications allow people to achieve much more than successfully completing nondiscretionary activities within the home. Access into, within, around, and out of the house can have a substantial impact on an individual's ability to participate actively. Increased independence, ease, and safety in undertaking daily activities within the home also afford people the time and energy to invest in family and community activities. Measures such as the *Activity Card Sort* (ACS; Baum & Edwards, 2001) allow therapists to compare the number of activities someone was able to participate in prior to the modification and following the intervention. This tool uses a Q-sort methodology to get clients to sort 80 photographs of instrumental, low-demand and high-demand, and social leisure activities into groups of never done, not done as an older adult, do now, do less, or given up (Law, Dunn, & Baum, 2005). It is available for older adults and children and has been developed for use in a number of countries. Although not used to date in research related to the outcomes of home modifications, this tool has great potential for examining the broader impact of home modifications on the person's participation.

The ICF also provides a checklist of activities (WHO, 2005). These include learning and applying knowledge; general tasks and demands; communication; mobility; self-care; domestic life; interpersonal relationships; major life areas such as work; and community, social, and civic life, which can evaluate an individual's performance in activities and participation domains. The performance qualifier measures the difficulty an individual experiences when undertaking various activities using scores that range from 0 (no difficulty in performance) to 4 (complete difficulty)—that is, there is a problem present more than 95% of the time with an intensity that totally disrupts the person's day-to-day life (WHO). This checklist is useful when comparing the person's level of activity engagement and participation pre- and postmodification.

A range of outcome tools has also been developed to measure the quality of activity engagement and level of participation in various aspects of community life. Global tools, such as OTFACT (Smith, 2002) and the *Assessment of Life Habits* (LIFE-H; Noreau, Fougeyrollas, & Vincent, 2002), examine people's level of engagement in an extensive range of activities and participation across life areas. OTFACT (Smith) and the developing ICFFACT software-based data collection system enable therapists to record performance in a range of activities. It uses the Trichotomous Tailored Sub-branching Scaling (TTSS) to customize the question set to the specific needs of the client (Smith). The TTSS system provides a mechanism for customizing scales to the needs of each individual. As issues are identified in an area, the software branches out, breaking the activity into subsections so that discrete aspects of the performance can be examined in detail (Smith). A percentage score is then calculated for activities, relevant to the individual where he or she is not able to fully participate. Therapists can then compare scores obtained prior to the modification with scores obtained post-modification.

Autonomy is another important aspect of participation and outcome of home modifications. The Impact of *Participation and Autonomy Questionnaire* (IPA) examines the extent of autonomy people experience in their day-to-day lives (Cardol, de Haan, de Jong, van den Bos, & de Groot, 2001). The IPA is a 39-item questionnaire that examines an individual's perceived participation and perceived problems in a range of domains, such as autonomy indoors and outdoors, family role, social situations, and paid work and education. Perceived participation is rated on a five-point scale, with 1 being very good and 5 being very poor (Cardol et al.). Perceived problems are rated from being no problem (0) to a severe problem (2). Although, to date, the IPA has been used to examine participation and perceived problems of people with spinal cord injuries (Lund, Nordlund, Nygard, Lexell, & Bernspang, 2005), it has not been used to examine the impact of home modifications.

Measures of the Home Environment

Many standardized measures of the environment have been developed with the purpose of identifying safety hazards—for example, the *Home Falls and Accident Screening Tool* (HOME FAST; Mackenzie, Byles, & Higginbotham, 2000), the *Home Environmental Assessment Protocol* (HEAP; Gitlin et al., 2002), and the *Westmead Home Safety Assessment* (WESHA; Clemson, 1997). Other developed standardized measures determine the accessibility of the environment—for example, the Americans with Disabilities Act (ADA) *Checklist for Existing Facilities* (Adaptive Environments, 1995). These tools evaluate the environment based on a recognized set of risks or an established standard, such as the ADA. Other tools, such as the *Safety Assessment of Function and the Environment for Rehabilitation* (SAFER; Oliver, Blathwayt, Brackley, & Tamaki, 1993) and the *Housing Enabler* (Iwarsson & Slaug, 2001), have been designed to evaluate the person-environment fit.

Although these tools are useful in identifying needs and confirming that identified risks or barriers have been removed, they are not suited to assessing the suitability or effectiveness of an environmental intervention in supporting or promoting occupational performance in the home or its impact on various dimensions of the home environment. Furthermore, they are not sufficiently sensitive to detect changes resulting from modifications. In recognition of the limitations of existing measures, Chiu and Oliver (2006) revised the SAFER to evaluate the effectiveness of intervention in addressing home safety concerns.

SAFER-HOME v.2 (Chiu & Oliver, 2006) allows therapists to use a combination of interviews, observation, and task performance to rate the safety of 93 activities. It consists of 10 domains: meal preparation (10 items), awareness of safety hazards (19 items), mobility and toileting (17 items), cognitive impairment (8 items), homemaking support (7 items), emergency communication (6 items), functional communication (6 items), personal care (6 items), family assistance (10 items), and medication (4 items). The binary scale in the original SAFER tool was expanded to a 4-point scale, where 1 = no identified concern and 4 = severe problem, high safety risk to client's function and/or environment (with 67% to 100% chance of negative consequences; Chiu & Oliver). Although this tool has not been used extensively in practice to date, it is well grounded in theory and has been carefully developed (Cooper, Letts, Rigby, Stewart, & Strong, 2005). Further, it has been found to be clinically useful, practical to administer, and sensitive in detecting changes (Chiu & Oliver). Using a factor analysis of 1,173 observations, Chiu and Oliver performed factor analysis and found the tools had an internal consistency coefficient alpha value of 0.86. Though test-retest reliability was established for the total score, only moderate reliability was established for the subscales. Weak correlation with another functional assessment supported the hypothesis that home safety was related, but not limited, to functioning (Chiu & Oliver).

Measures have been developed to assess the perceived quality of housing. These measures have been used in cross-cultural research to examine the relationship between perceived housing and healthy aging outcomes in very old age and could be useful in evaluating the impact of modifications on householders' perceptions of usability, meaning, and housing-related control beliefs. Usability in this instance is defined as the extent to which an individual's housing needs and preferences can be fulfilled with respect to activity performance in the home (Fänge & Iwarsson, 2005a). The *Usability in My Home* (UIMH; Fänge, 2002; Fänge & Iwarsson, 1999) is a self-administered questionnaire that asks clients to rate the usability of various aspects of the environment using a 7-point scale, with 7 indicating the most positive response alternative. Its 16 items target physical, activity, and personal/social aspects of the home environment. The authors of the UIMH have carefully developed this tool, establishing usability as a valid construct with three independent aspects (Fänge & Iwarsson, 2003, 2005b) and using an expert panel to establish content validity. The tool was also determined to have moderate to very good test-retest reliability with agreement for each item achieving correlation scores between 0.57 and 0.88 (Fänge & Iwarsson, 1999).

The meaning of the home concept incorporates subjective evaluations, values, goals, cognitions, and emotions of an individual in relation to his or her home (Marcus, 1995; Moore, 2000; Nygren et al., 2007; Oswald & Wahl, 2005). The *Meaning of Home Questionnaire* (MOH; Oswald et al., 2006) is another self-administered questionnaire that examines four different aspects of the meaning of home: physical (7 items), such as "being at home means for me living in a place that is well designed and geared to my needs"; activity (6 items), such as "being able to do whatever I please"; cognitive/emotional (10 items), such as "feeling comfortable and cozy"; and social (5 items), such as "being able to receive visitors" (Iwarsson, Horstmann, & Slaug, 2007; Nygren et al.). Factor analysis and structural equation modeling (SEM) techniques have been used to confirm four component models of perceived housing, which has held up in cross-cultural analysis of the same (Oswald et al.).

Another tool that has proved useful in examining perceptions of control in the home environment is the *Housing-Related Control Beliefs Questionnaire* (HCQ; Oswald, Wahl, Martin, & Mollenkopf, 2003). This 24-item questionnaire uses a five-point scale to measure agreement with statements based on the psychological dimensions of internal control (8 items); external control: powerful others (8 items); and external control: chance (8 items; Iwarsson et al., 2007). The Internal Control subscale examines housing events related to a person's own behavior, such as "I have been able to set up my home in accordance with my own personal ideas," "Everything in my home will stay the way it is; no one is going to tell me what to do," or "I myself decide whose help to accept within or outside my home" (Oswald, Wahl, Schilling, & Iwarsson, 2007). The two external control subscales examine events related to another person and chance, such as "Other people have told me how to arrange the furnishings in my home,"

"Whether I can stay in my home depends on luck and circumstance," or "Where and how I live has happened more by chance" (Oswald et al., 2007). To date, only internal consistency has been established for the external control dimensions of this tool (Iwarsson et al.).

CONCLUSION

This chapter has discussed the importance of evaluating the outcomes of home modifications. The rising costs of health and social care services, the aging population, inequities and inefficiencies in service delivery, practice errors, and inconsistencies in the quality of services have resulted in governments establishing accreditation systems to monitor service provision. The profession's ethical responsibilities and client-centered approach also require therapists to continually monitor their clients' outcomes and establish evidence to support their recommendations. Without adequate proof of the effectiveness of home modification interventions, occupational therapists and the services they provide are at risk of losing funding. A number of challenges to evaluating the outcomes of home modifications have been presented—namely, the complexities in the way home modification services are delivered, the unique approach and experience of each therapist providing advice, the diversity of people and households undertaking home modifications, and the variety of housing forms being modified—all of which combine to increase the complexity of this task.

The chapter reviewed four different purposes of outcome evaluation, each with a particular focus. Outcome evaluations can focus on monitoring the quality and consistency of service provision; determining whether service, client, or therapist goals have been met; building a body of knowledge/evidence; or demonstrating the efficiency and value of interventions. This chapter outlined the indicators of quality or effectiveness for each of these approaches and detailed how therapists can gather information to contribute to these evaluations in a way that informs day-to-day home modification practice.

A shift in the definition of health has resulted in traditional approaches to measurement being less appropriate in this community context. This chapter discussed the importance of choosing evaluation tools that are client centered and in line with occupational therapy's values and principles and conceptual frameworks. In particular, it highlighted the value of choosing tools that reflect an individualized perspective, focus on occupational performance, and recognize the dynamic interaction between person, occupation, and environment. The chapter also emphasized the value of using tools with sound psychometric properties. It described validity, reliability, responsiveness, and clinical utility and the role of each in ensuring the quality of the data gathered.

Finally, this chapter reviewed a range of outcome measures that are well suited to gathering information on the impact of home modification on the physical and mental health of clients, their occupational performance and participation, as well as their perceptions and experience of the home environment.

REFERENCES

Adaptive Environments. (1995). *Checklist for existing facilities.* Boston, MA: Author.

Allen, S., Resnik, L., & Roy, J. (2006). Promoting independence for wheelchair users: The role of home accommodations. *Gerontologist, 46*(1), 115-123.

Allison, P., Locker, D., & Feine, J. (1997). Quality of life: A dynamic concept. *Social Science Medicine, 45*(2), 221-230.

American Occupational Therapy Association. (2008). Occupational therapy practice framework: Domain and process (2nd ed.). *American Journal of Occupational Therapy, 62*, 625-683.

Andrich, R., & Caracciolo, A. (2007). Analysing the cost of individual assistive technology programs. *Disability and Rehabilitation: Assistive Technology, 2*(4), 207-234.

Andrich, R., Ferrario, M., & Moi, M. (1998). A model of cost-outcome analysis for assistive technology. *Disability and Rehabilitation, 20*(1), 1-24.

Arah, O. A., Westert, G. P., Hurst, J., & Klazinga, N. S. (2006). A conceptual framework for the OECD health care quality indicators project international. *Journal for Quality in Health Care, 18* (Suppl. 1), 5-13.

Backman, C. L. (2005). Outcomes and outcome measures: Measuring what matters is in the eye of the beholder. *Canadian Journal of Occupational Therapy, 72*(5), 259-261.

Barak, S., & Duncan, P. W. (2006). Issues in selecting outcome measures to assess functional recovery after stroke. *NeuroRx: The Journal of the American Society for Experimental NeuroTherapeutics, 3*, 505-524.

Baum, C., & Edwards, D. (2001). *Activity card sort.* St. Louis, MO: Washington University at St. Louis.

Beck, A. T., Ward C. H., Mendelson, M., Mock, J., & Erbaugh, J. (1961). An inventory for measuring depression. *Archives of General Psychiatry, 4*, 561-571.

Bieri, D., Reeve, R. A., Champion, G. D., Addicoat, L., & Ziegler, J. B. (1990). The Faces Pain Scale for the self-assessment of the severity of pain experienced by children: Development, validation and preliminary investigation for ratio scale properties. *Pain, 41*, 139-150.

Bottari, C., Dutil, E., Dassa, C., & Rainville, C. (2006). Choosing the most appropriate environment to evaluate independence in everyday activities: Home or clinic? *Australian Occupational Therapy Journal, 53*(2), 98-106.

Bowman, J. (2006). Challenges to measuring outcomes in occupational therapy: A qualitative focus group study. *British Journal of Occupational Therapy, 69*(10), 464-472.

Cardol, M., de Haan, R. J., de Jong, B. A., van den Bos, G. A., & de Groot, I. J. (2001). Psychometric properties of the questionnaire Impact on Participation and Autonomy Questionnaire. *Archives of Physical Medicine and Rehabilitation, 82*, 210-216.

Carr, A. J., Gibson, B. A., & Robinson, P. G. (2001). Is quality of life determined by expectations or experience? *British Medical Journal, 322*, 1240-1243.

Carswell, A., McColl, M. A., Baptiste, S., Law, M., Polatajko, H., & Pollock, N. (2004). The Canadian Occupational Performance Measure: A research and clinical literature review. *Canadian Journal of Occupational Therapy, 71*(4), 210-222.

Chiu, T., & Oliver, R. (2006). Factor analysis and construct validity of the SAFER-HOME. *Occupational Therapy Journal of Research: Occupation, Participation and Health, 26*(4), 132-142.

Clemson, L. (1997). *Home fall hazards: A guide to identifying fall hazards in the homes of elderly people and an accompaniment to the assessment tool the Westmead Home Safety Assessment.* Victoria, Australia: Co-ordinates Publications.

Cohen, M. E., & Kearney, P. J. (2005). Use of evaluation data to support evidence-based practice. In J. Hinojosa, P. Kramer, & P. Crist (Eds.), *Evaluation: Obtaining and interpreting data* (pp. 263-282). Bethesda, MD: AOTA Press.

Cooper, B., Letts, L., Rigby, P., Stewart D., & Strong, S. (2005). Measuring environmental factors. In M. Law, C. Baum, & W. Dunn (Eds.), *Measuring occupation performance: Supporting best practice in occupational therapy* (pp. 316-344). Thorofare, NJ: SLACK Incorporated.

Corr, S., & Siddons, L. (2005). An introduction to the selection of outcome measures. *British Journal of Occupational Therapy, 68*(5), 202-206.

Crepeau, E. (2003). Analysing occupation and activity: A way of thinking about occupational performance. In E. Crepeau, E. Cohn, & B. Schell (Eds.), *Willard & Spackman's occupational therapy* (10th ed., pp. 189-198). Philadelphia, PA: Lippincott Williams & Wilkins.

Crepeau, E., & Schell, B. (2009). Analysing occupations and activity: A way of thinking about occupational performance. In E. Crepeau, E. Cohn, & B. Schell (Eds.), *Willard & Spackman's occupational therapy* (11th ed., pp. 359-374). Philadelphia, PA: Wolters Kluwer Lippincott Williams & Wilkins.

Crist, P. (2005). Reliability and validity: The psychometric properties of standardized assessments. In J. Hinojosa, P. Kramer, & P. Crist (Eds.), *Evaluation: Obtaining and interpreting data* (pp. 175-194). Bethesda, MD: AOTA Press.

Davern, M. T., Cummins, R. A., & Stokes, M. A. (2007). Subjective wellbeing as an affective-cognitive construct. *Journal of Happiness Studies, 8*(4), 429-499.

de Jonge, D., Scherer, M. J., & Rodger, S. (2007). *Assistive technologies in the workplace.* St. Louis, MO: Mosby.

Dedding, C., Cardol, M., Eyssen, I. C., Dekker, J., & Beelen, A. (2004). Validity of the Canadian Occupational Performance Measure: A client-centred outcome measurement. *Clinical Rehabilitation, 18*(6), 660-667.

DeNeve, K. M. (1999). Happy as an extroverted clam? The role of personality for subjective well-being. *Current Directions in Psychological Science, 8*(5), 141-144.

DeRuyter, F. (2001). Outcomes and performance monitoring. In D. A. Olson & F. DeRuyter (Eds.), *Clinician's guide to assistive technology* (pp. 67-74). St. Louis, MO: Mosby.

Donnelly, C., & Carswell, A. (2002). Individualized outcome measures: A review of the literature. *Canadian Journal of Occupational Therapy, 69*(2), 84-94.

Donnelly, C., Eng, J. J., Hall, J., Alford, L., Giachino, R., Norton, K., & Kerr, D. S. (2004). Client-centred assessment and the identification of meaningful treatment goals for individuals with a spinal cord injury. *Spinal Cord, 42*(5), 302-307.

Douglas, H., Swanson, C., Gee, T., & Bellamy, N. (2005). Outcome measurement in Australian rehabilitation environments. *Journal of Rehabilitation Medicine, 37*(5), 325-329.

Duncan, R. (1998). Blueprint for action: The National Home Modifications Action Coalition. *Technology and Disability, 8*(1-2), 85-89.

Dunn, W. (2005). Measurement issues and practices. In M. Law, C. Baum, & W. Dunn (Eds.), *Measuring occupational performance: Supporting best practice in occupational therapy* (pp. 21-32). Thorofare, NJ: SLACK Incorporated.

Dutil, E., Bottari, C., Vanier, M., & Gaudreault, C. (2005). *ADL Profile: Performance-based assessment user's guide* (Version 5). Montreal, Quebec: Emersion.

Dutil, E., Forget, A., Vanier, M., & Gaudreault, C. (1990). Development of the ADL Profile: An evaluation for adults with severe head injury. *Occupational Therapy in Health Care, 7*, 7-22.

Fänge, A. (2002). *Usability in my home.* Lund, Sweden: Lund University, Division of Occupational Therapy.

Fänge, A., & Iwarsson, S. (1999). Physical housing environment: Development of a self-assessment instrument. *Canadian Journal of Occupational Therapy, 66*, 250-260.

Fänge, A., & Iwarsson, S. (2003). Accessibility and usability in housing: Construct validity and implications for research and practice. *Disability and Rehabilitation, 25*, 315-326.

Fänge, A., & Iwarsson, S. (2005a). Changes in ADL dependence and aspects of usability following housing adaptation—A longitudinal perspective. *American Journal of Occupational Therapy, 59*, 296-304.

Fänge, A., & Iwarsson, S. (2005b). Changes in accessibility and usability in housing: An exploration of the housing adaptation process. *Occupational Therapy International, 12*, 44-59.

Fisher, A. (1995). *Assessment of motor and process skills.* Fort Collins, CO: Three Star Press.

Fisher, A. G. (1998). Uniting practice and theory in an occupational framework. *American Journal of Occupational Therapy, 52*(7), 509-520.

Fisher, A. G. (2001a). *Assessment of motor and process skills: Vol. 1. Development, standardization, and administration.* Fort Collins, CO: Three Star Press.

Fisher, A. G. (2001b). *Assessment of motor and process skills: Vol. 2. User manual.* Fort Collins, CO: Three Star Press.

Frisch, J. (2000). *Some notes on the economics of disability.* Paper presented at Disability and Law Conference in Canberra, Australia, December 4, 2000. Retrieved from http://www.members.optushome.com.au/jackfrisch/EcsOfDisbltyNotes.pdf

Gelderblom, G. J., & De Witte, L. (2002). The assessment of assistive technology outcomes, effects and cost. *Technology and Disability, 14*, 91-94.

Gillespie, L., Gillespie, W., Robertson, M., Lamb, S., Cumming, R., & Rowe, B. (2003). Interventions for preventing falls in elderly people (Cochrane Review). *The Cochrane Database of Systematic Reviews, 4*, CD000340. DOI:10.1002/14651858. CD000340.

Gitlin, L. N. (2003). Next steps in home modifications and assistive technology research. In N. Charness & K. W. Schaie (Eds.), *Impact of technology on successful aging* (pp. 188-202). New York, NY: Springer.

Gitlin, L. N., Hauck, W. W., Winter, L., Dennis, M. P., & Schulz, R. (2006). Effect of an in-home occupational and physical therapy intervention on reducing mortality in functionally vulnerable older people: Preliminary findings. *Journal of American Geriatric Society, 54*, 950-955.

Gitlin, L. N., Luborsky, M. R., & Schemm, R. L. (1998). Emerging concerns of older stroke patients about assistive devices. *The Gerontologist, 38*(2), 169-180.

Gitlin, L. N., Schinfeld, S., Winter, L., Corcoran, M., Boyce, A., & Hauck, W. (2002). Evaluating home environments of persons with dementia: Inter-rater reliability and validity of the Home Environmental Assessment Protocol (HEAP). *Disability and Rehabilitation, 24*(1), 59-71.

Gitlin, L. N., Winter, L., Dennis, M., & Hauck, W. (2006). Assessing perceived change in the well-being of family caregivers: Psychometric properties of the perceived change index and response patterns. *American Journal of Alzheimer's Disease and Other Dementias, 21*(5), 304-311.

Gupta, A. (2008). *Measurement scales used in elderly care.* Oxford, UK: Radcliffe Publishing.

Haigh, R., Tennant, A., Biering-Sorenson, F., Grimby, G., MarinCek, C., Phillips, S., … Thonnard, J-L. (2001). The use of outcome measures in physical medicine and rehabilitation within Europe. *Journal of Rehabilitation Medicine, 33*(6), 273-278.

Hemmingsson, H., & Jonsson, H. (2005). An occupational perspective on the concept of participation in the International Classification of Functioning, Disability and Health: Some critical remarks. *American Journal Occupational Therapy 59*(5), 569-576.

Heywood, F. (2001). *Money well spent: The effectiveness and value of housing adaptations.* Bristol, UK: Policy Press.

Heywood, F. (2004a). The health outcomes of housing adaptations. *Disability and Society, 19*(2), 129-143.

Heywood, F. (2004b). Understanding needs: A starting point for quality. *Housing Studies, 19*(5), 709-726.

Heywood, F. (2005). Adaptation: Altering the house to restore the home. *Housing Studies, 20*(4), 531-547.

Heywood, F., & Turner, L. (2007). *Better outcomes, lower costs: Implications for health and social care budgets of investment in housing adaptations, improvements and equipment: A review of the evidence.* Leeds, UK: Department for Works and Pensions under license from the controller of Her Majesty's Stationery Office by Corporate Document Services.

Holm, M. B., & Rogers, J. C. (1999). Functional assessment: The Performance Assessment of Self-Care Skills (PASS). In B. J. Hemphill (Ed), *Assessments in occupational therapy mental health: An integrative approach* (pp. 117-124). Thorofare, NJ: SLACK Incorporated.

Hurstfield, J., Parashar, U., & Schofield, K. (2007). *The costs and benefits of independent living.* Norwich, UK: Office of Disability Issues, Department for Work and Pensions.

Iwarsson, S., Horstmann, V., & Slaug, B. (2007). Housing matters in very old age—Yet differently due to ADL dependence level differences. *Scandinavian Journal of Occupational Therapy, 14*, 3-15.

Iwarsson, S., & Slaug, B. (2001). *The Housing Enabler: An instrument for assessing and analyzing accessibility problems in housing.* Navlinge och Staffanstorp, Sweden: Veten & Stapen HB & Slaug Data Management. Retrieved from http://www.enabler.nu.

Jerosch-Herold, C. (2005). An evidence-based approach to choosing outcome measures: A checklist for the critical appraisal of validity, reliability and responsiveness studies. *British Journal of Occupational Therapy, 68*(8), 347-353.

Jette, A. M., & Haley, S. M. (2005). Contemporary measurement techniques for rehabilitation outcomes assessment. *Journal of Rehabilitation Medicine, 37*, 339-345.

Johansson, K., Lilja, M., Petersson, I. A., & Borell, L. (2007). Performance of activities of daily living in a sample of applicants for home modification services. *Scandinavian Journal of Occupational Therapy, 14*, 44-53.

Jones, A., de Jonge, D., & Phillips, R. (2008). *The role of home maintenance and modification services in achieving health, community care and housing outcomes in later life: Research report.* Melbourne, Australia: Australian Housing and Urban Research Institute.

Kjeken, I., & Lillemo, S. (2006). Exploration of the link between conceptual occupational therapy models and the International Classification of Functioning, Disability and Health: A response from colleagues in Norway. *Australian Occupational Therapy Journal, 54*, 142-143.

Klein, S., Barlow, I., & Hollis, V. (2008). Evaluating ADL measures from an occupational perspective. *Canadian Journal of Occupational Therapy, 75*(2), 69-81.

Larson, E. A. (2000). The orchestration of occupation: The dance of mothers. *American Journal of Occupational Therapy, 54*, 269-280.

Laver Fawcett, A. (2007). The importance of accurate assessment and outcomes measurement. In A. Laver Fawcett (Ed.), *Principles of assessment and outcome measurements for occupational therapists and physiotherapists: Theory, skills and application* (pp. 15-44). West Sussex, UK: John Wiley & Sons Ltd.

Law, M. (1998). *Client-centered occupational therapy.* Thorofare, NJ: SLACK Incorporated.

Law, M. (2005). Outcome measures rating form guidelines. In M. Law, C. Baum, & W. Dunn (Eds.), *Measuring occupational performance: Supporting best practice in occupational therapy* (pp. 396-409). Thorofare, NJ: SLACK Incorporated.

Law, M., Baptiste, S., Carswell, A., McColl, M. A., Polatajko, H., & Pollock, N. (1998). *The Canadian Occupational Performance Measure* (3rd ed.). Toronto: COAT.

Law, M., & Baum, C. (2005). Measurement in occupational therapy. In M. Law, C. Baum, & W. Dunn (Eds.), *Measuring occupational performance: Supporting best practice in occupational therapy* (pp. 3-20). Thorofare, NJ: SLACK Incorporated.

Law, M., Baum, C., & Dunn, W. (2005). Challenges and strategies in applying an occupational performance measurement approach. In M. Law, C. Baum, & W. Dunn (Eds.), *Measuring occupational performance: Supporting best practice in occupational therapy* (pp. 375-382). Thorofare, NJ, SLACK Incorporated.

Law, M., Dunn, W., & Baum, C. (2005). Measuring participation. In M. Law, C. Baum, & W. Dunn (Eds.), *Measuring occupational performance: Supporting best practice in occupational therapy* (pp. 107-126). Thorofare, NJ: SLACK Incorporated.

Luebben, A. J., & Royeen, C. B. (2005). Non-standardized testing. In J. Hinojosa, P. Kramer, & P. Crist (2005). *Evaluation: Obtaining and interpreting data* (pp. xi-xiv). Bethesda, MD: AOTA Press.

Lund, M. L., Nordlund, A., Nygard, L., Lexell, J., & Bernspang, B. (2005). Perceptions of participation and predictors of perceived problems with participation in persons with spinal cord injury. *Journal of Rehabilitation Medicine, 37*(1), 3-8.

Mackenzie, L., Byles, J., & Higginbotham, N. (2000). Designing the Home Falls and Accidents Screening Tool (HOME FAST): Selecting the items. *British Journal of Occupational Therapy, 63*(6), 260-269.

Mann, W. C., Ottenbacher, K. J., Fraas, L., Tomita, M., & Granger, C. V. (1999). Effectiveness of assistive technology and environmental interventions in reducing home care costs for the frail elderly: A randomized control trial. *Archives of Family Medicine, 8*(May/June), 210-217.

Marcus, C. (1995). *House as a mirror of self.* Berkeley, CA: Conrai Press.

McColl, M. A., & Pollock, N. (2001). Measuring occupational performance using a client-centered perspective. In M. Law, C. Baum, & W. Dunn (Eds.), *Measuring occupational performance* (pp. 81-91). Thorofare, NJ: SLACK Incorporated.

Melzack, R. (1975). The McGill Pain Questionnaire: Major properties and scoring methods. *Pain, 1*, 277-299.

Messecar, D. C., Archbold, P. G., Stewart, B. J., & Kirschling, J. (2002). Home environmental modification strategies used by caregivers of elders. *Research in Nursing and Health, 25*, 357-370.

Miller Polgar, J. (2009). Critiquing assessments. In E. Crepeau, E. Cohn, & B. Schell (Eds.), *Willard & Spackman's occupational therapy* (11th ed., pp. 519-536). Philadelphia, PA: Wolters, Kluwer, Lippincott, Williams, & Wilkins.

Moore, J. (2000). Placing home in context. *Journal of Environmental Psychology, 20*, 207-217.

Nikolaus, T., & Bach, M. (2003). Preventing falls in community-dwelling frail older people using a home intervention team. *Journal of the American Geriatric Society, 51*, 300-305.

Noreau, L., Fougeyrollas, P., & Vincent, C. (2002). The LIFE-H: Assessment of the quality of social participation. *Technology and Disability, 14*, 113-118.

Nygren, C., Oswald, F., Iwarsson, S., Fänge, J., Sixsmith, J., Schilling, O., ... Wahl, H-W. (2007). Relationships between objective and perceived housing in very old age. *The Gerontologist, 47*, 85-95.

Oliver, R., Blathwayt, J., Brackley, C., & Tamaki, T. (1993). Development of the Safety Assessment of Function and the Environment for Rehabilitation (SAFER) tool. *Canadian Journal of Occupational Therapy, 60*(2), 78-82.

Oswald, F., Schilling, O., Wahl, H. W., Fänge, A., Sixsmith, J., & Iwarsson, S. (2006). Homeward bound: Introducing a four-domain model of perceived housing in very old age. *Journal of Environmental Psychology, 26*, 187-201.

Oswald, F., & Wahl, H. W. (2005). Dimensions of the meaning of home in later life. In G. D. Rowles & H. Chaudhury (Eds.), *Home and identity in later life: International perspectives* (pp. 21-46). New York, NY: Springer.

Oswald, F., Wahl, H. W., Martin, M., & Mollenkopf, H. (2003). Toward measuring proactivity in person-environment transactions in late adulthood: The Housing-Related Control Beliefs Questionnaire. *Journal of Housing for the Elderly, 17*, 135-152.

Oswald, F., Wahl, H. W., Schilling, O., & Iwarsson, S. (2007). Housing-related control beliefs and independence in activities of daily living in very old age. *Scandinavian Journal of Occupational Therapy, 14*, 33-43.

Parker, D. M., & Sykes, C. H. (2006). A systematic review of the Canadian Occupational Performance Measure: A clinical practice perspective. *British Journal of Occupational Therapy, 69*(4), 150-160.

Patterson, D. R., Jensen, M., & Engel-Knowles, J. (2002). Pain and its influence on assistive technology use. In M. J. Scherer (Ed.), *Assistive technology: Matching device and consumer for successful rehabilitation* (pp. 59-76). Washington, DC: American Psychological Association.

Petersson, I., Fisher, A. G., Hemmingsson, H., & Lilja, M. (2007). The client-clinician assessment protocol (C-CAP): Evaluation of its psychometric properties for use with people aging with disabilities in need of home modifications. *Occupational Therapy Journal of Research: Occupation, Participation and Health, 27*(4), 140-148.

Petersson, I., Lilja, M., Hammel, J., & Kottorp, A. (2008). Impact of home modification services on ability in everyday life for people ageing with disabilities *Journal of Rehabilitation Medicine, 40*(4), 253-260.

Plautz, B., Beck, D., Selmar, C., & Radetsky, M. (1996). Modifying the environment: A community-based injury-reduction programme for elderly residents. *American Journal of Preventative Medicine, 12*(4), 33-38.

Polgar, S., & Thomas, S. (2000). *Introduction to research in the health sciences* (4th ed.). Edinburgh, UK: Churchill Livingstone.

Post, M. W. M., Festen, H., van de Port, I. G., & Visser-Meily, J. M. A. (2007). Reproducibility of the Caregiver Strain Index and the Caregiver Reaction Assessment in partners of stroke patients living in the Dutch community. *Clinical Rehabilitation, 21*, 1050-1055.

Pynoos, J. (2004). On the forefront of the ever-changing field of home modification. *Rehabilitation Management, 17*(3), 34-35, 50.

Pynoos, J., Rose, D., Rubenstein, L., Choi, H., & Sabata, D. (2006). Evidence-based interventions in fall prevention. *Home Health Care Services Quarterly: The Journal of Community Care, 25*(1/2), 55-72.

Pynsent, P., Fairbank, J., & Carr, A. (2004). *Outcome measures in orthopaedics and trauma* (2nd ed.). London, UK: A Hodder Arnold Publication.

Robinson, B. C. (1983). Validation of a Caregiver Strain Index. *Journal of Gerontology, 38*, 344-348.

Rogers, J. C., & Holm, M. B. (1994). *The performance assessment of self-care skills (PASS), Version 3.1.* Pittsburgh, PA: University of Pittsburgh.

Rogers, J. C., & Holm, M. B. (2007). The performance assessment of self-care skills (PASS). In I. E. Asher (Ed.), *An annotated index of occupational therapy evaluation tools* (3rd ed., pp. 102-110). Bethesda, MD: AOTA Press.

Rossi, P. H., Lipsey, M. W., & Freeman, H. E. (2004). *Evaluation: A systematic approach.* Thousand Oaks, CA: Sage Publications.

Sackett, D. L., Rosenberg, W. M. C., Gray, J. A. M., Haynes, R. B., & Richardson, W. S. (1996). Evidence-based medicine: What it is and what it isn't. *British Journal of Medicine, 312*, 71-72.

Salter, K., Jutai, J. W., Teasell, R., Foley, N. C., & Bitensky, J. (2005). Issues for selection of outcome measures in stroke rehabilitation: ICF body functions. *Disability and Rehabilitation, 27*(4), 191-207.

Sanford, J. A., Patricia C., Griffiths, P. C., Richardson, P. N., Hargraves, K., Butterfield, T., & Hoenig, H. (2006). The effects of in-home rehabilitation on task self-efficacy in mobility-impaired adults: A randomized clinical trial. *Journal of the American Geriatrics Society, 54*(11), 1641-1648.

Sbordone, R. J., & Guilmette, T. J. (1999). Ecological validity: Prediction of everyday and vocational functioning from neuropsychological test data. In J. J. Sweet (Ed.), *Forensic neuropsychology: Fundamentals and practice* (pp. 227-254). Exton, PA: Taylor & Francis.

Sells, C. H. (2005). Additional uses of evaluation data. In J. Hinojosa, P. Kramer, & P. Crist (Eds.), *Evaluation: Obtaining and interpreting data* (pp. 283-305). Bethesda, MD: AOTA Press.

Skidmore, E. R., Rogers, J. C., Chandler, L. S., & Holm, M. B. (2006). Developing empirical models to enhance stroke rehabilitation. *Disability and Rehabilitation, 28*(16), 1027-1034.

Smith, R. O. (2002). OTFACT: Multi-level performance-oriented software assistive technology outcomes protocol. *Technology and Disability, 14*, 133-139.

Stamm, T. A., Cieza, A., Machold, K., Smolen, J. S., & Stucki, G. (2006). Exploration of the link between conceptual occupational therapy models and the International Classification of Functioning, Disability and Health. *Australian Occupational Therapy Journal, 53*, 9-17.

Stark, S. (2004). Removing environmental barriers in the homes of older adults with disabilities improves occupational performance. *Occupation, Participation and Health, 24*(1), 32-40.

Thomas Jefferson University. (n.d.). *Center for Applied Research on Aging and Health.* Retrieved from http://www.jefferson.edu/jchp/carah/researchers.cfm

Tinetti, M. E., Richman, D., & Powell, L. (1990). Falls efficacy as a measure of fear of falling. *Journal of Gerontology: Psychological Sciences, 45*, 239-243.

Uniform Data System for Medical Rehabilitation. (1997). *Functional Independence Measure* (Version 5.1). Buffalo, NY: Buffalo General Hospital, State University of New York.

Ware, J., & Sherbourne, C. (1992). The MOS 36-Item Short Form Health Survey (SF36): Conceptual framework and item selection. *Medical Care, 30*(6), 473-481.

Ware, J. E., Snow, K. K., Kosinski, M., & Gandek, B. (1993). *SF-36 Health Survey Manual and Interpretation Guide.* Boston, MA: New England Medical Center, The Health Institute.

World Health Organization. (2001). *The International Classification of Function, Activity and Participation.* Geneva: Author.

World Health Organization. (2005). *ICF checklist.* Retrieved from http://www.who.int/classifications/icf/training/icfchecklist.pdf

Section III
Home Modification Applications

In this last section, the editors synthesize the theories, models, and applications presented by the authors through the presentation of case studies. These case studies highlight occupational performance issues arising from a range of environmental barriers, and information is not limited to the needs of people with physical disabilities. These cases highlight the unique role of occupational therapists working with clients with a range of home modification needs.

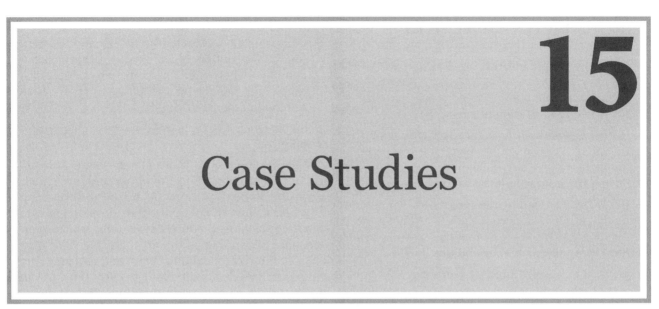

Case Studies

Elizabeth Ainsworth, MOccThy, Grad Cert Health Sci;
Kathy Baigent, Dip OT, Dip Hlth Prom;
Ruth Cordiner, DipCOT, Grad Cert OccThy;
Shirley de Wit, BOccThy; and May Eade, BOccThy

This chapter synthesizes the information from previous chapters by providing the reader with a range of case studies relating to older people and people with disabilities across the lifespan. Each case study highlights the home modification process. This chapter includes detail on a range of environmental interventions selected to enhance the health, safety, independence, and home and community participation of a range of clients. Additionally, it provides evidence of the value of postmodification evaluation to review client outcomes and to contribute to the occupational therapist's practice knowledge.

The first case study relates to a young man in a farming community who sustained a spinal injury, resulting in paraplegia. Home modifications were recommended to ensure thathis home was made wheelchair accessible and would meet his short- and long-term needs as he moved into adulthood.

The second case study involves a child with several rare conditions resulting in multiple disabilities. This child lives with her mother and sister in a large city but visits her friends who also provide care and support in another suburb. The case study highlights the changes made to a two-level home to ensure that the child is able to participate in all aspects of her friend's home and family life.

The third case study features the home modification requirements of an elderly man who lives alone in an apartment by the sea and is aging into disability.

The fourth case study describes the home modification needs of two men residing together and sharing 24-hour caregiver support. These two men have intellectual and physical disabilities and tend to damage property. This section discusses the home modifications required to improve the usability of the environment and to prevent ongoing damage.

The fifth case study provides information to the reader on a range of home modifications that have been considered for a person with a visual impairment living alone in her own home.

The sixth case study showcases the effect of housing types and home modifications on a young man with a psychiatric disability who has made the transition from an institution into the community. Changes discussed include home modifications that aim to prevent neighborhood disputes and improve the client's sense of safety and security in his own home.

The final case study describes the home modification requirements of an elderly couple where one partner is caring for a spouse who has dementia.

Ainsworth, E., & de Jonge, D..
An Occupational Therapists's Guide to Home Modification Practice (pp. 289-326)

CHAPTER OBJECTIVES

By the end of this chapter, the reader will be able to:

+ Explain the role of the occupational therapist in the home modification process

+ Recognize and discuss the application of the transactive approach to examining the person, his or her home environment, and occupations during the home modification process

+ Describe and apply the processes for home modification practice, including using clinical reasoning, for a range of people with varying health conditions and disabilities

+ Identify a range of products, designs, and solutions that could be considered when developing intervention options for individuals with specific housing requirements

CASE STUDY 1: A TEENAGER WITH A PHYSICAL DISABILITY

Client Interests and Daily Activities

Brett is a 15-year-old who lives with his parents and younger brother on a property outside a small country town. Brett catches the local bus to the high school where he is planning to complete his senior schooling. Outside of school, Brett assists his father on the small family farm that grows small crops and breeding cattle. His parents have lived on their property for at least 25 years. In addition to running the farm, Mr. G. also does part-time building work, and Mrs. G. is a homemaker. Brett has enjoyed growing up in the country and has a keen interest in repairing broken farm machinery, playing sports, and socializing with his friends.

Health Condition and Functional Performance

Brett sustained a spinal injury as a result of a motorcycle accident. He was transported to a city hospital spinal injuries unit for treatment and rehabilitation.

His T4 spinal injury resulted in the following:

+ Complete paralysis of the lower body and legs

+ Variation in upper body strength

+ Full neck and head movement with full muscle strength and shoulder movement

+ Full use of arms, wrists, and fingers

+ Compromise in sympathetic nervous system function resulting in autonomic dysreflexia, a condition where there is overactivity of the autonomic nervous system, resulting in an increase in blood pressure

+ Some compromise in respiratory capacity and endurance

Over the long term, there may be bone, soft tissue, and joint changes in the upper and lower limb joints and spine. Brett may be at risk of developing a syrinx, a fluid-filled cavity that develops in the spinal cord causing altered sensation, spasm, and weakness depending on the area affected. This may impact on his physical and functional capacity. His equipment needs might change over time as he grows and develops greater functional limitations.

Location and Description of the House

The occupational therapist visited the home in the small rural community outside the small country town. Brett lives in a low-set house situated on slightly sloping land. The home is set back a few miles from the main highway. The house is located in front of a large work shed where machinery is stored for the farm work. There are no fences around the house, but rather a sparse garden and a clothesline. The house looks out onto the surrounding fields.

The house has seven stairs at the side entry and five stairs at the rear entry. The rear entrance also includes a small tiled patio that is set a few stairs off of the ground. This is used as the main entry to the home.

The house has:

+ Four bedrooms

+ A partially renovated main bathroom with a shower over the tub, toilet, and pedestal sink

+ A large kitchen with ample storage above and below the counters, an upright stove, sink, island counter, and other standard fittings

+ A dining room off of the kitchen

+ A large living room area

+ A study next to the kitchen

+ A laundry located downstairs off of the rear tiled patio with a small wall-hung vanity and a laundry tub and space for a washing machine and a step at the entry

+ A second toilet located next to the downstairs laundry with a step at the entry

The house is of timber construction with polished floors, carpet on the bedroom floors, and vinyl in the kitchen and dining room areas. There are no significant changes in floor levels in the main areas of the home.

Client Goals

Brett indicated that his short-term goals included the following:

+ Gaining more confidence completing transfers on and off the toilet, a tub transfer bench, and furniture
+ Negotiating curbs and inclines in his wheelchair
+ Managing his own self-catheterization
+ Maintaining his health through prevention of urinary tract infections and pressure sores

His long-term goals included the following:

+ Recommencing his schooling
+ Participating in social activities with his friends
+ Returning to farm activities, including riding a motorbike and repairing farm machinery
+ Training to be a motor mechanic

Mrs. G. agreed with the goals set by Brett and indicated that she also wanted her son to:

+ Learn skills that would enable him to live by himself or with friends in the community when he was older
+ Pursue employment options after he had finished his schooling
+ Own and drive a car to ensure independent community access

Evaluating Occupational Performance and Identifying Needs

Prior to the home visit, the therapist reviewed the medical information and interviewed the treating rehabilitation staff to establish Brett's current physical and functional status.

During the home visit, the therapist interviewed Brett and his mother using the *Canadian Occupational Performance Measure* (COPM) to identify their goals and to ascertain Brett's capacity to function in the home. He was observed wheeling himself around in his wheelchair, undertaking transfers, and completing various activities in areas such as the bathroom and kitchen.

Mobility and Transfers

Brett reported that he uses his manual wheelchair to propel himself a long distance. He stated that he was learning to manage jumping curbs and could do this independently. He demonstrated his capacity to wheel up and down inclines during the time of the visit, including over dirt and paved areas. He reported that although he was able to manage side-on transfers on and off the toilet, and a chair and a tub transfer bench with ease in the hospital, he was struggling at home as a result of the inaccessible environment. Brett was also observed to transfer on and off the bed independently and demonstrated that he was able to transfer from the bed and then into a mobile over-toilet shower chair that he wheeled into the bathroom area.

Self-Care and Homemaker Activities

Brett indicated that he was able to manage some of his self-care activities independently, including dressing, bathing, and basic grooming. He showed the therapist where he undertook the various self-care tasks in the bathroom and bedroom. Brett reported that he needed assistance to get in and out of the bath and on and off the toilet because of the lack of space for equipment and positioning of the wheelchair for transfers. He also stated that he could not access the kitchen sink fully but that he could make light meals at home despite areas of the kitchen—the counters, oven, and sink areas—being inaccessible. He also has assistance in completing some basic cleaning tasks.

Anthropometric Measurements and Equipment

Brett's anthropometric measurements were taken while seated in his wheelchair, mobile over-toilet, shower chair, and tub transfer bench. This included his reach ranges while seated on the various pieces of equipment.

Purpose of Occupational Therapy Involvement

A home visit referral requested an occupational therapist visit to make home modification recommendations to ensure that Brett would be able to live in the home without having to rely on his family to assist him with transfers, mobility, self-care, or homemaker tasks. Home modifications were also required to enable him to return to participating in activities on the family property and local community.

During the interview and the process of observing Brett in his wheelchair negotiating spaces and environmental features, he and his mother discussed the layout of their existing home and the possible changes required to enable him to manage the built environment with ease. This discussion included the look and the possible cost of various modifications, given Brett's current and future roles, and the structure of the home. Consideration was also given to the changing nature of his disability over time and his current and future equipment needs. The therapist used a combination of narrative, scientific, ethical, and pragmatic reasoning approaches in examining Brett's access to, and performance in, each area of the home and the external areas of the property, including the rear shed. The therapist used the information gathered at the time of the hospital visit, the advice of a technical advisor, and the views of Brett and his parents to formulate options for discussion.

A technical advisor with a building background attended the home visit with the therapist to provide advice on the proposed structural modifications and compliance and building approval considerations associated with any such work. The therapist recorded equipment dimensions and Brett's anthropometric and reach range measurements to use in developing the modifications. Photos were also taken, and measurements of the built environment were recorded by the technical advisor and therapist.

Other considerations included the cost of the work, ensuring the home modifications were designed in keeping with the look of the home without creating an institutional appearance, and the needs of other household members.

Environmental Issues and Intervention Options

Various environmental issues and intervention options were discussed during the walk-through of the home with Brett and his parents.

Access to the Property

Wheelchair Access to the Home

Brett required assistance to negotiate the stairs in his wheelchair. Options considered included the installation of an elevator or a ramp at one or both external entries. The elevator was considered too costly compared with the installation of one or two ramps.

The final recommendation included the removal of the side stairs on the home and the installation of a wheelchair-accessible ramp from the rear of the home to the new, large covered deck on the side of the home. This ramp was set out from the side of the home to ensure the windows of the house did not open over the ramp (Figure 15-1). These modifications enabled the client to have access in and out of the home from the rear yard area (drop-off point for car parking and location of large work shed). As well, the ramp was installed in such a way that it would not be an obvious structural addition to the home when approaching the house along the driveway.

Wheelchair Access to the Rear Clothesline and Shed

There was no path leading to the clothesline, and there were uneven pavers on a small path leading to the rear work shed. Options considered included leaving the areas in their existing state, with the client negotiating the grass and pavers. This was considered unsuitable because the ground and pavers were not level and access would be difficult during wet weather. In addition, the tires of the wheelchair would become muddy and trail dirt into the house.

The final recommendation included the installation of a wheelchair-accessible path to the rear clothesline and the rear shed area to enable access to these areas from the home (Figure 15-2). Additionally, some of the uneven and unstable existing pavers on the small path were relaid.

Access Into the Downstairs Laundry and Toilet Areas

The downstairs laundry and toilet doorways lacked adequate clearance for Brett's wheelchair, which caused him to often scrape his knuckles on the doorframes as he wheeled through the doorways.

One option considered included Brett using the upstairs facilities for washing his hands after doing work in the shed. This option was considered inappropriate because the client required quick and easy access from the shed to an area to clean his hands before entering the home. He would also be putting grease and dirt on door fittings and fixtures and his wheelchair if wheeling upstairs to the bathroom. As well, easy access to the downstairs toilet would save time and be more convenient than using the upstairs toilet in the main bathroom.

The final recommendations included the widening of the laundry door and downstairs toilet door (Figure 15-3).

Outdoor Areas

Covered Area

Brett did not have a cool area where he could undertake outdoor activities, such as hobbies and farm work, and socialize with friends. Options

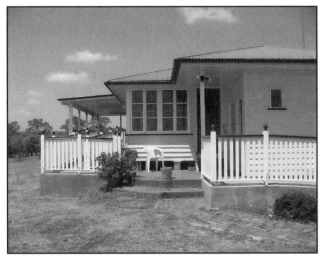

Figure 15-1. Ramp access at the side of the home.

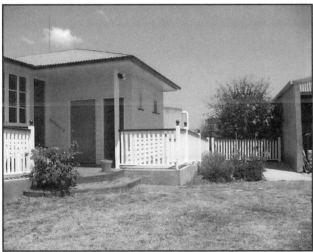

Figure 15-2. Ramp access to the rear clothesline and shed.

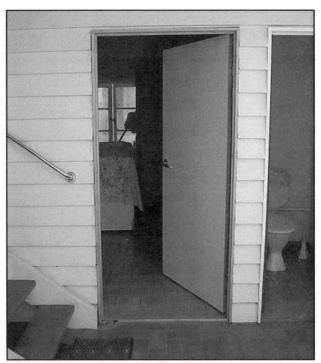

Figure 15-3. Widened laundry door and toilet door.

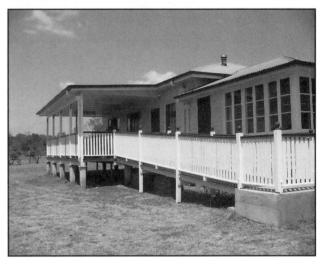

Figure 15-4. New deck.

considered included Brett continuing to use the shed and specific areas in the house during the year, but only when the weather was favorable or if there was air-conditioning installed or the installation of a deck on the side of the home to catch the breezes and provide an area for work and social activities.

The most cost-effective option was the installation of a large deck on the side of the home closest to the living and dining room areas (Figure 15-4).

Access to the New Deck Area From the Living and Dining Room Areas

A ramp to the deck and a door leading into the home off of the deck were required to provide an access point into the home for Brett in his wheelchair and for visitors requiring similar access.

The final recommendation included the creation of a new doorway off of the side deck, leading into the side room and dining room (Figure 15-5).

Internal Access

Adequate Door Widths

Brett experienced difficulty wheeling through the narrow hallways and doorways leading into the laundry, lounge room, bathroom, and his bedroom and was damaging his knuckles using the wheel rims to maneuver through the house.

Options considered included limiting the client's access to specific areas of the home or completing some structural modifications to the timber frames in the home along the hallways and at the doorways.

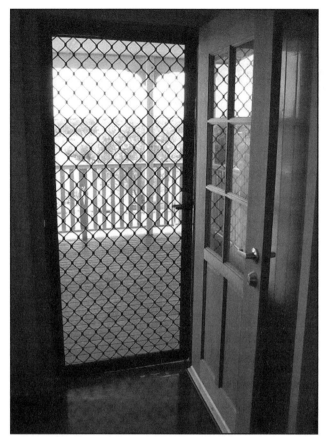

Figure 15-5. New doorway off of the side deck.

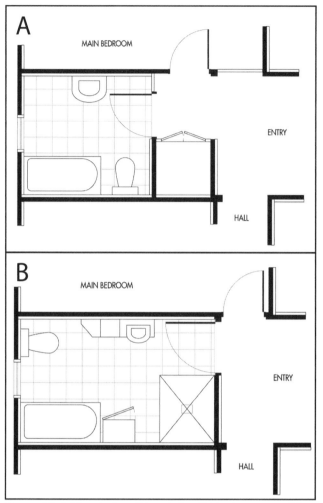

Figure 15-6. Plans before (A) and after (B) bathroom modifications.

The final recommendation included widening the doorways leading from the hallway into the living room and Brett's bedroom. The bathroom modifications included extending the bathroom by using the floor area just outside of this room. The extra floor area was gained by removing the linen closet and using this space as part of the extended bathroom (Figure 15-6). A swing door could be installed, in keeping with the look of the rest of the home, and the linen closet could be relocated to another area of the home, ensuring that this storage space was not lost.

Altered Door Swings on the Bedroom Door and Wardrobe Doors

Brett was experiencing difficulty accessing his bedroom because of the swing of the door and the floor space it took up in his room in relation to the location of his bed. The wardrobe doors swung out 90 degrees, and he frequently wheeled into them.

Options considered included not modifying the area, which would result in the client experiencing difficulty negotiating the features, or completing a structural change.

The final recommendation included reswinging the bedroom door to enable it to open more fully

for ease of access to the bed and other areas of the bedroom. As well, changing hinges on the wardrobe enabled the doors to swing open to 170 degrees to ensure greater wheelchair access to the drawers and shelves.

Access Within the Bathroom

Wheelchair Access Problems

Because of the presence of a low bath, inaccessible vanity, high mirror, narrow storage cupboard, and a step into the bathroom, Brett experienced difficulty in the bathroom. He had trouble getting into the bathroom and having sufficient space to the side or in front of various features. He was overreaching to access the sink, and there was no space to do a side-on transfer on and off the tub transfer bench. The mobile over-toilet shower chair was not sitting over the toilet properly, resulting in his need for alternative ways to transfer on and off the toilet with help.

Options considered included leaving the features with their current location and design, resulting in Brett having limited use of the facilities, or redesigning the area to include an accessible vanity, larger and lower mirror to suit the needs of the whole family, a large waterproof storage cupboard with shelves at various heights, and eliminating the step at the entry to the bathroom. Further, the tub transfer bench could continue to be used over the bath if other fittings were relocated to make space. To provide greater flexibility, the wheel-in shower area was considered as an alternative option to the bath to enable Brett easier use of the bench and the mobile over-toilet shower chair.

The final recommendation included the redesign and relation of the features to ensure that Brett had better wheelchair access. This included the removal of all existing features, except the bath, and the redesign to include the installation of a wheel-in shower, handheld shower, standard capstan taps, and recessed soap holder; a semi-recessed basin set into a vanity counter with storage above and below the counter, a new mirror, and waterproof power point; a waterproof storage cupboard; a new slip-resistant when wet floor covering with no step at the doorway; and the relocation of the existing toilet suite.

Adequate Storage for Catheter Equipment in the Bathroom

The vanity area did not have a storage shelf, and the small linen closet was located near the toilet and was difficult to access in a wheelchair. Brett had to balance items for toileting on his lap and, at times, he placed them on top of the toilet or in the sink. Reaching for these items was difficult. Options considered included the installation of a shelf near the toilet or the redesign of the vanity area to incorporate shelving.

The final recommendation included installing the storage area as part of the vanity to enable Brett to lift and carry items from just one area near the toilet.

Temperature Control

Installing Temperature Regulation Mechanisms

Because of Brett's difficulty in regulating his body temperature, options considered for Brett's bedroom included the installation of floor-based or wall-based fans or the installation of air-conditioning. Fans were not considered effective enough to reduce the heat in the bedroom.

The final recommendation included preparing the wall area by installing a power point for an air-conditioner.

Options for regulating the temperature in the rest of the home included installing fans or air-conditioning or building a deck that would be an outdoor area to catch the breezes and provide a venue in which Brett could work and socialize in hot weather. It was determined that fans would not be an effective option, and air-conditioning the whole home would be very expensive on an ongoing basis because of the large size and number of rooms in the home.

The final recommendation, considered the most beneficial for Brett, included the installation of a deck area to catch the breezes during summer, where he could sit under cover while working or socializing with friends and family.

Options for regulating the temperature in the bathroom during Brett's self-care routine included having someone assist him with showering or installing a temperature regulation device to limit the hot water. The final recommendation included the installation of a thermostatic temperature control device to regulate water temperature and to enable Brett to retain his independence during self care activities.

Access Within the Kitchen

Adequate Preparation Space and Wheel-Under Access

Options considered included leaving the kitchen in its current state, modifying part of the kitchen, or modifying the entire kitchen. It was determined that Brett would experience difficulty accessing the counters and would have to overextend when reaching for items on countertops and in cupboards and when accessing the power outlets. Further, his capacity to make meals would be limited, resulting in him being reliant on others to assist him during these activities. A full modification of the kitchen would prove costly, given that the area had been recently renovated by the family.

The final recommendation included modifying parts of the kitchen, including altering the island counter to allow wheel-under access, installing a pantry to provide height-adjustable shelving, and installing a short wall above a kitchen counter to provide an area close to the counter's edge for a new power outlet (Figure 15-7). These modifications would enable Brett to continue making snacks and to participate in basic meal preparation activities, including using a kettle and a microwave rather than the upright stove. The counter heights were not altered because Brett was tall enough to manage the standard height. It was envisaged that Brett would move out of the home in the future, and the family requested that only the basic features be altered. This modification was also considered more cost-effective in the short- to medium-term than a full renovation of the kitchen.

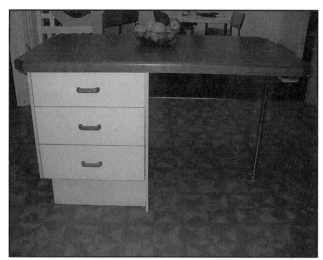

Figure 15-7. Modified island bench.

Clinical Reasoning, Evaluation, and Justification for Recommendations

Clinical reasoning began once information was provided by the referrer at the time of initial contact, documentation from the medical service was received, and through discussion and observing Brett in the home.

Scientific reasoning was used to interpret information regarding Brett's health condition. Because Brett is continuing to physically grow, acquire new equipment, and experience various health conditions because of his spinal injury, it is anticipated that he will continue to encounter changing environmental demands and barriers. Scientific reasoning was used to collect cues throughout the assessment process as to how Brett's skills and deficits were likely to affect his performance and when evaluating the effectiveness of each solution in addressing his occupational performance needs.

Narrative reasoning assisted the occupational therapist to understand and interpret information relating to past and present life and Brett's goals for the future. The therapist became aware, for example, that he had yet to complete his schooling and had to consider work options either on the home farm or in the community. Brett had a strong interest in undertaking outdoor activities with his friends and participating in all aspects of community life. Such preferences and lifestyle choices would continue to impact on his future goals.

Pragmatic reasoning was used to consider contextual factors, choice of materials and relevant measurements for modifications, as well as funding issues. For example, the age of the house and whether the client would continue to reside there

after finishing his schooling was considered in recommending the extent of the home modifications in various areas of the home. Funding for the home modifications had become available through an insurance claim and, though limited, it was allocated on the basis of his housing needs for the rest of his life. Brett was seriously considering his accommodation options for his adult years and recognized that funding would be required for an alternative solution to the family home.

Pragmatically, the choice of materials was considered. For example, an external timber ramp was selected because it was considered a reasonable cost compared with hiring a portable ramp for the short- to medium-term. The timber ramp also matched the look of the home and did not appear out of place in the design of the property. Anthropometric and equipment measurements were considered in planning clearances and circulation space and for positioning fittings and fixtures in all areas of the home.

Ethical reasoning was used in considering alternative decisions for each issue, including those that were not addressed and the consequences of recommendations made. Ethical reasoning was also considered in relation to the appropriate use of funding for a short- to medium-term planning of home modification solutions. For example, despite the client receiving funding through an insurance claim, the therapist did not make home modification recommendations that might have been considered extravagant or wasteful of resources.

The technical advisor provided samples of products and finishes and sketched preliminary designs to be discussed with Brett and his family. After concluding the home visit, the therapist and technical advisor, over a period of several weeks, developed design options for the family to consider. The therapist visited the home for a second time to show Brett and his mother the plan options and to trial the layouts drawn. These options were finalized, and the final therapy report, including the technical advisor's plans and specifications, was forwarded to the family.

Outcomes

Quotes were obtained from three building firms who specialized in home modification installations, and a builder was chosen to proceed with the work. The modifications were installed, and the therapist visited Brett in his home to complete a postmodification evaluation. The therapist conducted an interview and structured observation of Brett in the various areas of the home. The interview included the review of the original occupational therapy report to determine whether there had been any changes in Brett's capacity to manage the various activities in the home and community. The therapist observed that he had clearly improved in general health and functional capacity, being able to manage all activities with greater confidence. He could manage accessing all areas of the home that were modified with safety and ease. The home modifications were installed as per the original occupational therapy report. The products and finishes appeared to be coping with wear and tear and were reported to suit the needs of all of the family.

Since this postmodification visit, the therapist has kept in contact with family members who report that Brett continues to make progress with respect to resuming his schooling, hobbies, and interests. His family members are currently working to enhance wheelchair access in the community and to enhance the public's awareness of spinal injury. It is anticipated that further planning will occur in the future for the construction of a house designed with universal and adaptable design features to enable Brett to live independently in the community at a later stage.

CASE STUDY 2: A YOUNG GIRL WITH MULTIPLE DISABILITIES

Client Interests and Daily Activities

Suzie is a 9-year-old girl who lives with her parents, two brothers, and sister in a quiet suburban area of a large city. She is a sociable girl who enjoys being with close family and friends. She loves listening to music, going to the beach with her family, and playing with friends. Suzie attends her local special school 5 days a week. She also stays overnight regularly at the house of her best friend, Brittany Fisher. Brittany's family has offered informal respite support, and Suzie lives at their house approximately 2 weeks out of every 4.

Health Condition and Functional Performance

Suzie has a rare genetic condition resulting in microcephaly (a small head size as a result of the failure of the brain to develop) and microphthalmia (underdevelopment of the eyes), resulting in physical and intellectual disabilities, including blindness. She was born with dislocated hips and has undergone osteotomy on the left hip to construct the joint so it falls into a more normal position.

Suzie also has had a stroke, resulting in right-sided hemiplegia, and has a history of pneumonia, bronchitis, stomach ulcers, and esophagitis. She has undergone fundoplication surgery to minimize any ongoing reflux.

Suzie has a local doctor; a physiotherapist at her school, whom she sees intermittently; and biannual contact with various medical specialists at the local children's hospital. When at home, Suzie is visited daily by government-funded support workers, who assist with her bathing routine. No additional caregiver support is provided when Suzie stays with Brittany.

Location and Description of the House

Brittany's family own a four-bedroom detached house located on a quiet suburban street. The house is high-set, with an internal staircase of 14 stairs. Downstairs, there is Suzie's bedroom, a small bathroom (shower, vanity, and toilet), a separate laundry (located off of the garage), a living area, and a double garage used as a play area and to store household items and Suzie's mobility equipment. There are large doors enclosing the double garage, which leads out to the covered carport, located at the front of the house. Upstairs, there are three bedrooms, a small study, a bathroom (separate bath, shower, and vanity), a toilet, a kitchen, and a dining room. There is no wheelchair access to the various areas around the home.

Client Goals

Suzie's mother's goals for her daughter are to:
+ Stay safely for extended periods at her friend's home to provide her with respite
+ Access the external and internal areas of the home for family, self-care, and play activities
+ Receive appropriate assistance with her daily self-care and after-school routine
+ Be involved in all aspects of family life at her friend's home
+ Be involved in community life in her friend's neighborhood

Mr. and Mrs. Fisher's goals are to:
+ Provide a safe environment in their home for Suzie when she visits and stays for extended periods
+ Provide Suzie with safe access from the street to and through the front door into the home

+ Provide Suzie with safe access to all areas within the home, including upstairs and downstairs areas—the bedrooms, bathroom, and living and dining areas

+ Have a safe environment for Suzie's transfer, mobility, and self-care activities and for play, minimizing risk of injury to Suzie and to those who assist her in these tasks

+ Incorporate Suzie into all family and community activities

Evaluating Occupational Performance and Identifying Needs

The occupational therapist reviewed health information and school reports prior to the visit to establish Suzie's current physical and functional status.

During the home visit, the therapist interviewed both Suzie's mother and Mr. and Mrs. Fisher to investigate Suzie's capacity to function within their home. Suzie was also observed playing on the floor and sitting in her wheelchair. She was also observed being wheeled by Mr. and Mrs. Fisher through the various entrances to the home and accessing features of rooms within the downstairs portion of the home. The COPM was used to guide the discussion and formulate Suzie's goals for the short and long term.

Mobility and Transfers

Suzie spends a considerable amount of time seated on the floor in the living room area, engaging in play activities. She is unable to assist with transfers, weight-bear, or walk and is fully dependent on others to propel and navigate her attendant-propelled manual wheelchair.

Suzie sleeps on a mattress on the floor, because of previous falls from a bed, despite the installation of a bed rail to act as a barrier. She is moved from her bed into her wheelchair or mobile over-toilet shower chair by caregivers using a floor-based electric hoist.

Mr. and Mrs. Fisher transfer Suzie manually because of the lack of appropriate access for hoist equipment in some areas of their home. The lifts include transfers in and out of chairs, on and off the bed that has been lowered onto the floor (to prevent injury if the client rolls off of the mattress), and from bath to wheelchair. Mr. Fisher carries Suzie up 14 stairs to access the upper level of the home. On occasions, Brittany also lifts Suzie in and out of the upstairs bath. Suzie was observed sitting on the

floor, using her left arm for support, demonstrating good static sitting balance. She could also "bottom shuffle" short distances on the floor.

Suzie travels in a bus, modified to be safe to transport children in wheelchairs, to school. Her mother and Brittany's family drive Suzie in their own private cars to access the community. Suzie also uses a taxi service that has vehicles that have been modified for wheelchair use.

Self Care Activities

Suzie has a tendency to aspirate when eating her food, and she has a gastrostomy button for all feeding. She is incontinent and wears incontinent aids, which are changed by caregivers on her bed. It is anticipated that Suzie will not require wheelchair access in a toilet area. At home, her mother uses a hoist to transfer her from bed into a mobile over-toilet shower chair (attendant propelled), which is then wheeled into a stepless shower. Her mother uses a handheld shower hose to control water direction in the shower. At the conclusion of the routine, she takes Suzie back to her bedroom, where she is lifted onto her bed for dressing activities. Because of the severity of Suzie's physical and intellectual disabilities, she receives full physical assistance for all other self-care tasks, such as dressing, changing incontinence aids, and grooming.

When at the Fishers' home, her caregivers lift Suzie in and out of the bath without a hoist, and all dressing tasks are completed on her bed.

Suzie was observed to have full range of movement in her upper limbs; however, she is generally hypotonic. She is able to swipe and bat using whole arm movement, reach and grasp medium-sized objects—for example, a tennis ball—during play using a power grasp; however, she is unable to grasp objects with fine precision or at the request of caregivers. For example, she is unable to hold a handheld shower hose on request. Two-handed manipulation or transfer of objects from one hand to the other was not observed.

Anthropometric Measurements and Equipment

Suzie and her current equipment were measured (Table 15-1). It is anticipated that, as she grows, she will require larger equipment. Suzie's reach ranges were not measured because of her lack of upper limb function and her capacity to reach and operate features in the built environment. Her physical stature is similar to girls her own age.

Table 15-1. Approximate Anthropometric Measurements of Suzie in Her Wheelchair

	MANUAL WHEELCHAIR	*MOBILE OVER-TOILET SHOWER CHAIR*	*HOIST (ELECTRIC, FLOOR-BASED)*	*BED*
OCCUPIED WIDTH	22 in (560 mm)	23.5 in (600 mm)	22.75 in (580 mm)	78.75 in (2,000 mm)
OCCUPIED LENGTH	33.75 in (860 mm)	29.5 in (750 mm)	43.25 in (1,100 mm)	41.25 in (1,050 mm)
TURNING CIRCLE DIAMETER	47.25 in (1,200 mm)	<43.25 in (<1,100 mm)	Can fit through a 30.75-in (780 mm) door clearance off a 47.25-in (1,200 mm) wide corridor	N/A
FLOOR TO TOE WITH FOOT ON FOOTPLATE	11.75 in (300 mm)	11.5 in (290 mm)	N/A	N/A
FLOOR TO TOP OF ARMREST	28.25 in (720 mm)	31.5 in (800 mm)	N/A	N/A

Occupational Therapy Involvement

The service agency privately contracted the occupational therapist to provide advice on home modifications to enable Suzie to stay in the Fishers' home with greater safety and to ensure that she is included in all aspects of family life. Suzie's own home environment had been modified to provide wheelchair access to enable her and her caregivers to manage with safety and ease.

During the interview and in the process of observing the client in her wheelchair negotiating spaces and environmental features, Suzie's mother and Mr. and Mrs. Fisher discussed the layout of the Fishers' home and the possible changes required to enable those assisting Suzie to manage the built environment with ease. This discussion included the look and the possible cost of various modifications given Suzie's current and future roles and the structure of the home. Consideration was also given to the changing nature of her disability over time and her current and future equipment needs. A combination of narrative, scientific, ethical, and pragmatic reasoning approaches was used as the therapist examined the client's access to, and performance in, each area of the home and the external areas of the property. The therapist used the information gathered at the time of the hospital visit, the advice of a technical advisor, and the views of all people in attendance at the time of the visit to formulate options for discussion.

A technical advisor with a building background attended the home visit with the occupational therapist to provide advice on the proposed structural modifications and compliance and building approval considerations associated with any work. The therapist took Suzie's anthropometric measurements to use in developing the modifications. Photos were also taken, and measurements of the built environment were recorded by the technical advisor and occupational therapist.

Other considerations included the cost of the work, ensuring that the home modifications were designed in keeping with the look of the home without creating an institutional appearance, and the needs of other household members.

Environmental Issues and Intervention Options

Various environmental issues and intervention options were discussed during the walk-through of the home with Suzie's mother and Mr. and Mrs. Fisher.

Wheelchair Access to the Home

Because of the presence of a step at the front door, various intervention options were considered, including using portable ramps or installing a new concrete landing and short ramp to connect the front door to the carport, underneath the existing awning. A portable ramp was considered too heavy to relocate when accommodating the needs of other pedestrians walking in and out of the home and would not provide under-cover access.

The final recommendation was to create a landing and ramp design that would enable under-cover access and that would not detract from the look of the home. It was proposed that soil and turf be laid to the edges of the landing and path areas to ensure that the client would not wheel off a steep edge but would have a flat surface on which to roll. The ramp was designed to suit all pedestrians and, as a permanent feature, was a cost-effective alternative for the long term compared with installing a portable ramp.

More Suitable Location of Mr. and Mrs. Fisher's Bedroom

Suzie currently stays in a small room on the ground level of the home, which is adjacent to a bathroom, and the garage is converted into a storage room and playroom. Mr. and Mrs. Fisher's bedroom is upstairs at present, and they need to be closer to Suzie's bedroom to ensure that they can monitor her at night. Mr. and Mrs. Fisher identified the adjoining double garage as a suitable space to create their new bedroom. Other alternatives included Suzie residing upstairs, but this was considered problematic because the first level hallway and bathroom were not accessible. The option of converting some of the downstairs area into a bedroom for Mr. and Mrs. Fisher was considered the most viable solution, because it would create the least disruption to other family members who occupy bedrooms upstairs. Further, other areas of the home downstairs could be modified to create a completely accessible ground-level area to suit Suzie's self-care routine and play activities.

A new downstairs floor plan was designed to include a new bedroom, an accessible bathroom, and a two-way vestibule to allow for complete privacy when Suzie is moving from the bathroom into her own bedroom (Figure 15-8).

Access to the Downstairs Shower Area

A raised shower tray did not allow a mobile over-toilet shower chair to wheel into the recess easily. Further, there was inadequate space for caregivers to stand beside Suzie as they showered and dried her. It was noted that access to the toilet and vanity were not required. Caregivers assisted Suzie to wash her face and brush her teeth by holding a bowl under her chin.

It was determined that the overall dimensions of the existing bathroom were adequate, and the toilet and vanity would remain in their current positions to minimize renovation costs. Entry to the room was relocated by blocking the existing door and installing

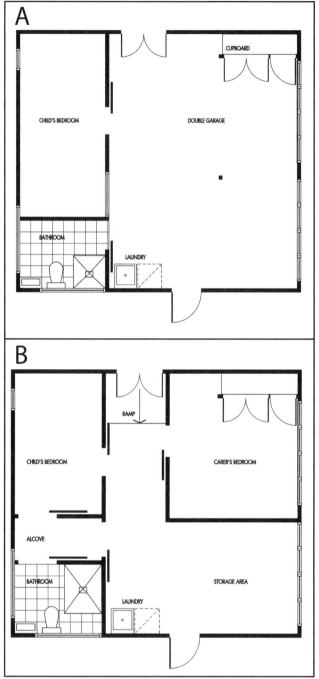

Figure 15-8. Plans before (A) and after (B) bathroom and bedroom modifications.

a new sliding door on the adjacent wall. This would create more floor space at the shower entry, so the over-toilet shower chair could be maneuvered with ease. The shower tray was removed, and a stepless shower was installed, with shower curtain and handheld shower to enable caregivers to complete the self care routine with Suzie with safety and ease. A handheld shower was recommended to ensure that water could be directed as required.

Wheelchair Access to Double Garage Area From Downstairs Living Area

An internal, short ramp was considered the most cost-effective means to achieve wheelchair access at this entry with the high step. Options considered included a temporary ramp or a permanent ramp. The temporary ramp was regarded as unsuitable because it could be unstable and dangerous if Suzie happened to shuffle on her bottom over to this area and negotiate the slope.

Access to the First-Floor Level

This was seen to be desirable to enable Suzie to participate in family meals and social activities. Options considered included the following:

+ Installing a ramp at the rear of the home, leading from ground level to the first level of the home

+ Installing an elevator on the outside of the home and creating a new doorway at the first level of the home

+ Providing a stair-lift on the 14 internal stairs

Installing a ramp at the rear of the home to the study or rear patio to comply with current US access standards requires a specific gradient (1:12). To achieve this, the ramp run would be lengthy, costly, and exposed to the weather, posing a safety risk, especially as Suzie increases in stature and weight. The long run would require numerous turns and take up at least half of the backyard area—space that is used for play by other children in the home. Access around to the rear was also problematic, and there was no area at the front of the home to install a ramp. The ramp option was discounted as a costly and inappropriate solution.

It was determined that installing an elevator would require significant building and earthworks to the area where it would need to be positioned. Access to the side of the home or the rear of the home where it could be located was problematic because of lack of space and the slope of the land. Although an elevator could be removed later and the area repaired to its former state, it was nonetheless considered an expensive and inappropriate solution.

The final option considered included installing a stair-lift on the internal stairs, which would allow Suzie to be transported up and down the stairs without being carried. Currently, Mr. Fisher lifts and carries her up and down the stairs, and he is experiencing back pain. The stair-lift could still enable others to use the stairs, because it would still allow adequate clearance in the stairwell. The stair-lift can be folded and positioned around the corner of the stairs at the top and bottom of the flight to minimize the amount of floor space occupied.

To ensure that the stair-lift would be the safest option and to check the technical requirements for installation, the therapist arranged for the supplier of the stair-lift to provide a trial. Suzie maintained her position on the seat on the stair-lift and, with the seat belt in place, was assessed as being safe when it moved. The pace of the stair-lift can be adjusted to suit Suzie, and the caregiver can walk beside her as she travels up the stairs. Having a back-up battery, this would be suitable to use during any power failure.

Installing a stair-lift was recommended as a cost-effective and safe solution for Suzie and her caregivers for the short-and long term, compared with the other options reviewed. It would be easy to remove from the stairs when no longer required and the area repaired to its former state.

Clinical Reasoning, Evaluation, and Justification for Recommendations

Clinical reasoning began once information was provided by the referrer at the time of initial contact, documentation from the medical service was received, and through discussion and observing Suzie in the home.

Scientific reasoning was used to interpret information regarding Suzie's health conditions. Because Suzie is continuing to physically grow, acquire new equipment, and experience various health conditions because of having multiple health disorders, it is anticipated that she will continue to encounter changing environmental demands and barriers. Scientific reasoning was used to collect cues throughout the assessment process as to how Suzie's skills and deficits were likely to affect her performance and when evaluating the effectiveness of each solution in addressing her occupational performance needs.

Narrative reasoning assisted the occupational therapist to understand and interpret information relating to past and present life and Suzie's goals for the future. The occupational therapist was advised, for example, that Brittany's family had previously befriended Suzie's mother and had offered to provide informal occasional support. As a result of the development of strong friendships and trust over time, Suzie will now continue to visit Brittany and her family in the long term and participate in all aspects of their home and community life. Such community links and support arrangements will continue to impact on her future goals for her lifestyle and involvement with others in the community.

Pragmatic reasoning was used to consider contextual factors, choice of materials, and relevant measurements for modifications, as well as funding issues—for example, the age of the house, the specific use of particular areas of the home for various activities, the flexibility of the family to change location of activities to suit Suzie, and whether she would continue to reside there on a part-time basis or whether the support would conclude when she reached adulthood. Funding for the home modifications had become available through a support program and, though limited, it was allocated on the basis of her support needs for the long term with the Fisher family. In particular, there was a focus on ensuring that the modifications suited the family, who undertook heavy lifting in the absence of suitable modifications. The support arrangements were not sustainable if a practical approach was not considered in relation to addressing the problems with caregivers lifting Suzie and carrying her between areas in the home.

Pragmatic reasoning was used when considering Suzie and her caregiver's anthropometric and equipment measurements when planning clearances and circulation space and for positioning equipment, fittings, and fixtures in the specific areas of the home. It was also important in designing the solution that the therapist factor in the growth of the child and ensure the well-being of the caregivers in the long term.

Ethical reasoning was used in considering alternative decisions for each issue, including those that were not addressed, and the consequences of recommendations made. Ethical reasoning was also used when considering the appropriate use of funding for short- to long-term planning of home modification solutions. For example, despite the client receiving funding through the home modifications program, the therapist was mindful that the program had limited funding and specific criteria for the provision of home modifications. The therapist made recommendations that did not compromise Suzie's health or safety and that also fit the guidelines of the program. This involved a process of negotiation between all parties.

At the initial home visit, the technical advisor provided samples of products and finishes and sketched preliminary designs for discussion with Mr. and Mrs. Fisher and Suzie's mother. Subsequent to the visit, the therapist and technical advisor refined the design options and presented these to Mr. and Mrs. Fisher and Suzie's mother during a second home visit. The proposed solutions were discussed and finalized. The occupational therapy report, including the technical advisor's plans and specifications, was forwarded to the family, who proceeded to obtain three quotes from building firms specializing in home modifications.

Outcomes

A preferred builder was chosen by the clients in consultation with the service providing funding for the work, and the modifications were installed.

The occupational therapist visited Suzie in the Fishers' home to complete a postmodification evaluation. An interview and structured observation of Suzie in the various areas of the home were conducted. The original occupational therapy report was reviewed during the interview to identify any changes in Suzie's functional status or her caregiver's capacity to manage the various activities in the home and community. Suzie and her caregivers were observed to manage with safety and ease accessing all areas of the home that were modified. The home modifications were installed as per the original occupational therapy report. The products and finishes appeared to be coping with wear and tear and were reported to suit the needs of all of the family. Caregiver well-being was established by questioning Mr. and Mrs. Fisher about whether they had sustained any injuries because of assisting Suzie with her mobility around the home.

The occupational therapist identified that the installation of a ceiling track hoist might be required in the upstairs area as Suzie grows, to eliminate the need for caregivers to lift her on and off the stair-lift.

Since this postmodification visit, the therapist has kept in contact with the Fisher family and Suzie's mother, who have reported that Suzie continues to make progress with respect to undertaking her schooling and hobbies and continues to be fully included in the family's activities when staying with Brittany. Neither Mr. nor Mrs. Fisher have sustained an injury while caring for Suzie since the modifications were installed, and Brittany is no longer required to assist with manual transfers. Mr. and Mrs. Fisher report that they feel safe assisting Suzie through self-care routines in the new environment.

CASE STUDY 3: AN ELDERLY MAN AGING INTO DISABILITY

Client Interests and Daily Activities

Walter is a 69-year-old pensioner who lives by himself in an apartment in a small seaside suburb. Walter moved from a large city to this suburb about

40 years ago after separating from his wife. He has had no contact with his wife or children since that time.

Walter completes a daily walk to access local shops and services located within a 0.62-mile (1 km) radius of his apartment. He enjoys this daily outing because it provides him with social contact and exercise and allows him to complete his community-based errands. Walter does not drive. He also enjoys listening to the radio, and he shares the daily newspaper with a neighbor.

Health Condition and Functional Performance

Walter has the following health conditions:

+ Cerebellar degeneration: The most characteristic symptom experienced by Walter is a wide-legged, unsteady walk, with a mild back-and-forth tremor in the trunk of his body. Other symptoms demonstrated include slow, unsteady, and jerky movements of his arms and legs and slowed and slurred speech. Walter was diagnosed with this condition 20 years ago with a slow progression of symptoms, and he has reviews by a neurologist every 6 months.

+ Colectomy secondary to colon cancer: This surgery (removal of part of the colon) occurred 23 years ago, and Walter takes medication to help him manage symptoms of the condition, which include urinary urgency and bowel irregularity. Walter is monitored by his doctor every 3 years.

+ Osteoarthritis in his back, hips, knees, and shoulders: Walter experiences pain and stiffness and loss of range in these joints.

Location and Description of Home

Walter lives in a rented, one-bedroom, ground-level apartment within a complex of 12 apartments in a small bayside suburb. The apartment is located within 0.6 mile (1 km) of local shops and the bay. Curb cuts, sidewalks, and seats facilitate good community access with a wheeled walker within the local area. The apartment complex is landscaped with low-maintenance shrubs and bushes and has lawn areas that are maintained by a hired gardener.

The complex is located on a block of land that has a slight downward incline from the road. A pathway with one 23.5-in (600 mm) step leads directly from a path at the street level to Walter's apartment. There is a 1.5-in (40 mm) step at the front and back doors of his apartment. Walter has an individual clothesline located in a courtyard at the back of his apartment. The garbage bins and mailboxes are located in a communal area that is accessed via a level pathway.

The accommodation is fitted with low-pile carpet in the living room, and there are non-slip tiles in the kitchen and the combined bathroom and laundry areas. The bathroom contains a 39.25-in by 39.25-in (1,000 mm by 1,000 mm) shower recess, the toilet, a sink, and the laundry area. The shower has a 2-in (50 mm) step down into the recess and is enclosed by a shower curtain. The kitchen contains an upright electric stove, pantry, and cupboards below the kitchen counter.

Client Goals

Walter indicated that his short-term goals are to maintain independence and improve safety in completing his daily routine and living activities despite deterioration in his balance and coordination. In particular, he identified showering, toileting, and access to the bathroom and local community as activities in which he was currently experiencing safety concerns.

Walter's long-term goal is to remain within his current accommodation and local community. He stated that, if possible, he did not want to move from his apartment.

Evaluating Occupational Performance and Identifying Needs

Prior to the home visit, the occupational therapist reviewed Walter's health information. This review served not only to inform the therapist of Walter's health history and symptoms, but also of likely progression of his illnesses.

During the home visit, the therapist interviewed Walter to identify his goals and ascertain occupational performance difficulties from his own perspective. The interview was followed by observation. He was observed mobilizing, negotiating steps, completing transfers, and simulating showering. The therapist tested the validity of performance difficulties reported during the interview and hypothesized as to the underlying causes of the problems by analyzing Walter's performance in identified activities.

Sufficient time was allocated for Walter's assessment so that he could articulate his concerns and for the therapist to observe functional performance. The assessment was undertaken within Walter's home, which was the context of identified occupational performance difficulties.

Mobility and Transfers

Walter walked independently indoors without the use of a walking aid; however, he used a four-wheeled walker for mobilizing outdoors. He had difficulty negotiating stairs, including single steps.

Walter was having increasing difficulty with standing balance and reported that he became more unsteady when fatigued. He said that he had difficulty with bending, particularly as he experienced arthritic pain in his lower extremities doing so. He also reported dizziness and unsteadiness once he stood up, stating that he was fearful of falling. Walter demonstrated difficulty transferring from the toilet seat height of 15.75 in (400 mm) above floor level and low-seated surfaces.

Self-Care and Homemaker Activities

Walter was lifting his walker over threshold steps and the step in the front path and, although he had not sustained a fall, he was anxious that this might occur as a result of his decreased balance.

Walter had difficulty negotiating the door in the bathroom to access the toilet and shower areas. He has to access the bathroom facilities numerous times during the day and night; however, he accesses the laundry area only once per week on average. When accessing the bathroom, Walter has to mobilize around the door, which impedes direct access.

He reported that he was independent with his self-care activities. He indicated that he stands to shower; however, he is feeling increasingly anxious when showering because of his reduced balance. The therapist observed Walter leaning against the wall to assist him when standing, and he stated that he sits on the toilet during showering to rest. He also identified that he was no longer showering on a daily basis, despite this being his preference, and that he was not satisfied with his ability to wash his hair and his legs due to a fear of falling.

The toilet is located directly beside the shower. Walter sits for all toileting. He demonstrated difficulty getting on and off the toilet and used the toilet seat and wall beside the toilet as supports to assist with transfers.

He reported that he does his own shopping, accessing the shops twice a week and transporting his groceries home with his wheeled walker.

Walter also does his own cooking, reporting that he enjoys preparing his own meals and prefers to eat at home rather than eating out. He generally cooks in an electric frying pan and uses a microwave to reheat food. He stated that he rarely uses the oven; however, he receives help from his neighbor on occasions when he does use the appliance because he experiences difficulty placing items on, and retrieving them from, low surfaces. Walter stated that his neighbor was happy to assist, and he is pleased with this arrangement. He avoids bending by putting regularly used items within easy reach in the pantry and on the shelves of the cupboards.

Walter receives assistance from a community-based cleaning service every second week to assist with cleaning, ironing, and laundry. He does his own personal laundry using a fold-up clothes-drying stand that he keeps on his back courtyard area.

Anthropometric Measurements

Walter's anthropometric measurements were taken to determine the best height for seated surfaces and reach ranges.

Purpose of Occupational Therapy Involvement

A home visit referral requested home modification recommendations to ensure Walter's safety and independence in his home environment. Home modifications were also required to enable Walter to safely access the community from his home environment. A combination of narrative, scientific, ethical, and pragmatic reasoning was used to assess the appropriate intervention options.

Environmental Issues and Intervention Options

Various environmental issues and intervention options were discussed during the walk-through of the home with Walter.

Facility for Sitting in Shower Recess

Options reviewed included the installation of a freestanding shower seat versus a fixed shower. Because of space restrictions in the shower area, the installation of a foldaway, wall-mounted shower seat was recommended.

The possibility of installing a handheld shower hose to allow Walter to direct the flow of water while seated was discussed with Walter, as were the various styles available.

Cost implications, the shower recess size, and factors including Walter's mobility and ability to transfer, sitting balance, anthropometric measurements, and reach range were considered in the final recommendations, which included the following:

+ Installing a space-saving foldaway, wall-mounted shower seat in the shower recess at a height of 18.5 in (470 mm) above floor level. The shower seat size recommended was 38.5 in (980 mm) wide by 15.75 in (400 mm) deep and mounted centrally on the shower wall so that the taps would be located on the left side when seated.

+ Removing the existing shower head and replacing it with a handheld shower that has a flexible nylon hose. The handheld shower was fit to a friction-sliding mount on a vertical rail configuration was recommended.

Supports at the Toilet for Transfers

Options considered included the use of an over-toilet frame, toilet raiser, and installing grab bars. Due to the potential trip hazard presented by the legs of an over-toilet frame in the confined bathroom area, installing a grab rail and toilet raiser were selected as the most appropriate options. Walter indicated a preference to initially trial a grab bar only, because he had personal concerns about cost, aesthetics, and the hygiene of a raised toilet seat.

The final recommendations included installing an L-shaped grab rail on the left side of the toilet when seated. The grab rail is to be installed as per the access standards, with the horizontal component of the grab rail to be located 27.5 in (700 mm) above floor level. The bend of the grab began 5.75 in (150 mm) forward of the datum point of the toilet.

Bathroom Access

The bathroom door is hinged on the right side and swings into the combined laundry and bathroom. The shower recess and toilet are located to the right when entering the bathroom, the vanity sink is directly opposite the doorway, and the laundry is situated to the left side of the room. The bathroom door impedes direct access into the bathroom area. Options of removing the door and hanging a curtain were discussed; however, Walter preferred to retain the door. It could not be reswung to open out into the hallway because of the confined space within the apartment, nor could a sliding door be fitted because of inadequate wall space.

The final recommendations included rehinging the bathroom door so that it would open to the left side toward the laundry area when entering the bathroom. A ceiling doorstop was recommended to prevent the rehung door from hitting the laundry light. The double light switch was to be relocated to the outside of the bathroom because of access issues that would occur following the rehanging of the door.

Steps a Barrier to Community Access

A step in the front pathway leading to Walter's apartment and a step at both the front and back entrances of the apartment were identified as hazards to Walter accessing the local community. In recommending the installation of a ramp at each of these separate entries, considerations, such as the gradient and length of the ramp, as well as construction material, were taken into account. Factors including Walter's reach range for accessing door handles when standing at the base of the ramp, level of mobility, type of walking aid used, and future deterioration of health condition were considered in the final recommendations, which were:

+ Construction of a brushed concrete ramp with side splays at the 1.5-in (40 mm) step at the front and back doors. The ramp was recommended to be 1:8 gradient and to extend the full width of the step at both the front and back entrances (width of finished ramp 52.75 in (1340 mm); length of finished ramp 12.5 in (320 mm).

+ Construction of a brushed concrete path at the 2.25-in (60 mm) step in the front path. The finished path was recommended to extend 91.25 in (2320 mm) forward from the step to an existing joint in the path, resulting in the gradient of the finished section to be approximately 1:35. Topsoil and turf were recommended beside the new ramped section to form a level verge of approximately 23.75 in (600 mm) wide on both sides.

Clinical Reasoning, Evaluation, and Justification for Recommendations

Clinical reasoning began once information was provided by Walter at the initial referral, documentation provided by Walter's local doctor was received, and knowledge of Walter's local area was gained.

Scientific reasoning was used to interpret information regarding Walter's health condition. Considerations that Walter was likely to have progressively deteriorating symptoms of decreased balance, incoordination, weakness, and pain, together with fewer internal resources and less energy due to aging, led to the reasoning that he would become more susceptible to environmental influences. Scientific reasoning was used to collect cues throughout the assessment process as to how Walter's skills and deficits were likely to affect his performance and, when evaluating the effectiveness of each solution, in addressing Walter's occupational performance needs.

Narrative reasoning assisted the therapist to understand and interpret information relating to Walter's life. The therapist became aware, for example, that Walter had lived within the bayside suburb for approximately 40 years and that his life focused around the local community and his home. He had a good relationship with neighbors that he valued.

Pragmatic reasoning was used to consider contextual factors, choice of materials, and relevant measurements for modifications, as well as funding issues. For example, the compact size of the accommodation was considered in recommending the installation of fixtures rather than equipment, because it was reasoned that freestanding equipment would present greater risk of trip hazards. In addition, because Walter was living in a state-owned property, funding was available for fixtures and structural changes. If, however, Walter had to purchase equipment, there would be cost implications given that he is a pensioner.

Pragmatically, choice of materials was considered. For example, a concrete ramp is not as susceptible to weathering as a wooden ramp, and a brushed concrete finish minimizes risks of slipping. Anthropometric measurements and reach ranges were considered in positioning grab bars, the shower hose, and the shower seat. They were also considered when calculating the length of the ramps at the entrances to the apartment.

Ethical reasoning was used when considering alternative decisions for each issue, including those not addressed, and the consequences of recommendations made. For example, Walter indicated that he was not able to access his oven but depended on a neighbor to assist him when he used it. Although Walter's solution to the issue may not be sustainable long term and there was a high risk of injury should Walter attempt to retrieve hot items from the oven, it was reasoned that Walter had sufficient insight into his limitations and the potential consequences. Hence, his inability to access the oven independently was not addressed as an area of concern.

Outcomes

Quotes were obtained from building firms who specialize in home modification installations, and a builder was chosen to proceed with the work. Following completion of the modifications, the therapist visited Walter in his home to complete a post-modification evaluation. The therapist conducted an interview and structured observation of Walter in the various areas of the home. The interview included the review of the original occupational therapy report to determine whether there had been any changes in Walter's capacity to manage the various activities in the home and community. He had clearly improved in general functional capacity, being able to manage all activities with greater confidence. The products and finishes recommended appeared to be coping with wear and tear.

CASE STUDY 4: TWO MEN WITH INTELLECTUAL AND PHYSICAL DISABILITIES SHARING A HOME

Client Interests and Daily Activities

Tony and Dean are 31-year-old men who have lived together in a house with 24-hour support for the past 11 years. Prior to living together, the two men lived with three other people in a shared housing arrangement in the same city suburb. They receive an additional 5 hours of support funding to enable them to access the community.

Tony enjoys going to the local park and the beach. His family members live on the opposite side of the city from him, but they visit on a monthly basis. Tony's mother assists him as his informal decision maker in relation to lifestyle and financial matters.

Dean enjoys drives in the country and visiting his family. His family members live locally, and he sees them on a regular basis. Dean's father acts as Dean's informal decision maker on matters relating to his lifestyle. A government service acts as the administrator of finances for Dean.

Both clients rely on support staff to drive them to facilities in the community.

Health Condition and Functional Performance

Both men have an intellectual disability. Tony has also been diagnosed as having

+ Epilepsy, controlled by medication
+ Urinary incontinence, particularly at night
+ Flexion deformity of the spine (a significant static scoliosis)
+ Internal rotation of hips secondary to cerebral palsy

Tony tends to be impulsive and likes to climb fences or benches and grab at items during meal preparation and other activities in the home. He has had a history of falls both inside and outside of the home, and he has damaged the walls inside of the home by chipping away at the sheeting. He also tends to fiddle with taps if left alone in the bathroom and has been known to drink the hot tap water from the bath spout when bathing unsupervised.

Dean has been diagnosed as having:

+ Autism
+ Temporal lobe epilepsy, controlled by medication
+ Occasional incontinence

He demonstrated difficulty with fine motor control in the upper limbs.

Over the long term, both clients might require more equipment as they age. This could include a mobile over-toilet shower chair, particularly to suit Tony's needs.

Location and Description of the House

The two men live in a standard three-bedroom brick home that is slab on ground (one step into the property) in a quiet city suburban area. There are detached houses located on either side of the property, in close proximity. Their house was purchased specifically for Tony and Dean, and it is typical of other detached houses in their city suburb. It has not been built specifically for people who use mobility equipment, such as wheelchairs.

The garage is located at the front of the property, and the front entry is at the side of the home. This entry is accessed by a path that has gardens planted on either side. There is a step at the front door. The spacious backyard is enclosed by a 3-foot-high (1,000 mm) timber fence. The rear yard contains a rotary clothesline. The rear entry includes a sliding glass door that leads in from a covered patio area. There is a step up into the house from this area.

The three bedrooms are located at the front of the dwelling. The kitchen is U-shaped and located to the side of the combined kitchen and living room area at the rear of the home. The laundry is located at the side of the home. The bathroom is separate from the toilet, and both areas are located along a hallway toward the front of the home. The bathroom includes a bath, vanity bench, and shower with a shallow tray floor. The home is carpeted throughout the living room, dining room, hallway, and bedrooms. The bathroom and laundry are tiled, and the kitchen area has vinyl flooring.

Client Goals

When Tony and Dean moved into their new home, their short-term goals, established with their parents as informal decision makers and staff helpers, were to:

+ Establish a familiar routine of daily activities with staff in their new home
+ Manage the new environment during these daily activities

Longer-term goals were to enable the men to:

+ Become familiar with the neighborhood and its residents
+ Participate in local community activities

At the time of interview, the men had established their routine of household activities, undertaking their self care routines in the morning and hobbies or resting at the house during the day. They also had a well-established routine for participating in activities in the community on a regular basis. Some features in the home were presenting as barriers to Tony and Dean.

The overall goal of the home modification was to accommodate the changing activity and access and mobility requirements of the two men (and their caregivers) as they age.

Evaluating Occupational Performance and Identifying Needs

Prior to the home visit, the therapist reviewed the medical information available to establish Tony and Dean's functional statuses prior to being housed and their current abilities.

During the home visit, the therapist interviewed staff and family representatives using the COPM to identify the goals that they felt were important for the men to achieve and to ascertain their capacity to manage safely in the home. The therapist also observed the two men as they moved around the various areas of the home and interacted with the staff and visitors.

Mobility and Transfers

Tony was observed to walk short distances independently; staff reported that he relied on the use of an attendant-propelled manual wheelchair to manage long distances, particularly outdoors. He demonstrated that he was able to manage transfers on and off the bed, a chair, and the toilet by himself without assistance. He was reported to have had falls in the past, both indoors and outdoors, as a result of his unsteady gait and tripping over uneven surfaces or small steps. He frequently moved from standing to sitting on the floor during the visit, and staff helped him to move up from the floor into the standing position. Despite such mobility difficulties, he was able to scale the rear fence.

Dean was observed to have difficulty managing transfers in and out of the bath and shower as a result of his reduced balance. He, too, was tripping in areas where there were small changes in floor levels. Staff provided physical assistance during these activities.

Self-Care and Homemaker Activities

Staff reported that both men relied on them for assistance during self-care activities. During dressing activities, Tony requires full assistance, whereas Dean relies on verbal prompting. Staff indicated that they wanted to leave the men unsupervised during some activities to ensure that they maintained their dignity and to enhance their independence. This has resulted in Tony damaging the built environment or injuring himself through fiddling with the taps, drinking the scalding hot water, and hitting the toilet cistern with his back. Tony's urinary incontinence resulted in ongoing spillage on the carpet in his bedroom, which was creating an unhealthy environment.

Staff also reported that they complete all household tasks for the two men, because they are not able to participate safely in these activities. They indicated that they have been experiencing difficulty managing the two men when preparing meals because Tony and Dean tend to interrupt the activities by grabbing at the various cooking items and accessing the kitchen cupboards. This is of particular concern to the staff, who indicated that only one member of their team works in the household at any one time.

Anthropometric Measurements and Equipment

Tony and Dean's physical stature and reach ranges were reviewed as well as the wheelchair that Tony uses. There was no need to take measurements of the wheelchair because it is not being used indoors at present. Thought was given to the future use of a mobile over-toilet shower chair in the bathroom, and measurements for this equipment were considered when planning various modifications.

Purpose of Occupational Therapy Involvement

A home visit referral requested home modification recommendations to ensure that Tony and Dean would be able to use the bathroom and other areas of the home with greater safety. A technical advisor with a building background attended the home visit with the therapist to provide advice on the proposed structural modifications and compliance and building approval considerations associated with this work.

During the interview and the process of observation of Tony and Dean in their home, the caregivers and family representatives discussed the existing layout of the home and the possible changes required to enable them to manage the built environment with greater safety and ease. This included a discussion about the possible cost of various modifications, given the current and future care requirements of the two men and the structure of the home. Consideration was also given to the changing nature of their disabilities and their current and future equipment needs. A combination of narrative, scientific, ethical, and pragmatic reasoning was used to assess the appropriate intervention options as each area of the home and the external areas of the property were examined. The therapist used the information gathered at the time of the home visit, the advice of the technical advisor, and the views of the staff and the clients' families to formulate options for discussion.

Photos were taken and measurements were recorded by the technical advisor and therapist. The anthropometric measurements of the clients and the caregivers, and those of future equipment to be used in the various areas of the home, were also used in the redesign. Other considerations included the cost of the work and ensuring that the home modifications would be in keeping with the look of the home without creating an institutional appearance. Of importance was ensuring that the home modifications were appropriate from a short- and long-term health, safety, and quality of life perspective for both men. The safety of the caregivers as they worked with the two men was another important consideration.

Environmental Issues and Intervention Options

External Access

Safe Fenced Area

Tony could scale the 39.25-in-high (1,000 mm) fencing easily. Options discussed included increasing the current level of supervision while the men were using the yard or changing the style of fence to ensure that if Tony attempted to climb the structure, he would be slowed down by its height and style of construction. Extra funding from the support service was not available to provide more hours of support staff supervision. The final recommendation included the construction of a 70.75-in-high fence (1,800 mm) that had no gaps in the palings or horizontal support beams on the inside of the fence that would act as footholds.

Safe Surface on the Rear Concrete Patio

Staff reported that Tony was having falls on the rear concrete patio and injuring himself. Options discussed included limiting the time Tony spent outdoors, restricting his access to the rear patio, laying carpet, or installing a more permanent outdoor ground cover that was cushioned. The final recommendation included installing the cushioned cover, which was funded by Tony's family. This was considered the best option rather than restricting Tony's use of the area and laying carpet that would not suit the outdoor conditions.

Internal Access

Easy-to-Grasp Door Handles

Dean was experiencing difficulty using the door handles and accessing the various areas of the home. The main recommendation considered was removing the existing door handles and replacing them with lever handles. This modification would enhance Dean's level of independence in the home.

Durable and Safe Flooring

Tony had urinary incontinence, and the ongoing spillage on the carpet in his bedroom was creating an unhealthy environment. The options considered included trialing medication with him, new continence products to be worn under his clothes, and removing the existing carpet and replacing it with a vinyl that was slip-resistant when wet and did not absorb the spillages so readily. All three options were recommended to enhance Tony's current health status and to ensure a clean environment for him and others in the household. Vinyl in other areas of the home, such as the kitchen and hallway, had holes and were slippery when wet. It was recommended that these areas be laid with new vinyl that was also slip-resistant when wet.

Safe Access to the Outdoors

Tony was having difficulty stepping over the sill of the rear sliding glass door and down onto the patio unsupported. Staff reported that he had fallen on this patio. Options considered included restricting Tony's access to the rear patio, allowing him access only with staff supervision, installing a grab rail on the inside and outside of the door wall for him to hold onto when stepping in and out of the area, and raising the level of the outside patio to the level of the sill. Restricting Tony's access to the outdoor area was considered inappropriate, because it did not encourage ongoing independence. As well,

monitoring and helping Tony was time-consuming for staff. Raising the level of the outside patio was considered too costly. The recommended option included installing grab bars on either side of the door entry to encourage the client to manage this area with greater safety and independence.

Kitchen

Switch Control Safety at the Stove

Both men tended to fiddle with switches. It was recommended that the stove be connected to an isolation switch that allowed it to be deactivated. This switch needed to be located in an inaccessible area. This modification was recommended to enhance the men's safety in the kitchen area.

Easy-to-Use Tap Handles

Dean was experiencing difficulty managing the taps in the various areas of the home. The main option considered was to remove the existing tap handles and replace them with short lever handles. This was recommended to enhance Dean's current level of independence in the home.

Fixed Kitchen Sink Spout

The spout over the kitchen sink tended to rotate and hit the splash back and spray water onto the counter and over the drainage area when turned by the men, who enjoy the activity. The recommendation made by the therapist included installing a fixed spout to direct the water flow into the sink.

Bathroom and Toilet

No Circulation Space in the Bathroom and Toilet for Future Wheelchair Access

The separation of the two areas did not allow future ease of access to a mobile over-toilet shower chair. It was also perceived to be undignified to be wheeled between the two rooms during their self-care routines. Further, the men appeared agitated when in the bathroom, and there was little space to move between the shower, bath and vanity, and caregivers. Options considered included leaving the current layout and relocating the men to another home in the future or combining the toilet and bathroom into one room to create more space. Relocating the men was considered disruptive and costly, and there might not be a suitable home available in the short or medium term. Combining the two rooms was recommended, because it was a home modification that could be done quickly and address immediate behavioral concerns.

Safe Flooring in Toilet and Bathroom Areas

The men and the caregivers alike experienced difficulty negotiating the flooring in the toilet and bathroom because it was not slip-resistant when wet. Options included either applying a slip-resistant coating or etching to the floor or replacing the existing floor covering with a better-quality product. The preferred option was to remove the existing flooring and replace it with a product that was slip-resistant in wet areas, as indicated in the access standards. The etching or coating of the floor would need ongoing maintenance over time; and the finish might ruin the look of the existing tiles and not provide as much grip.

Level Access Into the New Bathroom

There is a small step leading into the toilet and bathroom areas, which the men were tending to trip over. It was determined that this could be eliminated by combining the bathroom and toilet into one area rather than installing a small ramp, ensuring that the entry had a neat, level finish. The presence of a small ramp intruding into the hallway could still create a trip hazard.

Grab Rails for Transfers on and off the Toilet or in and out of the Shower Recess

Options included the men using a toilet surround frame or over-toilet frame in the toilet area and shower chair in the shower or the use of a drop-down shower seat in the shower combined with the installation of grab bars. The use of freestanding equipment was discounted, being considered less stable and safe than the grab bars and a drop-down shower seat as permanent fixtures.

Safe Style of Toilet Roll Holder

The current toilet roll holder protruded from the wall and was a hazard, particularly if the men had falls in the toilet area. Options considered included removing this feature completely or installing a semi-recessed toilet roll holder. The final recommendation included installing the semi-recessed toilet roll holder to enhance the men's safety, especially in the event of a fall in the area.

Safe Style of Soap Holder

The soap holder in the shower recess protruded and could cause an injury if one of the men fell in this area. Options considered included removing of this feature completely or installing a semi-recessed soap holder. The final recommendation included installing the semi-recessed soap holder to enhance the men's safety, especially in the event of a fall in the area.

Presence of Grab Bars

The men tended to lean heavily on the towel rails on the bathroom wall. They are not designed to take the weight of a person and are a hazard. Options considered included removing the rails completely or installing grab bars that could act as towel rails and also support the clients as they completed their self-care routine. The final recommendation included installing grab bars to enhance the men's safety, especially in the event of a fall in the area.

Robust Toilet Cistern and Toilet Seat

The toilet cistern and toilet seat were broken repeatedly by the rocking motion of Tony when he was seated on the toilet. Options included applying rubber foam on the existing cistern or removing the existing cistern and pan and installing an in-wall concealed cistern and new heavy-duty pan.

Various options were considered, including implementing various behavior modification strategies and the partial modification and full modification of the bathroom and toilet areas. Given the future access requirements of the men and the time taken and varying success of the behavior modification strategies, it was recommended that the bathroom be redesigned to include the toilet area and to enable full wheelchair access. It was also proposed that the toilet be removed and replaced with a concealed cistern and a heavy-duty bowl that matched the color of the rest of the room.

Bedrooms

Easy-to-Grasp Wardrobe Handles

Dean was experiencing difficulty managing the wardrobe handles in the various areas of the home. The main option considered included removing the existing wardrobe handles and installing D-shaped handles. This was recommended to enhance Dean's current level of independence in the home.

Electrical

Larger Light Switches

Dean was experiencing difficulty managing the small light switches in the various areas of the home. The main option considered included removing the existing small light switches and installing large rocker switches. This was recommended to enhance Dean's current level of independence in the home.

Other

Controlling Water Temperature

Options considered included staff providing constant supervision of the men around water or providing a thermostatic control device. The latter option was recommended to ensure the safety of the two men at all times, regardless of the level of supervision they were receiving around water.

Clinical Reasoning, Evaluation, and Justification for Recommendations

Clinical reasoning began once information was provided by the referrer at the time of initial contact and through discussion with staff and observing Tony and Dean in the home.

Scientific reasoning was used to interpret information regarding the two men's disabilities and health conditions. Scientific reasoning was used to collect cues throughout the interview, to observe how the men's skills and deficits were likely to affect their performance, and when evaluating the effectiveness of each solution in addressing their occupational performance needs.

Narrative reasoning assisted the therapist to understand and interpret information relating to the men's past and present lives and their goals for the future. The therapist relied on the client information presented by the caregivers because the men were not able to verbally communicate this detail.

Pragmatic reasoning was used to consider contextual factors, choice of materials, and relevant measurements for modifications, as well as funding issues. For example, the size of the home, the space and the finances available for various home modifications, and the look of the final solutions proposed were considered in home modification planning. Limited funding had become available through a home modification program, and recommendations had to focus on enhancing the health, safety, and independence of recipients.

Pragmatically, the clients' and caregivers' anthropometric and equipment measurements were considered in planning clearances and circulation space and for positioning the clients and caregivers as they worked together during self-care and homemaker activities in the specific areas of the home. It was also important when designing the solution that the therapist ensured that the home would be able to withstand possible ongoing damage from the men in the future. The therapist discussed the possibility of the men requiring future wheelchair access as they aged into disability.

Ethical reasoning was used in considering alternative decisions for each issue, including those that were not addressed, and the consequences of recommendations made. Ethical reasoning was also considered in relation to the appropriate use of funding for short- to long-term planning of home modification solutions. For example, despite the clients receiving funding through the home modifications program, the therapist was mindful that the program had limited funding and specific criteria for proving home modifications. The therapist made recommendations that did not compromise the clients' or caregivers' health or safety and that fit the guidelines of the program. This involved a process of negotiation between all parties.

The technical advisor provided samples of products and finishes and sketched preliminary designs for discussion with the caregivers. After concluding the home visit, the therapist and technical advisor then, in a short timeframe, developed design options for the various stakeholders to consider. The therapist visited the various stakeholders a second time to show them the plan options and to discuss the various products. These options were finalized, and the final occupational therapy report including the technical advisor's plans and specifications was forwarded to the home modification program for approval.

Outcomes

Quotes were obtained from three building firms that specialize in home modification installations, and a builder was chosen to proceed with the work. The modifications were installed over a period of several weeks, and the therapist visited the two men in their home to complete a postmodification evaluation. Staff members were interviewed, and structured observation of the two men in the various areas of the home was conducted. The interview included the review of the original occupational therapy report to determine whether there had been any changes in the clients' capacities to manage the various activities in the home and community.

Feedback from support staff indicated that both clients had learned to manage their self-care routines with assistance in the modified bathroom. They reported that both men were not as agitated in the bathroom area, possibly because the combined bathroom and toilet provided greater space for movement and activities with the caregivers. The combined bathroom and toilet area had fewer fittings and fixtures (that is, the bath was removed and the shower cubicle opened up to become wheelchair accessible), and there was greater light in the area.

Other outcomes included the clients experiencing fewer falls at the doorways and greater independence managing doors, taps, and light switches.

The home modifications were installed as per the original occupational therapy report. The products and finishes appeared to be coping with wear and tear and were reported to suit the needs of the two men.

CASE STUDY 5: AN ELDERLY WOMAN WITH A VISION IMPAIRMENT

Client Interests and Daily Activities

Olive is a 69-year-old woman who lives alone in a one-bedroom ground-floor apartment in a beachside suburb of a regional city. Olive has a daughter, living approximately 2 miles (4 km) away, who assists as necessary with some transport and general support. Olive walks along the beach promenade using a long white cane and often uses the bus to return home. When accessing the shopping precinct, she uses local council-subsidized taxicabs or the cab-charge subsidy vouchers supported by the state government. Twice monthly, Olive has access to a community transport service to attend medical appointments anywhere in the city. She states that she goes to the movies twice a month using public transport.

Olive likes to maintain her apartment independently as much as she is able, doing her own cooking, light household cleaning, and laundry tasks. She spends most of the time in her bedroom, especially in the winter months, because this room receives the most sunlight, which helps her limited sight and minimizes heating costs. In the evenings, she watches television in the lounge room. She has a large-screen television, which compensates for her limited sight.

Health Condition and Functional Performance

In 2005, Olive was traveling in California when she had a cerebral hemorrhage. She was hospitalized in Los Angeles for 2 months, and her family was advised that she was critically ill. However, she recovered to be well enough to be flown back home to begin rehabilitation. Prior to this event, Olive experienced good health.

Because of the cerebral hemorrhage, Olive has significant visual field loss, with vision in the upper left quadrant only, but has enough vision not to be declared legally blind. To be legally blind, a person must have visual acuity of 20/200 or less or a visual field of 20 degrees or less. Wearing glasses will not improve Olive's vision.

Physically, Olive recovered well, experiencing some balance problems when she moves quickly, which may be more related to the vision loss, and having a slow deliberate speech pattern. Olive shows no significant cognitive impairment. Other than the white cane to assist mobility, it is anticipated she will not need any other equipment in the future.

During her rehabilitation, Olive was taught how to adapt to her limited visual field by moving her head to scan the environment to avoid bumping into people and objects. Olive can read large print; however, her reading time is limited to a maximum of 15 minutes because of the concentrated effort required.

Olive states she is managing well with all activities of daily living, but adds she does not feel as confident when walking alone as she used to, especially in crowded areas. She states she is not "as sure on my feet, as if I might stumble." Olive is proficient at using the long white cane for mobility and orientation and turning her head to scan the entire surrounding environment, but states she has an intangible uncertainty in recent months. She prefers to use buses rather than taxis to access community facilities, stating that the bus drivers are more helpful than the taxi drivers.

Olive is concerned that she may have further neurological problems and is regularly monitored by a neurologist.

Location and Description of the Home

Olive's apartment is one of 18 in a complex of brick construction situated on a busy four-lane arterial road. There is a bus stop outside of the complex and a pedestrian crossing with audible traffic light controls that enable her to cross the road safely to access the beach promenade.

The apartment has one step at the entry and one step from the lounge area to the outdoor patio at the rear of the apartment. A previous tenant had installed a timber wedge and handrail at this entry. There is a small combined lounge and dining area, a separate kitchen, one bedroom large enough to accommodate a queen-sized bed, and a closet-style laundry. The bathroom has a toilet, vanity unit, and shower recess with a curb. There was originally a bath with a shower over it, but this was removed by a previous tenant, and a shower recess was installed. There is a shower curtain around the perimeter of the recess.

There is a small fenced private courtyard outside of the lounge room. Unfortunately, given the position of the apartment in the middle of an L-shaped block, there is very little sunlight in the courtyard or lounge area of the apartment. Some western sun filters into the bedroom on the opposite side of the unit. This influences the luminance in all rooms of the apartment.

Client Goals

Olive's primary goal is to live safely and independently in her own home for as long as possible. She has concern about having to move into an aged residential care facility if she cannot manage at home.

Olive's short-term goals are to:

+ improve her independence within the home

+ improve her safety by increasing the lighting and modifying the step access to the apartment

Her long-term goal is to remain living alone for as long as possible, using community services to assist if necessary.

Olive's daughter would like her mother to maintain her independence living alone and to improve her safety by minimizing the risk of falls.

Evaluating Occupational Performance and Identifying Needs

The referral for occupational therapy intervention from the orientation and mobility officer was supported by health reports from the local doctor and Olive's neurologist updating Olive's health status and functional ability.

The therapist conducted a home visit and used the COPM to interview Olive to ascertain her goals. The therapist observed her doing tasks in various areas of her apartment to determine her functional limitations.

Mobility and Transfers

Indoors, Olive does not use any mobility aid, and she was observed to be independent in transfers to and from the chair and bed and to move independently around the apartment.

Olive reported that she uses a long white cane to assist outdoor mobility. She was instructed in its use during her rehabilitation by an orientation and mobility trainer from a community agency specializing in training people in mobility activities.

Olive leaves the lights on in all rooms of her apartment to compensate for her poor vision and to assist her in daily activities.

Self-Care and Homemaker Activities

Olive is fully independent in all personal care activities. She does her own shopping, cooking, and laundry activities, and she has help once a fortnight with the heavier household cleaning, such as vacuuming and washing the floors.

Purpose of Occupational Therapy Involvement

The occupational therapy referral requested an assessment of the home environment to minimize possible safety risks so Olive could maintain her independence with minimal reliance on her daughter. Falls prevention was the primary concern. Since her cerebral hemorrhage, Olive has experienced significant vision loss, causing limitations in negotiating the general environment and increasing her risk of falls. Olive had recently moved to her apartment and was unfamiliar with the new surroundings and was having trouble with access into the apartment and the shower.

During the assessment interview and in the process of observing Olive performing activities in her home, she described and demonstrated the limitations and difficulties she was experiencing.

Olive discussed her vision loss and the impact it had on her daily activities and safety. The therapist pointed out options for adaptation and modification and discussed Olive's plans for future care and assistance in the home. The therapist used a combination of narrative, scientific, ethical, and pragmatic reasoning to assess the appropriate intervention options.

It was particularly important for the therapist to discuss with Olive how her limited visual field, vision acuity, and light sensitivity affected her functional ability. It was also important to have her demonstrate how she used contrast and light to assist her in reading tasks and activities, such as using the telephone and kitchen appliances. It was essential that the modifications provided would be appropriate for short- and long-term outcomes.

Environmental Issues and Intervention Options

External Areas

Access to the Front of the Unit

Olive stated that she found the height of the front step (5.5 in, 140 mm) very difficult to negotiate. Options considered included the installation of a ramp and landing or a half-step and landing at the entry. There was inadequate space to install an appropriate ramp and landing without impeding the public walk space.

The final recommendation was to provide a concrete landing at the height of the step and then a half-step (Figure 15-9). This provided two 2.75-in (70 mm) steps, which had a 2-in (50 mm) wide highlighted strip on each tread, and a handrail on the left side ascending. This modification enabled the client to safely negotiate the smaller step risers and use the handrails for extra support.

Risk of Falls at Doorway From the Lounge Onto Patio

The condition of the timber ramp was excellent and not assessed as needing replacement. The timber surface was coated with a slip-resistant paint, and a handrail was in place on the right side descending from the lounge door. The paint surface was a dark green and blended with the shadows of the patio overhang. The outer edges were not clearly distinguishable.

Options considered were to install an extra handrail on the left side to match that on the right or highlight the outer edges of the ramp. The position of the glass sliding patio door prevented installation of the rail in an appropriate position.

The final recommendation was to paint a contrasting highlighted strip on the outer edges of the ramp. Because the concrete and the timber wedge were a dark green, yellow was chosen as the most appropriate color.

Bathroom

Difficult Access Into Shower With a Curb Step

The corner of the existing curb step into the shower had a sharp tiled corner and had caused Olive to trip on many occasions. The floor tiles and those of the curb step were the same pastel color so there was little distinction to highlight the hazard.

Options considered included complete removal of the curb step or modification to the curb. The entire bathroom floor would need to be removed and relaid to track to the shower waste if the curb step was eliminated. This was considered a complex and costly modification that would result in Olive needing to move out of the unit for several days until the work was completed. Olive was not willing to relocate to enable this work to be completed.

The modification to the curb was considered the most appropriate option. This included work to bevel the corner of the shower curb near the vanity and retile the entire curb step in a contrasting color (Figure 15-10). A dark tile color was requested so it could be distinguished against the lighter toned floor tiles. This would ensure that the edge would not be a trip hazard and the contrasting color would provide a visual highlight to the area, ensuring that the edges could be seen. An additional handgrip in the shower and a handheld shower were also recommended to improve Olive's general safety and independence when she was showering.

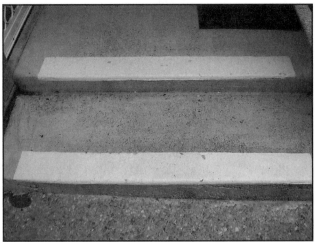

Figure 15-9. Concrete landing and highlighted strip on each tread.

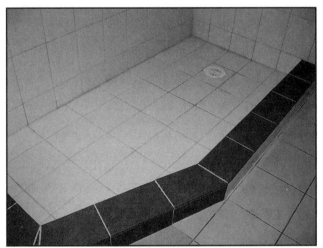

Figure 15-10. Contrasting tiled shower curb.

Internal Areas

Poor Lighting Throughout the Apartment

The therapist observed that the lighting in the apartment was very dim. Except in the bedroom, there was no sunlight entering the apartment because of the overhang from the apartments above. Olive had no task lighting in the kitchen or bathroom but did have direction lamps in the lounge and bedroom to assist reading. When asked if she considered the lighting poor, she stated she was unaware it could be improved. All lighting in the apartment was incandescent globes providing a maximum of 60 lux (100-watt incandescent standard bulb). The client reported that she had difficulty with her personal grooming activities in the bathroom and difficulty seeing to prepare meals at night in the kitchen.

Small halogen spotlights can be used for task lighting when placed in strategic positions, but they have to be inserted into the ceiling space or alternatively as track lighting. Because Olive's apartment was on the ground level with a solid concrete slab as the ceiling, it was difficult to install inset lighting. Track lighting can be expensive and unsuitable to achieve light in specific positions. Another less expensive option is the use of fluorescent lighting with triphosphor tubes. Triphosphor fluorescent tubes, often called daylight tubes, provide a clear white light similar to the daylight on a clear day and cast a softer shadow than incandescent globes or halogen lighting.

The final recommendation was to install a circular fluorescent light fitting (60 lux) to improve luminance at the front entry and 47.25-in (1,200 mm) long double fluorescent light fittings in the bathroom and kitchen (240 lux with standard 36 watt tubes) because these were the areas where Olive needed light to assist in her daily activities, such as personal grooming and meal preparation. A double fluorescent light fitting was also recommended for the lounge/dining area to help Olive see better when eating her meals or reading. Triphosphor fluorescent tubes were requested because these increased the luminance to 320 lux.

Clinical Reasoning, Evaluation, and Justification for Recommendations

From information provided by Olive at the initial referral, documentation provided by Olive's local doctor, and the therapist's extensive knowledge of the effect of visual impairment and intervention options, a process of clinical reasoning began.

Narrative reasoning and scientific reasoning assisted the therapist to understand and interpret information relating to Olive's life and the presentation of her condition.

Scientific reasoning was used to interpret information regarding Olive's health condition, and it was used to collect cues throughout the assessment process as to how Olive's condition was likely to affect her performance. In order to understand Olive's functional vision, the therapist asked her to explain the limitations of her vision and how it affected her day-to-day tasks and mobility. She explained that she had vision on her left side only and that she had to be aware of her environment to avoid bumping into objects or people. She reported that lighting was important so she could better determine the outline of objects within the environment and that, even though she kept the lights on in the apartment, they did not seem to give enough light to complete her tasks to her satisfaction. Olive indicated that contrast was important for her to distinguish one object from another or changes in the

environment—for example, distinguishing steps or changes in ground level. In the kitchen, she stated that she had difficulty distinguishing the control knobs on the stove because the dim lighting did not allow her to distinguish the white knobs against the white enamel of the stovetop, saying, "It all looks the same."

Olive indicated that she could see better on a clear sunny day than she could on a dull, cloudy day. Although she was unaware of the various lighting options and modifications to the environment available to assist her, she was open to suggestions that helped guide the decision-making process during the home visit. Pragmatic reasoning was used to consider contextual factors, choice of materials, and relevant measurements for modifications, as well as funding issues.

The therapist had a comprehensive knowledge of environmental issues relevant to people with visual impairment to apply to this scenario. For example, sufficient lighting and contrast are two important elements in the environment of a client who has significant vision loss. Each client has individual needs concerning the extent of lighting improvement, so it is important to allow the client to explain how he or she sees his or her environment and how light and glare impacts his or her vision. In select instances, "more lighting is better than less lighting" but glare from bright light will lessen contrast and cause difficulty in distinguishing colors of similar tones or hues. Contrast can be improved by reducing glare and improving luminance. The color spectrum can be used to create contrast or improve luminance. Light pastel colors will reflect light and help improve the ambient luminance in a room, whereas dark colors absorb light. White or yellow are often used to highlight step edges or indicate changes in ground level because these reflect light well and provide an exaggeration of contrast against most other colors.

Ethical reasoning was used in considering alternative decisions for each issue, including those that were not addressed, and the consequences of recommendations made. The final recommendations were agreed to at the time of the home visit, and the occupational therapist documented this information in a written report, for consideration by the organization approving the work.

Outcomes

Quotes were obtained from three building firms that specialize in home modification installations, and a builder was chosen to proceed with the work. The modifications were installed, and the therapist visited Olive in her home to complete a postmodification evaluation. Olive was observed in her home environment and an interview was conducted, which included the review of the original occupational therapy report to determine whether there had been any changes in the client's capacity to manage the various activities in the home and community.

Olive was enthusiastic in her appreciation of the improvements in the environment. She reported that the bathroom was a major improvement with better lighting and the installation of the contrast shower curb step. She was observed in the bathroom using the new grab bar in the shower and stepping over the curb step without hesitation. She reported that she has not had a fall since the modifications were installed and, subsequently, is less fearful in the shower.

Olive was observed going in and out of the front entry using the handrail and negotiating the smaller steps. It was noted she could find the key in the door lock more easily. She stated that the front entry was easier to access, and she no longer feared falling while entering her apartment. She also stated that the improved lighting generally enabled her to see, especially on cloudy days when the apartment was very dim. It is now only on these days that she leaves the lights on all day.

It is anticipated that Olive might require future intervention as her health status changes or if she has any deterioration in her mobility. Olive is cognizant of the services available and indicated that she would contact the occupational therapist when she requires further assistance.

CASE STUDY 6: A YOUNG MAN WITH A PSYCHIATRIC DISABILITY

Client Interests and Daily Activities

Chris is a 31-year-old man who shares a three-bedroom detached house with another young man. His mother, who is his formal adult guardian, lives 5 miles (approximately 8 km) away but visits three to four times a week to ensure that her son is managing with daily activities. Chris's main interest is watching television or DVDs and listening to music. He is not involved in community groups or activities. His support worker takes him shopping, or his mother drives him to community facilities as required.

Health Condition and Functional Performance

In 1998, at the age of 22, Chris was diagnosed with schizophrenia and spent many months in the psychiatric ward of the local hospital. His behavior was aggressive, and he exhibited significant symptoms of his schizophrenic illness, such as constant voices in his head, a delusional state of mind, and antisocial behaviors. His mother was unable to care for him in her home.

In 1999, he applied to a social housing provider for a one-bedroom apartment. In the ensuing 6 years, Chris was relocated three times before being housed in his current accommodation. In each of the three locations, Chris had difficulty maintaining his tenancy because of his overt unacceptable behavior, constant loud music, and offensive language. Chris stated that he needed the music to drown out the voices in his head.

Attempts to encourage him to use earphones or to govern the volume of the stereo failed. Other residents in the apartment complexes made many complaints about the music and his antisocial behavior.

In each of these properties, Chris lived alone, with his mother visiting daily to try to keep the peace and to support her son. There were other supports provided for Chris: a case manager from the community mental health unit visited twice weekly, and he had daily visits from the mental health intervention team (MIT) to provide daily medications. Additionally, a worker from the community home care service visited fortnightly to assist with household cleaning.

In 2004, the social housing provider decided to provide a detached house for Chris. At that time, he had a friend, who also had a diagnosis of schizophrenia, staying in his apartment from time to time. The two men decided to try a shared accommodation arrangement. It was anticipated that the house would provide space away from neighbors so the music and behaviors would not have as great of an impact.

Location and Description of the Home

The detached house is situated in a densely populated suburb with older couples and families. There are neighbors on two sides of the home and a park area at the rear boundary. The neighbor on one side is separated by a driveway between the homes.

The house has five steps at the front and eight at the back. There is a small bathroom consisting of a shower over the bath and a vanity. The toilet is separate and adjacent to the bathroom. There is a large backyard and several feet from the house to each side boundary. The front entry faces the street. There is a 6-foot-high fence on three boundaries but no fencing at the front of the property.

Client Goals

Chris's primary goal is to live safely and independently in his own home and to be able to live in harmony with his community.

His short-term goals are to have safety and privacy in his home and not feel as if others are always watching him.

His long-term goal is to remain living in his own home, using community services to support him and minimize his admissions to hospital.

Chris's mother would like her son to maintain his tenancy and increase his independence so she can reduce her visits to once-weekly and limit her involvement in his day-to-day life.

Evaluating Occupational Performance and Identifying Needs

The referral for occupational therapy intervention was the result of a case conference with the mental health community workers, Chris's mother, and staff of the social housing provider. It was felt that the house required some modifications to enable Chris to feel comfortable, safe, and secure.

During a home visit from the therapist, where Chris, his mother, and case manager were present, Chris was observed doing tasks in the home and was asked how the home environment affected symptoms of his illness. The therapist used the COPM with the case manager and Chris's mother, who could provide insight into the issues and difficulties experienced by Chris and the community workers.

Mobility and Transfers

Chris does not have any mobility problems. He is a tall man, about 6'2" (1,880 mm) in height and weighing 196 lbs (approximately 89 kg or 14 stone).

Self-Care and Homemaker Activities

Chris is independent in all personal care activities, but needs prompting to bathe and groom himself regularly. He uses water, either in the shower or bath, to reduce his anxiety and symptoms of his illness.

He relies on help for cooking and shopping, household cleaning, and laundry. His mother or caseworker provides transport to community facilities.

Purpose of Occupational Therapy Involvement

The occupational therapy referral requested an assessment of the home environment to provide privacy from the neighbors and to improve hygiene in the home. The community home care workers had complained that the habits of the two men in the home were such that workers were at risk. The toilet was always in an unclean state with urine all over the floor and around the crevices of the toilet pan.

During the assessment, interview, and observation process, the caseworker and Chris's mother raised their concerns that the home care workers had refused to clean the home until the bathroom and toilet areas were improved. The other area of concern was the front entry being open to the street and having limited privacy from the neighbors opposite.

The therapist used a combination of narrative, scientific, ethical, and pragmatic reasoning to assess the appropriate intervention options. It was particularly important to discuss with Chris's mother and the caseworker the options to modify behaviors and interventions attempted in the past.

Environmental Issues and Intervention Options

External Areas

Privacy at the Front of the Home

The front door was exposed to the neighbors opposite, causing Chris to feel that he was being watched constantly. Neighbors also needed privacy from Chris's overt behaviors.

A lattice screen had been installed across the front entry but Chris still felt that he was being watched. Several other homes on the street had fences and gates across the front boundary, so a similar installation would be in keeping with the streetscape and look to fit in.

The final recommendation was to provide a 6-ft-high (1,830 mm) timber fence across the front boundary.

Toilet Area

Cleaning the Toilet Area

The problem arose because both men have difficulty urinating into the toilet bowl, causing urine to contaminate the floor and risking it being walked throughout the house (Figure 15-11A).

The options considered included modifying the behavior by providing a target, such as a ping-pong ball, in the toilet pan. However, other such devices had been tried several times without success.

Although the vinyl floor covering had been changed to tiles at the case manager's request, because it was felt that the tiles were easier to scrub, it was also unsuccessful.

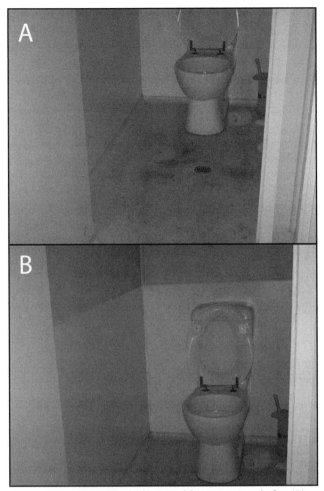

Figure 15-11. The toilet before modification (A) and after (B).

The final recommendation was to install a toilet pan with fully enclosed plumbing to minimize areas in which the urine could collect. It was also recommended that lamipanel sheeting be installed around the walls of the toilet to provide a water-resistant surface to clean or scrub (Figure 15-11B) and to install vinyl flooring cover 4 in (100 mm) up the wall to provide a water-impervious seal. A floor waste drainage was also installed so the floor could be sluiced with water and contaminated water could be washed away. Chris and his co-tenant were happy to use a portable toilet during the time the work was in progress and tolerated the inconvenience for that short time.

Bathroom Area

Flow of Water on the Bathroom Floor

Because Chris showers for a long time, is a big man, and does not use a shower curtain, excess water flows onto the bathroom floor. The floor is not profiled to drain the water away and so the water pools, causing a slip hazard.

Options considered included installing a shower screen on the bath edge, but this suggestion was rejected because it could be broken easily if Chris became aggressive. A shower curtain was also refused because of Chris's intolerance to using one. Floor mats posed another hazard as well as creating added laundry.

The final recommendation was to remove the existing flooring in the bathroom and profile the floor so that the water would drain to the floor waste and not pool into the center of the floor.

Clinical Reasoning, Evaluation, and Justification for Recommendations

The process of clinical reasoning began once information was provided by the service at the initial referral, documentation was provided by the doctor, local information about the various neighborhoods was considered, and the occupational therapist's knowledge of the effects of a psychiatric disability and institutionalization on Chris's behavior was assessed.

Narrative reasoning assisted the therapist to understand and interpret information relating to Chris's life. The therapist became aware, for example, that Chris had lived in an institution for a long time and needed time to adapt to community living. He expressed a desire to establish good relationships with neighbors and to participate in community life, despite having moved several times.

Scientific reasoning was used by the therapist to understand the nature of the behaviors involved and the impacts of Chris's symptoms on his ability to learn new skills or change old habits. Chris's behaviors had caused problems for him over a number of years. The new environment of a detached house enabled him to enjoy a freedom he had not had for many years, and the neighbors on the street were tolerant of his music and behaviors. It was necessary to be flexible in approaching the issues presented by this client with a severe mental illness. Consultation with family, case managers, and community workers, as well as the client, enhanced the understanding of the specific problems and the triggers that provoked the behaviors.

Ethical reasoning was used in considering alternative decisions for each issue, including those that were not addressed, and the consequences of recommendations made. Consideration had to be given to those neighbors living in close proximity to Chris and their acceptance of people whose behaviors might become challenging. There was a duty of care to both the client and the community as a whole throughout the process of finalizing the location of the housing and the types of modifications made to the home.

The modifications enabled Chris to feel in control of his environment and enabled the caregivers to feel safe when having to clean a contaminated area.

Outcomes

A technical adviser visited the home with the therapist to determine the exact floor specifications so that the contracted builder could understand the unusual request for the floor drainage in the toilet area and the need for drainage in the bathroom.

Quotes were obtained from three building firms that specialize in home modification installations, and a builder was chosen to proceed with the work. The modifications were installed, and the therapist visited Chris in his home to complete a postmodification evaluation. The therapist observed Chris in his home environment and conducted an interview with him, which included a review of the original occupational therapy report, to determine if there had been any changes in Chris's capacity to manage the various activities in the home and community.

Chris enthusiastically showed the therapist the improvements in the environment. He reported that the bathroom was a major improvement with the floor being much safer and the cleaners happier being able to sluice the toilet floor.

Chris was also appreciative of the privacy at the front of the home, which he stated gave him a greater feeling of security.

His caseworker reported that the home care workers were much happier now that the modifications were completed. Chris's mother also reported that she is not visiting as often to supplement the cleaning when the community agency does not visit.

It is anticipated that Chris might require future intervention as his symptoms change. The community mental health service continues a close liaison with the occupational therapist and the property owner to ensure that Chris is able to maintain his tenancy with minimal impact on his surrounding community into the future.

CASE STUDY 7: SPOUSE SUPPORTING A PERSON WITH DEMENTIA

Client Interests and Daily Activities

Eighty-two-year-old Alan and his 80-year-old wife Doris live in a house in a regional city suburb. The house has been Alan and Doris's home for the past 50 years, where they raised two sons and a daughter. Their daughter Jenny lives with her family in the local community and their sons live in nearby suburbs. One grandson also lives in close proximity. Alan and Doris's daughter, son-in-law, or grandson visits them 4 to 5 days a week, providing them with ongoing emotional and physical support.

Alan was a mechanic by trade prior to his retirement and was the main provider for the family. He continues to enjoy reading automobile magazines, as well as helping his son-in-law to restore an old car. Alan and Doris played lawn bowls together for years but, since the onset of her dementia, Doris is no longer able to participate in this activity. She has spent most of her married life as a homemaker, raising the children, and looking after the home. Her hobbies included gardening, knitting, and crocheting.

Health Condition and Functional Performance

Doris was diagnosed with dementia 2 years ago. Since then, she has shown increased symptoms of the disease, including memory loss and repeated questioning, wandering at night, pacing, decreased visual perception, incontinence, poor sleep routine, disorientation, confusion, and agitation.

She is capable of completing her daily living activities of showering, dressing, and toileting with assistance and prompting but has been susceptible to falls in the home because of her reduced visual perception and loss of good dynamic balance when standing and walking. Doris also has a medical history of osteoporosis. She is currently on medication for this condition and experiences occasional back pain. Doris is no longer capable of independently completing homemaker tasks or activities previously of interest to her, such as gardening, knitting, and crocheting.

Alan has a medical history of arthritis, particularly affecting his knees and shoulders; reduced vision as a result of his poorly controlled diabetes; and clinical depression. He has experienced increased physical and emotional distress over the past 2 years as the symptoms of Doris's dementia have worsened and as he has had to take on the role of caregiver. He regularly consults his local doctor, who has prescribed medication for his depression.

Location and Description of the Home

Alan and Doris's home is a four-bedroom detached brick house, located on level land on a quiet suburban street. The house is high set with external staircases of 12 stairs at both front and back entrances. All living areas of the house are located upstairs. Downstairs houses a double garage, the laundry, and storage and work areas Alan uses to store car components and workshop tools and materials. There is a pathway leading from the base of the external stairs to the driveway. The backyard has a well-established lawn with garden beds and a 4-ft-high (1,200 mm) wooden paling fence around the perimeter. There is a path at the rear of the building, as well as a pathway leading from the laundry door to the clothesline located in the middle of the backyard.

The home has a living room, dining room, and kitchen located at front of the house and a narrow hallway leading to the bathrooms and bedrooms at the rear. There is low-pile carpet on the floor in the living areas, linoleum on the floor in the kitchen, and tiles on the floor in the bathroom and toilet. The bathroom contains a bath, separate shower, and a vanity basin with a mirror and towel rails. The shower recess has a 60-mm-high curb and is enclosed by a shower screen that has a pivoting door. The toilet is located in a separate room adjacent to the bathroom.

With Alan and Doris having lived in the home for 50 years, the living room has become cluttered with personal items and furniture to accommodate family who visit frequently. The home is fitted with smoke detectors. The interior of the home is dim during the day.

Client Goals

Alan indicated that his short-term goals included the following:

+ Gaining increased understanding and acceptance of his wife's dementia and developing strategies to better manage her symptoms, including her incontinence, poor sleep routine, disorientation, confusion, and agitation

+ Improving the safety of both himself and his wife when assisting her with transfers, mobility in and around the home, and her showering and toileting routine

+ Managing his increased anxiety and stress associated with ensuring his wife's safety in the home day and night

Alan stated that his long-term goals included the following:

+ Maintaining his own physical and emotional health in his role as a caregiver

+ Safely and effectively assisting his wife in her daily self care activities and supporting her for as long as possible in the family home

Evaluating Occupational Performance and Identifying Needs

The occupational therapist had reviewed Alan and Doris's health information prior to the visit to establish Doris's current physical, emotional, cognitive, and functional status. Because of Alan's overwhelming sense of loss, change in lifestyle and roles in the home, and feelings of anxiety about how he would manage in the future, the therapist conducted a series of four visits spread over a month. During the home visits, the therapist interviewed Alan to gather information on the functional status and daily routines of both Alan and Doris. They were also observed walking in and around the home environment and demonstrating how they managed Doris' self-care activities. The therapist used the COPM to identify the couple's goals and to ascertain their capacity to function in the home.

Doris and Alan's daughter was present during some of the home visits. She reported that she and her family provided regular assistance with tasks such as shopping, meal preparation, caring for the yard, and driving Alan and Doris to community facilities. Alan reported that he no longer drives because of his poor vision. The daughter indicated that the extended family provided emotional support and cared for Doris one day a week to enable Alan to have a break and go shopping or visit the doctor.

Mobility and Transfers

Doris walked around independently both in- and outdoors. The therapist noted that Doris tended to lean on Alan or on nearby walls and furniture to maintain her balance, particularly when negotiating a change in level or when moving from sitting into the standing position. Doris was also observed to lean heavily on Alan when transferring on and off the toilet.

Alan indicated that Doris required increasing physical support when negotiating the front and back stairs. The stairs at the back and front entrances have one handrail on the left side when ascending. The handrail at the back stairs has deteriorated and is an unstable support. Doris experiences decreased visual perception, and Alan indicated that she frequently "catches" her foot on the nosing when ascending the stairs. She supports herself using the handrail and holds onto Alan for support. Alan has reduced vision and balance; consequently, the couple is at risk of falling on the stairs.

Alan indicated safety concerns when assisting Doris to transfer in and out of the shower recess and when helping her with showering, particularly because she tends to become agitated and move around unpredictably. Doris stands as she showers. Alan stated that Doris clings to him during showering because of a fear of falling and that she strikes out at him when agitated. The physical space available to allow the caregiver to access the shower recess to assist Doris during her showering routine was observed to be limited by the fixed shower screen and the pivoting door. There were no grab bars in the recess, and Alan indicated that Doris frequently leaned on him or used the taps for support when transferring in and out of the area and when standing in the shower. The shower recess had a fixed shower head, limiting the control of the water flow. The shower curb is white, providing little differentiation between the white shower tray and white floor tiles. This raised step is a trip hazard for both Alan and Doris.

Alan reported that Doris spends many hours of the day and night pacing and wandering around the house. He stated that his wife also liked to wander around the backyard and look at the garden; however, he keeps external entrances locked because he is anxious about Doris's safety should she attempt to negotiate the back stairs independently. The backyard has uneven areas between the pathways, landings, and the turf. Alan noted that Doris frequently stumbles when stepping off of the pathways onto the turf because of the change in surface heights. He expressed concern that she may fall if this were not rectified. Alan reported that, if he felt confident that Doris was safe in the yard, he would be able to sit down on the back landing and look through his magazines, allowing time for relaxation.

Alan walked independently around the house but used a single-point stick to assist with maintaining his balance when mobilizing outdoors. In addition to the arthritic pain in his knees, Alan indicated that his mobility has been affected by his lack of confidence walking over uneven terrain or negotiating change in levels and surfaces. He stated that his vision had deteriorated over time and that he had nearly fallen a few times. Alan indicated that neither he nor his wife had fallen in the home. He is independent with transfers; however, he reported increased difficulty transferring from low-seated surfaces, particularly when tired or experiencing knee pain.

Self-Care and Homemaker Activities

Alan reported that Doris was capable of undertaking her daily living activities of showering, dressing, and toileting with prompting and assistance but that she required an increasing amount of attention and monitoring.

Alan indicated that he organizes Doris's clothes for her and that she sits on the bed to dress. He has to prompt and assist Doris to orient her clothing during the dressing routine.

Doris is no longer capable of completing homemaker tasks; however, she wanders into the kitchen and rummages through doors and cupboards, turns on the stove and other switches, and fills the sink to wash the dishes. At times, she wanders off, leaving the stove or oven on or the water overflowing from the sink onto the floor.

Alan stated that he does the laundry, vacuuming, and mopping and cleans the bathroom and toilet on a regular basis. His family assists with preparing meals that the couple freezes until required. Their daughter does most of the shopping, and their grandson mows the lawn and maintains the yard.

Alan reported difficulty coping with homemaker tasks, which were always completed by Doris previously. He stated that a combination of emotional and physical stress, as well as reduced sleep, contributes to his diminishing capacity to cope with these tasks as well as monitor and care for his wife.

Anthropometric Measurements and Equipment

Alan and Doris's anthropometric measurements were taken in the seated and standing positions, including reach range. It was important that both clients' measurements were taken because they both use the same areas of the home and will both use specific interventions, such as grab bars and handrails, as they continue to age.

Purpose of Occupational Therapy Involvement

A home visit referral from Alan and Doris's local doctor indicated the need for the occupational therapist to review the existing home environment. The referral indicated a need for equipment, home modification, support service recommendations, and practical advice to enable Alan to provide Doris with ongoing support.

The couple has lived in the same home for 50 years and, despite increasing stress, Alan wished to continue supporting Doris there for as long as possible. He acknowledged Doris's deteriorating function and indicated that he continued to struggle with the personal loss of relationship and intimacy with his wife and his changing role and routines.

The therapist used a combination of narrative, scientific, ethical, and pragmatic reasoning to assess the appropriate intervention options. Various recommendations were made at the conclusion of each visit. In addition to environmental modifications, Alan and his wife were referred to the local Alzheimer's Association Support Group and to other community services for respite, nursing and social work support, and caregiver assistance with domestic tasks. Given the nature of Doris's dementia, a team approach and ongoing support were seen as fundamental to the intervention planning process.

The recommendations were discussed with Alan and his family and were presented in writing to ensure that they had a record of the discussion and proposed actions arising out of each visit. This considered and paced approach allowed Alan and his family time to review and discuss the proposals and to prioritize recommendations in collaboration with the various stakeholders, including staff from community agencies. It was envisioned that this process would provide Alan with a reasonable sense of control over the intervention planning process and would ensure that he would not become overwhelmed by the number of recommendations or the effort involved in coordinating the introduction of further changes into their lifestyle.

Environmental Issues and Intervention Options

External Access

Improved Handrail Support at Front and Back Entrances

Relocation to ground-level accommodation was not considered a viable option for Alan and Doris because it would be expensive. Alan indicated that he wished to remain in the family home becuase they were both familiar with the environment and it contained a lot of memories associated with them raising their family.

Options of installing a lift or stair-lift were considered; however, Doris would not be able to independently operate these devices. They were also considered too costly for Alan and his wife.

The final recommendations included the following:

+ Repairing the existing handrail at the back stairs. The handrail had deteriorated with the weather and was no longer stable.

+ Providing an additional handrail on the right side ascending at both the front and back stairs, so that the clients could use the bilateral rails. This would also eliminate the need for Alan to support Doris when she ascends and descends the stairs.

+ Providing strips of contrasting color to the nosing of each stair tread to improve visibility. Because the stair treads were dark brown, a contrasting white strip was seen as an appropriate application for the nosing of each step.

Level Adjacent Surface Areas in the Backyard to Eliminate Trip Hazards

The option of fencing off a large section of even yard to allow Doris to safely wander was discussed; however, Alan indicated a preference to allow as much access for Doris to available yard space. The recommendation made was to raise the turf and soil adjacent to all the paths and landings around the home to ensure smooth transitions between the lawn and paths and reduce trip or fall hazards.

Bathroom

Enhance Space and Design of the Shower Recess

Options reviewed included remodeling the bathroom to reprofile the bathroom floor to allow installation of a curb-free shower recess, providing color-contrasting strips to the existing curb to improve visibility, and installing grab bars to provide the couple with support as they stepped over the curb. The installation of a fixed shower seat or a freestanding chair was also discussed.

In making final recommendations, the cost of the changes, the potential disruption to routines, and the impact of works completion on Alan's stress levels were considered.

The final recommendations included:

+ Removing the existing shower screen with its pivot door and replacing it with a rod and shower curtain to open up the area and provide more space for Doris and her caregiver

+ Applying color-contrasting strips to the curb at the entrance of the shower to highlight the edges and to reduce the trip hazard

+ Installing a vertical and horizontal grab bar on the tap wall of the shower recess to provide Doris with support when she stands in the shower and transfers in and out of the area. It was recommended that the vertical grab rail be fitted with a friction-sliding mount on which the handheld shower could be positioned, to enable the caregivers to better direct water flow. A handheld shower was seen as a safer alternative to retaining the shower head.

+ Installing a temperature-control device for the hot water to reduce the risk of Doris burning herself if left unsupervised in the shower

+ Providing a freestanding shower chair for trial to allow Doris to sit during her showering routine

Enhance Safety of the Towel Rail Fittings

The towel rail in the bathroom area has come loose, and Alan indicated that Doris supported herself on the rail when moving around the bathroom. It was recommended that the towel rail be replaced with a grab bar that could be used as a towel rail but that could also take her weight if she leaned on it for support.

Enhance Safety in the Toilet Area During Transfers

Doris tends to lean heavily on her husband when moving from sitting to standing in the toilet area. Options considered included Doris using an over-toilet frame or a toilet raiser and grab bars. Due to the potential trip hazard presented by the legs of an over-toilet frame in the confined toilet area, installing grab bars and a toilet raiser were selected as the most appropriate options. Alan indicated a preference to initially trial grab bars only, because of concerns about Doris potentially becoming confused about the change to the toilet setup and the general aesthetics of a raised toilet seat.

The final recommendation was to install vertical and horizontal grab bars on both sides of the toilet, because this configuration would ensure that Doris would not hold onto Alan for support and she could complete transfers safely and independently.

Kitchen

Reduce Risk of Injury and Potential for Electrocution, Water Damage, or Fire

Because Doris tends to wander and turn switches and taps on and off, various options were considered for the kitchen area. These included closing off the kitchen with a lockable door to restrict Doris from accessing the kitchen or installing locks on cupboards, removable tap heads on taps, and isolating switches linked to the stove, oven, and refrigerator.

Because Doris previously completed homemaker tasks in the kitchen, Alan felt reluctant to completely restrict her from there.

The final recommendations included the following:

+ Installing an isolation switch to the oven, stove, and refrigerator

+ Removing appliances, such as the toaster and electric jug, from the kitchen countertops and placing them in lockable cupboards

+ Installing a lock on one kitchen cupboard in which to store of knives, medications, cleaning fluids, and electrical devices. Sink plugs are to be stored in the cupboard also to reduce the risk of flooding the kitchen

Bedroom

Reduce Visual Cues That May Stimulate Activity During Sleeping Hours

Alan noted that Doris frequently gets up during the night and tends to undertake activities such as dressing, toileting, or wandering to the kitchen to turn on taps and switches. These activities tend to be triggered by visual cues, such as leaving clothing at the end of the bed or a cup being left on the bedside table. Alan continues to sleep in the same room as Doris because of the need to monitor her movements and activities. He indicated that, although he is frequently awakened during the night, he wants to continue sharing a room with Doris.

It was recommended that Alan remove distracting items in the bedroom, particularly at night, in order to reduce visual cues that may stimulate activity. It was also recommended that nightlights be installed in the hallway and toilet to assist Doris with finding the toilet at night.

Internal Access

Improve Lighting Throughout the Home to Reduce Risk of Tripping and Falling

The therapist observed that the lighting in the home was very dim, causing particular concern for client safety in high-risk areas, including the bathroom, hallway, bedroom, and kitchen.

Installing daylight tone fluorescent lighting with diffuser shields was recommended in these areas to improve illumination and minimize glare and a shadowing effect.

Security External Doors

Alan indicated increasing anxiety that Doris might wander outdoors, particularly at night. The use of various alarms that could alert Alan to Doris's movements through one of the external doorways was discussed. Alan expressed concern that an alarm may agitate and upset Doris.

The final recommendation was that a deadbolt lock be installed on both the front and back doors and for Alan to keep the keys on him at all times, especially in the event of the couple needing to make a quick exit from the home.

Improve Doris's Safety When Pacing and Wandering

The living room was cluttered with personal items, including photographs of Alan and Doris' extended family and additional furniture items to accommodate the increasing size of family that visited over the years. Doris frequently paced within the living room, and it was recommended that a glass table within the room and two lounge chairs that are rarely used be removed. Alan was also encouraged to consider reducing clutter within the room by hanging some of the family photos on a wall or asking his daughter to place the photos in a memory album for him and his wife.

The therapist also made referrals to various services to ensure that Alan would receive adequate support in the home. This included referral to:

+ An incontinence specialist for education about night toileting and incontinence

+ The nursing service to recommence assistance with self-care activities

+ Physical therapy regarding mobility device options and to provide a freestanding height-adjustable shower chair

+ A rheumatologist to monitor the current integrity of Alan's joints and effectiveness of pain control measures

+ An ophthalmologist for an assessment of Alan's vision

+ A respite service for regular respite care

Clinical Reasoning, Evaluation, and Justification for Recommendations

Information received at the initial referral from the doctor, detail provided by Alan and his family, observation of the couple at the time of the home visit, and the occupational therapist's knowledge of dementia and other health conditions assisted the process of clinical reasoning.

Narrative reasoning was used by the therapist to interpret information relating to Doris and Alan's life, the involvement of their family in their day-to-day routines, and how they participate in their home and in the community. When making the recommendations about interventions, it was important to allow Alan and his family to prioritize the suggestions. It was recognized that Alan was seeking to exert some level of control over his immediate environment and over the process of introducing changes into the home. His aim was to keep things "normal" and to maximize quality of life for both Doris and himself. It was acknowledged that Alan struggled with continually adjusting his personal goals and daily routines, coping with the profound personal loss of relationship with his wife, and recognizing and adapting to what Doris was no longer able to do.

The therapist used scientific, pragmatic, and ethical reasoning as she considered the impact of the dementia process on the couple and whether the clients could realistically continue to live in their home in the medium to long term with support and minor modifications. It was anticipated that both Doris and Alan would continue to encounter changing environmental demands and barriers as they age and as their health conditions decline.

Pragmatic reasoning was used to consider contextual factors, choice of materials, and relevant measurements and funding for equipment, services, and home modifications.

Outcomes

Following a number of visits and discussions on the range of suitable interventions, Alan was provided with a written list of identified environmental issues and final recommendations. Once these were prioritized and Alan felt comfortable that the recommendations would assist him to better manage his wife within the home, he arranged quotes from building firms specializing in the installation of home modifications. Doris was placed in respite for a 2-week period while the environmental modifications were completed.

Referrals to other services were initiated by the occupational therapist, in consultation with the doctor. Support services were introduced, including cleaning and respite services.

The therapist visited Alan and Doris to complete a postmodification evaluation in the form of an interview and structured observation. The home modifications and changes were completed as per the final recommendations, with Alan reporting increased ease in assisting his wife and decreased anxiety over safety. He continued to experience sleepless nights and concern about his wife's safety around the home but reported that she had not had any falls or accidents. He indicated that he has felt less overwhelmed with the housekeeping activities since the introduction of support services.

Because of the ongoing decline of Doris' health as a result of her dementia and Alan's ongoing physical and mental health issues, the therapist has kept in regular contact with the couple. It is anticipated that the environment will need to be modified again in the future because of the ongoing changes in the couple's health conditions. It is also likely that their support and equipment needs will change periodically. Intersectorial collaboration with a range of services will be required to ensure that the clients can remain at home for as long as possible.

CONCLUSION

Each scenario in this chapter has highlighted the difference that occupational therapy-based home modification practice can make in the lives of a range of people encountering barriers to occupational performance in the home environment. The case studies have demonstrated that much information can be gained from undertaking a home visit to hear the client's story and observe his or her ability to manage in the home. The therapist can then use this information and use the clinical reasoning process to plan and negotiate interventions. This includes the therapist engaging in professional reasoning—using knowledge of the functional impacts of health conditions (scientific reasoning), the understanding of the client's life story and his or her perspective as an "expert" in his or her own life (narrative reasoning)," and assessment of the practical limitations and ethical considerations of the situation (pragmatic and ethical reasoning)—to determine the best outcome for a client.

This chapter has shown that an occupational therapist can introduce the client to a range of interventions, in addition to home modifications, including providing equipment, finding alternative ways of undertaking activities, and referring to service providers who can provide a further support and advice. Further, the therapist has a role in working with design and construction professionals to evaluate proposed home modification designs to ensure that alterations meet the client's needs effectively.

The case studies have emphasized that clients may present with a range of occupational performance issues at the time of the home visit. Issues discussed in this chapter include ensuring physical access to the home, completing self-care and homemaker tasks, ensuring safe performance of caregiving, maintaining tenancy and neighborhood relationships, establishing community integration, and being able to age in place.

Further, a range of types of interventions have been showcased to help maintain or improve the person's occupational performance, including relocating, refitting or replacing fittings and fixtures, redesigning spaces, and ensuring adjustability and usability of the home modifications by a range of users. The types of interventions elected in these case studies included products and designs that would suit the current and long-term needs of the client and the household, including changes in equipment and caregiver support over time.

While this case study information can guide future occupational therapy practice, it is important that occupational therapists not overgeneralize this information when dealing with other clients but continue to take an individualized approach to evaluating the needs of individuals and the effectiveness of home modification interventions. This will ensure that solutions are tailored to achieve the best possible outcomes for each person, his or her family, caregivers, the various roles and activities he or she undertakes, and the home environment in which he or she lives.

Outline Shapes of Occupied Wheelchairs

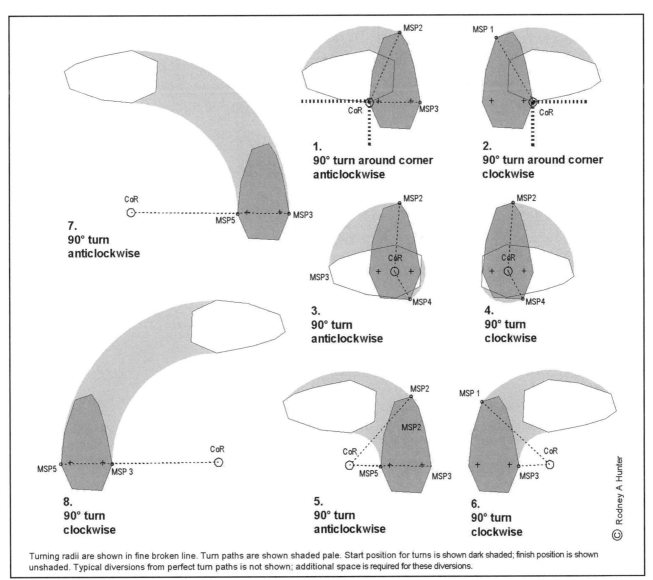

Turning radii are shown in fine broken line. Turn paths are shown shaded pale. Start position for turns is shown dark shaded; finish position is shown unshaded. Typical diversions from perfect turn paths is not shown; additional space is required for these diversions.

(Reprinted with permission from Rodney A. Hunter.)

B

Fundamental Types of Compact Turns

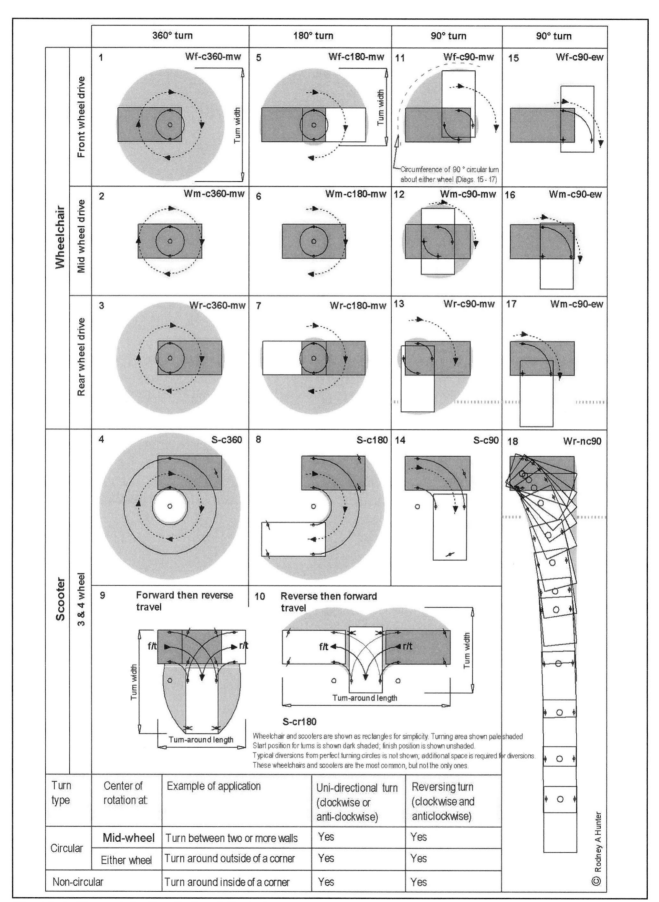

(Reprinted with permission from Rodney A. Hunter.)

Ramp Installation Considerations

Ramps are often provided as an alternative to stairs and can be permanent or temporary installations. Permanent installations are those that are fixed in place; temporary ramps are usually modular and adjustable. Ramps are suitable for people who use wheeled mobility equipment, such as wheelchairs or wheeled walkers, but they also have practical applications for a range of people. For example, they help where access to the home is needed for pushing shopping carts or prams or people moving furniture on wheels (Center for Accessible Environments, 2009). Because some older people and people with disabilities can find ramps difficult to use, they should always be in close proximity to steps where possible (Center for Accessible Environments; Center for Universal Design, 2004).

The following discussion provides broad design principles in relation to the design of ramps and detail about tailoring ramps to suit the needs of individuals, their equipment, and caregivers. There are also practical instructions on how to design an external ramp for a home.

BUILDING ADVICE AND ACCESS STANDARDS

To ensure the most appropriate ramp design for a home, occupational therapists might need to consult with companies that manufacture or supply ramps or seek advice from builders or design professionals who have had experience installing them. Information discussed among therapists and the ramp company representatives and/or builders can include the following:

+ Ramp design and construction requirements as indicated in local building codes and the relevance and application of access standards

+ Alternative ramp configurations to suit the space available, the desired direction of travel, and the slope of the land—that is, whether the ramp needs to be straight, L-shaped, U-shaped, switchback, or curved

+ Types of building materials suitable for construction

+ The appearance of the ramp in relation to the home, garden, fencing, and other features in the yard

+ The cost of ramp design options and associated works, such as paths leading to the bottom of the ramp

+ Product warranty

+ The source and level of availability of technical assistance for repairs and maintenance over time

Local building codes and access standards are used to guide the design of public buildings and spaces. Therapists can also make use of them when designing domestic ramps. The public access standards provide important measurements and detail on essential features and design elements to ensure ramps are safe to use by people who can walk unaided or those who use mobility equipment. Such information includes, for example, detail on the minimum gradient, ramp width, ramp length dimensions between landings, and rail height.

Occupational therapists need to ensure that the dimensions in the standards suit the relevant client's measurements, his or her equipment, and other people who might assist the client with the equipment, including caregivers or other household members. If the dimensions that are listed in access standards do not suit the measurements and function of the person and his or her equipment and caregivers, they will need to be altered. This might include, for example, decreasing the ramp gradient (to make it less steep), increasing the ramp width (to make it wider), or altering the size of the landing at the turns (to make it longer and wider).

Local building codes and access standards can serve as ramp design guides where there is little or no information on the characteristics and requirements of the ramp user or if there is likely to be a range of ramp users (Hunter, 1992).

The quality and structural integrity of the ramp will be guided by compliance with industry standards and local code requirements. There might be a range of design or manufacturing standards existing in various countries that relate to the construction of ramps—for example, standards relating to slip resistance, loads, the construction of aluminum and steel structures, and the construction of fixed platforms and walkways.

PEOPLE, THEIR MOBILITY, AND THEIR EQUIPMENT

A ramp might suit someone who uses a manual wheelchair and has sufficient upper-limb strength and endurance to push the equipment along a gradual slope, or it might suit an individual using an electric wheelchair or scooter to travel distances. It can also prove a more appropriate alternative to stairs for a client who uses a wheelie walker or walking aid or who can walk without a mobility device. In these instances, the client needs to demonstrate the required endurance and capacity to manage the gradient and walk the length of a ramp without adversely affecting his or her health, safety, and independence.

Therapists need to observe and measure the person with the disability and his or her equipment and caregivers to ensure the correct design of the ramp. If a person with a disability is to walk along a similar ramp, with or without mobility equipment, to trial it, therapists should observe the person's capacity to negotiate distances on a slope, noting whether he or she has a safe stride and good balance and endurance. Therapists should also note whether the person needs to hold on to the rail for support and whether he or she requires frequent level landings to rest. Further, all ramp users, especially people who have a visual impairment, might need enhanced lighting at the entry and exit to the ramp and along its length.

Clients might use a ramp in a range of ways and hence the design can vary to suit its use (Goldsmith, 2000). For example, a client may wheel along the ramp in his or her wheelchair or scooter and use the rails more as a physical barrier to prevent the equipment from rolling off of the edge of the structure, rather than holding onto them for support. Other clients might use both handrails to pull themselves up the ramp run to provide a change of strain on the shoulder joints as an alternative to pushing themselves in the wheelchair.

The types of measurements relating to the clients, their equipment, and their caregivers that determine the design of the ramp and whether the access standards are applicable include the following:

+ The overall occupied length and width of the equipment, influencing the length and width of the level landings and the width of the ramp

+ The turning space of the equipment (from 90 degrees to 360 degrees), impacting on the length and width of the landings on entry and exit and the width of entry landings

+ The reach range of the person, influencing the height of the rails

+ Space for the caregiver standing behind or beside the client and his or her equipment, determining the width of the ramp, and the width and length of landings

Therapists can establish these measurements by using a large indoor or outdoor area to mark out the space required, or they can set up obstacle courses to test their final dimensions. For example, chalk or adhesive tape can be used on a level surface to set out the diameter measurement of a turning circle of a person in a wheelchair or scooter.

Therapists will also need to check the weights of clients and their wheelchairs or scooters to ensure that the builder constructs ramps that are able to withstand the load. Further, therapists might need to contact the manufacturers or suppliers of scooters and wheelchairs to determine the maximum safe gradient that the equipment can negotiate.

SUITABILITY OF THE HOME

Ramp design and materials need to reflect the overall look of the dwelling rather than appear as an addition that stands out from the rest of the home (Center for Universal Design, 2004). Therapists should give consideration to the type of materials used and choose colors that make the ramp design blend with the home and its surrounding garden area. For example, if there is a wooden house requiring modification, the therapist might consider recommending the installation of a wooden ramp painted in the same colors as the home.

Using a screen, such as a decorative wall or foliage, can serve to disguise the area and prevent highlighting that a person with a disability lives in the home (Center for Universal Design, 2004). In other cases, it might be more aesthetically pleasing to place the ramp at the side or rear of the premises.

The homeowner will also need to consider whether expenditure on the ramp is cost effective, given the age and condition of the home. Further, the location and size of the ramp might affect the use of yard area and how the client, other members of the household, and visitors use the various entries of the home. Other factors that might influence the final design of the ramp are permanent structures, such as car parking facilities, the location of outdoor sheds, meters, hot water units, or tanks, or the style of windows near the proposed ramp location. Extra expenditure might be required to change some of the permanent fittings and fixtures to accommodate the ramp. If there is an extreme level change that requires a long, circuitous ramp or if space is limited, a lift may be a more appropriate design solution (Center for Accessible Environments, 2009).

RAMP DESIGN FEATURES AND ELEMENTS

The following features and design elements are important for occupational therapists to consider when designing a ramp.

Length

The ramp run is the horizontal distance the ramp must travel from entrance threshold to the surface or level of the ground (grade; NAHB Research Center, 2006).

If a short and long ramp are placed on the same height step or rise (the vertical distance the ramp must rise from the grade to the entrance threshold; NAHB Research Center, 2006), the shorter wheelchair ramp will increase in steepness, whereas a longer wheelchair ramp will be less steep. Ramps with long runs might be fatiguing for people to negotiate and more hazardous to descend compared with shorter ramps (Hunter, 1992). It is best to design a ramp that will result in the shortest length possible by taking advantage of the high points on the existing site grade (Center for Universal Design, 2004).

Gradient or Running Slope

The ramp gradient or running slope is the rate of incline expressed in a ratio or in degrees (NAHB Research Center, 2006). Ramp gradient should be constant between landings or changes in direction. If the characteristics and requirements of the ramp user are not known or if the ramp is to be used by a range of people, the gradients recommended in the access standards should be used as a guide (Hunter, 1992).

A ramp gradient of 1:3 is steeper than a ramp gradient of 1:12. The steeper the gradient, the harder to wheel up and down the slope. A shallow ramp gradient might be suitable for people who push themselves in their wheelchair. A steeper gradient might be more appropriate for someone who uses a scooter or electric wheelchair manufactured to suit steeper inclines and long distances. Further, there might be space restrictions limiting the run length of the ramp, resulting in the need for a short, steep ramp, but this would only be provided if the client is able to safely manage this type of design. As indicated earlier, therapists will need to consider manufacturers' information regarding the maximum safe gradient that the equipment can negotiate. The shallower the gradient, the more likely it will suit a large range of people with different disabilities and equipment (Hunter, 1992).

The therapist will also need to consider the age- and disease-related deterioration of the person over time, because the gradient can become one of the most significant features of the ramp, influencing a person's mobility over time. For example, a person in a wheelchair might experience upper limb joint deterioration and pain over time, impacting on his or her capacity to wheel up and down a ramp. Older people and people with a disability who are ambulant may experience fatigue as they ascend a ramp and joint pain in the lower limbs on descent, depending on their heath condition or disability.

The transition between a ramp and landing needs to be smooth to ensure that wheelchairs do not have to negotiate changes in surface levels. The gradients of the two surfaces that are transitioning should be shallow enough to ensure that wheelchair footplates do not catch when moving from one surface to another (e.g., from the landing onto the ramp).

Further, the angle of the transition from the ramp to the landing and vice versa needs to be such that the four wheels on a wheelchair are always on a surface. This is important to ensure that there is no twist or instability or displacement of the person's center of gravity, which can result in the individual falling out of his or her equipment as the equipment transitions across the surfaces.

When compared with curved ramps, straight runs are preferred for easier maneuverability and landing construction (NAHB Research Center, 2006). On a curved ramp, the gradient might need to be shallower than that of a straight ramp to ensure the equipment does not roll off of the ramp edge on the turns. There will need to be a reduction in the curved ramp gradient in proportion to the decreasing radii of the curvature so that a ramp with a smaller curve has a shallower gradient than a ramp with a larger curve (Hunter, 1992).

Ramps can be L-shaped, switchback, or U-shaped with landings at the changes in direction (Center for Universal Design, 2004). Ramps can be configured in these arrangements as a result of limitations of space and the presence of permanent structures (Center for Universal Design).

Cross Slope or Cross Fall

The slope perpendicular to the direction of travel is the cross slope (NAHB Research Center, 2006). A shallow slope, rather than a flat surface, is required on the ramp to ensure water drains away or small particles or loose objects run off of the area. If the cross slope is too steep, it is difficult to control the direction of the wheelchair or scooter, and the person may tip over in his or her equipment. On curved ramps, the cross slope should fall toward the center of the curvature of the ramp (Hunter, 1992).

Vertical and Horizontal Clearance

The ramp width provides horizontal clearance for the person and his or her equipment. The ramp might need to be wider than the measurements in the access standards along its run or at the landings where the wheelchair turns to ensure that long and wide equipment can fit on the turns and through doorways that open off of landings.

The space above the ramp surface provides vertical clearance, and it is to be free of obstructions to ensure people who might vary in height and who might use a range of equipment are safe mobilizing along the ramp. For example, windowsills, windows, window shades, light fittings, or trees might need to be altered to ensure that the necessary vertical clearance is attained.

Landings

Landings are the intermediate platforms between sloped segments of a ramp (NAHB Research Center, 2006). They are also required at the top and bottom of the ramp run and at any point where there is a change in direction.

Landings should be level or have a very shallow gradient and be large enough to accommodate the length of the person using his or her mobility equipment. Landings provide a flat surface on which people can rest. If designed wide enough and long enough, landings can provide a surface on which wheelchairs and other equipment can change direction safely without any wheels leaving the ramp surface.

The interim landing should be as wide as the widest ramp run leading to this landing. The length dimension may vary, depending on the turning space requirements of the person with a disability and his or her equipment.

Therapists will need to examine the path of travel leading up to and away from the landing areas to ensure that the ramp is suitably positioned for ease of access from other areas of the yard. Landings should not intrude or terminate in areas that do not provide sufficient space for the person and his or her equipment to exit or enter the ramp.

The door circulation space on landings needs to be considered where a ramp leads to a landing that has a doorway. A door might swing inward or outward, which can influence the size of the landing required near this area. It is useful to refer to access standards to guide the design of the landing in relation to the door clearance, the direction of door swing, and approach.

Rails

Rails are the horizontal member supported by vertical posts and include top, mid-rails, and curbs; the mid-rail is a rail positioned midway between the top railing member and the deck of the ramp or the ramp surface; and the curb is positioned near the decking at the edge of the ramp (NAHB Research Center, 2006).

Rails act as a barrier to prevent individuals and their equipment from falling off of the edge of the ramp. They are also used as a support to help people maintain their balance as they ascend or descend the ramp. Clients who might benefit from the use of rails on ramps include people with sensory impairment or those who lack stamina.

Rails should begin in the ramp approach and departure zones to act as an indicator of the start and finish of the ramp. They should be located on both sides of a ramp and be continuous. They should not, however, protrude into a person's path of travel, particularly when there is a 90 degree approach to a ramp. The ends of the rails should turn to the side or down, close to the final balustrade. These types of terminations to the rails will ensure that people are not injured when approaching or passing the landing area at the top or bottom of the ramp.

Rails can provide support for people making the transition onto or from a level landing area (Hunter, 1992). Bilateral rails provide better support than just one rail, especially if people have the use of only one arm when ascending and descending the ramp or if a person needs support on both sides of the ramp.

Clients might not use the rail or they might use it only as a guide, without holding onto it firmly. But if clients hold the rails for support, they should be rounded to ensure their hand can grasp them easily. They can be made of wood, metal, or polyvinyl chloride (PVC) supported at intervals by brackets (NAHB Research Center, 2006).

Rails with a round diameter should have fittings attached to the underside that allow the hand to run freely along the rail length. The fixture adjoining the rail to a wall or a support post should be supportive enough to allow the rail to take significant body weight as indicated in the access standards.

Any bends in the rails need to have a smooth finish to ensure there are no sharp edges on which people can hurt themselves if they run their hands along the surface.

Curb or Edge Protection

In some countries, curbs are required on ramps and are installed directly underneath rails to ensure the wheels on mobility equipment do not roll off of the edge of the ramp. Curbs should be installed on each side of ramp runs and at each side of ramp landings. They might not be required if there is a wall adjacent to the ramp that can act as a curb or, if the landing adjacent, and extending out for a distance, is level with the ramp edges. This level edge ensures that if someone rolls off of the edge of the ramp, he or she is still on a safe, flat surface.

Curbs can aid people who are blind or who have a visual impairment and who use a cane to guide their mobility. This edge protection provides a surface along which the cane can run as the person walks along the ramp.

Curbs should be installed so that they are flush with the inside face of the rail and should not intrude into the horizontal circulation space of the ramp. They are to be high enough to prevent footplates catching on them or riding over the top of them.

Construction Materials

A range of materials can be used to construct a ramp, and the materials selected might depend on a client's budget and the type of finish he or she wishes to achieve. The choice of ramp material might be determined by maintenance requirements and how well it can withstand weather conditions and manage loads. Further, it is important that the ramp is able to be used in all weather conditions, so chosen materials should guarantee traction and slip resistance when wet.

Additionally, ramps might require specific materials and finishes to prevent termite damage. This is an issue that will need to be discussed with the builder, particularly if they are prevalent in the client's residential area.

Weight Limit

Lightweight materials make the ramp easier to transport and for builders to install, although the final construction will need to take the weight of a range of loads. The supplier or builder of any ramp should state the maximum load limit.

Therapists working with a designer or builder of a ramp will need to consider, for example, the following:

+ The weight of the client in the wheelchair or scooter
+ The weight of the person's caregiver, if the client requires assistance to wheel up and down ramps
+ The weight of a number of people standing on the ramp
+ The weight being taken by the ramp if it is used during the process of moving furniture in and out of the home

Adaptability

It is useful to question whether the ramp can be installed in such a way as to allow it to be dismantled and the ramp modified in the future—for example, if the ramp is to be stored and reconstructed at a later date or at an alternative location or if the landings and ramp surfaces need to be widened to accommodate larger equipment. The ramp might need to be dismantled, stored, and reconstructed again in an alternative location. Simple and easy assembly and installation can contribute to reduced transport and building labor costs and increased adaptability.

In situations where a permanent ramp cannot be installed, a temporary ramp might be the preferred solution (Center for Accessible Environments, 2009). The longer the temporary ramp, the heavier and more awkward it might be to manage, depending on the materials used for its construction (Center for Accessible Environments). It might be difficult to provide a landing at the top of the ramp, depending on the design of the home. Further, the temporary ramp needs to be installed in such a way that ensures that it is positioned firmly and securely on two surfaces (Center for Accessible Environments).

Lighting

Adequate lighting of an external ramp is required to ensure that the features of the ramp are easily distinguished day or night in varying weather conditions. A sensor light at the door to activate the outdoor lighting prevents having to consider the location of switches along the path leading to the ramp.

Obstacles

The ramp should extend into areas where there are no obstacles—for example, clotheslines, garden sheds, driveways, garages or carports, garden beds, push-out windows, or brick sills on windows. If there are obstacles in the area of the proposed ramp, these will need to be removed or modified or the ramp redesigned to accommodate the obstructions.

When planning the ramp design and location, therapists will also need to consider the location of in-ground drainage or sewer pipes for easy access by tradesmen. A ramp should not sit over ground pipes because it will be difficult for plumbers to gain access to undertake repair work.

Local Building Codes and Permit Issues

In the United States, local building codes might have requirements for ramps based on safety, health, and welfare rather than access. Safety issues might include information about the slope of the ramp, the amount of weight that the rail has to withstand, landing size, and the distance between the balusters on a ramp railing. Local code and permit requirements need to be considered and federal codes consulted for guidance, rather than for compliance information (Center for Universal Design, 2004; NAHB Research Center, 2006). The therapist might need to consult with the builder or local inspection or planning office for advice (Center for Universal Design).

Other countries, such as Australia, have a range of design or manufacturing standards relating to the construction of permanent or temporary ramps, including standards for slip resistance of surfaces, loads, the construction of aluminum and steel structures, and the construction of fixed platforms and walkways. This information can be used in discussions with design and building professionals on the design of ramps.

Cost of Installation

It is important to compare the cost-effectiveness of providing a ramp in relation to the installation of a stair-lift, lift, or relocation of the client to alternative accommodation. The longer the ramp, the more expensive it will be and the greater the area it will occupy. It might be more costly than a lift or stair-lift, but it is also more aesthetically pleasing, easier to manage, and take up less space. A lift or stair-lift can be removed and sold or relocated and the external area of the home restored to its original design.

CONSIDERATIONS WHEN LOCATING AN EXTERNAL RAMP

Location of the Ramp

A home may have one step up from ground level or a set of stairs. There could be one or a number of entries into the home. When siting a ramp, all access points to the home and access areas around the home, including the slope of the land, need to be investigated. It is important to determine where the person enters the property—for example, through the front gate and path or always through the garage. Ramps might be installed to provide access to and from the house to the area where the car might be parked or they can run to and from a path that leads out of the property and onto the street.

Establishing the Ramp Design

Rise of the Ramp

The first step to determining the length of a ramp in a specific location is to measure the rise, or the vertical distance from the ground level to the height of the landing. The height of the landing at the door is usually the starting point for measuring the ramp. The end point of the ramp will be the grade or ground where the features of a landing are needed. There might already be a path or concreted area at the end of the ramp that can act as the landing; consequently, a separate landing might not need to be installed.

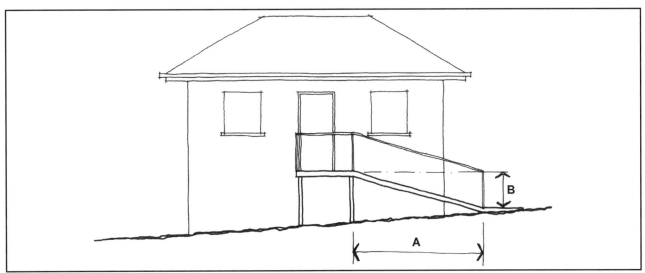

Figure C-1. Land sloping up away from the home and running a ramp toward the slope. (Reprinted with permission from Paul Coonan.)

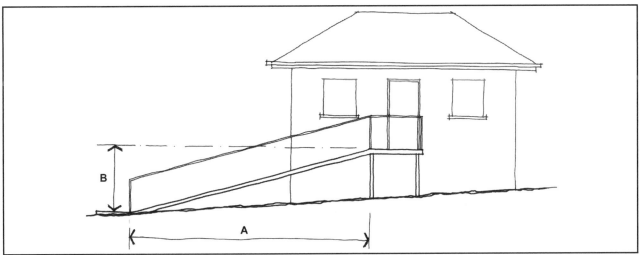

Figure C-2. Land sloping down away from the home and running a ramp along the slope. (Reprinted with permission from Paul Coonan.)

Ramp Gradient, Length, and Direction

The measurement of the rise and information about the slope direction of the land will influence the run length and the direction of the ramp. If the land slopes up away from the home, running the ramp away from the house will result in a short ramp (Figure C-1). If land slopes down away from the home, running the ramp away from the house will result in a very long ramp (Figure C-2).

Essential Measurements That Guide the Design

As indicated previously, important measurements for the ramp design include the following:

+ The overall occupied length and width of the equipment, influencing the length and width of the level landings and the width of the ramp

+ The turning space of the equipment (from 90 degrees to 360 degrees), impacting on the length and width of the landings on entry and exit and the width of entry landings

+ The reach range of the person, influencing the height of rails

+ Space for the caregiver standing behind or beside the client and his or her equipment, determining the width of the ramp, and the width and length of landings

Equipment and Resources

The equipment required to measure up for a ramp includes the following:

+ Tape measure (at least 16 feet/5000 mm long) to measure dimensions

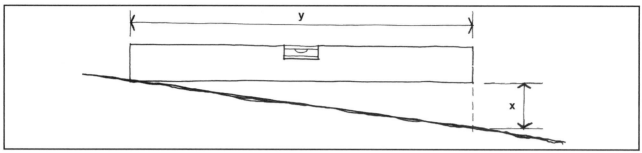

Figure C-3. Measuring the gradient of the land with a spirit level. (Reprinted with permission from Paul Coonan.)

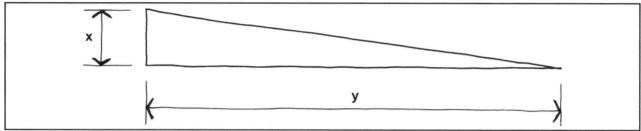

Figure C-4. The rise in relation to length. (Reprinted with permission from Paul Coonan.)

+ Small spirit level that can hang on string or a clinometer

+ String to use to show the length of the ramp from the start of the ramp to the point of termination

+ Tent pegs for tying the string to at ground level

+ Access standards and design guides to direct the design of the ramp

Measuring the Gradient of the Land

The therapist can measure the gradient of land with a spirit level or two uprights placed a distance apart and a horizontal line to measure the distance between them (Figure C-3). The bubble in the spirit level is to be located centrally to denote a horizontal position.

The gradient in the diagram is the X measurement in relation to the Y measurement.

Alternatively, Figure C-4 shows the rise in relation to the length and the resulting gradient.

Units are usually expressed in inches or in metric measurement (Tables C-1 and C-2).

Calculating the Length of a Straight Ramp in Relation to the Gradient of the Ramp and the Fall of the Land

1. Identify the height, length, and width dimensions of the landing required at the entrance to the home.

2. Fix the end of the string to the outer edge of the proposed landing where the ramp will start (Figure C-5).

3. Extend the string to the proposed point of termination of the ramp and place the spirit level in the middle of the extended string line.

4. At the point of the proposed termination of the ramp, pull the string tight and ensure that it is level by checking the small spirit level. The most accurate reading will be achieved by placing the spirit level in the middle of the total length of the string. The bubble needs to be located at the center of the spirit level to indicate that the string is level. Alternatively, the clinometer can be held on the string to judge whether it is level.

5. At the point of proposed termination of the ramp, measure the distance from the string to the ground. Multiply this measurement by the gradient you wish to achieve (e.g., 1:12 or 1:14) to determine the required length of the ramp. Once you know the length needed to cover the fall, measure the length of the string and extend it to the required ramp length. Then, remeasure the drop from the string to the ground and calculate the ramp length again.

6. Alternatively, divide the measurement of the string to the ground into the length dimension of the string line to determine the gradient of the ramp and whether ending the ramp at this point would result in it being shallower or steeper than the desired gradient.

Table C-1. Gradient Table for 1:12 Gradient

	X:Y	*GRADIENT*
IMPERIAL	$3\frac{7}{8}$ in:$47\frac{1}{4}$ in	1:12
METRIC	100 mm:1,200 mm	

Table C-2. Gradient Table for 1:14 Gradient

	X:Y	*GRADIENT*
IMPERIAL	$3\frac{7}{8}$ in:$55\frac{1}{4}$ in	1:14
METRIC	100 mm:1,400 mm	

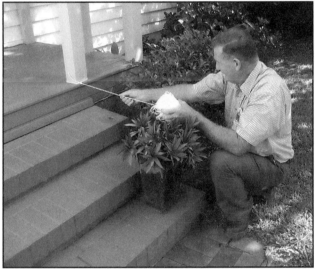

Figure C-5. Fixing the string to the outer edge of the proposed landing.

For example, for a 1:12 gradient, the string should be dropped 1 in per ft length toward the ground. If the distance from the string to the ground is 14.1875 in (or 360 mm) and the length of the string from the starting point of the ramp is 168.75 in (or 4,286 mm), the gradient of the ramp will be 1:12 (Table C-3).

Calculating the Length of a Straight Ramp With a Switchback or Return in Relation to the Gradient of the Ramp and the Fall of the Land

If there is insufficient room for a straight ramp or if the ground falls away from the home, increasing the fall and the length of the ramp, it may be necessary to incorporate a switchback or turn that has a level landing to have a more appropriate length and end point (Figure C-6).

1. Identify the height, length, and width dimensions of the landing required at the entrance to the home.

2. Fix end of string to the outer edge of the proposed landing where the ramp will start.

3. Extend the string, pull it tight, and ensure that it is level by checking the small string level that is hung centrally on the string or using a spirit level to measure the level (Figure C-7).

4. Divide the calculated ramp length and add the landing dimension to determine where the ramp would be located as it turns. Adjust the ramp length to suit the location of the landing but maintain a consistent gradient on the slope (Figure C-8).

5. Pull the string level to the point where the interim landing would start and measure from this point back to the edge of the first landing. Measure the distance of the string to the ground and lower the string the required distance to achieve the desired gradient. For example, if there is a 15.75-in-high (400 mm) landing and there is a need to install a 1:12 gradient ramp, this measurement of the landing is multiplied by 12. The total length of the ramp will then be 189 in (4,800 mm). Divide the 189 in (4,800 mm) measurement and have the ramp-run sections sit between the location of the three sets of landings.

Table C-3. Examples of Gradient Calculation

	GRADIENT = 1:12		GRADIENT = 1:14	
EXAMPLE 1	Imperial	Metric	Imperial	Metric
A	$168\frac{3}{4}$ in	4,286 mm	$196\frac{7}{8}$ in	5,000 mm
B	$14\frac{3}{16}$ in	360 mm	$14\frac{3}{16}$ in	360 mm
EXAMPLE 2				
A	$234\frac{1}{4}$ in	5,952 mm	$275\frac{5}{8}$ in	7,000 mm
B	$19\frac{3}{4}$ in	500 mm	$19\frac{3}{4}$ in	500 mm

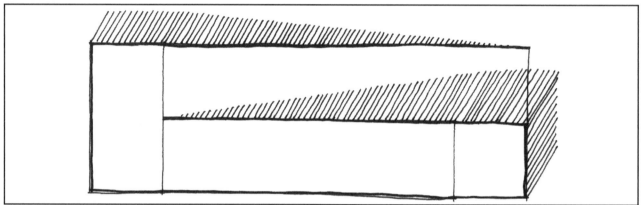

Figure C-6. Site plan view of a ramp with a switchback or turn that has a level landing. (Reprinted with permission from Paul Coonan.)

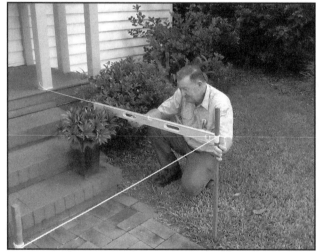

Figure C-7. Checking the level of the landing section.

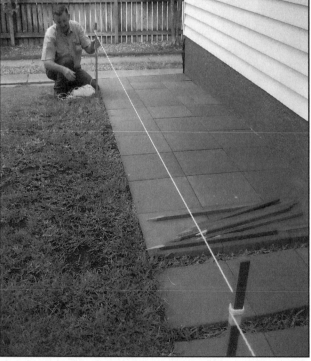

Figure C-8. Determining the size and position of the middle landing

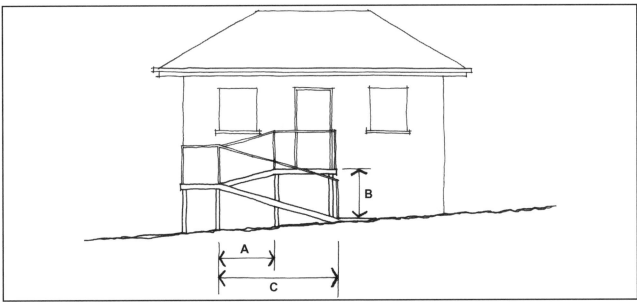

Figure C-9. Ramp with a switchback or turn that has a level landing (refer to Table C-5). (Reprinted with permission from Paul Coonan.)

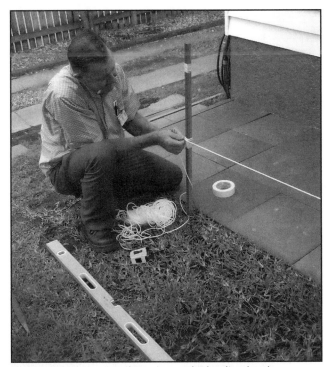

Figure C-10. Lowering the string to the landing level.

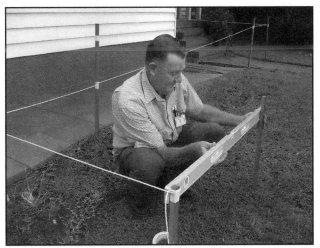

Figure C-11. Measuring the level of the landing.

Alternative Options to Ramps

A ramp might not suit someone who cannot manage the gradient and length of the ramp or who requires stairs to ensure intentional foot lift and placement on a surface. In these instances, there might be other cost-effective solutions available. For example, a no-step entry or zero-level entry can be created that allows a person to enter the home without negotiating steps. This type of entry may be created by regrading the yard and landscaping and adding a path or new landing over the existing level area at the bottom of the step at the entry (Center for Universal Design, 2004; NAHB Research Center, 2006). Landscaped options can be expensive but can have a longer lifespan and need less maintenance than ramps (Center for Universal Design).

When dividing the ramp, it is not necessary to split the measurement for the ramp length evenly between the landings. Rather, the location of the interim landing is dependent on how the client wants the landing to look in relation to the rest of the home and the presence of available space and permanent structures (Figures C-9 through C-13; Table C-4).

Ramps may be designed in a range of configurations as illustrated in Figures C-14 through C-16.

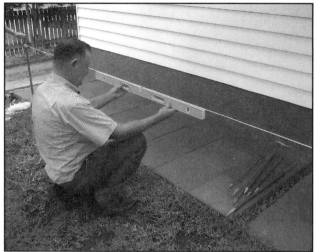

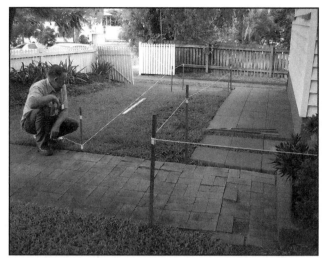

Figure C-12. Measuring the level of the line.

Figure C-13. The final proposed ramp set out with string.

Table C-4. Example of Calculations for a Ramp With a Switchback or Turn That Has a Level Landing

	GRADIENT – 1:12		GRADIENT – 1:14	
	Imperial	Metric	Imperial	Metric
A	$78\frac{3}{4}$ in	2,000 mm	$78\frac{3}{4}$ in	2,000 mm
B	$15\frac{3}{4}$ in	400 mm	$15\frac{3}{4}$ in	400 mm
C	$110\frac{1}{4}$ in	2,800 mm	$141\frac{3}{4}$ in	3,600 mm

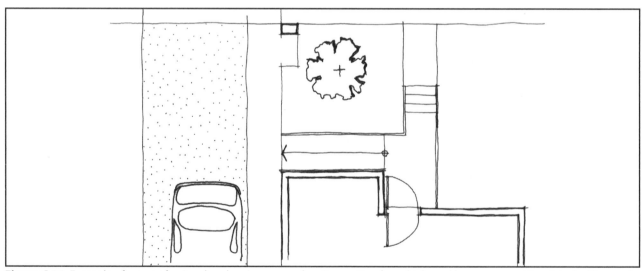

Figure C-14. Example of a part of a site plan showing a ramp location option for vehicle and house access. (Reprinted with permission from Paul Coonan.)

If a house is high-set and located on flat land, it may be more appropriate to install a lift or stair-lift than an excessively long ramp with a number of turns, which could be difficult to negotiate and expensive to install (Center for Universal Design, 2004). The choice of lift or stair-lift will depend on the client's budget, the availability of space and vertical height for travel of the device, and the person's capacity to use the device, including operating the controls and maintaining a safe body position during its use.

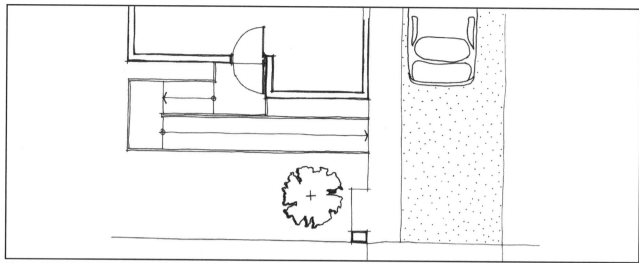

Figure C-15. Example of a part of a site plan showing a ramp location option for vehicle and house access. (Reprinted with permission from Paul Coonan.)

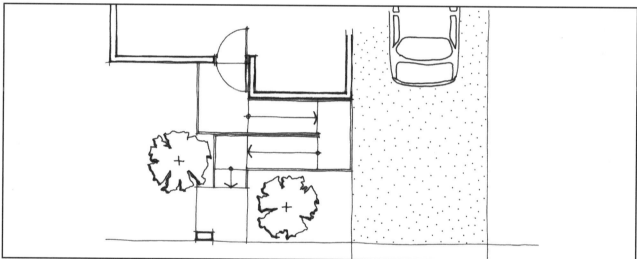

Figure C-16. Example of a part of a site plan showing a ramp location option for front entry access. (Reprinted with permission from Paul Coonan.)

Lifts vary in style and finishes and features, such as single or double entries, laminated mirrors, rails, an intercom, forced ventilation, and a fold-down chair. Lifts have rated weight loads, and cabin and landing doors can be automatically or manually operated.

Safety devices might also be fit to lifts. These can include safety switches, automatic return of the car to the ground floor, followed by automatic door opening in the event of power failure, accurate leveling at the floor, door protection devices, and an auto call emergency communicator (for a bidirectional communication between the assistance center and the passengers in an emergency).

Stair-lifts can be installed on internal or external stairs, depending on the type and style of construction of the stairs and the clearance along the length and top and bottom of the stairs for egress. Features include remote control or switch operation, swivel seats, arm rests, seat belts, battery back-up in the event of power failure, automatic shut-off if there is a collision with an obstruction, and the capacity to pace the rate of travel. They might have a platform design rather than a fold-down seat to accommodate a wheelchair.

Both vertical lifts and stair-lifts are required to comply with industry standards in a range of countries, which ensures the quality of the manufactured item and the safety of the client using the equipment.

Occupational therapists need to consider whether one option is more suitable than the other by examining the ramp, stair-lift, or lift in relation to various factors including the following:

+ The client's capacity to manage each of these alternatives

+ How his or her mobility equipment will be accommodated by each option

+ The access needs of other household members

+ Whether each option suits the style and condition of the home

+ The cost of installing each option as well as the associated building works

+ Whether there is sufficient space to incorporate each of the options

+ The appearance of the home from the street with respect to each option

+ Local building code regulations for installation

To assist therapists in the assessment process, manufacturers and suppliers of stair-lifts and lifts can provide advice on client factors and the possible structural changes to the home when incorporating the item as a home modification.

REFERENCES

Center for Accessible Environments. (2009). *Design guidance: Ramps*. Retrieved from http://www.cae.org.uk/guidance_ramps.html

Center for Universal Design. (2004). *Wood ramp design: How to add a ramp that looks good and works too*. Retrieved from http://www.design.ncsu.edu/cud/pubs_p/docs/rampbooklet296final.pdf

Goldsmith, S. (2000). *Universal design: A manual of practical guidance for architects*. Woburn, MA: Architectural Press.

Hunter, R. A. (1992). *More accessible housing for independent living: A guide to designing and adapting dwellings for the aged and people with disabilities*. City of Sale, Australia: McPherson's Printing.

NAHB Research Center. (2006). *Safety first: A technical approach to home modifications*. Washington, DC: Author.

Home Modification Resources

Please note that most of these sites are located in the United States. Although some of the information is applicable to home modification practice in other locations, some information is specific to the U.S. context.

DEDICATED AGING, DISABILITY, HOME MODIFICATION, AND REMODELING RESOURCE SITES AND GUIDES

American Association of Retired Persons (AARP) Policy and Research

http://www.aarp.org

A nonprofit organization dedicated to addressing the needs and interests of people 50 years old and older. This Web site provides links to information and resources on home design and modification, home and community livability, falls prevention, financing home improvements, and the Fair Housing Act.

Department of Housing and Urban Development (HUD)

http://portal.hud.gov/portal/page/portal/HUD/groups/disabilities

This site has a section dedicated to providing people with disabilities with information about renting, buying, making homes accessible, and funding options as well as details of people's fair housing rights.

Disability.gov

http://www.disability.gov

This site provides access to information about disability programs, services, housing, laws, and benefits. Resources can be located within each state using the Find State and Local Resources map located in each of the topic areas.

Homemods.org

http://www.homemods.org

This Web site, a university-based and nonprofit effort, is dedicated to promoting aging in place and independent living for people of all ages and abilities. It also serves as an information clearinghouse on home modification to equip professionals and consumers with a comprehensive inventory of resources. It provides information on training and education opportunities for professionals who wish to respond to the increasing demand for home modification services.

Home Modification Resource Guide, 4th Ed., 2003

http://www.homemods.org/resources/library.shtml

The comprehensive guide provides information on a range of resources related to home modifications, including the following:

+ General resources that discuss the relationship between the functional capabilities of the elderly and their need for home modifications

+ Assessment procedures and instruments that can be used to assess the competency of an individual, problems that the environment presents, and the need for modifications

+ Financing mechanisms to develop programs and pay for modifications

+ Products/programs and services pertaining to home modifications

+ Home modification program development and implementation

+ Product development and implementation

+ Research and education

National Directory of Home Modification Resources

http://www.usc.edu/dept/gero/nrcshhm/directory
This Web site provides state-by-state information on home modification activity in the United States and links to products, programs, services, and organizations related to home modification, independent living, and aging in place. It also provides information on publications and research projects from the National Resource Center on Supportive Housing and Home Modification (NRCSHHM) on home modification delivery, home modification funding, universal design (UD) ideas, aging in place, access to home modification programs and services, new tools to better home modification, and housing frail elders.

National Kitchen and Bath Association

http://www.nkba.org
This Web site provides consumers and professionals with tips and guidelines on kitchen and bath designs and remodeling projects.

The National Resource Center on Supportive Housing and Home Modification (NRCSHHM)

http://www.usc.edu/dept/gero/nrcshhm/aboutus
The National Resource Center on Supportive Housing and Home Modification is a university-based and nonprofit Web site dedicated to promoting aging in place and independent living for people of all ages and abilities. The center is associated with the University of Southern California Gerontology Department, and its mission is to make supportive housing and home modification a more integral component of successful aging, long-term care, preventive health, and the development of elder-friendly communities. The Center also promotes practical strategies and materials for policymakers, practitioners, consumers, manufacturers, suppliers, and researchers.

ToolBase Services

http://www.toolbase.org/index.aspx
ToolBase Services is the housing industry's resource for technical information on building products, materials, new technologies, business management, and housing systems. It provides product descriptions, design and construction guides, best practices, performance reports, case studies, and other resources for builders and remodelers.

COMPANY CATALOGUES

The following catalogues offer products for enhancing ability in home design and modifications.

AliMed

http://www.alimed.com
AliMed is a designer, manufacturer, and master distributor of essential health care products. These include bariatric equipment and bathing, dressing, and toileting aids.

American Standard

http://www.americanstandard-us.com
American Standard is a manufacturer of bath and kitchen products including bathroom toilet and kitchen fixtures and furniture. UD- and Americans With Disabilities Act (ADA)-compliant designs are also available.

Architectural Products for Barrier Free Living

http://www.barrierfree.org
Accessible products including ADA roll-in wheelchair showers, shower pans, accessible assisted-living bathtubs, safety grab bars, shower seats, access ramps, and other unique bathroom and home accessories.

Best Bath

http://www.best-bath.com

Best Bath focuses on low-threshold safe bathing and showering options.

Black and Decker

http://www.blackanddecker.com

Black and Decker is a global manufacturer of quality power tools and accessories, hardware and home improvement products, access control, and technology-based systems.

Dynamic Living

http://www.dynamic-living.com

This searchable online catalogue provides information on a range of assistive devices and specialized products. It allows users to browse by use (function) or location (areas of the house). Use or function categories include moving around, sitting/standing, hands, vision, hearing communicating, caregiving, memory, generously sized, or reaching. Locations or areas of the house are bathroom, shower and tub, toilet, medicine cabinet, dressing room, bedroom, kitchen, dining room, family room, kid's corner, and tool shed.

Hewimd USA

http://www.hewimd.com

Hewimd USA supplies grab bars, shower seats, bath accessories, cabinet handles/pulls, cabinet knobs, recessed pulls, hooks, handrails, door stops, and hardware. Hewi products are available in various sizes, styles, and colors. They integrate clean design, high-quality materials and functional precision.

Kraftmaid Cabinets

http://www.kraftmaid.com/cabinets/home.aspx

Kraftmaid provides hundreds of custom cabinet options in a range of designs including UD cabinetry.

Kohler

http://www.kohler.com

Koehler is a manufacturer of kitchen and bath products.

Sammons Preston

http://www.pattersonmedical.com

Sammons Preston has a range of rehabilitation, assistive, and splinting products including grab bars, reachers, furniture risers, doorknob grippers and extenders, bath aids, and handheld shower hoses.

TRADE EXHIBITS/DISPLAY CENTERS

The following trade shows and centers offer opportunity for vendor contact and assistive technology (AT) product viewing.

Build Boston

http://www.buildboston.com/ResPlus/BuildBoston

New England's annual residential tradeshow and 2-day convention and tradeshow for the design and construction industry features more than 220 product exhibits, 85 workshops, and special events.

Institute for Human Centered Design (IHCD)/Adaptive Environments (AE)

http://www.adaptenv.org

IHCD/AE is an international nonprofit organization, based in Boston, committed to advancing the role of design in expanding opportunity and enhancing experience for people of all ages and abilities. AE's work balances expertise in legally required accessibility with promotion of best practices in human-centered or UD.

International Builders Show

http://www.buildersshow.com

This is an annual building exhibit in the United States for builders, architects, remodelers, developers, dealers, and distributors supported by more than 16,000 suppliers and manufacturers of building products.

National Association of Home Builders (NAHB)

http://www.nahb.org

NAHB is a trade association that helps promote policies that make housing a national priority. This site has a range of resources for consumers and building professionals.

DESIGN INFORMATION

American Society of Interior Design

http://www.asid.org

The American Society of Interior Design is a community of people driven by a common love for design and committed to the belief that interior design is a service to people. This site has a section dedicated to providing formation resources and links on UD and designing for accessibility and aging.

Design Linc

http://www.designlinc.com

Design Linc provide design tips for the exterior of the home as well as the bathroom, kitchen, bedroom, and laundry.

Home Free Home

http://homefreehome.org

Home Free Home is a national nonprofit organization that provides pro bono architectural design services to people who need to remodel their homes to accommodate a disability.

InformeDesign

http://www.informedesign.umn.edu

InformeDesign is a site dedicated to translating and disseminating research into an easy-to-read, easy-to-use format for architects, graphic designers, housing specialists, interior designers, landscape architects, urban designers and planners, and the public. Occupational therapists would also find the diverse research summaries of value, especially those reporting on design research related to spaces in residential environments, and characteristics of various occupants in terms of ability/disability, age, and type (renters and caregivers).

The Center for Universal Design

http://www.design.ncsu.edu/cud/index.htm

The Center for Universal Design (CUD) is a national information, technical assistance, and research center that evaluates, develops, and promotes accessible and UD in housing, commercial and public facilities, outdoor environments, and products. It provides information resources on UD and accessible housing and home modifications and residential remodeling.

Wheelchair-Accessible House Plans

http://www.homeplans.com/exec/action/psp/architectural_designs/wheelchair-accessible_house_plans/content/159/hsme/msnsrch/hspos/msn2net/section/homeplans

This site provides wheelchair-accessible house plans that feature sloping walkways to the main entrance; wider doorways, interior passages, and closet doors; lever-style hardware; and convenient heights for things such as thermostats and light switches.

DATABASES

The following databases offer resources related to home environment enhancement using equipment and AT.

Able Data

http://www.abledata.com

This site provides an online database of AT and environmental adaptations. It also features product reviews and information on designs and products related to the bathrooms, doors, floors, furniture, kitchens, public restrooms, storage, walls, windows, furniture, outdoor environment, vertical accessibility, lighting, and signs.

BUILDEASE

http://www.lifease.com/lifease-ease.html

This is a software program that integrates an assessment of the client and the home, with a database of more than 1,500 suggested solutions and building products, including where products can be obtained.

CATEA's National Public Web Site on Assistive Technology

http://assistivetech.net

The database provided by the Center for Assistive Technology and Environmental Access (CATEA) has information on a broad range of specialized and mainstream products that can be browsed by function, activity, or vendor. Alternatively, a basic or advanced search of the database can be undertaken using any or all of the search fields including keywords, vendor, functional limitation, activity, or product type as search options. This database also has a function that allows identified products to be compared by tabling the image, price, vendor, description, functions, features, options, considerations, and requirements of each option selected.

Directory of Accessible Building Products (DABP) for 2007

http://www.toolbase.org/PDF/DesignGuides/2007_DABP_complete.pdf

The DABP is a resource that contains information on more than 200 products available to individuals with disabilities and functional limitations. A search of the directory can be undertaken online by room/system, product, or manufacturer.

Toolbox Building Systems

http://www.toolbase.org/ToolbaseResources/level2.aspx?BucketID=1

This site provides information on selected products and processes that can assist with building or remodeling homes such as appliances; doors; electrical/electronics; exterior walls; floors; foundations; heating, ventilating, and air conditioning; interior partitions and ceilings; landscaping; plumbing; roofs; site work; whole-house systems; and windows.

PROFESSIONAL PUBLICATIONS AND RESOURCES

Industry Publications

http://www.cae.org.uk/abd.html

Access by Design is the United Kingdom's leading quarterly publication on inclusive design. The journal regularly features design sheets, building studies, updates on legislation and case law, reports on current research, and book reviews.

Books

+ *Accessible Bathroom Design: Tearing Down the Barriers, Second Edition*—Jacobs, J. C. (2007). San Jose, CA: JIREH Publishing Company. *Accessible Bathroom Design* provides a guide to remodeling bathrooms for people with disabilities.

+ *Accessible Home Design: Architectural Solutions for the Wheelchair User*—Davies, T. D., & Lopez, C. P. (2006). Washington, DC: Paralyzed Veterans of America. This book systematically addresses the accessibility of areas of the home including entrances, residential elevators and lifts, kitchen design, bath and toilet room plans, plumbing fixtures, grab bars, doors, windows and outdoor rooms, and garden paths.

+ *Aging in Place: Designing, Adapting and Enhancing the Home Environment*—Taira, E. D., & Carlson, J. L. (2000). New York, NY: Haworth Press. This book is a compilation of chapters contributed by various authors on older people's environmental needs and preferences with regard to modifications. Topics covered include the universally designed home, the role of occupational therapists in home modification programs, aging in place, and quality of life in different types of housing among older people.

+ *Complete Guide to Alzheimer Proofing Your Home*—Warner, M., & Warner, E. (2000). West Lafayette, IN: Purdue University Press. Written by a practicing architect and gerontologist, this book details how to create a home environment that will address the many difficulties associated with Alzheimer's. The book is divided into two sections. Section 1 discusses interior and exterior spaces, providing information on how to ensure that the person with Alzheimer's will be safe and secure, and section 2 provides a detailed list of potential problems related to Alzheimer's and practical information on how to cope with these in the home environment.

+ *ElderHouse: Staying Safe and Independent in Your Own Home as You Age*—Altman, A. (2008). White River Junction, VT: Chelsea Green Publishing. This book is a practical guide to preventing accidents, ensuring comfort, and maintaining independence in the home environment as its residents age. It explains basic interior design elements that can maximize living pleasure in a smaller living space.

+ *Remodeling for Easy Access Living*—Peters, R. (2006). New York, NY: Hearst. This book is a room-by-room guide from *Popular Mechanics* for older adults to assist them in remodeling their home to continue living independently. Some of the alterations can be completed by do-it-yourself remodelers, while others require a professional. It includes information on numerous projects, from creating multilevel countertops to installing grab bars in the bathroom. The book details options for flooring, sinks, tubs, appliances, windows, doors, and lighting that make the house more welcoming and discusses materials that work best, including nonskid floor options, antiscalding devices on sinks, and curbless showers. For complicated remodeling tasks, detailed information is provided on what the jobs entail, how long they might take, and typical costs.

+ *Residential Design for Aging in Place*—Lawlor, D., & Thomas, M. (2008). Hoboken, NJ: John Wiley & Sons. A useful reference for designing homes for aging people, if you seek to understand how to create effective spaces for the older people. This book examines various areas within the home and provides case study examples of good design solutions for designing for aging in place.

+ *Smart Technology for Aging, Disability, and Independence*—Mann, W. C. (2005). Hoboken, NJ: John Wiley & Sons. This book draws on the expertise of international specialists from multiple disciplines. It overviews important concepts, defines key terms, and provides detailed product descriptions, photographs and illustrations, and case studies. Some of the cutting-edge technologies discussed include wearable systems, smart wheelchairs, handheld devices and smart phones, visual sensors, home automation, assistive robotics, and in-room monitoring systems.

+ *Staying Put, Adapting the Places Instead of the People*—Lanspery, S., & Hyde, J. (1996). Amityville, NY: Baywood Publishing. This edited book features chapters from a number of experts on the issues of housing adaptation for older people. Parts 1 and 2 cover housing adaptations and users' perspectives, and Part 3 looks at implementing housing adaptation programs and housing adaptation policy.

+ *The Accessible Home: Updating Your Home for Changing Physical Needs*—Creative Publishing International. (2003). Chanhassen, MN: Author. This book provides practical information for homeowners who wish to make their homes convenient and accessible for people with physical impairments or aging relatives. The how-to instructions are clearly written and well illustrated. It includes a number of how-to projects and a planning guide for readers who are more likely to hire contractors for the work.

+ *The Rehab Guide, Volume 6: Kitchens and Baths*—Steven Winter Associates. (1999). Washington, DC: U.S. Department of Housing and Urban Development. Retrieved from http://www.toolbase.org/PDF/DesignGuides/rehab6_kitchen.pdf. *The Rehab Guides* are a series of nine guidebooks to inform the design and construction industry about materials and practices in housing rehabilitation. The series focuses on building technologies, materials, components, and techniques rather than projects, such as adding a new room. This volume includes an overview of kitchen and bath design considerations as well as details on repairing, renovating, and modifying cabinets, countertops, appliances, sinks and lavatories, tubs and showers, as well as toilets and bidets.

+ *Universal Design for the Home: Great-Looking, Great-Living Design for All Ages, Abilities, & Circumstances*—Jordan, W. A. (2008). Beverley, MA: Quayside Publishing. This book features a blend of beautiful projects, creative ideas, and substantive planning information. Highly visual, the book features projects showing room contexts, as well as detail shots. The mix of projects encompasses small and large houses; one-story and multi-story houses; and ideas for general accessibility and comfort as well as some targeted more directly at accessibility. There is an emphasis on remodeled projects, but new homes designed with an eye toward accessibility are also included. Chapters cover the spectrum of accessible home planning, from room arrangements to kitchens, baths, entries, and exterior areas. Basic specifications, how-to tips, and other technical content are featured throughout the book in easy-to-find boxes and sidebars.

TRAINING COURSES

Accessibility Consultation, Environmental Modifications, and Assistive Technology for Homes, Worksites, Schools, and Community Living

http://www.aotss.com

This program offers 2-day on-site seminars at various locations as well as Internet-based training/home study programs to health care professionals, case managers, building contractors, architects, designers, community service organizations, consumers, and caregivers. It includes training on home safety, home/job site modifications, UD, team building, marketing, and ADA consulting.

Certified Aging-In-Place Specialist (CAPS) Program

http://www.nahb.org/generic.aspx?sectionID=1389&genericContentID=9334

The NAHB Remodelors Council, in collaboration with the AARP, NAHB Research Center, and NAHB Seniors Housing Council, developed this program to provide comprehensive, practical, market-specific information about working with older and maturing adults to remodel their homes for aging-in-place. In a 3-day program, CAPS teaches the strategies and techniques for marketing, designing, and building aesthetically enriching, barrier-free living environments. Upon completion of the CAPS coursework, participants receive a graduation application. Participants must complete and submit the graduation application to the NAHB University of Housing before they can use the "CAPS" designation. Classes are offered through local and state home building associations and at national trade shows including NAHB's International Builders' Show and the Remodeler's Show.

Executive Certificate in Home Modification Program

http://www.homemods.org/online-courses/legal/certificate.shtml

This program is designed for professionals (e.g., remodelers/contractors, planners, personnel of organizations representing the elderly and people with disabilities, occupational and physical therapists, policymakers) who work directly or indirectly in the field of supportive home environments. Students can take one course or all five right from the comfort of their computer. By completing all five courses, students will obtain an Executive Certificate in Home Modification from the National Resource Center on Supportive Housing and Home Modification at USC. The program consists of five courses. Each course is approximately 2 to 3 weeks long. After completing all five courses, students take a final exam. CEUs are offered for various types of professionals.

IDEAS/USC Home Modification Practitioners Programs

http://www.ideasconsultinginc.com/store/products.asp

This set of four courses on home modifications was developed through a National Institutes of Health grant to I.D.E.A.S., Inc. The courses are designed for professionals (e.g., remodelers/contractors, planners, personnel of organizations representing the elderly and people with disabilities, occupational and physical therapists, policymakers) who work directly or indirectly in the field of supportive home environments. Each course follows a similar format, providing detailed information about the various causes of limitations that can make it difficult to perform everyday activities and the range of environmental modifications that can be implemented to compensate for these limitations. This program has modules on home modifications for people with dementia, sensory impairments, motor impairments, and those at risk for falls.

The Center for Inclusive Design and Environmental Access (IDEA) Program

http://www.udeworld.com/training/continuing-education.html

This program is designed for advocates, builders/contractors, planners, architects, occupational and physical therapists, and policymakers who are interested in learning about the UD of places, products, and systems with a particular focus on the implications of a lifespan perspective. The continuing education curriculum is divided into three sections. Part I contains two core courses. Part II covers human factors and has two courses. Part III comprises special topics and has five courses. Each course lasts 4 weeks and includes readings, quizzes, exercises, and discussion sessions. Students can take one course or all nine remotely. By completing six courses (three required and three elective), students can obtain a certificate of completion.

Workplace Accommodation and Home Modification Assessments

http://www.catea.gatech.edu/news/newsItem.php?id=4101&table=events&referringPage=courses

The course will provide an in-depth examination of workplace accommodation and home modification processes that address the needs of people with functional limitations. The course will focus on describing and implementing the assessment process, including the analysis of clients, environmental factors, and identification of barriers. The course will also review assessment products across a broad range of costs and technology levels, focusing on integrating accommodation examples from previous core courses into the assessment process. Multiple case studies will provide students with real-world examples of the methods of assessment and types of accommodation used to identify and overcome barriers to access. Students will learn the importance of addressing environmental factors, UD, compensatory strategies, and common technologies.

LISTSERVS

AccessibleHousing-L

LISTSERV@HANDINET.ORG

This listserv is intended to discuss the issues surrounding visitability, home modifications, and accessible apartments and the legislation and advocacy efforts that make accessible housing a reality. To subscribe to the list, send an email to LISTSERV@ HANDINET.ORG and in the body of the message type SUBSCRIBE AccessibleHousing-L. List Manager: Warren King.

Home Mods/Aging in Place

http://otconnections.aota.org/forums

This list is for occupational therapy practitioners to discuss issues related to home modification and aging in place. It is intended to assist occupational therapists to form partnerships with other community services providers such as home builders, contractors, remodelers, etc. List Manager: OT Connection.

Home Modifications Task Force List

HOMEMODIFICATIONS-LIST@LISTSERV.BUFFALO. EDU

This list is intended to provide communication among the Home Modifications Task Force and anyone interested in home modifications. Information disseminated through this list includes announcements of conferences and resource materials. Discussion of issues surrounding home modifications, their funding, and construction is also strongly encouraged. List Manager: Jordana Maisel.

CONFERENCES AND WORKSHOPS

The following list is a sample of professional training and conference opportunities and sponsors of organizations that hold training events and conferences in the areas of home modifications and AT.

International Conference on Aging, Disability, and Independence (ICADI)

http://www.icadi.phhp.ufl.edu

International conference held every other year (even years) and hosted by the University of Florida and the American Occupational Therapy Association. Community and home living and AT are areas of focus for the conference. Research-focused sessions and preconference workshops are offered.

American Association of Retired Persons (AARP)

http://www.aarp.org

AARP sponsors/co-sponsors several conferences yearly on aging issues in home and community as well as home modifications.

http://www.aarp.org/research

Research branch of AARP also offers resources and publications on local and global research.

American Occupational Therapy Association (AOTA)

http://www.aota.org/ConfandEvents

AOTA sponsors an annual conference and co-sponsors local and regional conferences.

NAHB National Association of Home Builders: CAPS

http://www.nahb.org/meeting_search.aspx?search= 1&sectionID=116&courses=1

Training program for aging-in-place home modifications. Offered as coursework taught by CAPS instructors. Taught in locations throughout the United States via local chapters of the NAHB.

Rehabilitation Engineering and Assistive Technology Society of North America (RESNA)

http://resna.org

RESNA offers professional development through continuing education, online and onsite workshops, skills training, as well as an annual conference.

Assisted Technology Industry Association (ATIA)

http://www.atia.org/i4a/pages/index.cfm?pageid=1

ATIA offers yearly events for training and continuing education in access and AT, including a national conference.

Appendix E

Access Standards Resources

United Kingdom Resources

British Standards Institution (BSI)—*http://www.bsigroup.com*

National Standards Authority of Ireland (NSAI)—*http://www.nsai.ie*

Australian Resource

Standards Australia (SA)—*http://www.standards.org.au*

Canadian Resource

Canadian Standards Association (CSA)—*http://www.csa.ca/cm/ca/en/home*

United States Resources

American National Standards Institute (ANSI)—*http://www.ansi.org*

ADA Accessibility Guidelines (ADAAG) (1991, as amended through 2002)—*http://www.access-board.gov/adaag/html/adaag.htm*

Uniform Federal Accessibility Standards (UFAS) (1984)—*http://www.access-board.gov/ufas/ufas-html/ufas.htm*

Revised ADA-ABA Guidelines (2004)—*http://www.access-board.gov/ada-aba/final.cfm*

Swedish Resource

Swedish Standards Institute (SSI)—*http://www.sis.se/defaultmain.aspx?tabid=740*

Norwegian Resource

Standards Norway—*http://www.standard.no/en/About-us/Standards-Norway*

Japanese Resource

Japanese Standards Association—*http://www.jsa.or.jp/default_english.asp*

Other International Resource

International Organization for Standardization—*http://www.iso.org/iso/about.htm*

Home Visit Checklist

HOME VISIT CHECKLIST

MAY BE PHOTOCOPIED AND USED ON HOME VISIT

Confidential

Name:

Address:

Phone Number:

Date of Birth:

File Number:

Request Made:

Date of Request:

Medical Documentation on File: YES   NO

Appointment Made:

Date of Visit:

Present at Visit:

Occupational Therapist:

Health Condition/Disability Specific Information:

Disability/Medical Condition (relevant to housing needs):

CLIENT: FILE NUMBER:

Level of Mobility (include community access):

- . . . . . Independently mobile—no assistive devices
- . . . . . Independently mobile using a single-point walking stick
- . . . . . Independently mobile using a four-point walking stick
- . . . . . Independently mobile using a walking frame
- . . . . . Independently mobile using a wheeled walking frame
- . . . . . Independently mobile using a manual wheelchair
- . . . . . Uses a manual wheelchair—dependent on others to push
- . . . . . Independently mobile using an electric wheelchair
- . . . . . Level of coordination
- . . . . . Dependent for mobility
- . . . . . Mobilizes on floor

Physical endurance: . . . .

Ability to manage stairs: . . . .
Ability to manage ramp: . . . .
Access to community: . . . .

Level of Independence:

Toilet:
- . . . . . Independent
- . . . . . Managing transfers with difficulty—benefit from grab bars
- . . . . . Uses over-toilet frame
- . . . . . Uses wheeled over-toilet chair

Shower:
- . . . . . Independent transferring in/out of bath to access shower
- . . . . . Managing to transfer in/out of bath/shower with difficulty
- . . . . . Has/requires grab bars
- . . . . . Has/requires bath board
- . . . . . Has/requires shower hose
- . . . . . Has/requires folding shower seat
- . . . . . Uses/needs shower recess
- . . . . . Can manage hob
- . . . . . Needs hob-free

Bath:
- . . . . . Independent
- . . . . . Problems getting in/out of bath
- . . . . . Grab bars
- . . . . . Bath board
- . . . . . Shower hose

CLIENT: FILE NUMBER:

Household Duties:

Heavy duties . . . .
. . . .
Light duties . . . .
. . . .
Shopping . . . .
. . . .
Meal preparation . . . .
. . . .
Laundry . . . .
. . . .

Use of Equipment:

. . . . .	Walking stick	. . . . . .	Walking frame
. . . . .	Wheeled walking frame	. . . . . .	Crutches
. . . . .	Manual wheelchair	. . . . . .	Electric wheelchair
. . . . .	Over-toilet frame	. . . . . .	Shower chair (static/wheeled)
. . . . .	Bathboard		

Measurements—Equipment/Client:

Support Services:

Current Housing Situation:

1. Size, layout, and construction of accommodation:

2. Details of existing tenants/occupants and the relationship between them (is the accommodation under-occupied?):

3. External Access:

Slope of land: . . . .
Access to street: . . . .
Paths: . . . .
Vehicle access: . . . .
Carport/garage: . . . .
Obstacles: . . . .

CLIENT: FILE NUMBER:

Front Door Access:
Description: ....
Stairs: Measurements .... Number .... Rails .... R .... L ....
Landing: ....
Door: ....
Ramps: ....
Obstacles: ....

Rear Door Access:
Description: ....
Stairs: Number .... Rails .... R. .... L ....
Landings: ....
Ramps: ....
Obstacles: ....

Comments:

4. Internal Access:

Hallway width: ....
Door entry: ....
Door widths: ....
Floor levels: ....
Room positions—for example, right-angled off hall: ....

Comments:

5. Bathroom: (separate diagrams required giving measurements)

Description: ....
....
Door width: ....
Floor covering: ....
Wall surface: ....

Bath:
Plunge: .... Hob height ....
Bath height: ....

Shower:
Shower cubicle: .... Hob height ....
Shower over bath: ....
Types of screening: ....
Dimensions: ....
Taps: Double: .... Single: ....
Shower hose: ....
Grab bars in situation: ....
Grab bars required: ....

CLIENT: FILE NUMBER:

Basin:

Description: ....

Taps: ....

Height: ....

Mirror: ....

Storage: ....

Toilet: (separate diagram required giving measurements)

Location: ....

Dimensions of room: ....

Door width: ....

Door opening: ....

Toilet heights in situation: ....

Grab bars required: ....

Floor covering: ....

Access to paper: ....

Has alternative equipment been trialed? ....

Comments:

6. Kitchen

Description: ....

....

....

Counter height and depth: ....

Sink access: ....

Taps: ....

Stove/oven: ....

Storage: ....

Floor coverings: ....

Comments:

7. Laundry

Location/access/description:

8. Miscellaneous

CLIENT: FILE NUMBER:

<u>Details of Home Modifications Request:</u>

<u>Proposals Discussed:</u>

Signed:

_____   _____

               Occupational Therapist   Date

CLIENT: FILE NUMBER:

Home Modification Report Template

OCCUPATIONAL THERAPY
HOME MODIFICATION REPORT

Client Information—Confidential

<u>Name:</u>

<u>Address:</u>

<u>Contact Phone Number:</u>

<u>File Number</u>

<u>Date of Birth/Age:</u>

<u>Date of OT Visit:</u>

<u>Present at Visit:</u>   Client,   Occupational Therapist (include name of organization and phone #)

<u>Client Profile:</u>

Health Condition or Disability Specific Information:
Client reported he/she has the following medical condition, which affects his/her daily function:
+ State source of information—for example, client/medical reports/family stated.
+ List medical conditions/disability in point form.
+ Be concise.
+ Avoid jargon.
+ Describe unfamiliar conditions in simple language.

Level of Mobility
Brief paragraph including the following:
+ Primary method of mobility
+ Walking and standing tolerances
+ Balance ability
+ Transfer ability/technique—on/off bed, chair, toilet; in/out bath, shower
+ Ability to use stairs and how many
+ Ability to manage ramps and hills
+ Community access—public transport options used, private vehicle use

Level of Independence
Brief paragraph including the following:
+ Independence with activities of daily living: personal and domestic
+ Information related to person (not to do with housing needs)—for example, carer assists client in shower because she is unable to safely transfer in/out of shower or turn taps on/off

CLIENT:

Use of Equipment
+ Currently used equipment
+ Future needs and clarification of how future needs were determined
+ Measurements for wheelchairs, hoists, etc., to be included

Wheelchair
+ Length (occupied or unoccupied)
+ Width (occupied or unoccupied)
+ Floor to top of toe with foot on footplate
+ Floor to top of knee with foot on footplate
+ Floor to armrest
+ Floor to hand on top of hand control on armrest
+ Turning circle
+ Diagram of wheelchair dimensions to be attached if required

Hoist
+ Width
+ Length
+ Height of feet above floor level
+ Turning circle

Anthropometric Measurements of Client

Support Services

+ Type of support services being used
+ Frequency of service
+ Include informal and family support

Brief Description of Property:

Include details of present housing situation.

This next section is to give the reader an understanding of the house layout and the problems the client is experiencing or likely to experience in the future so that he or she is able to understand the need for the modification and/or suitability of the property. The home audit checklist gives a guide for items to be included in each section but not all points will be necessary. Some areas may say, "No problems reported," but more detail is required if it relates to the client's request for modification.

If a problem is identified or is anticipated due to the nature of the disability/medical condition, the report should indicate how the client is coping with the problem. For example, if it is noted that the client has difficulty coping with stairs and the current accommodation has five steps, the report should indicate how the client is coping with the stairs or if a modification is required.

CLIENT:

External Access
   + Site of accommodation—for example, sloping block, busy road
   + Paths/driveways
   + Stairs—how many and if there are handrails
   + Security screens—any the department has installed
   + Access to mailbox, trash cans, and clothesline

Is the client experiencing problems with any of these areas or, because of the nature of the client's disability, does the occupational therapist expect that he or she would be experiencing difficulties?

Internal Access
   + Floor levels
   + Corridor and door widths

Is the client experiencing problems in this area?

Bathroom/Toilet
   + Type of facility—for example, shower over bath, square bath, separate shower and bath facilities
   + Is the toilet combined in the bathroom or in a room adjacent (future modification possible)?
   + Height of hob or bath
   + Type of flooring
   + Existing modifications

Is the client experiencing any problems with any of these areas?

Kitchen
   + General layout—for example, large kitchen used for dining as well as meal preparation
   + Type of stove—for example, upright electric

Is the client experiencing any problems with any of these areas?

Laundry
   + Location of laundry and if there are paths to clothesline

Is the client experiencing any problems with any of these areas?

Other issues

List any other issues arising.

Recommendations

Complete the following table to set out how problems identified in the housing situation section are to be solved and linked with the original request. Justify all modifications and show that the least expensive and easily achieved modifications have been considered before a modification has been requested—for example, before recommending a bath be removed, note that a bath board was trialed or not suitable for a stated reason.

CLIENT:

RECOMMENDATIONS	REASONING/OTHER OPTIONS CONSIDERED

The client was in agreement with the recommendations listed above at the time of the interview.

Signed: Approved by:

_____   _____
Occupational Therapist   Program Manager
Date: _____   Date: _____

CLIENT: _____

HOME MODIFICATIONS BRIEF TO CONTRACTOR

<u>Name</u>:

<u>Address</u>:

<u>Contact Phone Number</u>:

<u>File Number</u>:

MODIFICATIONS:

Note:
1. Modifications are based on specific client requirements. Any alteration to this brief should be checked with the Occupational Therapist,   , phone: .
2. Drawings (where provided) are not to scale and should be read in conjunction with the written brief.
3. Paint/repair all areas disturbed.

Signed: Approved by:

_____   _____
Occupational Therapist   Program Manager
Date: _____   Date: _____

CLIENT:

Appendix

Example of an Occupational Therapy Report

Section 1

Susan Taylor
Occupational Therapist
Central Home Modifications Program
PO Box 12AA
New York
Phone: (212) 925-2742
Fax: (212) 925-2745

OCCUPATIONAL THERAPY
HOME MODIFICATION REPORT

Client Information—Confidential

<u>Name:</u>	Mr. and Mrs. Alan Gray
<u>Address:</u>	8 Lakeside Close New York, NY 10012
<u>Contact Phone Number:</u>	(212) 925-2742
<u>File Number:</u>	AKH 13222555
<u>Date of Birth/Age:</u>	Mrs. Doris Gray—3 January 1929 (80 years old) Mr. Alan Gray—11 April 1927 (82 years old)
<u>Date of OT Visit:</u>	6 June 2009
<u>Present at Visit:</u>	Mr. and Mrs. Gray, their daughter Mrs. April Jones, Miss Susan Taylor (Occupational Therapist, Central Home Modification Program)

<u>Source and Reason for Referral:</u>

Peter Jones from Jones, Light, and O'Brien Attorneys provided a referral to the occupational therapist requesting a home assessment for Mr. and Mrs. Gray, with a view to making recommendations for home modifications. This information is to form part of Mrs. Gray's claim for damages following a motor vehicle accident on 1 January 2009. The referral was received on 5 May 2009.

<u>Client Profile:</u>

Information About Health Conditions or Disabilities:
Medical information reviewed prior to the home visit included the following:

A letter from Dr. Barrington dated 5 May 2009. This documentation states that the client was in her car, stopped at a traffic light, and was run into by a truck on 1 January 2009. Her car was described to have been pushed into an electric pole (light pole), and, as a result, she sustained a traumatic brain injury and multiple orthopedic and neurological injuries.

The injuries reported in this documentation include the following:
+ fractured right humerus
+ fractured left tibia
+ acquired brain injury (diffuse axonal injury, subarachnoid and subdural hemorrhage) resulting in left-sided hemiplegia with fluctuating upper limb and lower limb tone
+ aphasia

She was observed to be wearing a second skin-pressure garment on her left upper limb to reduce the tone in this arm. Mr. Gray indicated that he uses a communication board with his wife.

The medical documentation indicates that prior to her accident she had the following conditions:
+ urinary incontinence
+ urinary tract infections: June 2002, May 2003, May 2004

At the time of interview with this couple, Mr. Gray indicated that he is the main caregiver for his wife.

Mr. Gray reported that he has been diagnosed with the following conditions:
+ rheumatoid arthritis affecting the knees and shoulders—the client has pain, stiffness, and swelling of the joints, limiting his capacity to walk long distances and bend
+ non–insulin-dependent diabetes—poorly controlled; currently experiencing difficulty with his vision
+ clinical depression—managed by medication

Level of Mobility:

Mr. Gray stated that his wife relies on the use of a manual wheelchair to wheel short and long distances. He indicated that her fractures have healed but that she is not able to weight bear on her lower limbs and relies on the use of a floor-based electric hoist for all transfers. Mr. Gray reported that he has used the hoist with occasional caregiver assistance when transferring her on and off the bed, chair, and in and out of the mobile over-toilet shower chair.

At the time of the home visit, the occupational therapist observed Mr. Gray wheeling his wife around the home in her attendant-propelled wheelchair and attendant-propelled mobile over-toilet shower chair. He also demonstrated the various transfers on and off this equipment using the hoist. He indicated that he experiences joint pain as he undertakes this activity by himself without caregiver assistance due to the need to bend and reach to fit the sling around his wife and maneuver the hoist into position over the bed or other piece of equipment on carpet in the bedroom.

Mr. Gray reported that his wife is mainly confined to the upstairs area of the home, because of the presence of the external stairs that she is unable to negotiate.

Mr. Gray reported that he is experiencing joint pain and finds his own transfers on and off low seats, such as the toilet, quite difficult. He indicated that he is able to walk short distances indoors and uses a single-point stick when walking outdoors. Mr. Gray stated that his mobility has been affected by his arthritis and by his lack of confidence when walking over uneven terrain or when negotiating changes in levels. He indicated that his vision has deteriorated and that he has nearly had falls in outdoor areas.

Self-Care and Homemaker Tasks:

Mr. Gray indicated that the doctor had arranged for a nursing service to visit once a day to assist his wife as she was showered but this service discontinued after a few months when she returned home from rehabilitation.

Mr. and Mrs. Gray, 8 Lakeside Close, New York, NY 10012

Mr. Gray indicated that he completes all homemaker tasks, such as shopping, cooking, cleaning, and laundry, although his daughter has been providing meals for the freezer and his grandson has been mowing the yard and maintaining the garden. He demonstrated how he experiences difficulty reaching and bending during his own and his wife's showering activities and while in the kitchen undertaking meal preparation.

Community Access:

Mrs. Jones stated that she and her husband take her parents on drives and to appointments when required since her father no longer drives because of his diminishing eyesight. She indicated that both she and her husband physically lift Mrs. Gray down the stairs and into the vehicle. Mrs. Jones indicated that she worries that these transfers are often unsafe.

Equipment Dimensions:

Attendant Propelled Wheelchair

Occupied length:	43¼ in (1,100 mm)
Occupied width:	26½ in (670 mm)
Floor to top of toe with foot on footplate:	8 in (200 mm) above floor level (AFL)
Floor to top of seat cushion:	23½ in (600 mm) AFL
Floor to top of knee with foot on footplate:	25½ in (650 mm) AFL
Floor to top of armrest:	28½ in (720 mm) AFL
Turning circle:	59 in (1,500 mm) diameter
Turning capacity:	Can fit through a 33½-in-clear (850 mm) doorway and turn 90 degrees in a 47¼-in-wide (1,200 mm) corridor

Mobile Over-Toilet Shower Chair

Occupied length:	43¼ in (1,100 mm)
Occupied width:	23¾ in (600 mm)
Floor to top of toe with foot on footplate:	9¾ in (250 mm) AFL
Floor to top of knee with foot on footplate:	25½ in (650 mm) AFL
Floor to top of armrest:	31½ in (800 mm) AFL
Turning circle:	59 in (1,500 mm) diameter
Turning capacity:	Can fit through a 33½-in-clear (850 mm) door and turn 90 degrees in a 47¼-in-wide (1,200 mm) corridor

Floor Based Electric Hoist

Unoccupied width:	27½ in (700 mm)
Unoccupied length:	43¼ in (1,100 mm)
Floor to top of legs:	4¾ in (120 mm)
Turning capacity:	Can fit through a 30¾-inch-clear (780 mm) door but needs 51¼ in (1,300 mm) clearance in front of the door for turning 90 degrees or 180 degrees

Bed (hospital style, height adjustable)

Width:	41¼ in (1,050 mm)
Length:	82¾ in (2,100 mm)

Mr. and Mrs. Gray, 8 Lakeside Close, New York, NY 10012

Other Issues:

Mr. Gray indicated that his wife is now no longer able to undertake any of her hobbies (gardening, knitting, and sewing). He stated that he is finding it increasingly difficult to care for his wife and he feels that his own mental and physical health is declining. He indicated that he used to be a motor mechanic but is now retired and enjoys reading his automobile magazines and helping his grandson restore an old car. He reported that he barely has time to engage in these leisure activities due to his need to monitor his wife all day. Mr. Gray indicated that he and his wife do not want to move out of their home because they have lived there for more than 50 years, raising their family and enjoying the relationships they have established in the neighborhood. Mr. Gray stated that his wife was very unsettled when in rehabilitation after her accident, and he reported that she showed an improvement in her mood when she returned home.

Assessment Tools:

A combination of interview and observation was used during the assessment phase. As well, the *Canadian Occupational Performance Measure* was used with Mr. Gray to establish outcomes to be measured after the interventions were introduced. Mr. Gray rated all of his daily activities as to importance. The five top-rated activities are listed below, with ratings of performance ("How well I do this activity") and satisfaction ("How satisfied I am with this activity"). All ratings are on a scale of 1 (lowest rating) to 10 (highest rating).

Occupation	Importance (1-10)	Performance (1-10)	Satisfaction (1-10)
Caring for his wife—showering, dressing, toileting, transfers	10	4	4
Homemaker tasks	10	6	3
Self-care routine	10	5	5
Going shopping at least once a week	8	10	10
Reading	7	10	10
Restoring the car with his grandson	8	5	10

Mr. Gray indicated that his short-term goals included the following:
+ Gaining an increased understanding and acceptance of his wife's condition and developing strategies to better manage her symptoms, including her ongoing incontinence.
+ Improving the safety of both him and his wife when providing her with assistance with her transfers and mobility in and around the home and during her showering and toileting routine.
+ Managing his increasing anxiety and stress associated with ensuring his wife's health and well-being.

Mr. Gray stated that his long-term goals included the following:
+ Maintaining his own physical and emotional health in his role as a caregiver.
+ Safely and effectively assisting his wife in her daily self care activities and supporting her for as long as possible in the family home.

Mr. and Mrs. Gray, 8 Lakeside Close, New York, NY 10012

Brief Description of Property:

Mr. and Mrs. Gray live in a 4-bedroom detached brick house that is high-set with the following features:

+ Twelve brick stairs at the front and rear of the home with a wooden handrail on the left side ascending
+ Living and dining room, kitchen, four bedrooms, bathroom, and separate toilet located on the first level of the home
+ Double garage, laundry, and storage areas located on the ground level of the home
+ Pathway leading from the base of the external front stairs to the driveway
+ 47.25-in-high (1,200 mm) wooden paling fence around the perimeter of the yard
+ Pathway along the rear wall of the home
+ Pathway leading from the laundry to the clothesline
+ Flooring—low-pile carpet in the living and dining rooms and bedrooms; linoleum in the kitchen; tiles in the bathroom, toilet, and laundry areas
+ Bathroom upstairs—vanity with mirror above; bath; separate shower with a fixed shower screen and pivoting door, and a curb; and towel rails

The client's movements and capacity to access various features of the home was assessed at the time of the visit, and the following home modification items are recommended to suit the client. These recommendations take into consideration the client's current health status and his or her present level of safety, independence, and quality of life. The features are relevant for the client's current and future physical status. This report concentrates on the most essential home modification features required by the client, the options considered (if any), and the reasoning for the home modification recommendations. The performance criteria of the various features have been described rather than specific brands of products.

RECOMMENDATIONS	REASONING/OTHER OPTIONS CONSIDERED
Provide a wheelchair-accessible lift from the ground level to the first level of the home at the rear of the home. Lift to be installed at the rear of the home and a wheelchair-accessible path that is at least 47¼ in (1,200 mm) wide to be installed from the rear garage door to the lift. The path that is to adjoin the garage door is to have no step at the entry.	The house is too high to ramp from the ground level to the first level, and Mrs. Gray would not be able to maintain safe static balance perched on a stair lift. The couple is not willing to relocate to ground-level accommodation, despite their deteriorating mobility. There is also insufficient area under the home to create a living, bedroom, and bathroom area for Mrs. Gray, to prevent the need for her to go upstairs. The lift is recommended to enable the client to move between the two levels with ease in her wheelchair. The pathway is also recommended to ensure the clients have a level path of travel from the garage door area to the lift in all weather conditions.
Extend the width of the pathways around the home so that they are at least 47 in (1,200 mm) wide. Raise the turf and soil by all the paths and landings around the home to ensure that the various surfaces are level.	Mr. Gray reported that he is experiencing difficulty wheeling his wife on the narrow paths and uneven terrain. Installing wider paths and leveling the turf and soil with the paths will eliminate any hazards and improve their current level of safety.
Remove the bath, shower, vanity, and toilet in the upstairs bathroom and re-lay the floor to remove the step at the door and install a wheelchair-accessible shower, vanity, and toilet areas and a slip-resistant flooring.	The current bathroom is not wheelchair accessible. Mr. Gray is showering his wife over the floor waste and is experiencing difficulty positioning the mobile over-toilet shower chair over the toilet. There is limited space, and the floor appeared slippery when wet. The installation of a wheelchair-accessible bathroom with no step at the door and slip-resistant flooring will ensure a more spacious layout that suits the size of the equipment, the client, and Mr. Gray as they use the area during Mrs. Gray's self-care routine.

Remove the existing carpet in the main bedroom and replace with vinyl.	Mr. Gray indicated that his wife continues to experience incontinence and that there have been "accidents" in the bedroom on occasions. He also reported that the hoist and other equipment are difficult to maneuver on the carpet. The removal of the carpet and replacement is recommended to enable Mr. Gray to clean the floor and move the equipment with greater ease and safety.
Remove the rear entry, main bedroom and bathroom doors, and door frames. Install sliding doors that achieve 33½ in (850 mm) clearance. Relocate light switches to adjacent wall at standard height to suit location of new doors.	Mr. Gray stated that the entries into the rear door, main bedroom, and bathroom are narrow and that the mobility equipment is scraping the door frames. The door clearances are approximately 30¼ in (770 mm). It is recommended to provide wider door clearance and changing the style of the doors from swing doors to sliding doors to give more space through which the equipment can safely move. The wider doorways will also accommodate wider equipment if this is required in the future.
Install a vertical grab bar on the tap wall of the shower recess. Vertical grab bar to be fit with a friction-sliding mount. Remove and replace shower head with a handheld shower that is to attach to the friction sliding mount.	The vertical grab bar that is to be fit with a friction-sliding mount on which the handheld shower could be positioned will enable Mr. Gray to better control water flow. A handheld shower was seen as a safer alternative than retaining the shower head.
Install daylight-tone fluorescent lighting with diffuser shields in the kitchen, living room, dining room, and corridor areas.	At the time of the home visit, the occupational therapist noted that the interior of the home required enhanced lighting because it was quite dark. The installation of stronger lighting is required to ensure the safety of the clients as they wheel through the various areas of the home and undertake activities. It will also improve illumination and minimize glare and a shadowing effect in the home.

Additional Recommendations:

Mr. Gray will:

- Reduce the clutter within the various rooms by hanging some of the family photos on a wall or asking his daughter to create a memory album he and his wife can use.

Services required:

- Referral to incontinence specialist for education about toileting/incontinence.
- Referral to the nursing service to recommence immediate assistance with self-care activities.
- Referral to rheumatologist to monitor the current integrity of Mr. Gray's joints and effectiveness of pain control measures.
- Referral to ophthalmologist for an assessment of Mr. Gray's vision.
- Referral to a social worker for assessment for regular respite care.

Mrs. Gray was in agreement with the recommendations listed above at the time of the interview.

Signed: _____

Approved by: _____

Occupational Therapist

Date: _____

Program Manager

Date: _____

Mr. and Mrs. Gray, 8 Lakeside Close, New York, NY 10012

Section 2

HOME MODIFICATIONS BRIEF TO CONTRACTOR

<u>Name</u>:	Mr. and Mrs. Alan Gray
<u>Address</u>:	8 Lakeside Close New York, NY 10012
<u>Contact Phone Number</u>:	(212) 925-2742
<u>File Number</u>:	AKH 13222555

MODIFICATIONS:

<u>External Access</u>
+ Extend the rear landing on the first level of the home to suit the installation of a wheelchair-accessible lift with outward swinging doors with 33.5-in (850 mm) clearance.
+ Landing dimension to be 98.5 in (2,500 mm) long x 78.75 in (2,000 mm) wide.
+ Widen rear entry door to achieve 33.5-in (850 mm) clearance and ensure that there is no change in level between the landing and the internal floor greater than 0.25 in (6 mm).
+ Install wheelchair-accessible lift with wheelchair carriage size to accommodate standard wheelchair and caregiver.
+ Install a wheelchair-accessible path that is at least 48 in (1,200 mm) wide and extend from the rear garage door to the lift. The path that is to adjoin the garage door is to have no step at the entry.
+ All paths to be 48 in (1,200 mm) wide (excluding obstacles) with a slip-resistant finish.
+ Abutting surfaces to have a smooth transition with maximum tolerance of 0.25 in (6 mm) with the protruding surface having a rounded end.
+ Paths level with adjoining turfed edges, and turfed edges to extend horizontally for at least 23.5 in (600 mm) before ramping away due to a slight gradient in the land.
+ Vertical clearance of 78.75 in (2,000 mm) required along full length of path.
+ Maximum cross fall of 1:40.
+ Paths adjoining grass—no abutments between the two surfaces greater than 0.25 in (10 mm).

<u>Internal Access</u>
+ Remove the main bedroom and bathroom doors and doorframes.
+ Install sliding doors that achieve 33.5 inches (850 mm) clearance.
+ Relocate light switches to adjacent wall at standard height to suit location of new doors.

Bathroom/Toilet
+ Remove the flooring, fittings, and fixtures in the existing bathroom.
+ Remove the existing sliding door, and install a face of wall-sliding door that achieves 33.5 in (850 mm) clearance.
+ Door to have 2.5 in (60 mm) clearance on either side of D-shaped handles.
+ Flooring to be "slip resistive when wet."
+ Install 2 x 23.5 in (600 mm) long towel rails at standard height on the walls of the bathroom.

Wheel-in shower with no hob

+ Install large shower recess with continuous curtain track that is located 71 in (1,800 mm) to the underside and weighted shower curtain that extends to the floor—shower recess size to be 47.25 in (1,200 mm) x 59 in (1,500 mm).
+ Install handheld shower on a friction slide mount on a vertical grab rail—base of the rail to be located 35.5 in (900 mm) AFL.
+ Fall in bathroom floor to drain to the shower—1:50 to 1:60 fall within the shower and 1:70 to 1:80 fall from the door to the shower edge.
+ Shower fixtures configuration to include handheld shower on a friction-sliding mount on a vertical grab rail, recessed soap holder, and lever tap.
+ Recessed soap holder and lever tap to be located between 35.5 in (900 mm) and 43.25 in (1,100 mm) AFL and to be positioned so that the tap is on the open side of the shower and the soap holder is on the other side of the grab bar that is located centrally on the wall.
+ Shower hose to be non–heat-conducting.

Vanity

+ Vanity unit to have a bench top and drawers located in the corner area—to be on easy-glide runners with stops and to have D-shaped handles.
+ Bench width to be 13.75 in (350 mm).
+ Clearance under counter at least 32.25 in (820 mm) wide; pipe work not to intrude into knee space.
+ Datum point of semi-recessed basin in the vanity to be 33.5 in (850 mm) AFL.
+ Corners of vanity to be rounded and ends truncated.
+ Large mirror to be installed above the vanity to start 2 in (50 mm) above the level of the bench.

Toilet

+ Center line of toilet to be located 17.75 in (450 mm) to 18 in (460 mm) from adjacent wall.
+ 450-mm clearance required from the center line of the toilet to the open side.
+ Toilet height to be 18 in (460 mm) to 18.75 in (480 mm) AFL including solid seat but not lid.
+ Front of toilet to be located 31 in (790 mm) to 31.75 in (810 mm) from cistern wall.
+ Toilet roll holder to be recessed in style and to be located 27.5 in (700 mm) AFL and 33.5 in (850 mm) from the rear cistern wall.
+ Solid toilet seat and lid with metal hinges to be installed.

Temperature Control

Install a temperature control device to be on line to the bathroom, kitchen, and laundry.

Lighting

Remove existing lighting in the kitchen, living room, dining room, and corridor areas, and install daylight-tone fluorescent lighting with diffuser shields.

Please note that modifications are based on specific client requirements. Any alteration to this brief should be checked with the occupational therapist.

Signed: Approved by:

_____   _____
Occupational Therapist   Program Manager
Date: _____   Date: _____

Mr. and Mrs. Gray, 8 Lakeside Close, New York, NY 10012

Financial Disclosures

Elizabeth Ainsworth has no financial or proprietary interest in the materials presented herein.

Kathy Baigent has no financial or proprietary interest in the materials presented herein.

Ruth Cordiner has no financial or proprietary interest in the materials presented herein.

Desleigh de Jonge has no financial or proprietary interest in the materials presented herein.

Shirley de Wit has no financial or proprietary interest in the materials presented herein.

May Eade has no financial or proprietary interest in the materials presented herein.

Andrew Jones has no financial or proprietary interest in the materials presented herein.

Barbara Kornblau has no financial or proprietary interest in the materials presented herein.

Rhonda Phillips has no financial or proprietary interest in the materials presented herein.

Jon Pynoos has no financial or proprietary interest in the materials presented herein.

Jon Sanford has no financial or proprietary interest in the materials presented herein.

Bronwyn Tanner has no financial or proprietary interest in the materials presented herein.

Index

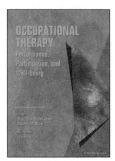
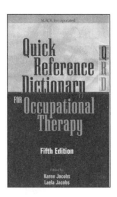

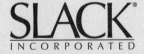